LIPPINCOTT'S REVIEW SERIES

Medical-Surgical Nursing

FOURTH EDITION

LIPPINCOTT'S REVIEW SERIES

Medical-Surgical Nursing

FOURTH EDITION

Ray A. Hargrove-Huttel, RN, PhD
Instructor
Trinity Valley Community College
Kaufman, Texas

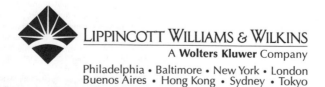

LIPPINCOTT WILLIAMS & WILKINS
A **Wolters Kluwer** Company
Philadelphia • Baltimore • New York • London
Buenos Aires • Hong Kong • Sydney • Tokyo

STAFF

Executive Publisher
Judith A. Schilling McCann, RN, MSN

Acquisition Editor
Elizabeth Nieginski

Editorial Director
H. Nancy Holmes

Clinical Director
Joan M. Robinson, RN, MSN

Senior Art Director
Arlene Putterman

Art Director
Mary Ludwicki

Editorial Project Manager
William Welsh

Copy Editor
Scott Etkin

Designer
Lynn Foulk

Digital Composition Services
Diane Paluba (manager), Joyce Rossi Biletz
Donna S. Morris

Manufacturing
Patricia K. Dorshaw (director), Beth J. Welsh

Editorial Assistants
Megan L. Aldinger, Tara L. Carter-Bell,
Josh Levandoski, Linda K. Ruhf

Indexer
Barbara Hodgson

The clinical treatments described and recommended in this publication are based on research and consultation with nursing, medical, and legal authorities. To the best of our knowledge, these procedures reflect currently accepted practice. Nevertheless, they can't be considered absolute and universal recommendations. For individual applications, all recommendations must be considered in light of the patient's clinical condition and, before administration of new or infrequently used drugs, in light of the latest package insert information. The authors and publisher disclaim any responsibility for any adverse effects resulting from the suggested procedures, from any undetected errors, or from the reader's misunderstanding of the text.

LRSMS011004—030606

Library of Congress Cataloging-in-Publication Data

Hargrove-Huttel, Ray A.
  Medical-surgical nursing.—4th ed. / Ray A. Hargrove-Huttel.
      p. ; cm.—(Lippincott's review series)
  Includes bibliographical references and index.
  ISBN 1-58255-348-3 (hardcover, pbk. : alk. paper)
  1. Nursing—Outlines, syllabi, etc. 2. Surgical nursing—Outlines, syllabi, etc. 3. Nursing—Examinations, questions, etc. 4. Surgical nursing—Examinations, questions, etc. 5. National Council Licensure Examination for Registered Nurses. I. Title. II. Series.
  [DNLM: 1. Nursing Care—Examination Questions. 2. Perioperative Nursing—Examination Questions. WY 18.2 H279m 2005]
  RT52.H366 2005
  610.73'076—dc22
                                                    2004012388

REVIEWERS

Judy Callicoatt, RN, MS
ADN Instructor
Trinity Valley Community College
Kaufman, TX

Kathryn Colgrove, RN, MS, CNS, OCN
ADN Instructor
Trinity Valley Community College
Kaufman, TX

Jolyne McGregor, RN, PHD
ADN Instructor
Trinity Valley Community College
Kaufman, TX

INTRODUCTION

Lippincott's Review Series is designed to help you in your study of the key subject areas in nursing. The series consists of eight books, one in each core nursing subject area:

> Critical Care Nursing
> Fluids and Electrolytes
> Maternal-Newborn Nursing
> Medical-Surgical Nursing
> Mental Health and Psychiatric Nursing
> Pathophysiology
> Pediatric Nursing
> Pharmacology

Lippincott's Review Series was developed in response to your requests for comprehensive outline review books that address each major subject area and also contain a self-test mechanism. These books meet the need for strong and weak areas of knowledge. Each book is a complete source for review and self-assessment of a single core subject. Together, all eight provide a comprehensive review of entry-level nursing.

Each book is all-inclusive of the content addressed in major textbooks. The content outline review uses a consistent nursing process format throughout and addresses nursing care for well and ill clients. Also included are necessary teaching and other concepts, such as nutrition, pharmacology, body structures and functions, and pathophysiology. Special features include the following:

• **Nursing process overview sections** review each step of the nursing process for the system or group of disorders in discussion. These overviews improve your ability to apply principles to practice by highlighting common assessment findings, diagnoses, goals, interventions, and outcomes.

• **Nursing process overview icons** ✦ remind you to refer back to the nursing process overview section for in-depth discussion of relevant nursing interventions.

• **Nursing alert icons** ✋ are fundamental guidelines you can follow to ensure safe and effective care.

• **Drug charts** provide quick reference for medications that are commonly used in treating the disorders discussed within a given chapter. The drug classification, indications, and selected nursing interventions are provided.

• **Client and family teaching boxes** detail health teaching information, which may be applied in the clinical setting.

• **Chapter study questions** help you chart your progress through each chapter. Answer keys are provided with rationales for correct and incorrect responses. New to this edition are questions designed after the NCLEX's alternate-format questions.

• **The comprehensive examination** mimics the NCLEX and allows you to assess your strengths and weaknesses. An answer key is provided with rationales for correct and incorrect responses. New to this edition are questions designed after the NCLEX's alternate-format questions.

• **A list of referral organizations,** complete with telephone numbers and Web sites, helps you quickly provide your clients with the referral information they need.

• **The glossary of terms,** presented at the end of the book, highlights noteworthy terms not covered in-depth within the text.

• **The accompanying CD-ROM** provides more than 200 additional NCLEX-style questions (including alternate-format questions) so you can practice computer adaptive test-taking skills. Answers are provided with rationales for correct and incorrect responses.

You can use the books in this series in several different ways. Overall, you can use them as subject reviews to augment general study throughout your basic nursing program and as a review to prepare for the NCLEX. How you use each book depends on your individual needs and preferences and on whether you review each chapter systematically or concentrate only on those chapters whose subject areas are particularly problematic or challenging. You may instead choose to use the comprehensive examination as a self-assessment opportunity to evaluate your knowledge base before you review the content outline. Likewise, you can use the study questions for pre- or post-testing after study, followed by the comprehensive examination as a means of evaluating your knowledge and competencies of an entire subject area. Regardless of how you use the books, one of the strengths of the series is the self-assessment opportunity it offers in addition to guidance in studying and reviewing content. The chapter study questions and comprehensive examination questions have been carefully developed to cover all topics in the outline review.

Unlike the NCLEX examination that tests the cumulative knowledge needed for safe practice by an entry-level nurse, these practice tests systematically evaluate the knowledge base that serves as the building block for the entire nursing educational process. In this way, you can prepare for the NCLEX examination throughout your course of study. Good study habits throughout your educational program are not only the best way to ensure ongoing success, but also will prove the most beneficial way to prepare for the licensing examination.

Keep in mind that these books are not intended to replace formal learning. They cannot substitute for textbook reading, discussion with instructors, or class attendance. Every effort has been made to provide accurate and current information, but class attendance and interaction with an instructor will provide invaluable information not found in books. Used correctly, these books will help you increase understanding, improve comprehension, evaluate strengths and weaknesses in areas of knowledge, increase productive study time and, as a result, help you improve your grades.

MONEY-BACK GUARANTEE — Lippincott's Review Series will help you study more effectively during coursework throughout your educational program, and help prepare you for quizzes and tests, including the NCLEX exam. If you buy and use any of the eight volumes in Lippincott's Review Series and fail the NCLEX exam, simply send us verification of your exam results and your copy of the review book to the address below. We will promptly send you a check for our suggested list price.

Lippincott's Review Series
Marketing Department
Lippincott Williams & Wilkins
530 Walnut Street
Philadelphia, PA 19106

ACKNOWLEDGMENTS

Thank you to the Lippincott Williams & Wilkins team, and especially Joan Robinson, for their continued support in my endeavor to improve and update the fourth edition of *Lippincott's Review Series: Medical-Surgical Nursing*.

I also want to acknowledge and thank the faculty, staff, students, and graduates of Trinity Valley Community College Health Science Center's Associate Degree Nursing program for making this book possible. Without their support and encouragement, I would not have been able to complete this edition. After 25 years of nursing — including 15 years of teaching — I still love this wonderful profession. I am grateful to the nursing students and faculty who have enriched my professional and personal lives. I hope that I have made a difference in their lives, as well.

This endeavor could not have been attempted and completed without the support and encouragement of my family. I dedicate this book to my husband, Bill, and my parents T/Sgt. Leo R. Hargrove and Nancy A. Hargrove. I want to thank my sisters, Gail and Debbie; my nephew, Benjamin; and Paula for their continued love, encouragement, and support in everything I do in my life. To my children, Teresa and Aaron, thank you for a wonderful life and for your unconditional love. Good luck as you both embark on new chapters of your life.

CONTENTS

1 *Nursing health assessment*

I. OVERVIEW OF NURSING HEALTH ASSESSMENT

A. Definition

1. Assessment, the first step of the nursing process, refers to the systematic appraisal of all factors relevant to a client's health.
2. Health-assessment components
   a. Collecting information through the health history, physical examination, records and reports, and laboratory and diagnostic studies
   b. Analyzing information by comparing client data with baseline data
   c. Synthesizing information from all sources to form a complete clinical picture and discover relationships among data

B. Purposes

1. Surveying the client's health status and risk factors for particular health problems
2. Identifying latent or occult (undetected) disease
3. Screening for a specific disease, such as diabetes or hypertension (i.e., case finding)
4. Identifying risks for particular health problems
5. Determining functional impact of disease (i.e., human response to actual or potential health problems)
6. Evaluating the effectiveness of the health care plan

II. HEALTH HISTORY

A. Purposes

1. Through the health history, the nurse elicits a detailed, accurate, and chronological health record as seen from the client's perspective.
2. The health history helps the nurse connect with a client and develop good rapport, provides insight into the client's functional status, and helps focus and guide subsequent physical examinations.

B. Data-collection techniques

1. Provide privacy and comfort for the client.
2. Greet the client, and introduce yourself.
3. Establish a verbal contract with the client that delineates the purpose of the history-taking session, the client's role, and a time limit for the interview.
4. Ask open-ended questions to explore the problem area, such as "Tell me about the problems you are having with your breathing."
5. Ask progressively more specific questions after identifying a particular problem (i.e., symptom analysis).
6. Guide the interview to obtain essential information without discouraging the client's discussion.
7. Ensure that all information remains confidential. The Health Insurance Portability and Accountability Act prevents the sharing of a client's private information and ensures safeguards to guarantee that only those individuals or entities that have a real need for protected health care information have access to it.

C. Reliability of data

1. During the health history interview, it is important to observe and document behaviors that lead you to believe the client is a reliable, partially reliable, or unreliable source of

information (i.e., "responded promptly to all questions, maintained eye contact, and dates consistent: client reliable").

   2. Reliability may come into question for clients who change their minds about their history, cannot recall certain events, do not know why they take certain medications, and are generally uncertain about their responses.

D. Components

   1. Biographic information. Document the following information, but do not repeat it if the information is already in the client's record:

   a. date and time of the interview

   b. client's name, address, telephone number, and Social Security number

   c. name, address, and telephone number of a person to contact in case of emergency or other situation

   d. gender, race, ethnic origin, and religious preference

   e. age, birth date, birthplace, and marital status

   f. occupation and level of education

   g. health insurance, usual sources of health care, and source of referral

   h. information regarding an advance directive and durable power of attorney for health care.

   – Determine whether the client has these documents, ascertain where the originals are located, and obtain copies for the client's chart.

   – If the client does not have these documents, encourage him to obtain them or to provide information about how to obtain these vital documents.

   2. Chief complaint. Identify the client's reason for seeking health care and obtain:

   a. a brief statement, usually in the client's own words, of the overriding problem for which he is seeking help

   b. a description of the onset and duration of the problem.

   3. Current health history. Elicit a detailed description of the chief complaint, including:

   a. a detailed chronologic statement of the problem, beginning with when the client last felt well and ending with a description of the current condition

   b. an individual description of each health problem (in cases of multiple problems)

   c. a symptom analysis of each problem that includes:

   – bodily location and radiation of pain (e.g., pain in the lower right abdomen)

   – quality (e.g., sharp pain)

   – quantity (e.g., pain of about 6 on a 10-point scale)

   – chronology, including onset, duration, and constant or intermittent nature

   – setting, including precipitating circumstances, place, activity, and persons present

   – aggravating and alleviating factors (e.g., "When I stand up straight, the pain is worse; when I curl up, it goes away.")

   – associated manifestations (e.g., vomiting, headache).

   d. information on possible exposure or incubation period in case of acute infections

   e. observations about whether and when the client stopped working or went to bed or about any change of activity level

   f. the client's perception about whether the problem is getting better or worse

   g. information on previous treatments, including medications, the prescribing practitioner, and treatment setting (e.g., hospital, clinic)

   h. information on current medication status, including prescription drugs, over-the-counter remedies, folk remedies, and any type of alternative health care (e.g., herbs)

i. identification of the problem as acute, chronic, or an acute exacerbation of a chronic problem.

4. **Past health status.** Obtain a description of the client's health history. Elicit information not specifically associated with the current problem, which is usually considered to be any problem occurring more than 6 months to 1 year earlier. Ask the client to describe:

    a. general health and strength compared with 1 year ago, including the stability of weight and appetite

    b. past illnesses, including childhood illnesses, acute infectious diseases, illnesses not requiring hospitalization, and illness requiring hospitalization or surgery

    c. accidents and injuries

    d. sexual history, including sexual performance, sexual preference (i.e., heterosexual, homosexual, or bisexual), menstrual history, and pregnancies (*Note:* This information may also appear in the review of systems.)

    e. immunizations

    f. allergies (with a description of the reaction), including eczema, hives, and itching; and allergy treatments

    g. geographic exposure, including areas of residence and foreign travel

    h. psychiatric history, including a history of "nervous breakdown," anxiety, and depression.

5. **Family health history.** Obtain information regarding grandparents, parents, brothers, sisters, spouse, and children. Collect information on:

    a. age and health status or age at death and cause of death of relatives and adopted relatives (e.g., adoptive parents who smoked may help identify problems related to smoking)

    b. family history of blood relatives with heart disease, hypertension, stroke, diabetes, gout, kidney disease or calculi, thyroid disease, asthma or other allergic disorders, blood problems, cancer, epilepsy, mental illness, arthritis, alcoholism, and obesity

    c. hereditary diseases such as hemophilia or sickle-cell disease

    d. family history presented as a genogram (see *Figure 1-1*) or diagram of the "family tree" with added notation regarding family negatives (e.g., diseases not present in the family).

6. **Review of body systems.** Elicit subjective information on the client's perceptions of major body-system functions. Note current status, any related past symptoms (i.e., positives) or lack of symptoms (i.e., negatives), and add a symptom analysis of any positive findings. The important information collected for each body part or system is described in section III of this chapter.

    a. **General:** weakness, fatigue, malaise, fever, chills, and recent weight loss or gain

    b. **Integumentary:** pruritus, pigmentary and other color changes, bleeding and bruising tendencies, lesions, excessive dryness, change in texture or character of hair or nails, and use of hair dyes or any possibly toxic agent

    c. **Head:** headache, head injury, scope, and dizziness

    d. **Eyes:** pain, recent change in appearance or vision, eyeglasses or contact lenses and recent change in prescription, diplopia, photophobia, blind spots, itching, burning, discharge, conjunctivitis, infection, glaucoma, cataracts, diabetes, and hypertension

    e. **Ears:** hearing acuity, earaches, tinnitus, vertigo, discharge, infection, and mastoiditis

    f. **Nose and sinuses:** sense of smell, sinus pain, epistaxis, nasal obstruction, discharge, postnasal drip, frequency of head colds, sneezing, and use of nose drops or sprays

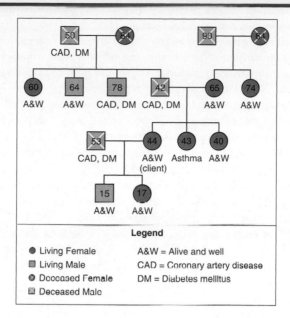

FIGURE 1–1
Genogram

g. **Oral cavity:** toothache; recent extractions; state of dental repair; dry mouth; soreness or bleeding of lips, gums, mouth, tongue, or throat; disturbed taste sensation; hoarseness; tonsillectomy; and history of smokeless tobacco

h. **Neck:** pain, limitation of motion, and thyroid enlargement.

i. **Lymph nodes:** tenderness or enlargement of neck, axillary, epitrochlear, or inguinal nodes; and duration and progress of abnormality

j. **Breasts:** pain, lumps, nipple discharge, surgery, any change in appearance of a breast, mammography and breast self-examination, timing of self-examination with regard to menstrual cycle, and estrogen-replacement therapy

k. **Respiratory system:** chest pain and its relationship to respiration, pleurisy, frequent sneezing, cough, sputum production (character and amount), hemoptysis, wheezing and its location in the chest, stridor, asthma, bronchitis, pneumonia, tuberculosis or contact therewith, night sweats, date of recent chest radiograph, and smoking history

l. **Cardiovascular system:** precordial or retrosternal pain or discomfort, palpitations, dyspnea, dyspnea on exertion, orthopnea, paroxysmal nocturnal dyspnea, edema, cyanosis; history of heart murmur, rheumatic fever (and its manifestations), hypertension (and usual blood pressure, if known), or coronary artery disease; and most recent electrocardiogram and results

m. **GI system:** appetite, food intolerance, dysphagia (with solids and liquids), heartburn, postprandial pain or distress, biliary colic, jaundice, other abdominal pain or distress, belching, nausea, vomiting, hematemesis or flatulence, change in character or color of stools (e.g., bleeding, melena, clay colored, diarrhea, constipation) or change in bowel habits; use of laxatives (type and frequency), rectal conditions (e.g., pruritus, hemorrhoids, fissures, fistula), ulcers, gallbladder disease, hepatitis, appendicitis, colitis, parasites, hernia, and radiographs (where and when obtained and results)

n. **Renal and urinary systems:** renal colic, frequency of urination, nocturia, polyuria, oliguria, urine retention, hesitancy, urgency, dysuria, narrowing of urine stream, dribbling, incontinence, hematuria, albuminuria, pyuria, kidney disease, facial edema, renal calculi, and results of cystoscopy if indicated

o. **Male reproductive system:** testicular pain and change in scrotum; puberty (e.g., onset, voice change, erections, emissions); libido and satisfaction with sexual relations; and history of sexually transmitted disease, such as gonorrhea, syphilis, herpes, and human immunodeficiency virus infection or acquired immunodeficiency syndrome, including date of onset, treatments and their effectiveness, and any complications

p. **Female reproductive system:** menstrual history (e.g., menarche, last period, cycle and duration, amount of flow, premenstrual pain, dysmenorrhea, intermenstrual bleeding), vaginal discharge, dyspareunia, obstetric history (e.g., gravida/para, miscarriages, abortions, complications), menopause and associated symptoms, contraceptive methods used, libido, satisfaction with sexual relations, and history of sexually transmitted diseases as described in the previous section

q. **Peripheral vascular system:** intermittent claudication, varicose veins, and thrombophlebitis

r. **Musculoskeletal system:** joint pain, stiffness, or edema (e.g., location, migratory nature, relation to known cardiac involvement); rheumatoid arthritis, gout, or bursitis; limitations in function or range of motion; flat feet, osteomyelitis, or fractures; muscle pain or cramps; and back pain (i.e., location and radiation, especially to extremities), stiffness, limitation of motion, and sciatica or disk disease

s. **Neurologic system:** loss of consciousness, convulsions, meningitis, encephalitis, stroke, seizures, or other neurologic problems; use of medication for seizure control; cognitive disturbances (e.g., recent or remote memory loss, hallucinations, disorientation, speech and language dysfunction, inability to concentrate); change in sleep pattern; motor problems (e.g., gait, balance, coordination), tics, twitching, or tremors; muscle weakness or spasms; paralysis, muscle wasting, or activity intolerance; sensory disturbances (e.g., pain, insensitivity to temperature or touch, paresthesias); and neuralgic pain in the head, neck, trunk, and extremities

t. **Hematopoietic and immune systems:** bleeding tendencies of skin or mucous membranes, anemia, blood type, transfusions and reactions, blood dyscrasias, low platelet count, exposure to toxic agents or radiation, and unexplained systemic infections and lymph node edema

u. **Endocrine and metabolic systems:** nutritional and growth history; thyroid dysfunction (e.g., goiter), adrenal problems, or diabetes; changes in tolerance to heat and cold; relationship between appetite and weight; excessive voiding or excessive thirst; change in skin (i.e., pigmentation, texture); changes in body contour, hair distribution, and shoe or glove size; and unexplained weakness

7. **Developmental considerations.** Obtain an overview of the client's growth history, including pertinent physical and cognitive developmental milestones and factors.

8. **Lifestyle practices.** Obtain information about the client's activities of daily living and ability to care for himself and his family, including:

a. status of client's mobility in relation to activities and demands of daily living (e.g., "Can you go out of doors? Can you walk up and down stairs? Can you get out of the house? Can you wash and bathe yourself? Can you dress yourself? Can you put on your shoes? Can you cut your toenails?")

CLIENT AND FAMILY TEACHING 1-1
Guidelines for health promotion

- Explain to the client that taking responsibility for himself is the key to successful health promotion.
- Discuss the necessity of ensuring an adequate amount of sleep; this is individualized, but 6 to 8 hours are recommended.
- Discuss the importance of a properly balanced diet that supplies all of the essential nutrients and an awareness of the relationship between diet and disease.
- Encourage the necessity of managing stress appropriately to include such techniques as relaxation training, exercise, and modification of stress-producing situations. Always include quality family time and recreational time.
- Explain that a regular exercise program can promote health by improving the function of the circulatory system and the lungs, decreasing cholesterol and low-density lipoproteins, and lowering body weight by increasing caloric expenditure.
- Discuss the importance of using safety devices, such as seat belts or helmets, and of following precautions when using pesticides or fertilizers.
- Discuss the importance of obtaining examinations to include annual health checkups, eye examinations, gynecologic checkups, mammograms, prostate examinations, and digital rectal examinations.
- Discuss the importance of self-examinations, including breast, testicular, and skin examinations.
- Discuss the importance of avoiding smoking, excessive alcohol intake, and substance abuse of any kind.
- Discuss the importance of safety conditions in the home, work, and community settings.

   b. client's preferred lifestyle (e.g., "Is there anything you cannot do now compared with last year? Do you travel now? Did you in the past? Where did you travel?")
   c. client's home and neighborhood environment (e.g., "Who buys and carries the groceries? Who cooks? Who does the housekeeping? Do you feel safe in and around your home?").

9. **Health promotion and maintenance activities.** Obtain information concerning the client's practices that promote healthy living. Take this opportunity to provide client and family teaching relative to health promotion and maintenance. (See *Client and family teaching 1-1*.)
   a. Health beliefs
      - Expectations of health care
      - Promotive, preventive, and restorative practices (e.g., breast self-examination, use of safety devices)
      - The meaning of illness
      - Cultural implications of health and illness
      - Alternative health care (e.g., use of herbs, massage therapy, aroma therapy)
   b. Personal habits
      - Use of tobacco, alcohol, and street drugs
      - Use of prescribed and over-the-counter medications
      - Use of caffeine
      - Hygiene
      - Elimination patterns
   c. Sleep and wake patterns
   d. Exercise and activity
   e. Recreation
   f. Nutrition
      - Height, weight, and anthropometric measurements
      - 24-hour dietary recall, including number of portions and portion sizes
   g. Stress and coping patterns
   h. Socioeconomic status

- Educational level
- Financial status

  i. Environmental health patterns
  - Home conditions, including living arrangements, housing, others in the home (i.e., family and nonrelatives), and the health of others in the home
  - General environmental conditions, including neighborhood and region

  j. Occupational health patterns
  - Exact nature of work or of previous work if retired
  - Exposure to toxic agents, fatigue, and abnormal surroundings

10. **Role and relationship patterns.** Obtain information about family roles, work roles, and interpersonal relationships. Collect information on:

    a. self-concept
    - self-expectations (short- and long-range goals)
    - perceived strengths and weaknesses

    b. cultural influences

    c. spiritual and religious influences

    d. family role and relationship patterns

    e. sexuality and reproductive patterns
    - menstrual history and puberty history
    - sexual activity (i.e., past and present)
    - pregnancies (i.e., miscarriages and live births)

    f. social support patterns (e.g., family, friends, and agencies)

    g. emotional health status.

11. **Conclusion.** Complete the health history by asking, "Is there anything else you would like to tell me?" This allows the client to end the interview by discussing his feelings and concerns.

12. **Gerontologic consideration.** When obtaining a health history from an elderly client, determine his ability to hear and comprehend the questions, and allow sufficient time for a response.

III. PHYSICAL EXAMINATION

A. General principles

1. Physical examination is the second component of a complete nursing health assessment. Perform a complete or partial physical examination after obtaining a careful comprehensive or problem-related history. History findings help focus the physical examination.

2. Examine the client in a quiet, warm, well-lighted room. Consider privacy and comfort needs. Use appropriate draping, exposing only the portions of the body being examined.

3. Practice and adhere to standard precautions throughout the entire physical assessment.

4. Explain what you plan to do, what the client can expect to feel, and what you expect from the client.

5. Always compare body sides for symmetry and, when appropriate, compare distal to proximal areas.

6. Visualize underlying structures and organs when performing the examination. Use anatomic landmarks to locate specific structures and to report significant findings (e.g., thorax, heart, abdomen).

7. During the physical assessment of an elderly person, prioritize the physical examination with special attention to positioning, comfort, and mobility to prevent fatigue.

B. **Assessment techniques.** The nurse uses four basic techniques in physical assessment: inspection, auscultation, palpation, and percussion.

1. **Inspection**
   a. An important assessment point (but one that is commonly forgotten) is that inspection starts at the initial client encounter.
   b. Beginning with each portion of an examination, inspection employs the senses of vision and smell to observe the client.

2. **Auscultation**
   a. This technique involves listening (usually through a stethoscope) to sounds produced in the body, particularly in the heart, lungs, blood vessels, stomach, and intestines.
   b. A Doppler ultrasonic stethoscope and an acoustic stethoscope can be used to amplify body sound.

3. **Palpation**
   a. In this technique, different parts of the hand are used to detect characteristics of pulsations, vibrations, texture, shape, temperature, and movement.
   b. Palpation can confirm and amplify findings observed during inspection.
   c. Light palpation is always done first. Using the finger pads, provide superficial (0.4" [1-cm] deep) and delicate palpation to explore skin texture and moisture; overt, large or superficial masses; and fluid, muscle guarding, and superficial tenderness. With deep palpation, use the hands to explore the internal structures (1.6" to 2" [4- to 5-cm] deep).

4. **Percussion**
   a. Sharply tapping the body surface with the fingers, hands, or a rubber reflex hammer produces sounds whose quality depends on the density of underlying structures (e.g., organ borders, fluid, gas).
   b. Percussion is used to elicit tenderness and to assess reflexes.

C. **Components.** The physical examination involves the assessment of vital signs, height and weight, general appearance, and body systems.

1. **Vital signs**
   a. Normal ranges for temperature, pulse, respiratory rates, and blood pressure depend on the situation and the particular health care institution. (See *Table 1-1*, page 10.)
   b. In blood-pressure measurements, several distinctions are common:
      - A difference of 5 to 10 mm Hg between arms is common; systolic pressure usually is 10 mm Hg higher in the legs than in the arms.
      - Changing positions from recumbent to standing can cause a 10 to 15 mm Hg drop in systolic pressure and a slight rise (about 5 mm Hg) in diastolic pressure. The client may complain of dizziness or lightheadedness because of this change. Remember to institute safety precautions.
      - In elderly clients, check blood pressure in the lying, sitting, and standing positions to detect excessive postural orthostatic hypotension related to antihypertensive drugs or age-related physiologic changes.
   c. When assessing a client's vital signs, keep in mind that they normally vary with the time of day.
      - Diurnal body temperature varies from 0.5° to 2° F (-17.5° to -16.7° C); it is lowest during sleep and highest from noon to early evening.

TABLE 1-1
Normal vital signs in adults

Sign	Range
Pulse rate	60 to 100 beats/minute (regular, full, strong)
Respiratory rate	12 to 20 breaths/minute
Blood pressure (BP)	Less than 140/85 mm Hg
BP*	Normal: ■ Systolic BP (SBP): < 120 mm Hg *and* ■ Diastolic BP (DBP): < 80 mm Hg Prehypertension: ■ SBP: 120 to 139 mm Hg *or* ■ DBP: 80 to 89 mm Hg Stage 1 hypertension: ■ SBP: 140 to 159 mm Hg *or* ■ DBP: 90 to 99 mm Hg Stage 2 hypertension: ■ SBP: ≥ 160 mm Hg *or* ■ DBP: ≥ 100 mm Hg
Temperature	96.4° to 99.2° F (35.8° to 37.3° C)

Note: Subnormal readings are common in elderly clients.

*Source: National Institutes of Health. *The Seventh Report of the Joint National Committee on Detection, Evaluation, and Treatment of High Blood Pressure* (NIH Pub No.; 03-5233), May 2003. Available at *www.nhlbi.nih.gov/guidelines/hypertension/jncintro.*

- Blood pressure may decrease during sleep and fluctuate throughout the day with no predictable pattern.
- Pulse rate may decrease during sleep and increase during the day in response to activity and stress.

2. **Height and weight**
   a. Weight is related to body frame size: small, medium, or large.
   b. Adipose tissue measurements (e.g., triceps skinfold thickness) help determine body fat percentage.
   c. Aging clients, particularly females, commonly lose height because of osteoporotic kyphosis.
3. **General appearance**
   a. Race
   b. Gender
   c. General physical development (stature)
   d. Nutritional status
   e. Mental alertness
   f. Evidence of pain and restlessness
   g. Body position
   h. Age versus apparent age
   i. Clothing, hygiene, and grooming

4. **Integument**
   a. **Inspection**
      – Observe the skin's color, complexion, and mucous membranes. Note jaundice, cyanosis, polycythemia, carotenemia, vitiligo erythema, and clubbing of fingers or toes.
      – Assess for evidence of bleeding, ecchymosis, or increased vascularity.
      – Assess pigmentation.
      – Look for lesions and scars (e.g., distribution, type, configuration, size) and superficial vascularity.
      – Inspect the skin for moisture.
      – Note edema.
      – Inspect hair distribution.
      – Observe the nails.
   b. **Palpation**
      – Assess temperature.
      – Palpate the skin for texture, consistency, elasticity, turgor, and mobility.
      – Note any tenderness.
   c. **Normal findings**
      – Lesions (except freckles, birthmarks, or moles) and rashes are not found. Areas of increased vascularity, ecchymosis, or bleeding are not seen.
      – The skin is warm, slightly moist, smooth, and finely textured. Skin turgor is elastic.
      – Hair distribution is characteristic for gender and age.
      – Nails are smooth and slightly rounded or flat (angle of nail base should be approximately 160 degrees). Nails have a pink cast in light-skinned individuals and a brown cast in dark-skinned individuals.
      – Mucous membranes are moist and pink.
   d. **Gerontologic considerations**
      – Skin is wrinkled, drier (from loss of subcutaneous fat, diminished sweat-gland activity, and diminished secretion of natural oils), and increasingly fragile in elderly clients.
      – Turgor decreases with aging. Do not use turgor to assess level of hydration.
      – Hair is grayer and sparser on the head, axilla, extremities, and pubic area. Elderly women have increased facial hair. Bristly hair grows in the nose and ears of elderly men.
      – Mucous membranes may be drier and paler in elderly clients.
      – Nails are possibly horny and tough in response to decreased peripheral circulation.
      – Common benign lesions, such as senile lentigines (i.e., age spots or liver spots), seborrheic keratoses (i.e., yellowish or brownish wartlike lesions with oily scale), and cherry angiomas (i.e., small bright or dark red papules), may occur with aging.
      – Decreased total body weight with an increase in body fat is common in elderly clients.

5. **Head**
   a. **Inspection**
      – **Skull.** Observe the size and shape.
      – **Face.** Observe for symmetry.
      – **Scalp.** Observe for flaking, lesions, masses, deformities, edema, and tenderness.
      – **Hair.** Notice color, distribution, and nits on hair shafts.

  b. **Palpation**
  - **Skull.** Palpate for bony overgrowths and symmetry.
  - **Face.** Palpate the temporomandibular joint for pain and tenderness.
  - **Hair.** Notice the texture.

  c. **Normal findings**
  - The skull is normocephalic.
  - The face is symmetric.
  - No signs of alopecia or foreign bodies in the hair are observed on the scalp.
  - Hair is shiny and resilient when traction is applied. It does not come out in clumps.

  d. **Gerontologic considerations.** In elderly clients, the nose and ears commonly appear larger in proportion to head size.

6. **Eyes and vision**

  a. **Inspection**
  - **Globes.** Observe for protrusion.
  - **Palpebral fissures.** Assess symmetry and width.
  - **Lid margins.** Observe for scaling, secretions, erythema, and position of lashes.
  - **Conjunctivae.** Inspect for congestion and note color.
  - **Sclerae and irises.** Observe color.
  - **Pupils.** Note the size, shape, symmetry, and reaction to light and accommodation.
  - **Eye movement.** Assess extraocular movements (i.e., cover/uncover test), and note nystagmus or convergence.
  - **Inner eye.** Perform a fundoscopic examination (with an ophthalmoscope), and locate the red reflex. Check the transparency of the anterior and posterior chambers, cornea, and lens. Examine the retina, optic disk, macula, and blood vessels.

  b. **Palpation**
  - **Upper lids.** Evaluate strength by attempting to open the client's closed lids against her resistance.
  - **Eyeballs.** Assess tenderness and tension.

  c. **Vision testing**
  - Test visual acuity with a Snellen chart. Test a client wearing corrective lenses with and without the lenses.
  - Test visual peripheral fields.

  d. **Normal findings**
  - Central vision is 20/20 in both eyes. Visual fields are unrestricted.
  - Eyes appear symmetric with no ptosis, lid lag, or infections or tumors of the eyelids.
  - Eyes move in conjugate fashion.
  - The cover/uncover test reveals no movement of either eye.
  - The anterior and posterior chambers, lens, and cornea are transparent. The sclera and conjunctiva are clear.
  - The lacrimal system is unobstructed, with no enlargement, edema, redness, or exudate.
  - Pupils are equal, round, and reactive to light and accommodate.
  - Red reflex is symmetrically seen in the center of each cornea.
  - Bilateral well-marginated disks are revealed on funduscopic examination.
  - No signs of arterial narrowing, venous engorgement, atrioventricular nicking, hemorrhages, or exudate are seen.

  e. **Gerontologic considerations**
  - Assess for entropion, ectropion, lens opacity, and eye dryness, which are common in elderly clients. Entropion can cause discomfort and damage to the eye.

- Funduscopic examination may be difficult in an elderly client because the pupil commonly is small (1.2″ [3 cm]), with limited ability to dilate without a medicinal dilator.
- Elderly clients generally experience diminished ability to focus on close objects, decreased ability to distinguish colors, and difficulty adjusting to changes in light intensity.

7. **Ears and hearing**
   a. **Inspection**
   - **Pinna.** Assess size, shape, placement on head, and color. Note any lesions or masses.
   - **External canal.** With an otoscope, check for discharge, impacted cerumen, inflammation, masses, and foreign bodies.
   - **Tympanic membrane.** With an otoscope inserted inferiorly into the distal portion of the tympanic canal, assess color, luster, shape, position, transparency, and integrity; note any scarring; and locate landmarks (e.g., cone of light, umbo, handle and short process of malleus, pars flaccida, and pars tensa). The adult client's ear should be pulled up and back with the examiner's hand braced against the client's head.

   b. **Palpation.** Examine the pinna for tenderness, consistency of cartilage, edema, and pain.

   c. **Auditory testing**
   - Test gross hearing acuity with whispered words or a watch.
   - With a tuning fork, perform Weber's test (i.e., bone conduction) and the Rinne test (i.e., air conduction to bone conduction ratio).

   d. **Normal findings**
   - The Weber's test result is not referred (or lateralized).
   - The Rinne test result is positive (e.g., air conduction is greater than bone conduction).
   - Appearance of external ear is normal.
   - Canals are clear without discharge.
   - Tympanic membranes are pearly gray and intact, with visible landmarks.

   e. **Gerontologic considerations.** Moderate hearing loss (especially of high-frequency sounds) and difficulty discriminating sounds are common in elderly clients. These changes may interfere with the ability to follow instructions associated with testing. The elderly client may need more time to respond or react to verbal stimuli.

8. **Nose and sinuses**
   a. **Inspection**
   - **Nose.** Observe the position of the nose on the face, and note any discharge.
   - **Nasal passageway.** Assess airway patency, and note any nasal obstruction. Perform a speculum examination of interior structures, including the nasal septum (assessing position and noting any bleeding or perforation), mucous membranes (noting hydration and color), and turbinates (assess color and note any edema).

   b. **Palpation.** Apply fingertip pressure to the frontal and maxillary sinuses to assess for tenderness.

   c. **Normal findings**
   - Nose is symmetrically placed on face.
   - Nasal passages are patent with septum in midline.
   - Mucous membranes are moist and dark pink without perforation or bleeding.
   - Sinuses are nontender.

d. **Gerontologic considerations.** Elderly clients generally have pale nasal mucosa and a decreased ability to taste and smell.

9. **Mouth and pharynx**

   a. **Inspection.** Use a penlight and tongue depressor when examining inside the client's mouth.
   - **Lips.** Observe color and moisture, and note abnormal pigmentation, masses, ulcerations, or fissures.
   - **Teeth.** Note the number, arrangement, and general condition.
   - **Gingivae.** Assess color and texture. Note discharge, edema, retraction, or bleeding.
   - **Buccal mucosa.** Assess for discoloration, vesicles, ulcerations, or masses.
   - **Pharynx.** Note any inflammation, exudate, or masses.
   - **Tongue** (at rest and protruded). Assess size, color, moisture, and symmetry. Note any lesions, deviations from midline, fasciculations, or tremors.
   - **Salivary glands.** Assess patency.
   - **Uvula.** Assess the position on phonation, which should be midline.
   - **Soft palate.** Observe symmetry on phonation and intactness.
   - **Tonsils.** Note the presence or absence, size, ulcerations, exudate, or inflammation.
   - **Breath.** Note the odor.
   - **Voice.** Assess voice volume, and note any hoarseness.
   - **Swallow.** Check the client's ability to swallow.

   b. **Palpation** (*Note:* Wear gloves when putting your fingers inside the client's mouth.)
   - **Oral cavity.** Palpate for masses and ulcerations.
   - **Tongue.** Retract and palpate the tongue by grasping it with a gauze sponge. Inspect its undersurface and the floor of the oral cavity.
   - **Gag reflex.** Attempt to elicit it bilaterally.

   c. **Normal findings**
   - No lesions are present on the lips, gums, tongue, or buccal mucosa.
   - Tongue is pink, moist, well papillated, and in midline when at rest and on protrusion.
   - Salivary glands are unobstructed.
   - Pharynx is not injected.
   - Tonsils are nonobstructing.
   - Uvula is in the midline.
   - Palate elevates symmetrically on phonation.
   - Gag reflex is present bilaterally.
   - Teeth are present with no caries.
   - Gums are clear.

   d. **Gerontologic considerations.** Elderly clients are at risk for mouth lesions, untreated caries, periodontal disease, tooth loss, decreased saliva production, shinier and thinner mucosa, and pale gums. To prevent this, assess hydration status by looking for a small saliva pool under the tongue. If the client wears dentures, be sure to remove them before examining the mouth.

10. **Neck**

    a. **Inspection**
    - **All areas of neck anteriorly and posteriorly.** Assess muscle symmetry and range of motion. Note any masses, unusual edema, or pulsations.
    - **Thyroid.** Observe for enlargement.
    - **External jugular veins.** Note distention.

    b. **Palpation**
- **Cervical nodes and salivary glands.** Palpate for enlargement and tenderness.
- **Trachea.** Note deviation from midline.
- **Thyroid.** Palpate for nodules, masses, or irregularities.
- **Carotid arteries.** Note amplitude and symmetry of pulsations.

    c. **Auscultation.** Listen for bruits over the carotid arteries and the thyroid.

    d. **Normal findings**
- Neck is symmetric without tenderness or limitation of movement.
- Trachea is positioned in the midline.
- Thyroid is not palpable.
- Bruits are not auscultated.

    e. **Gerontologic considerations.** Elderly clients are at risk for heart irregularities (i.e., reflex drop in pulse rate or blood pressure if carotid arteries are palpated at level of carotid sinuses); to prevent this, palpate well below the upper border of the thyroid cartilage.

11. **Lymph nodes**

    a. **Inspection.** Note observable nodes.

    b. **Palpation**
- Feel for palpable nodes. Assess size, shape, mobility, and consistency of nodes. Note tenderness or inflammation.
- Locations to palpate include cervical, supra, and infraclavicular; axillary central, lateral, subscapular, and pectoral groups; inguinal (horizontal and vertical); and epitrochlear.

    c. **Normal findings.** Nodes are neither palpable nor tender.

    d. **Gerontologic considerations.** Any palpable or tender lymph nodes should warrant further investigation.

12. **Female breasts**

    a. **Inspection**
- With the client sitting with her arms at her side, inspect the nipples and areola for position, pigmentation, inversion, discharge, crusting, and masses. Note any supernumerary nipples.
- Observe the size, shape, color, symmetry, surface contour, skin characteristics, and level of breasts. Note any retraction or dimpling of skin or nipples, new pigmentation, engorged veins, edema, or any tendency of a breast to cling to the thorax.
- Repeat these observations with the client's hands above or behind her head, with the hands pressed firmly on the hips, while leaning forward from the hips, and while in the supine position.

    b. **Palpation**
- Palpate the breasts with the client sitting and supine. When the client is supine and for a client with large breasts, place a pad under the ipsilateral scapula of the breast being palpated, and raise the arm on that side over the head.
- Palpate one breast at a time, using the palmar aspects of the fingers in a rotating motion and moving in concentric circles from the periphery of the breast to the nipple.
  - Assess skin texture, moisture, and temperature.
  - Note any masses.
  - Be sure to include the tail of Spence (i.e., breast tissue extending into the axillary region in the upper outer quadrant of the breast).

- Gently squeeze, milk, and then invert the nipple to check for any expressible discharge and to detect any mass beneath the nipple.
- Repeat these steps for the other breast, and compare findings for both sides.
- Conclude by applying lotion for lubrication. Using the palmar surface of the fingers and sweeping both breasts superiorly to inferiorly, compress them against the thorax. Note any masses.

c. **Normal findings**
- Nipples are symmetric with no signs of erosion, discharge, or recent inversion.
- Breasts are symmetric, although they may vary in size.
- Breast tissue is soft, lobular, and homogenous.

d. **Gerontologic considerations**
- In postmenopausal women, the breasts may feel nodular or stringy on palpation.
- Breast tissue is denser in younger women. Breast tissue thins with age.

13. **Male breasts.** Although this examination is brief, it should not be omitted.
   a. **Inspection.** Observe the nipples and areola for ulceration, nodules, edema, or discharge.
   b. **Palpation.** Palpate the areola, noting nodules and tenderness.
   c. **Normal findings**
   - Nipples are symmetric with no erosion or discharge.
   - Masses, discharge, and tenderness are not noted.

14. **Thorax and lungs**
   a. **Inspection**
   - **Posterior chest.** With the client seated:
     - Observe the spine for mobility and structural deformity.
     - Inspect symmetry, posture, mobility of thorax, and intercostal spaces (e.g., bulges or retraction) on respiration.
     - Assess anteroposterior diameter in relation to the lateral diameter of the chest.
   - **Anterior chest.** With the client supine:
     - Inspect for structural deformities.
     - Assess the width of the costal angle.
     - Notice the rate and rhythm of breathing. Observe for respiratory abnormalities (e.g., bulging or retraction of intercostal spaces, and use of accessory muscles) and asymmetry.
   b. **Palpation**
   - **Posterior chest.** With the client seated:
     - Palpate the ribs and costal margins for symmetry, mobility, and tenderness.
     - Palpate the spine for tenderness and vertebral position.
     - Assess respiratory excursion (notice the distance that the thumbs part) and symmetry of motion and fremitus with the client's arms crossed and scapulae separated.
   - **Anterior chest.** With the client supine, assess as for the posterior chest, comparing symmetric areas and gently displacing female breasts if necessary.
   c. **Percussion**
   - **Posterior chest**
     - With the client seated with arms across the chest and the scapulae separated, percuss symmetric areas, comparing sides. (See *Figure 1-2.*) Begin across the top of each shoulder, and proceed downward between the scapulae and under the scapulae, moving medially and laterally in axillary lines; detect and localize abnormal percussion sounds. (See *Table 1-2,* page 18.)

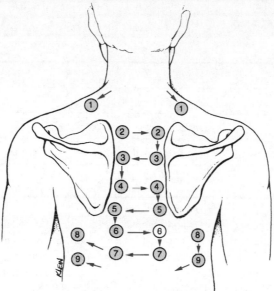

FIGURE 1–2

Percuss the posterior chest progressively from the shoulder tops to the costal margins at the midclavicular lines.

Adapted from Bickley, L.S., and Szilagyi, P.G. *Bates' Guide to Physical Examination and History Taking,* 8th ed. Philadelphia: Lippincott Williams & Wilkins, 2003.

- Percuss for diaphragmatic excursion on complete exhalation and inhalation, marking points where resonance changes to dullness; notice symmetry and levels.
 - **Anterior chest.** With the client supine and arms at sides, percuss from just below the clavicles along the midclavicular line (displacing female breasts as necessary) and then move laterally. Note intercostal spaces where hepatic dullness on the right side and cardiac dullness and gastric air bubble tympany on the left side are detected.

  d. **Auscultation**
   - **Posterior chest.** With the client seated as for percussion, ask him to breathe more deeply than normal with his mouth open. With a stethoscope, listen over the same areas and in the same pattern as for percussion, comparing from side to side and moving from apices to lung bases. (See *Figure 1-2.*)
   - **Anterior chest.** Auscultate over the same areas and in the same pattern as for percussion, comparing sides and proceeding from lung apices to bases. Notice the distribution of vesicular and bronchovesicular sounds posteriorly and anteriorly (See *Table 1-3*, page 19.)

  e. **Normal findings**
   - Respiratory rate ranges between 16 to 20 breaths per minute.
   - The thorax is symmetric. Costal angle is less than 90 degrees. Transverse diameter is 1:2 to 5:7 (healthy adult is wider from side to side than from front to back). Expansion is 1.2″ to 2″ (3 to 5 cm), symmetric, and free and easy; no bulges or retractions are detected in intercostal spaces.

TABLE 1-2
Review of percussion sounds

Sound	Description
Flat	Soft, high-pitched, short duration (e.g., thigh)
Dull	Medium intensity, pitch, and duration (e.g., liver)
Resonant	Loud, low-pitched, long duration (normal lung)
Hyperresonant	Very loud, lower pitched, longer duration (e.g., emphysematous lung)
Tympanic	Loud, musical (e.g., gastric air bubble, intestine)

- Diaphragm position and excursion is 1.2″ to 2.4″ (3 to 6 cm).
- Fremitus can be felt throughout lung fields, diminishing near the periphery.
- Percussion is resonant over symmetric areas of the lung to expected lung borders (fifth intercostal space [ICS] anteriorly, seventh ICS laterally, and T10 posteriorly); dullness is noted between the third and fifth left intercostal spaces (LICS).
- Adventitious sounds (i.e., crackles, gurgles, wheezes, and friction rubs), enhanced voiced sounds (i.e., egophony, bronchophony, and whispered pectoriloquy), or bronchial breath sounds are not present.

f. **Gerontologic considerations**
- The anteroposterior chest diameter is increased in elderly clients.
- Crackles may be auscultated at the lung bases in the absence of heart failure. Such crackles should clear with deep breathing or coughing; however, elderly adults tend not to breathe as deeply or cough as productively as younger adults because of decreased rib mobility and reduced vital capacity.
- A decrease in gas exchange and diffusing capacity is noted in elderly clients.
- A decrease in forced vital capacity is noted in elderly clients.

15. **Heart**
    a. **Inspection**
    - **Precordium.** Look for lifts, heaves, thrusts, or pulsations.
    - **Apical impulse.** Observe for visible pulsations, which occur in about 50% of clients.
    b. **Palpation**
    - **Auscultatory areas.** Using the palms, palpate all auscultatory areas, noting vibrations or thrills.
    - **Apical impulse.** Locate and assess the rate and strength of pulsations.
    c. **Percussion.** Percuss the heart's borders in the third to fifth LICS, noting areas of cardiac dullness.
    d. **Auscultation**
    - In each auscultatory area, listen with the stethoscope's diaphragm (best for high-pitched sounds) and bell (best for low-pitched sounds). (See *Figure 1-3*, page 20.)
      - The aortic area (A) is the second ICS to the right of the sternum.
      - The pulmonic area (P) is the second ICS to the left of the sternum.
      - The midprecordial area (E), Erb's point, is located in the third ICS to the left of the sternum.
      - The tricuspid area (T) is the fifth ICS to the left of the sternum (also known as the *right ventricular area* or the *septal area*).

TABLE 1-3
Review of lung sounds

Sound	Description
Breath sounds	
Vesicular	Longer on inspiration than expiration; low pitch, soft intensity on expiration; heard over most of the peripheral lung
Bronchovesicular	Equal duration on inspiration and expiration; medium pitch and intensity on expiration; heard near the mainstem bronchi (anteriorly, below the clavicle at sternal borders to near the level of the second intercostal space; posteriorly, between the clavicles and between T1 and T4)
Bronchial	Shorter on inspiration than expiration; high-pitched and loud intensity on expiration; heard over the trachea (the presence of bronchial sounds over a lung is always abnormal.)
Adventitious sounds	
Crackles	Formerly called rales or crepitations; discrete noncontinuous sounds usually heard on inspiration in dependent right and left lung bases; may clear on coughing; two types: fine crackles (soft, short, high-pitched), and coarse crackles (louder, longer, lower-pitched)
Gurgles	Loud gurgling, bubbling; heard during inspiration and expiration; may result from secretions in the trachea and large bronchi
Wheezes	Continuous, lengthy, musical; heard during inspiration or expiration
Pleural rub	Loud, low pitched; confined to small area of chest wall; result from inflamed pleura
Altered vocal sounds (sound transformed through airless lung tissue)	
Bronchophony	Unusually loud and clear voiced sound (e.g., "99")
Egophony	Nasal bleating quality: "ee" sounds like "ay"
Whispered pectoriloquy	Unusually loud and clear whispered sounds (e.g., "1, 2, 3")

- The mitral area (M) is the fifth ICS at the left midclavicular line (also known as the *left ventricular area* or the *apical area*).
- Identify S1 and S2 (i.e., lub-dub sound).
- Determine which sound is louder. Normally, S2 is loudest in the aortic and pulmonic areas; S1 is louder than or equal to S2 in the tricuspid area; and S1 is loudest in the mitral area.
- Listen for physiologic split in S2.
- Determine systolic phase (between S1 and S2) and diastolic phase (between S2 and S1). Diastolic should be longer than systolic at a heart rate of 120 beats per minute or less.
- Note extra sounds or murmurs.
- Determine the heart rate and rhythm.
  e. **Normal findings**
- Regular apical pulse rate ranges between 60 to 100 beats per minute.
- Thrills, heaves, or abnormal pulsations are not present.

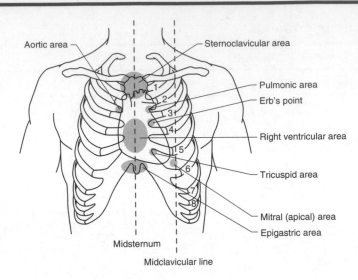

Aortic area — Sternoclavicular area

Pulmonic area
Erb's point

Right ventricular area

Tricuspid area

Mitral (apical) area
Epigastric area

Midsternum

Midclavicular line

FIGURE 1–3
Areas of the precordium to be assessed when evaluating heart function

- Apical impulse is the fifth LICS, at or medial to the midclavicular line (palpated within one ICS and no more than 0.4″ to 0.8″ [1- to 2-cm] wide; 2.8″ to 3.5″ [7- to 9-cm] from the sternal border).
- Left cardiac border dullness is percussed 3.5″ to 4.7″ [9 to 12 cm] from the sternal border.
- S1 and S2 are heard in expected locations with expected intensities (S2 split is common in the supine position on inspiration); no extra sounds or murmurs are present.

f. **Gerontologic considerations**
- Arrhythmias become more common with aging. They may or may not indicate stenosis or myocardial insufficiency.
- Stiffened sclerotic heart valves may cause murmurs or S4 ("Ten-nes-see") in the elderly client.
- S3 ("Ken-tuck-y") in elderly clients usually is pathologic.
- An increase in the systolic blood pressure (normal blood pressure of 160/90 mm Hg) may be noted in the elderly client.
- A decrease in cardiac output, heart-rate response to stress, and stroke volume may be noted in the elderly client.

16. **Peripheral circulation**
a. **Inspection**
- **Jugular veins**
  - With the client supine, observe the neck for internal jugular venous pulsations; if present, note the characteristics and relationship to inspiration.
  - With the client sitting, observe for distended jugular veins.
- **Carotid arteries.** Observe for pulsations (timed with apical impulse).

     – **Extremities (arterial)**
- Observe color, noting pallor or rubor.
- Inspect hair distribution, noting abnormal absence.
- Observe skin characteristics, noting shiny or thin skin and any circumscribed lesions on feet and toes.

     – **Extremities (venous)**
- Observe color, noting abnormal brown pigmentation.
- Look for skin lesions on the lower legs, varicosities, edema, and Homans' sign.

b. **Palpation**

     – **Extremities (arterial)**
- Assess the temperature of the skin.
- Palpate pulses (i.e., radial, femoral, posterior tibial, dorsalis pedis), comparing sides: 0, absent pulse; 1+, thready/weak; 2+, normal; 3+, increased or strong; 4+, bounding.
- Check capillary refill times in fingernails and toenails.
- Perform Allen's test to determine arterial patency.

     – **Extremities (venous)**
- Palpate the skin over the tibia and at the medial malleoli for pitting edema.
- Compress the calf between two hands placed anteriorly and posteriorly; note any pain that this maneuver elicits.

c. **Auscultation.** Listen over the carotid, abdominal, and femoral arteries for bruits.

d. **Normal findings**
- Jugular veins are soft and undulating. When the individual is supine, jugular veins decrease on inspiration. When the individual is sitting, jugular veins are not observable.
- Carotid artery pulsations are synchronous with apical impulse.
- In the extremities, skin is warm without discoloration, lesions, varicosities, or edema.
- Pulses are 2+ bilaterally on a scale of 0 to 4+
- Capillary refill is less than 3 seconds. Hands are pink immediately in response to Allen's test.
- Calves are not tender. Homans' sign is negative bilaterally.
- Bruits are not auscultated over the carotid, abdominal, or femoral arteries.

e. **Gerontologic considerations**
- Elderly people commonly experience thickening, hardening, and loss of elasticity in vessel walls, resulting in an increase in peripheral vascular resistance.
- Gradual pink or purple discoloration on the toes and feet is common in elderly people.

17. Abdomen

a. **Inspection**
- Observe for scars, striae, and rashes.
- Note general contour and symmetry.
- Observe for visible peristalsis, aortic pulsations, and hernias (i.e., umbilical, inguinal, and incisional).

b. **Auscultation.** Auscultate the abdomen before percussing and palpating to avoid stimulating intestinal activity and altering bowel sounds.
- In all quadrants, listen to bowel sounds, noting frequency, pitch, and duration. It is necessary to listen for at least 5 minutes in an abdominal quadrant before concluding that bowel sounds are absent.

– Over the abdominal aorta and the renal, iliac, and femoral arteries, auscultate for bruits.

c. **Percussion**
   – **All quadrants.** Percuss, noting areas of tympany or dullness.
   – **Right midclavicular line.** Percuss starting below the umbilicus and moving upward to locate the liver borders.
   – **Left upper quadrant.** Percuss for gastric air bubbles.
   – **The back.** With the client sitting, strike at the costovertebral angles, noting tenderness or pain.

d. **Palpation**
   – **Abdomen.** Palpate lightly in all quadrants; follow with deep palpation. Assess organ location and abdominal muscle tone. Note unusual masses, pulsations, tenderness, or pain.
   – **Kidney.** Palpate kidneys bimanually, slightly below the umbilicus. Note size, shape, and any tenderness.
   – **Abdominal aorta.** Palpate for contour and pulsations.
   – **Lymph nodes.** Palpate inguinal and femoral areas bilaterally. Note enlargement.

e. **Normal findings**
   – No scars are evident. The client does not have incisional, umbilical, or inguinal hernias. The abdominal wall is flat symmetric with no masses or tenderness.
   – Bowel sounds are intermittent (every 5 to 35 seconds) and gurgling with no hyperactive or tinkling sounds. Rushing sounds over the ileocecal valve (in the right lower quadrant) are heard 4 to 7 hours after eating. Abdominal bruits are not auscultated.
   – Liver dullness is noted 2.4" to 4.7" (6 to 12 cm) at right midclavicular line. Tympany of gastric air bubble is noted over left anterior lower border of thorax. Tympany in all quadrants is noted.
   – Costovertebral angle tenderness is not evident.
   – The aorta is 1" to 1.6" (2.5- to 4-cm) wide, soft, and pulsatile.
   – Pole of right kidney may be palpable.

f. **Gerontologic considerations**
   – Elderly clients commonly exhibit diminished salivation and peristalsis.
   – In the elderly client, the liver may be 0.4" to 0.8" (1- to 2-cm) below the right costal margin because of an enlarged lung field.
   – Elderly clients exhibit delayed esophageal and gastric emptying and delayed pancreatic insulin release.
   – Elderly clients have difficulty swallowing food and a decreased basal metabolic rate.

18. **Male genitalia.** Wear gloves during the examination.

a. **Inspection**
   – **Pubic hair.** Assess distribution, and note any nits or lice.
   – **Penis.** Retract the foreskin, if present. Note any ulcerations, masses, or scarring on the glans penis. Inspect the urethral meatus for location, lesions, and discharge.
   – **Scrotum.** Inspect anterior and posterior aspects, assessing size, contour, and symmetry. Note ulcerations, masses, redness, or edema.
   – **Inguinal areas.** Look for bulges, with and without the client bearing down, or when raising his head off the bed.

    b. **Palpation**

- **Penis.** Palpate the shaft for lesions, nodules, or masses; if present, note tenderness, contour, size, and degree of induration.
- **Scrotum.** Palpate each testis and epididymis, assessing size, shape, and consistency. Note any masses or unusual tenderness. Look for any nodules or tenderness of the spermatic cord and vas deferens.
- **Inguinal and femoral areas.** Assess for hernias.

    c. **Normal findings**

- Normal male pubic hair distribution is noted. Pubic hair is free of infestation.
- Penile lesions, masses, or discharge are not present.
- Testes are symmetric without masses or undue tenderness. The left testis may be slightly larger and hang lower than the right testis.
- Inguinal or femoral hernias are not present.

    d. **Gerontologic considerations**

- In elderly men, pubic hair commonly thins, and scrotal skin loses tone, causing the scrotum to appear more pendulous.
- Some degree of testicular atrophy and softening commonly occurs with aging.
- Elderly men experience a decreased penis size and a slower sexual response.
- Elderly men may experience decreased bladder capacity, delayed voiding sensation, and benign prostatic hypertrophy.

19. **Female genitalia.** Wear gloves during the examination.

    a. **Inspection and palpation.** These examinations are performed almost simultaneously. Place the client in the lithotomy position and drape properly.

- **External genitalia.** Assess pubic hair distribution. Note any nits or lice. Inspect the labia majora, mons pubis, and perineum. Note skin color and integrity.
- **Internal genitalia.** Separate the labia majora, and inspect the clitoris, urethral meatus, and vaginal opening. Note abnormal color, ulcerations, edema, nodules, or discharge.

    b. **Normal findings**

- Female pubic hair distribution is normal. Pubic hair is free of infestation.
- The outlet, vagina, and perineum are free of masses, edema, tenderness, nodules, lesions, and discharge.
- Urinary discharge or odor is not present.

    c. **Gerontologic considerations**

- In elderly women, pubic hair becomes gray, more sparse, and brittle.
- External genitalia typically atrophy somewhat in elderly women.
- Weakened perineal muscle tone with aging increases the likelihood of cystocele.
- Elderly women generally experience vaginal narrowing, decreased vaginal elasticity, decreased vaginal secretions, and a slower sexual response.
- Elderly women may experience a decreased bladder capacity.

20. **Rectum.** Wear gloves during the examination.

    a. **Inspection.** Examine the anus and the perianal and sacral regions, with the client lying in the left Sims' position and properly draped. If necessary, use an alternative position for the examination. Male clients may stand and bend over the table; female clients may assume the lithotomy position.

- Spread the buttocks, and note any inflammation, nodules, scars, lesions, ulcerations, rashes, bleeding, fissures, or hemorrhoids.
- Check for bulges when the client bears down.

b. **Palpation**
- **Sphincter.** Ask the client to bear down. Slowly insert the lubricated index finger of the gloved hand through the anal sphincter. Assess sphincter tone.
- **Rectum and rectal walls.** Gently rotate the index finger to palpate the rectum and rectal walls anteriorly and posteriorly. Note any nodules, masses, or tenderness. Palpate for fecal impaction.
- **Prostate.** In a male client, anteriorly palpate the two lateral lobes of the prostate gland for irregularities, nodules, edema, or tenderness.
- **Fecal material.** Withdraw the finger gently. Test any fecal material on the glove for occult blood.

c. **Normal findings**
- Sphincter closes around finger.
- Wall of rectum is smooth and moist. Soft stool may be present.
- No hemorrhoids, fissures, or fistulas are evident.
- Stool guaiac test result is negative.
- Male prostate is 1″ to 1.6″ (2.5 to 4 cm) in diameter, with a small groove separating the lobes. It feels firm, smooth, nonmovable, nontender, and rubbery.

d. **Gerontologic considerations.** Most older men exhibit some degree of prostatic enlargement.

21. **Musculoskeletal system**
    a. **Inspection**
    - Observe the client's ability to perform functional tasks of daily living (e.g., performing personal hygiene, rising from sitting to standing, walking up and down stairs, walking on a level surface). Note any pain the client experiences while performing functions or being examined.
    - **Extremities.** Examine the arms and legs. Note the size, symmetry, muscle mass, and any deformities.
    - **Spine.** Assess for range of motion (i.e., flexion, extension, lateral flexion, and rotation) and lateral or anteroposterior curvature.
    - **Joints.** Assess all major joints, noting any limitations to active range of motion, edema, or redness.
      - **Neck.** Assess flexion, extension, and lateral rotation.
      - **Shoulders.** Assess flexion, extension, and rotation.
      - **Elbows.** Assess flexion, extension, supination, and pronation.
      - **Wrists.** Assess flexion, extension, and ulnar and radial deviation.
      - **Fingers.** Assess flexion, extension, abduction, and adduction.
      - **Hips.** Assess flexion, extension, and rotation.
      - **Knees.** Assess flexion and extension.
      - **Ankles.** Assess dorsiflexion, plantar flexion, inversion, and eversion.
      - **Toes.** Assess flexion, extension, abduction, and adduction.

    b. **Palpation**
    - **Joints of the neck and upper and lower extremities.** Palpate while noting tenderness, edema, temperature, limitations to passive range of motion, and crepitation.
    - **Muscles.** Palpate to assess size, tone, and any tenderness.
    - **Spine.** Palpate, noting bony deformities and crepitation.

    c. **Percussion.** Directly percuss the spine from the cervical to lumbar region, using the ulnar surface of the fist. Note any pain or tenderness.

d. **Normal findings**
  - Functional limitations are not evident.
  - Gross deformities and abnormal postures are not present.
  - Range of joint motion is unrestricted in extremities and spine.
  - Muscle mass is symmetric without hypertrophy or atrophy. The tone is normal.
  - Joint pain, crepitus, bony overgrowths, and tenderness in the extremities or spine are not evidenced.

e. **Gerontologic considerations**
  - Elderly clients commonly exhibit diminished joint flexibility and decreased muscle and bone mass and strength.
  - Other common age-related musculoskeletal problems include degenerative joint changes, mild scoliosis or kyphosis, stooped body posture, and some degree of functional limitation.
  - Elderly clients have a decrease in deep tendon reflexes and a decrease in height.

22. **Neurologic system**

  a. **Components** of the neurologic examination
    - Mental status
    - Cranial nerve function
    - Cerebellar function
    - Motor function
    - Sensory function
    - Reflexes

  b. **Mental status.** During history taking, assess:
    - **state of consciousness,** noting whether the client is alert, somnolent, stuporous, or comatose
    - **orientation** to person, place, and time
    - **memory,** including immediate, recent, and remote
    - **cognition,** including calculations, current events, and response to proverbs
    - **judgment and problem solving ability**
    - **emotion,** including mood, affect, and congruence of responses.

  c. **Cranial nerve (CN) function**
    - **Olfactory (CN I).** With the client's eyes closed, present various odors, occluding one nostril at a time. Note the client's ability to identify the odors.
    - **Optic nerve (CN II).** Test visual acuity and visual fields, and examine the optic disk with an ophthalmoscope.
    - **Oculomotor (CN III), trochlear (CN IV), and abducens (CN VI) nerves.** Assess extraocular motion.
      - Evaluate the six cardinal positions of gaze. Look for parallelism, and note nystagmus (involuntary movement).
      - Perform the cover/uncover test (i.e., movement of eye when uncovered or opposite eye when contralateral eye covered).
      - Assess corneal light reflex (i.e., symmetry of reflection of light on pupil); check size and shape of pupils and pupillary reaction to light and accommodation.
    - **Trigeminal nerve (CN V)**
      - **Motor.** Assess the client's ability to chew and the strength of his bite.
      - **Sensory.** Assess the client's ability to distinguish light touch and pain. Lightly stroke his face with a cotton wisp, and gently prick the skin with a sterile pin or toothpick on the forehead (to assess the ophthalmic branch), cheek (to assess the maxillary branch), and chin (to assess the mandibular branch).

- **Facial nerve (CN VII)**
  - **Motor.** Assess symmetry of facial movements as the client smiles, frowns, grimaces, clenches his teeth, and other facial movements.
  - **Sensory.** Ask the client to identify various distinct flavors placed on the anterior two-thirds of the tongue.
- **Acoustic nerve (CN VIII)**
  - **Cochlear branch.** Assess hearing acuity.
  - **Vestibular branch.** Perform Romberg's test to evaluate equilibrium. Have the client stand with feet together and eyes closed for 20 to 30 seconds without support. Note excessive swaying.
- **Glossopharyngeal nerve (CN IX).** Test for the gag reflex by gently touching the posterior pharyngeal wall with a tongue blade.
- **Vagus nerve (CN X).** As the client speaks, check movement of the uvula (noting any deviation from midline) and palate (noting asymmetric elevation).
- **Spinal accessory nerve (CN XI).** Assess the strength of the sternocleidomastoid and upper trapezius muscles by asking the client to move his head against the resistance of your hand. Observe and palpate the contraction of the sternocleidomastoid muscle on the opposite side. Ask the client to shrug his shoulders against the resistance of your hands.
- **Hypoglossal nerve (CN XII).** Test strength and articulation of the tongue by having the client push his tongue to the side of the mouth against resistance applied to the cheek. Ask him to stick out his tongue and then return it to his mouth while you observe for deviation, asymmetry, tremors, and fasciculations.

d. **Cerebellar function** (i.e., coordination and balance)
- Assess **posture, gait,** and **balance.** Have the client walk forward and backward in a straight line.
- Assess **coordination in the upper extremities** by having the client perform the finger-to-nose test.
- Assess **coordination in the lower extremities** by having the client tap his toes and slide his heel down the contralateral shin.

e. **Motor function**
- **Muscle mass.** Assess symmetry and distribution distally and proximally, and the circumference of the extremities.
- **Tone.** Evaluate resistance of muscles in response to passive motion during flexion and extension of extremities.
- **Strength.** Assess hand squeeze and evaluate muscle strength in each extremity against resistance during flexion and extension (also abduction and adduction when appropriate), comparing bilaterally.
- **Observe for involuntary movements** (e.g., tics, fasciculations, tremors, twitching) and **abnormal postures** (e.g., fetal, decorticate, decerebrate).

f. **Sensory function.** With the client's eyes closed, assess the following:
- **Light touch.** Have the client indicate response to a cotton wisp lightly stroked on his skin at representative dermatomes (i.e., backs of hands, forearms and upper arms, torso, thigh, tibia, and dorsal portion of foot). Compare bilaterally and distal to proximal.
- **Pain.** Repeat the pattern of light-touch assessment, using a sterile safety pin to elicit sharp sensation. Alternate with the pin's rounded end for contrast.
- **Vibration**
  - Place a vibrating low-pitched tuning fork over the sternum.

- On the distal interphalangeal joint of a finger, quickly ask the client to identify whether vibration sensation in the finger is 100%, 75%, 50%, or 25% of that felt in the sternum. Ask the client to indicate when vibration is no longer felt.
  - Repeat this procedure on a great toe.
  - If vibration sense is impaired in the finger or toe, proceed to assessment in more proximal bony prominences (e.g., wrist and elbow or medial malleolus, patella, anterior iliac spine, and spinous processes).
- **Position sense.** With your finger placed on the lateral surface of the client's digit (finger or great toe), move it up or down. Ask the client which direction the digit is pointing.
- **Stereognosis.** Ask the client to identify small objects placed in the hand, one hand at a time (e.g., key, paper clip).
- **Graphesthesia.** Ask the client to identify a number that the nurse traces with the fingertip in the palm of the client's hand.

g. **Deep tendon reflexes.** Striking with a reflex hammer, compare reflex amplitude bilaterally, grading on a 4-point scale: 4+, hyperactive; 2+ or 3+, average; 1+, diminished; 0, no response.
- **Brachioradialis (C5, C6).** Strike the radius tendon about 1″ to 2″ (2.5 to 5.1 cm) above the wrist; observe for flexion and supination of the forearm.
- **Biceps (C5, C6).** Place your thumb or forefinger at the base of the biceps tendon, and strike it. Observe for flexion of the arm at the elbow.
- **Triceps (C7, C8).** Strike the triceps tendon just above the elbow. Observe for slight elbow extension.
- **Patellar or quadriceps (L2, L3, L4).** Sharply strike the patellar tendon. Observe for extension of the knee.
- **Achilles or ankle jerk (S1, S2).** Support the client's foot in the dorsiflexed position; tap the Achilles tendon, and observe for plantar flexion.

h. **Superficial cutaneous reflexes**
- **Abdominal.** Stroke the abdomen above (T8, T9, T10) and below (T10, T11, T12) the umbilicus bilaterally. Observe for contraction of abdominal muscles and deviation of the umbilicus toward the stimulus.
- **Cremasteric (L1, L2).** In a male client, stroke the inner surface of the thigh. Observe for prompt elevation of the testis on the ipsilateral side.
- **Plantar (L4, L5, S1, S2).** Extend the client's legs with the feet relaxed; stroke the lateral aspect of the sole from the heel to the ball of the foot, curving medially across the ball. Observe for flexion of toes.

i. **Normal findings**
- **Mental status.** The client is alert, quiet, and able to follow three-step instructions. He is oriented to person, place, and time. Judgment and intellectual performance are within normal limits.
- **Cranial nerve function.** CN I through XII responses are present, including absence of abnormal muscle movement; no vertigo; ability to shrug shoulders; normal eye movement; and normal sensation.
- **Cerebellar function.** Romberg's test is negative, movement is not clumsy, and coordination is normal.
- **Motor.** Atrophy, tremors, or weakness are not evident.
- **Muscle tone.** Flaccidity, rigidity, and spasticity are not evident.
- **Muscle strength** is strong and equal.

- **Sensory function.** Light touch, pain, vibration, and position sense are normal. Stereognosis and graphesthesia are intact, as evidenced by the ability to identify object and number.
- **Reflexes.** Deep tendon reflexes (e.g., brachioradialis, biceps, triceps, patella, and ankle) score 2+ (on a scale of 0 to 4+); superficial reflexes (i.e., abdominal and cremasteric) are present; and plantar reflexes (i.e., toes flex) are normal.

j. **Gerontologic considerations**
  - Many elderly clients exhibit moderate recent memory loss.
  - The sense of smell tends to become less keen with aging.
  - Age-related changes in cerebellar function may include drifting during Romberg's test; wide-based, slowed gait; diminished sense of equilibrium, especially when moving rapidly; and a slowed reaction time.
  - Elderly clients commonly exhibit some degree of muscle atrophy and decreased muscle strength.
  - Age-related sensory changes may include diminished pain perception and diminished sense of touch, temperature, vibration, and position.
  - Reflexes commonly diminish or subside with aging.

IV. SUPPORTIVE STUDIES

A. **Laboratory studies.** The third part of a complete health assessment, laboratory study results fall into three basic categories: urinalysis, hematology, and blood chemistry. Normal value ranges may vary according to a health care institution's policies and standards. (See *Table 1-4.*)

B. **Diagnostic studies.** Diagnostic tests are performed during routine physical examinations (e.g., electrocardiogram, stress test, mammogram, digital rectal examination) and assist in diagnosing disease (e.g., endoscopy, biopsy, radiography). Specific diagnostic tests are discussed in each chapter, and abnormal results are discussed with each disease process.

C. **Nurse's responsibility.** The nurse is responsible for caring for the client during pretest, intratest, and posttest periods. Facility policies, procedures, and protocols for collecting, handling, and transporting specimens should be followed at all times. The nurse must educate the client concerning preparation for the diagnostic test (e.g., fasting, activity restrictions, withholding medications); obtain written consent if necessary; ensure the client's safety during the procedure; assist with the procedure if necessary; and monitor for complications after the diagnostic test (e.g., monitoring vital signs, assessing return of gag reflex). Standard precautions must be adhered to at all times.

TABLE 1-4
Common laboratory studies

Test	Normal values	Gerontologic considerations
Urinalysis		
Protein	Negative	Normal values rise slightly with aging.
Glucose	Negative	Normal values decline slightly with aging.
Specific gravity	1.015 to 1.025	Normal value declines to 1.024 by age 80.
Ketones	Negative	Normal values should not change with aging.
Hematology		
Hemoglobin	Men: 13 to 18 g/100 ml Women: 12 to 16 g/100 ml	Normal value drops by 1 to 2 g/100 ml in elderly men; no change documented in elderly women.
Hematocrit	Men: 42% to 50% Women: 40% to 48%	Specific changes in elderly persons are not documented to date; a slight decline has been hypothesized.
White blood cells	5,000 to 10,000/mm^3	Total count drops to 3,100 to 9,000/mm^3 with aging.
Platelets	100,00 to 400,000/mm^3	No changes in platelet number have been detected in elderly clients, but changes in platelet characteristics have been documented.
Prothrombin time	11 to 15 seconds	No change has been identified in healthy elderly clients.
International Normalized Ratio	1	No change has been identified in healthy elderly clients.
Partial thromboplastin time	20 to 45 seconds	No change has been identified in healthy elderly clients.
Blood chemistry		
Albumin	3.5 to 5 g/100 ml; the level tends to be higher in men than in women	After age 65, values equalize and decline at the same rate.
Total serum protein	6 to 8.4 g/100 ml	No change has been identified in elderly clients; increased beta-globulin balances decreased albumin.
Sodium	135 to 145 mEq/L	No change has been identified in elderly clients.
Potassium	3.5 to 5.5 mEq/L	Normal value increases slightly in elderly clients.
Chloride	95 to 105 mEq/L	No change has been identified in elderly clients.
Blood urea nitrogen	Men: 7 to 18 g/100 ml	Values increase in elderly clients, sometimes as high as 69 mg/100 ml.
Creatinine	0.2 to 0.8 mg/100 ml	Value increases in elderly men are sometimes as high as 1.9 mg/100 ml.

(continued)

TABLE 1-4

Common laboratory studies *(continued)*

Test	Normal values	Gerontologic considerations
Blood chemistry *(continued)*		
Creatinine clearance	100 to 150 ml/min	The formula for calculating age-referenced interval in men is 140 minus age times body weight (in kg), divided by 72 and times serum creatinine. In women, the age-referenced interval is 85% of this figure.
Glucose tolerance	Fasting: 60 to 110 mg/dl Nonfasting: 85 to 140 mg/dl	In elderly clients, an elevated fasting glucose level may indicate diabetes mellitus.
Triglycerides	40 to 150 mg/100 ml	Normal values in elderly clients range from 20 to 200 mg/100 ml.
Cholesterol	120 to 200 mg/100 ml	In men, values tend to increase up to age 50 and then decrease. In women, values tend to be lower than those in men until age 50 and then higher up to age 70; values decrease after age 70.
High-density lipoproteins	Male: 32 to 70 mg/dl Female: 38 to 85 mg/dl	Differences among men and women diminish with age.
Thyroxine	4.5 to 11.5 µg/100 ml	Values decrease by about 25% in elderly clients.
Triiodothyronine	75 to 200 mg/100 ml	Values decrease by about 25% in elderly clients.
Thyroid-stimulating hormone	0.5 to 5 µU/ml	Values increase slightly in elderly clients.
Alkaline phosphatase	30 to 115 IU/L	Values increase by 8 to 10 IU/L in elderly clients.
Acid phosphatase	0 to 10 ng/ml	No age-related changes have been identified.
Aspartate aminotransferase	7 to 56 U/L	No age-related changes have been identified.
Creatinine phosphokinase	Male: 50 to 325 mU/ml Female: 50 to 250 mU/ml	Values increase slightly in elderly clients.
Lactate dehydrogenase	100 to 225 U/L	Values increase slightly in elderly clients.

Study questions

1. Which assessment data should the nurse include when obtaining a review of body systems?
   1. The client's name, address, age, and phone number
   2. Brief statement about what brought the client to the health care provider
   3. Information about the client's sexual performance and preference
   4. Client complaints of chest pain, dyspnea, or abdominal pain

2. A client has come to the nursing clinic for a comprehensive health assessment. Which statement would be the best way to end the history interview?
   1. "What brought you to the clinic today?"

2. "Would you describe your overall health as good?"
3. "Do you understand what is happening?"
4. "Is there anything else you would like to tell me?"

3. For which time period would the nurse notify the health care provider that the client had no bowel sounds?
1. 2 minutes
2. 3 minutes
3. 4 minutes
4. 5 minutes

4. Which is the *best* area for auscultating the apical pulse?
1. Aortic arch
2. Pulmonic area
3. Tricuspid area
4. Mitral area

5. Which scientific rationale should the nurse remember when performing a breast examination on a female client?
1. One half of all breast cancer deaths occur in women ages 35 to 45.
2. The tail of Spence area must be included in self-examination.
3. The position of choice for the breast examination is supine.
4. A pad should be placed under the opposite scapula of the breast being palpated.

6. To prevent client discomfort and injury during an otoscopic examination, which action should be avoided?
1. Tipping the client's head away from the examiner and pulling the ear up and back
2. Inserting the otoscope inferiorly into the distal portion of the external canal
3. Inserting the otoscope superiorly into the proximal two-thirds of the external canal
4. Bracing the examiner's hand against the client's head

7. Which intervention should the nurse perform when assessing the lower extremities for arterial function?
1. Assessing the medial malleoli for pitting edema
2. Performing Allen's test
3. Assessing for Homans' sign
4. Palpating the pedal pulses

8. Which assessment examination requires the nurse to wear gloves?
1. Oral
2. Ophthalmic
3. Breast
4. Integumentary

9. To ensure a client's safety during Romberg's test, which intervention should the nurse implement?
1. Standing close to provide support
2. Allowing the client keep his eyes open
3. Letting the client spread his feet apart
4. Having the client hold on to furniture

10. During an abdominal examination, the nurse performs the four physical-examination techniques in which sequence?
1. Auscultation immediately after inspection and then percussion and palpation
2. Percussion, followed by inspection, auscultation, and palpation
3. Palpation of tender areas first and then inspection, percussion, and auscultation
4. Inspection and then palpation, percussion, and auscultation

11. Which data would be of *greatest* concern to the nurse when completing the nursing assessment of a 75-year-old client hospitalized with pneumonia?
1. Alert and oriented to date, time, and place
2. Clear breath sounds and nonproductive cough
3. Buccal cyanosis and capillary refill greater than 3 seconds
4. Hemoglobin concentration of 13 g/dl and leukocyte count of 5,300/mm^3

12. During the nursing assessment, which data represent information concerning health beliefs?
1. Use of prescribed and over-the-counter medications
2. Promotive, preventive, and restorative health practices
3. Educational level and financial status
4. Family role and relationship patterns

13. Which is an example of biographic information that may be obtained during a health history?
1. The chief complaint
2. Past health status
3. History of immunizations
4. Location of an advance directive

14. When percussing a client's chest, the nurse would expect to find which assessment data as a normal sign over the client's lungs?
1. Tympany
2. Resonance
3. Dullness
4. Hyperresonance

15. Which laboratory result would warrant *immediate* intervention by the nurse caring for a patient diagnosed with dehydration?
1. Serum sodium level of 138 mEq/L
2. Serum potassium level of 3.1 mEq/L
3. Serum glucose level of 120 mg/dl
4. Serum creatinine level of 0.6 mg/100 ml

16. Which interventions are the nurse's responsibility when caring for a client having multiple diagnostic and laboratory studies? (Select all that apply.)
1. Educating the client concerning preparation for the diagnostic test
2. Obtaining written consent when needed for the diagnostic test
3. Escorting the client to the appropriate room for the procedure
4. Delegating responsibility for client assessment for postprocedure complications
5. Notifying the health care provider when the diagnostic test is complete
6. Adhering to standard precautions at all times when caring for the client

Answer key

1. The answer is **4.**
Client complaints about chest pain, dyspnea, or abdominal pain are considered part of the review of body systems. This portion of the assessment elicits subjective information on the client's perceptions of major body system functions, including cardiac, respiratory, and abdominal. The client's name, address, age, and phone number are biographic data. A brief statement about what brought the client to the health care provider is the chief complaint. Information about the client's sexual performance and preference addresses past health status.

2. The answer is **4.**
By asking the client if there is anything else, the nurse allows the client to end the interview by discussing feelings and concerns. Asking about what brought the client to the clinic is an ambiguous question to which the client may answer "my car" or any similarly disingenuous reply. Asking if the client describes his overall health as good is a leading question that puts words in his mouth. Asking if the client understands what is happening is a yes-or-no question that can elicit little information.

3. The answer is **4.**
To completely determine that bowel sounds are absent, the nurse must auscultate each of the four quadrants for at least 5 minutes; 2, 3, or 4 minutes is too short a period to arrive at this conclusion.

4. The answer is **4.**
The mitral area (also known as the *left ventricular area* or the *apical area*), the fifth intercostal space (ICS) at the left midclavicu-

lar line, is the best area for auscultating the apical pulse. The aortic arch is the second ICS to the right of sternum. The pulmonic area is the second intercostal space to the left of the sternum. The tricuspid area is the fifth ICS to the left of the sternum.

5. The answer is **2.**

The tail of Spence, an extension of the upper outer quadrant of breast tissue, can develop breast tumors. This area must also be included in breast self-examination. One half of all women who die of breast cancer are older than age 65. The correct position for breast self-examination is not limited to the supine position; the sitting position with hands at sides, above head, and on hips is also recommended. A pad is placed under the ipsilateral (e.g., same side) scapula of the breast being palpated.

6. The answer is **3.**

In the superior position, the speculum of the otoscope is nearest the tympanic membrane, and the most sensitive portion of the external canal is the proximal two thirds. It is important to avoid these structures during the examination. Tipping the client's head away from the examiner, pulling the ear up and back, inserting the otoscope inferiorly, and bracing the examiner's hand against the client's head are all appropriate techniques used during an otoscopic examination.

7. The answer is **4.**

Palpating the client's pedal pulses assists in determining if arterial blood supply to the lower extremities is sufficient. Assessing the medial malleoli for pitting edema is appropriate for assessing venous function of the lower extremity. Allen's test is used to evaluate arterial blood flow before inserting an arterial line in an upper extremity or obtaining arterial blood gases. Homans' sign is used to evaluate the possibility of deep vein thrombosis.

8. The answer is **1.**

Gloves should be worn any time there is a risk of exposure to the client's blood or body fluids. Oral, rectal, and genital examinations require gloves because they involve contact with body fluids. Ophthalmic, breast, or integumentary examinations normally do not involve contact with the client's body fluids and do not require the nurse to wear gloves for protection. However, if there are areas of skin breakdown or drainage, gloves should be used.

9. The answer is **1.**

During Romberg's test, the client is asked to stand with feet together and eyes shut and still maintain balance with a minimum of sway. If the client loses his balance, the nurse standing close to provide support, such as having an arm close around his shoulder, can prevent a fall. Allowing the client to keep his eyes open, spread his feet apart, or hang on to a piece of furniture interferes with the proper execution of the test and yields invalid results.

10. The answer is **1.**

With an abdominal assessment, auscultation always is performed before percussion and palpation because any abdominal manipulation, such as from palpation or percussion, can alter bowel sounds. Percussion should never precede inspection or auscultation, and any tender or painful areas should be palpated last.

11. The answer is **3.**

Buccal cyanosis and capillary refill greater than 3 seconds are indicative of decreased oxygen to the tissues, which requires immediate intervention. Alert and oriented, clear breath sounds, nonproductive cough, hemoglobin concentration of 13 g/dl, and a leukocyte count of 5,300/mm^3 are normal data.

12. The answer is **2.**

The health-beliefs assessment includes expectations of health care; promotive, preventive, and restorative practices, such as breast self-examination, testicular examination, and seat-belt use; and how the client perceives illness. Use of medications provides information about the client's personal habits. Educational level, financial status, and family role and relationship patterns represent information associated with role and relationship patterns.

13. The answer is **4.**

Biographic information may include name, address, gender, race, occupation, and location of a living will or a durable power of attorney for health care. The chief complaint, past health status, and history of immunizations are part of assessing the client's health and illness patterns.

14. The answer is **2.**

Normally, when percussing a client's chest, percussion over the lungs reveals resonance, a hollow or loud, low-pitched sound of long duration. Tympany is typically heard on percussion over such areas as a gastric air bubble or the intestine. Dullness is typically heard on percussion of solid organs, such as the liver or areas of consolidation. Hyperresonance would be evidenced by percussion over areas of overinflation such as an emphysematous lung.

15. The answer is **2.**

A normal potassium level is 3.5 to 5.5 mEq/L. A normal sodium level is 135 to 145 mEq/L, a normal nonfasting glucose level is 85 to 140 mg/dl, and a normal creatinine level is 0.2 to 0.8 mg/100 ml.

16. The answers are **1, 2, 6.**

Educating the client, obtaining written consent, and adhering to standard precautions are all the responsibility of the nurse when caring for a client undergoing a diagnostic test. The client can be escorted by unlicensed personnel, the nurse cannot delegate assessment, and the health care provider does not need to be notified when the diagnostic test is complete.

2 *Homeostasis*

I. ESSENTIAL CONCEPTS

A. Cellular composition

1. The nurse must be aware of cellular structure, composition, and function to understand the body's reaction to cell injury and ability to maintain homeostasis.
2. Cells are composed of protoplasm (75% water, electrolytes, proteins, lipids, and carbohydrates).
3. A cell has three major parts (see *Figure 2-1*):
   a. The **nucleus** is the control center for the cell. It contains deoxyribonucleic acid, which comprises chromosomes.
   b. The **cytoplasm,** which surrounds the nucleus, is where the work of the cells takes place. Embedded in the cytoplasm are organelles: ribosomes, endoplasmic reticulum, Golgi complex, mitochondria, lysosomes, microtubules, and filaments.
   c. The **cell membrane** is a semipermeable structure that separates intracellular and extracellular environments. It provides receptors for hormones and other chemical messengers that regulate cellular activity, participates in the electrical events that occur in nerve and muscle cells, and aids in regulating cell growth and proliferation.

B. Principles of homeostasis

1. Homeostasis refers to the state of equilibrium in the body's internal environment — the cells, tissues, organs, and fluids.
2. Cellular activities related to homeostasis include:
   a. energy production
   b. reproduction
   c. intracellular digestion.
3. Maintenance of homeostasis (i.e., steady state) depends primarily on normal cellular function. Through a process of negative feedback, deviations from a predetermined range of adaptability triggers a response aimed at correcting for the deviation. This process is regulated primarily by the autonomic nervous system and the endocrine system.
4. When stress or change occurs that causes the normal cellular function to deviate from its normal range, compensatory mechanisms are initiated to restore or maintain homeostasis.
5. Homeostasis is constantly being threatened by physical, psychological, and environmental stress. Health represents successful adaptation to that stress.

C. Cellular repair.
Stress is a state resulting from a change in the environment that is perceived as threatening homeostasis. A stimulus that evokes this state is known as a stressor. During times of stress, the cell undergoes cellular repair — change that permits survival, maintenance of function, and maintenance of homeostasis.

1. **Mechanisms of cellular repair**
   a. **Cellular adaptation** occurs when cells undergo changes in size, number, and type. Adaptation is the desired outcome in managing actual or perceived stress to reestablish equilibrium.
   b. **Regenerative healing** occurs when damaged cells and tissues are replaced by identical new cells and tissues (e.g., GI mucosal cells, epithelial cells of the skin, liver cells, renal tubule cells) after injury.
   c. **Replacement healing** occurs with replacement cells, such as connective tissue, and results in scar formation.

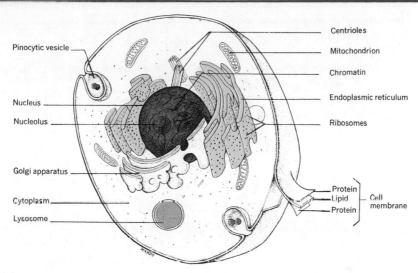

FIGURE 2–1

Cell composite representing the various components of the nucleus and cytoplasm

Source: Porth, C.M. *Pathophysiology: Concepts of Altered Health States,* 6th ed. Philadelphia: Lippincott Williams & Wilkins, 2002.

2. **Factors affecting cellular repair**
   a. **Age.** Elderly clients may have decreased blood flow to skin, organ atrophy and di- minished function, and altered immunity. These effects slow cellular repair and in- crease the risk of infection.
   b. **Nutritional status.** Adequate protein and caloric intake is essential to optimal cel- lular repair. A person with cellular injury has greater protein and calorie needs.
   c. **Infection** slows cellular repair.
   d. **Chronic illness.** Various chronic illnesses (e.g., uncontrolled diabetes mellitus) can predispose a client to cellular injury.
   e. **Nature of the wound.** Incisional wounds made under aseptic conditions are less prone to infection than traumatic wounds, which typically involve microorganism invasion.
   f. **Extent of the wound and associated blood loss.** The greater the extent, the slow- er the healing process is in most cases.
   g. **Tissue involved.** Tissues with adequate blood supply heal faster (e.g., wounds of the hands and head tend to heal more quickly than wounds of adipose tissue or lower extremities).
   h. **Psychosocial factors** (e.g., stress, fatigue) can impair healing.

II. CELLULAR DYSFUNCTION

A. **Description.** The inability of the cell to function normally may result in cell death (i.e., necrosis). Cell death can impede muscle contraction and nerve transmission; cells become edematous, and energy transformation ceases.

B. Etiology. Pathologic cellular adaptation results from excessive physiologic stress or pathologic stimuli in an effort to preserve the cell.

1. **Psychosocial sources of stress**
   a. **Daily stressors** (e.g., traffic jams, arguments, school difficulties)
   b. **Major complex occurrences involving large groups or nations** (e.g., war, terrorism, economic depression)
   c. **Major life events** (e.g., death, marriage, birth, divorce, retirement)

2. **Physiologic sources of stress**
   a. **Hypoxia** (i.e., inadequate cellular oxygenation). This leading cause of cell death may result from diminished blood supply to tissue, reduced oxygen-carrying capacity of blood (i.e., hemoglobin disorders), or ventilation-perfusion problems.
   b. **Temperature extremes** (heat or cold). Extreme heat increases metabolic activity of cells, subsequently destroying enzymes and coagulating cytoplasmic protein. Cold temperatures cause vasoconstriction, which decreases blood supply to tissues, and blood stasis, which may lead to thrombus formation.
   c. **Trauma.** Wounds can disrupt cells and tissues. The outcome of wound healing is related to the type and extent of injury, tissue involved, and mechanism of injury (e.g., blunt versus penetrating wounds).
   d. **Radiation.** Exposure to ionizing radiation can cause cell mutation, damage enzymes, and interrupt cell division.
   e. **Chemical agents** can injure or destroy cells. Damage depends on the nature of the exposure and on cellular susceptibility to the chemical.
   f. **Infectious agents.** Viruses, bacteria, rickettsiae, mycoplasma, fungi, and protozoa may cause disease.
   g. **Nutritional imbalances.** Deficiency or excess of one or more essential nutrients increases stress on cells and tissues.
   h. **Immune-system dysfunction.** Immunodeficiency occurs with hypoactivity; hypersensitivity occurs with hyperactivity.

C. Pathophysiology. Insults at the cellular or organ level may result in pathologic (disease) processes. Cell death causes the cell membrane to become impaired, resulting in a nonrestricted flow of ions. Responses of the internal environment to diseases are called pathophysiologic processes.

1. The inflammatory response occurs when limits of adaptive capability are exceeded or when no adaptive response is possible. It may be reversible or irreversible if cell death occurs.
2. Transient vasoconstriction occurs immediately after injury, followed by vasodilation.
3. Blood flow increases to the injury site, resulting in local heat and redness.
4. As vascular permeability increases, plasma leaks into inflamed tissues, producing edema.
5. Edema causes pressure on nerve endings or possibly direct irritation of nerve endings by chemical mediators, such as histamines or kinins.
6. Loss of function usually is attributed to pain and edema.
7. Plasma elements left in tissue include white blood cells (WBCs), platelets, and red blood cells.
8. WBCs (i.e., leukocytes) migrate to the injury site; their primary purpose is phagocytosis (i.e., engulfing organisms and removing cellular debris).
9. Fibrinogen from leaked plasma coagulates, forming a fibrin wall that helps prevent the spread of infection.
10. Systemic responses to cellular injury include:

  a. temperature elevation, caused by endogenous pyrogens released from neutrophils and macrophages

  b. leukocytosis

  c. malaise, loss of appetite, aching, and weakness.

11. **Response to cellular injury is acute or chronic.**

  a. **Acute responses** usually last less than 2 weeks and are characterized by vascular congestion with inflammatory exudate.

  b. **Chronic responses,** which usually last weeks to months, are characterized by proliferative exudate. A continued cycle of cellular infiltration, necrosis, and fibrosis may cause scarring.

12. **Types of maladaptation**

  a. **Atrophy** is a decrease in cell size through loss of cell substances. Predisposing factors include aging, inadequate nutrition, and diminished workload, as can occur with paralysis and loss of neural innervation.

  b. **Hypertrophy** is an increase in cell size, resulting in an increase in organ size. Predisposing factors include increased functional demand (e.g., in hypertension, the heart muscle enlarges in effort to pump blood more efficiently through vasoconstricted or atherosclerotic arterioles).

  c. **Hyperplasia** is an increase in the number of cells in organ or tissue. Predisposing factors are related to hormonal influences and tissue removal or destruction (e.g., precancerous cervical changes and hepatocellular changes associated with liver failure or cirrhosis).

  d. **Metaplasia** is a reversible change in which one adult cell type (epithelial or mesenchymal) is replaced by another cell type. Predisposing factors include stress to highly specialized cells, as occurs with changes in epithelial cells of the trachea and bronchi in a habitual cigarette smoker.

NURSING PROCESS OVERVIEW

 ## III. THE CLIENT WITH ALTERED HOMEOSTASIS

A. Assessment

1. **Health history**

  a. **Elicit a description of the client's present illness and chief complaint,** including onset, course, location, duration, and precipitating and alleviating factors. Cardinal signs and symptoms indicating cellular injury include inflammation, redness, edema, and increased temperature.

  b. **Explore the client's health history for risk factors** associated with cellular injury:
  – Immobility
  – Physical and psychosocial stress
  – Chronic disease
  – Impaired nutritional status
  – Increased age
  – Noncompliance with required immunizations
  – Exposure to illness, animal or insect bites, and travel to disease-endemic areas.

2. **Physical examination**

  a. **Inspection**
  – Inspect the injured area for redness, heat, and edema.
  – Assess for pain or discomfort at the injury site.

– Assess for loss of function.
– Assess for involuntary cessation of movement.
– Assess vital signs (i.e., temperature, pulse, respirations).
– Monitor for weight loss.
– Assess for abnormal discharge from body openings.

   b. **Palpation.** Palpate for enlarged lymph nodes.
   c. **Auscultation**
   – Auscultate blood pressure.
   – Auscultate lung sounds.

3. **Laboratory and diagnostic studies**
   a. **Complete blood cell count** can detect changes in formed elements.
   b. **Culture and sensitivity** tests can determine growth of any microorganisms and evaluate appropriate antibiotic therapy.
   c. **Electrolyte, blood urea nitrogen,** and **creatinine levels** can determine imbalances that indicate altered cellular or organ function.

B. Nursing diagnoses
   1. Risk for infection
   2. Risk for imbalanced body temperature
   3. Acute or chronic pain
   4. Imbalanced nutrition: less than body requirements
   5. Deficient fluid volume or excess fluid volume
   6. Impaired skin integrity
   7. Impaired physical mobility
   8. Activity intolerance
   9. Impaired gas exchange
   10. Impaired bowel elimination
   11. Impaired urinary elimination
   12. Social isolation
   13. Impaired home maintenance
   14. Deficient knowledge

C. Planning and outcome identification. The major goals of the client with a cellular injury include absence of infection, maintenance of normothermia, pain relief, improved nutritional status and fluid and electrolyte balance, maintenance of skin integrity, absence of contracture and deformity, increased activity tolerance, improved gas exchange, normal bowel and bladder function, improved social interaction, ability to live independently, and understanding of the disease process and therapy.

D. Implementation
   1. **Promote infection control.**
      a. Use and promote correct handwashing technique (the most important procedure in preventing the spread of microorganisms). Wash hands properly after contact with urine, feces, blood, or other potential infection sources.
      b. Adhere to Centers for Disease Control and Prevention standard precautions.
      c. Maintain aseptic technique for all surgical wounds and all indwelling catheters.
      d. Monitor for signs and symptoms of inflammation (e.g., redness, odor, drainage) and infection (e.g., elevated temperature, elevated white blood cell count).
      e. Administer antibiotics as prescribed.
      – Assess for allergies.
      – Obtain cultures as ordered before administering antibiotics.

    – After the first dose, watch the client closely for an allergic reaction. After several doses, assess for signs of superinfection (i.e., thrush, diarrhea, and vaginal discharge).

2. **Maintain normothermia.**
   a. Monitor vital signs every 4 hours and as needed.
   b. Implement measures to decrease temperature.
       – Administer antipyretics.
       – Reduce the room temperature.
       – Provide tepid baths, cool compresses, and a cooling blanket if necessary.
   c. Encourage increased oral fluid intake to compensate for insensible losses.

3. **Provide pain relief.**
   a. Assess the type, intensity, and location of pain.
   b. Rule out complications that require independent nursing interventions or warrant immediate intervention by a health care provider. Pain may be expected in some situations, but pain is also a sign of a complication that requires immediate nursing intervention.
   c. Take action as appropriate based on the assessment data.
       – Administer appropriate nonopioid or opioid pain medication.
       – Administer nonsteroidal antiinflammatory drugs to reduce edema and relieve pressure on nerve endings.
       – Position the client to promote comfort.
       – Teach the client to splint the wound as appropriate.
       – Elevate the injured area to promote venous return.
       – After an injury, apply cool packs to the site; then apply warm packs to reduce edema.
       – Call the health care provider if complications occur.
   d. Evaluate pain-relief measures for effectiveness 30 minutes after nursing interventions or medication administration.

4. **Promote adequate nutritional intake.**
   a. Ensure a diet high in protein and calories with vitamin supplements, as needed, to optimize tissue repair.
   b. Monitor dietary intake to detect deficiencies.
   c. Monitor serum albumin and total protein levels to identify any nutritional deficits.
   d. Provide nutritional supplementation as necessary.

5. **Maintain normal fluid and electrolyte balance.** (See chapter 3, Fluids and Electrolytes.)
   a. Monitor intake and output, using an urometer if necessary.
   b. Weigh the client daily at same time and in same clothes.
   c. Encourage the client to increase his fluid intake (fill a 2-L bottle with water each night, and instruct him to drink it by the next night; he can drink any other fluids throughout the day).
   d. Assess mental status, vital signs, and laboratory values (i.e., potassium, sodium).
   e. Administer electrolyte supplements as indicated. Administer I.V. therapy.
   f. Inform the client of the need to wear appropriate clothing and to avoid excessive exposure to heat and sunlight.

6. **Maintain skin integrity.**
   a. Promote adequate blood supply to the injury area by turning the client every 2 hours and using the prone position.
   b. Perform active and passive range-of-motion exercises on all extremities.

    c. Avoid tourniquets and tight dressings.

    d. Elevate the injured area to increase venous return to the heart, aid wound drainage, and decrease the risk of thrombus formation.

    e. Use pressure-relieving devices (e.g., convoluted foam mattress, air-fluidized therapy, heel or elbow protectors).

    f. Keep the client's skin clean and dry. Keep linens dry and wrinkle-free.

    g. Assess the client's skin every shift for signs of breakdown.

    h. Do not massage reddened areas, because this may increase the damage to already damaged areas.

    i. Use a lift sheet to prevent dragging the client across the bed.

    j. Encourage the client to shift his weight every 15 minutes while sitting in a chair. Encourage him to get up and walk every hour and to stop every hour and get out of the car when on long car rides.

7. **Promote mobility and prevent contractures.**

    a. Maintain a normal functional body position.

      – Maintain correct body alignment at all times; use pillows and splints.

      – Use a foot board or pillows to keep the client's feet in correct position (prevents foot drop).

    b. Promote activity.

      – Perform active and passive range-of-motion exercises on all extremities at least four times daily and more if possible (also teach the client and his family how to perform the exercises).

      – Encourage active participation in activities of daily living; encourage and assist the client to maintain independence.

      – Instruct the client in the proper use of all assistive devices (e.g., walkers, canes, transfer devices, crutches).

8. **Promote adequate rest.**

    a. Cluster necessary activities to allow uninterrupted periods of rest.

    b. Teach the client energy-conservation techniques, such as maintaining good posture and avoiding overactivity.

    c. Provide bed rest, and limit physical activity.

    d. Limit visitors and long conversations.

9. **Promote gas exchange.**

    a. Instruct the client to cough, turn, and deep-breathe every 2 hours.

    b. Instruct the client to ambulate as tolerated.

    c. Auscultate lung sounds every shift and as needed.

    d. Assess respiratory rate and pattern and cough.

    e. Evaluate the color, odor, amount, and consistency of any sputum. Instruct the client on appropriate ways to discard contaminated tissues.

    f. Suction as necessary to clear secretions.

    g. Monitor arterial blood gas values and pulse oximeter readings.

    h. Monitor capillary refill time, buccal and peripheral cyanosis, and the client's level of consciousness.

10. **Maintain normal bowel function.**

    a. Assess the normal frequency, character, amount, and consistency of stool.

    b. Advise the client to increase roughage in his diet (e.g., salad, fruits, and bran).

    c. Increase fluid intake.

    d. Encourage the client to participate in a regular exercise program.

    e. Establish a regular bowel evacuation schedule.

f. Use stool softeners, bulk-forming agents, laxatives, and enemas as needed. Warn the client against becoming dependent on these medications.

g. Assess for fluid volume deficit.

h. Keep the perineal area clean and dry to prevent skin breakdown.

i. Reinforce the principles of handwashing (after each bowel movement).

j. Send stool specimens to the laboratory, maintaining enteric precautions.

11. **Maintain normal bladder function.**

a. Monitor intake and output (do not decrease intake to decrease frequency of urination).

b. Develop a toileting schedule based on normal urinary habits.

c. Encourage the client to perform Kegel exercises (i.e., tighten the pelvic floor muscles for 4 seconds 10 times, at least 20 times each day; stop and start urinary flow).

d. Avoid indwelling catheters if possible; you may use condom catheters.

e. Perform scrupulous Foley care twice daily.

f. Use incontinence pads or diapers as a last resort; change pads frequently, cleanse skin, and use a moisture barrier to protect the skin.

12. **Promote social interaction.**

a. Provide accurate information about disease transmission to allay fears or clarify misconceptions.

b. Assess the client's normal patterns of communication.

c. Observe the client for diminished interpersonal interactions, hospitality, or depression.

d. Encourage verbalization of feelings and concerns.

e. Collaborate with the client to identify available support systems and effective coping mechanisms.

f. Provide care in an accepting, nonjudgmental manner.

g. Provide diversionary activities to relieve boredom.

13. **Prepare the client for home maintenance management.**

a. Assess the home environment for adequacy of heating and cooling systems, availability of a stove and refrigerator, and the presence of stairs and their relation to the rooms used.

b. Ask about finances, including resources available to buy food, medications, and health insurance.

c. Discuss availability and reliability of the client's support system (e.g., family, friends, neighbors).

d. Evaluate self-care capabilities, including ability to prepare meals, bathe properly, administer medications, and ambulate with assistance.

e. Refer to social services, rehabilitation services, or home health care services as needed.

14. **Provide client and family education.**

a. Discuss the signs and symptoms of infection to watch for and report.

b. Explain specifics of any drug therapy. Use a medication calendar to clearly describe the drug, its dosage, and the time and length of therapy.

c. Define follow-up wound care. Instruct the client on dressing changes and whether it is appropriate to shower.

d. List activity limitations.

e. Discuss stress-reduction measures.

f. Encourage follow-up appointments with the health care provider.

g. Talk about maintenance of proper nutrition.

h. Point out the need to keep all immunizations up to date.

E. Outcome evaluation

1. The client displays no signs or symptoms of infection or inflammation.
2. The client is afebrile.
3. The client reports pain relief.
4. The client maintains adequate nutritional intake.
5. The client maintains adequate hydration, as evidenced by normal blood urea nitrogen and hematocrit values and by elastic skin turgor and moist mucous membranes.
6. The client displays no signs of skin breakdown and maintains adequate circulation as evidenced by warm, pink extremities with palpable distal pulses.
7. The client displays functional mobility and no signs of contractures.
8. The client is able to perform activity without exhaustion and verbalizes a sense of being rested.
9. The client's lungs are clear on auscultation and arterial blood gas values remain within normal ranges.
10. The client regularly passes stools of normal color and consistency.
11. The client is voiding adequately and has no urinary tract infection.
12. The client verbalizes diminished sense of social isolation.
13. The client verbalizes appropriate discharge teaching and appropriate referrals are made.
14. The client verbalizes signs and symptoms of infection, appropriate medication information, activity limitations, and stress-reduction measures.

Study questions

1. Which nursing intervention is appropriate when addressing the client's need to maintain skin integrity?
   1. Using a foot board to maintain correct anatomic position
   2. Monitoring intake and output accurately
   3. Instructing the client to cough and deep-breathe every 2 hours
   4. Keeping the linens dry and wrinkle free

2. Which should the nurse do *first* after assessing that a client has a reddened area over the left hip?
   1. Massage the reddened area for a few minutes.
   2. Turn the client to the right side for 2 hours.
   3. Notify the health care provider immediately.
   4. Arrange for a pressure-relieving device.

3. Which intervention should the nurse do after assessing a client's complaints of pain rated as 8 on a scale of 1 (no pain) to 10 (worst pain)?
   1. Administering the client's ordered pain medication immediately
   2. Attempting to rule out complications before administering pain medication
   3. Using guided imagery instead of administering pain medication
   4. Using therapeutic conversation to try to discourage pain medication

4. Which intervention is the *most* important factor in preventing the spread of microorganisms?
   1. Correct handwashing technique
   2. Maintenance of asepsis with indwelling catheter insertion
   3. Use of masks, gowns, and gloves when caring for clients with infection
   4. Cleanup of blood spills with sodium hydrochloride

5. Which nursing intervention should be included in the care plan for a client with

tented skin turgor, dry mucous membranes, and decreased urinary output?

1. Assessing the color, odor, and amount of sputum
2. Monitoring serum albumin and total protein levels
3. Administering I.V. and oral fluids
4. Clustering necessary activities throughout the day

6. When planning care for a client with cellular injury, the nurse should consider which scientific rationale?

1. Tissue with inadequate blood supply may heal faster.
2. The presence of infection may slow the healing process.
3. Nutritional needs remain unchanged for the well-nourished adult.
4. Age is an insignificant factor in cellular repair.

7. Which nursing intervention should be included for reducing pain due to cellular injury?

1. Administering anti-inflammatory agents as prescribed
2. Elevating the injured area to decrease venous return to the heart
3. Keeping the skin clean and dry
4. Applying warm packs initially to reduce edema

8. Which intervention is appropriate to include when developing a care plan for a client with altered urinary function because of urinary dribbling?

1. Having the client perform Kegel exercises
2. Inserting an indwelling Foley catheter
3. Encouraging trips to the bathroom every 8 hours
4. Using pads or diapers on the client

9. Which goal is *most* important for a client admitted with bacterial pneumonia who is febrile, diaphoretic, and short of breath and has asthma?

1. Maintenance of adequate oxygenation
2. Prevention of fluid volume excess
3. Pain reduction
4. Education about infection prevention

10. Which nursing intervention is *most* important to include in the care plan for a client who is about to be discharged from the acute care setting?

1. Home environment evaluation
2. Skin-care measures
3. Stress-reduction techniques
4. Participation in activities of daily living

11. Which nursing intervention is appropriate for maintaining normal bowel function?

1. Assessing dietary intake
2. Providing limited physical activity
3 Turning, coughing, and deep breathing
4. Decreasing fluid intake

12. Which nursing intervention should be included in the care plan for a client experiencing hyperthermia?

1. Antiemetic agent administration
2. Axillary temperature measurements every 4 hours
3. Fluid restriction of 2,000 ml/day
4. Room-temperature reduction

13. Which client statement indicates to the nurse that the client understands the discharge teaching about cellular injury?

1. "I do not have to see my health care provider unless I have problems."
2. "If I have any redness, drainage, or fever, I should call my doctor."
3. "I can stop taking all my antibiotics as soon as I am feeling better."
4. "I can return to all my normal activities as soon as I go home."

14. The nurse is caring for a client in a long-term–care facility. Which interventions would be appropriate when identifying nursing interventions aimed at promoting and preventing contractures? (Select all that apply.)

1. Clustering activities to allow uninterrupted periods of rest
2. Maintaining correct body alignment at all times
3. Monitoring intake and output, using an urometer if necessary
4. Using a foot board or pillows to keep feet in correct position
5. Performing active and passive range-of-motion exercises
6. Weighing the client daily at the same time and in the same clothes

15. Which intervention should be included in the home health care nurse's instructions about measures to prevent constipation?
   1. Instructing the client to fill a 2-L bottle with water every night and drink it the next day
   2. Discouraging the client from eating large amounts of roughage-containing foods in the diet
   3. Encouraging the client to use laxatives routinely to ensure adequate bowel elimination
   4. Instructing the client to establish a bowel evacuation schedule that changes every day

16. Which assessment data is the *priority* for the home health care nurse when assessing a client for the first time in the home?
   1. Current immunization status
   2. Availability of support systems
   3. Availability of diversionary activities
   4. Hourly rest stops when outside

Answer key

1. The answer is **4.**
Keeping the linens dry and wrinkle-free aids in preventing moisture and pressure from interfering with adequate blood supply to the tissues, helping to maintain skin integrity. Using a foot board is appropriate for maintaining normal body function position. Monitoring intake and output aids in assessing and maintaining bladder function. Coughing and deep breathing help to promote gas exchange.

2. The answer is **2.**
Turning the client to the right side relieves the pressure and promotes adequate blood supply to the left hip. A reddened area is never massaged, because this may increase the damage to the already reddened, damaged area. The health care provider does not need to be notified immediately. However, the health care provider should be informed of this finding the next time he is on the unit. Arranging for a pressure-relieving device is appropriate, but this is done after the client has been turned.

3. The answer is **2.**
When intervening with a client complaining of pain, the nurse must always determine if the pain is expected pain or a complication that requires immediate nursing intervention. This must be done before administrating the medication. Guided imagery should be used along with, not instead of, administration of pain medication. The nurse should medicate the client and not discourage medication.

4. The answer is **1.**
Handwashing remains the most effective procedure for controlling microorganisms and the incidence of nosocomial infections. Aseptic technique is essential with invasive procedures, including indwelling catheters. Masks, gowns, and gloves are necessary only when the likelihood of exposure to blood or body fluids is high. Spills of blood from clients with acquired immunodeficiency syndrome should be cleaned with sodium hydochloride.

5. The answer is 3.

The client's assessment findings would lead the nurse to suspect that the client is dehydrated. Administering I.V. and oral fluids is appropriate. Assessing sputum would be appropriate for a client with problems associated with impaired gas exchange or ineffective airway clearance. Monitoring albumin and protein levels is appropriate for clients experiencing inadequate nutrition. Clustering activities helps with energy conservation and promotes rest.

6. The answer is 2.

Infection impairs wound healing. Adequate blood supply is essential for healing. If inadequate, healing is slowed. Nutritional needs, including protein and caloric needs, increase for all clients undergoing cellular repair because adequate protein and caloric intake is essential to optimal cellular repair. Elderly clients may have decreased blood flow to the skin, organ atrophy and diminished function, and altered immunity. These conditions slow cellular repair and increase the risk of infection.

7. The answer is 1.

Anti-inflammatory agents help reduce edema and relieve pressure on nerve endings, subsequently reducing pain. Elevating the injured area increases venous return to the heart. Maintaining clean, dry skin aids in preventing skin breakdown. Cool packs, not warm packs, should be used initially to cause vasoconstriction and reduce edema.

8. The answer is 1.

Kegel exercises, which help strengthen the muscles in the perineal area, are used to maintain urinary continence. To perform these exercises, the client tightens pelvic floor muscles for 4 seconds 10 times at least 20 times each day, stopping and starting the urinary flow. Inserting an indwelling Foley catheter increases the risk for infection and should be avoided. The nurse should encourage the client to develop a toileting schedule based on normal urinary habits. However, suggesting bathroom use every 8 hours may be too long an interval to wait. Pads or diapers should be used only as a last resort.

9. The answer is 1.

For the client with asthma and infection, oxygenation is the priority. Maintaining adequate oxygenation reduces the risk of physiologic injury from cellular hypoxia, which is the leading cause of cell death. A fluid volume deficit resulting from fever and diaphoresis, not excess, is more likely for this client. No information regarding pain is provided in this scenario. Teaching about infection control is not appropriate at this time but would be appropriate before discharge.

10. The answer is 1.

After discharge, the client is responsible for his own care and health maintenance management. Discharge includes assessing the home environment for adequacy of heating or cooling; availability of a stove, refrigerator, and food supply; and the presence of stairs in the house. These areas are most important for determining the client's ability to maintain his health at home. Skin-care measures, stress reduction, and participation in activities of daily living are additional areas that may need to be addressed to maintain skin integrity, provide adequate rest, and maintain independence, depending on the client's exact situation.

11. The answer is 1.

Assessing dietary intake provides a foundation for the client's usual practices and may help determine if the client is prone to constipation or diarrhea. Limited physical activity, appropriate for promoting rest, decreases peristalsis and may contribute to constipation. Turning, coughing, and deep breathing helps to promote gas exchange. Fluid intake should be increased, not decreased, to aid in bowel elimination.

12. The answer is **4.**

For the patient with hyperthermia, reducing the room temperature may help decrease body temperature. Tepid baths, cool compresses, and a cooling blanket may also be necessary. Antipyretics, not antiemetics, are indicated to reduce fever. Oral or rectal temperature measurements are generally accepted as more accurate than axillary measurements. Fluids should be encouraged, not restricted, to compensate for insensible losses.

13. The answer is **2.**

Knowledge that redness, drainage, or fever — signs of infection associated with cellular injury — require reporting indicates that the client has understood the nurse's discharge teaching. As part of this discharge teaching, follow-up appointments should be encouraged along with an emphasis on completing the entire course of antibiotic therapy, even if the client feels better. After most cases of cellular injury, there are usually activity limitations.

14. The answers are **2, 4, 5.**

Correct body alignment, preventing footdrop, and range-of-motion exercises will help prevent contractures. Clustering activities will help promote adequate rest. Monitoring intake and output and weighing the client will help maintain fluid and electrolyte balance.

15. The answer is **1.**

Adequate fluids and fiber in the diet are key to preventing constipation. Having the client fill a 2-L bottle with water every night and drink it the next day is one method for ensuring that the client receives at least 2,000 ml of water daily. The client also should be instructed to drink any other fluids throughout the day. High fiber or roughage foods are encouraged. Laxatives should not be used routinely for bowel elimination. They should be used only as a last resort, because clients may become dependent on them. A regular bowel evacuation schedule should be established.

16. The answer is **2.**

Crucial to the client's home maintenance management is the availability and reliability of support systems. Family, friends, and neighbors who will be available to assist with the client should be identified and notified of the client's needs and situation. This is a priority. Immunization status, diversionary activities, and rest periods are also important but are not the priority for the first visit.

3

Fluids and electrolytes

I. ESSENTIAL CONCEPTS

A. Fluids

1. Fluids (i.e., electrolytes and proteins in a large volume of water) account for about 60% of an adult's total body weight.
2. Intracellular fluid (ICF) constitutes about two thirds of this amount; extracellular fluid (ECF) accounts for the other one third.
3. ECF is further divided into the intravascular space (i.e., fluid within the blood vessels) and the interstitial space (e.g., fluid that surrounds the cell).
4. Loss of ECF into a space that does not contribute to equilibrium between the ICF and ECF is referred to as a third-space fluid shift.

B. Electrolytes

1. An electrolyte is a substance that dissociates and forms ions when mixed with water.
2. Potassium and phosphate are the major electrolytes in ICF.
3. Sodium (Na) and chloride are the major electrolytes in ECF. The Na level is the primary determinant of ECF concentration.

C. Acid-base balance

1. An **acid** is any substance that ionizes in water and forms hydrogen ions and anions. An acid is a hydrogen donor.
2. A **base** is any substance that can bind to hydrogen ions. A base is a hydrogen acceptor.
3. The **pH** (e.g., hydrogen ion concentration in the blood) is a measure of acid-base balance. The more hydrogen ions, the more acidic the medium and the lower its pH; conversely, the fewer hydrogen ions, the more base and the higher its pH. Normal pH for humans is approximately 7.4.

D. Regulatory mechanisms. Various mechanisms regulate fluid distribution between intracellular and extracellular compartments.

1. **Osmosis** involves fluid shifting through membranes from an area of low solute concentration to an area of higher solute concentration in the attempt to achieve physiologic balance (i.e., homeostasis).
2. **Diffusion** involves fluid movement from an area of high solute concentration to one of lower solute concentration (i.e., exchange of oxygen and carbon dioxide in between the pulmonary capillaries and alveoli).
3. **Filtration** refers to removal of particles from a solution through the movement of fluid across a membrane or other partial barrier (i.e., passage of water and electrolytes from the arterial capillary bed to the interstitial fluid).
4. **Active transport** is an energy-requiring process that transports ions across the cell membrane against a concentration gradient (e.g., the sodium-potassium pump).

E. Sources of normal fluid loss

1. Fluid loss constantly occurs as a normal result of bodily functions.
2. The kidneys normally produce a fluid output of 1 to 2 L daily.
3. From the skin, sensible losses (i.e., visible perspiration) normally range from 0 to 1,000 ml/hour, depending on temperature. Insensible losses (i.e., water loss by evaporation) equal about 600 ml/day; these amounts increase with fever.
4. The lungs cause insensible loss (e.g., exhaled water vapor) of 300 to 400 ml/day, which increases with fever.
5. Losses from the GI tract normally range from 100 to 200 ml/day.

F.   Homeostatic mechanisms. Various organ systems and mechanisms interact to maintain homeostasis (e.g., optimal fluid and electrolyte balance).

1. **Renal system**

    a. The kidneys filter about 170 L of plasma daily.

    b. The kidneys reabsorb bicarbonate (HCO_3), secrete hydrogen ions (H^+) in proximal and distal tubules, and produce ammonia.

    c. The kidneys compensate for imbalances more slowly than the lungs. They may take up to several days to achieve balance.

2. **Cardiovascular system**

    a. The cardiovascular system maintains adequate renal perfusion.

    b. Normal arterial blood gas values reflecting homeostasis include:

    – pH: 7.35 to 7.45

    – partial pressure of oxygen (Po_2): 80 to 100 mm Hg

    – partial pressure of carbon dioxide (Pco_2): 35 to 45 mm Hg

    – HCO_3: 22 to 26 mEq/L .

3. **Pulmonary system**

    a. The lungs work to maintain acid-base balance by controlling carbon dioxide (CO_2) and carbonic acid (H_2CO_3) excretion.

    b. Pco_2 is the most powerful respiratory stimulant, followed by pH, then Po_2.

4. **Buffer system**

    a. Buffers are chemical systems that maintain body pH (acid-base balance) by inactivating or releasing H^+.

    b. The primary buffer system involves HCO_3 and H_2CO_3.

    c. The HCO_3 (base) buffer system is regulated by the kidneys; they can regenerate HCO_3 ions and reabsorb them from the renal tubular cells.

    d. The H_2CO_3 buffer system is regulated by the lungs; they do so by adjusting ventilation in response to the amount of CO_2 in the blood.

    e. An HCO_3 to H_2CO_3 ratio of 20:1 is necessary to maintain body pH; disruption of the ratio alters pH (normal, 7.35 to 7.45).

    f. Less important buffer systems are the phosphate buffer system (intracellular) and the protein buffer system.

5. **Endocrine system**

    a. The pituitary gland secretes antidiuretic hormone, which promotes water retention.

    b. The adrenal cortex produces aldosterone, which causes sodium retention and potassium loss.

    c. The parathyroid glands secrete parathyroid hormone, which regulates calcium and phosphate balance.

II. FLUID VOLUME DEFICIT

A.   Description. Fluid volume deficit, also called *hypovolemia*, is excessive loss of water and electrolytes in equal proportion; vascular, cellular, or intracellular dehydration.

B.   Etiology

1. Inadequate fluid intake

2. Increased output, as occurs with severe diarrhea, vomiting, and blood loss

3. Massive third-space fluid shift, as occurs with ascites caused by liver dysfunction, pancreatitis, or burns

C. Assessment findings
1. **Clinical manifestations**
   a. Tented skin turgor and dry mucous membranes
   b. Postural hypotension
   c. Increased heart rate
   d. Extreme thirst
   e. Dizziness, weakness, and change in mental status
   f. Renal shutdown and coma with severe fluid volume deficit
   g. Acute weight loss
2. **Laboratory and diagnostic study findings**
   a. Urine specific gravity is above 1.020.
   b. Blood urea nitrogen level is elevated disproportionately to that of serum creatinine.
   c. Hematocrit is elevated.

D. Nursing management
1. **Maintain normal fluid balance.**
   a. Monitor intake and output accurately. Use a urometer if necessary.
   b. Monitor urine specific gravity.
   c. Weigh the client daily at the same time and in the same clothes.
   d. Maintain adequate hydration through oral or I.V. fluid supplementation.
2. **Provide ongoing assessment.** Assess vital signs, level of consciousness, central venous pressure, breath sounds, and skin color to determine when therapy should be slowed to avoid volume overload.
3. **Maintain skin integrity.** Assess skin turgor, tongue turgor, and mucous membranes.
4. **Provide frequent oral care.**
5. **Teach the client to change positions slowly to minimize postural hypotension.**

III. FLUID VOLUME EXCESS

A. Description.
Fluid volume excess, also called *hypervolemia*, is excessive retention of water and electrolytes in equal proportion; increased local or total body fluid volume

B. Etiology
1. Excessive fluid intake
2. Impaired ability to excrete fluid, as in renal disease
3. Abnormal fluid retention, as occurs with heart failure or corticosteroid therapy
4. Excessive sodium intake (I.V. or oral)

C. Assessment findings
1. **Clinical manifestations**
   a. Weight gain
   b. Dependent edema (in feet, ankles, and sacrum)
   c. Dyspnea and crackles (particularly in clients with a history of cardiac problems)
   d. Change in mental status
   e. Bounding pulse
   f. Jugular vein distention
2. **Laboratory and diagnostic study findings.** Blood urea nitrogen and hematocrit values are decreased.

D. Nursing management

1. **Maintain normal fluid balance.**
   a. Monitor intake and output accurately. Use a urometer if necessary.
   b. Weigh the client daily at the same time and in the same clothes.
   c. Assess vital signs. Assess for peripheral and sacral edema.
   d. Closely monitor the rate of I.V. fluids.

2. **Prevent or minimize edema.**
   a. Assess lung sounds. If pulmonary edema occurs, elevate the head of the bed and have the client turn, cough, and deep-breathe every 2 hours.
   b. Turn the client every 2 hours; edematous tissue is more prone to skin breakdown.
   c. Administer diuretics as prescribed.

3. **Provide client and family teaching.**
   a. Teach the client the fundamentals of a sodium-restricted diet as ordered.
   b. Restrict sodium and water as ordered.
   c. Instruct the client to avoid over-the-counter medications without first checking with a health care provider, because they may contain sodium.

IV. HYPONATREMIA

A. Description.
Hyponatremia (i.e., sodium deficiency) is a serum sodium level below 135 mEq/L resulting from excessive sodium loss or excessive water gain.

B. Etiology

1. Fluid loss, such as from vomiting, diarrhea, fistulas, diaphoresis, diuretic therapy, and nasogastric suctioning
2. Adrenal insufficiency
3. Syndrome of inappropriate antidiuretic hormone (SIADH) excretion
4. Excessive water gain from intake of sodium-deficient parenteral fluids or compulsive water drinking
5. Water pulled into cells because of decreased extracellular sodium level and increased cellular fluid concentration

C. Assessment findings

1. **Clinical manifestations**
   a. Anorexia, nausea, and vomiting
   b. Muscle cramps
   c. Altered level of consciousness, including lethargy, disorientation, headache, confusion, and convulsions (with a serum sodium level less than 115 mEq/L)

2. **Laboratory and diagnostic study findings**
   a. Serum sodium level is less than 135 mEq/L.
   b. Urinalysis reveals urine sodium and specific gravity levels to be low if caused by sodium loss and high if caused by SIADH.

D. Nursing management

1. **Maintain fluid balance.**
   a. Monitor intake and output accurately. Use a urometer as necessary.
   b. Weigh the client daily at the same time in the same clothes.
   c. Assess for signs of fluid volume excess.
   d. Administer sodium supplements orally, by nasogastric tube, or parenterally.
   e. Infuse hypotonic solutions cautiously.

2. Prevent injury.

a. Assess neurologic (e.g., lethargy, confusion, muscular twitching, seizures) and GI status (e.g., anorexia, nausea, vomiting, abdominal cramping).

b. Maintain seizure precautions.

c. Monitor the serum sodium level (normal, 135 to 145 mEq/L).

d. Maintain strict water restriction when hyponatremia is present with normal or excess fluid volume excess.

V. HYPERNATREMIA

A. Description. Hypernatremia (i.e., sodium excess) is a serum sodium level greater than 145 mEq/L caused by a gain of sodium in excess of water or a loss of water in excess of sodium.

B. Etiology

1. Water loss from:

   a. diarrhea

   b. fever

   c. hyperventilation

   d. diabetes insipidus

2. Inadequate water replacement, most commonly caused by decreased intake by elderly, cognitively impaired, or comatose clients

3. Inability to swallow

4. Rarely, seawater ingestion or excessive oral or parenteral sodium intake

5. Water pulled from cells because of increased extracellular sodium level and decreased cellular fluid concentration

C. Assessment findings

1. **Clinical manifestations**

   a. Thirst

   b. Tented skin turgor

   c. Edematous dry tongue and sticky mucous membranes

   d. Elevated body temperature

   e. Lethargy and restlessness

   f. Peripheral and pulmonary edema

2. **Laboratory and diagnostic study findings**

   a. Serum sodium level is greater than 145 mEq/L.

   b. Serum osmolality is greater than 295 mOsm/kg.

   c. Urinalysis reveals an elevated urine specific gravity and urine osmolality.

D. Nursing management

1. **Maintain normal fluid balance.**

   a. Monitor intake and output accurately; use a urometer if necessary.

   b. Weigh the client daily at the same time and in the same clothes.

   c. Encourage increased fluid intake as appropriate.

   d. Infuse hypertonic solutions cautiously.

   e. Monitor the serum sodium level (normal, 135 to 145 mEq/L).

2. **Protect the client from injury.**

   a. Assess the client's vital signs, skin turgor, and neurologic status; also assess for thirst.

   b. Monitor the serum sodium level (normal, 135 to 145 mEq/L).

   c. Reposition the client frequently.

d. Keep the bed side rails up, the bed in low position, and the call light within reach.

e. Secure all invasive lines.

f. Obtain a medication history, because some medications may have a high sodium content.

VI. HYPOKALEMIA

A. **Description.** Hypokalemia (i.e., potassium deficiency) is a serum potassium level below 3.5 mEq/L.

B. **Etiology**
1. Inadequate dietary potassium intake
2. Excessive loss from:
   a. treatments, such as carbenicillin, amphotericin B, diuretics, or steroid therapy; parenteral fluid therapy without potassium replacement; gastric suctioning; colostomy and ileostomy
   b. GI disorders, such as diarrhea, vomiting, or fistula
   c. diaphoresis and renal disorders
3. Metabolic alkalosis
4. Hyperaldosteronism

C. **Assessment findings**
1. **Clinical manifestations**
   a. Anorexia, nausea, and vomiting
   b. Fatigue
   c. Muscle weakness, leg cramps, or paresthesia
   d. Cardiac arrhythmias
   e. Decreased bowel motility, ileus, or abdominal distention
2. **Laboratory and diagnostic study findings**
   a. Serum potassium level is below 3.5 mEq/L.
   b. Electrocardiogram (ECG) reveals a flattened T wave, prominent U wave, ST-segment depression, and prolonged PR interval.

D. **Nursing management**
1. **Prepare for and assist with therapies as prescribed.**
   a. Administer oral potassium daily; assess the client for abdominal distention, pain, or GI bleeding, which may indicate bowel lesions that require intervention.
   b. Infuse parenteral potassium supplement. Always dilute in at least 100 ml of solution, administer on an infusion pump, and monitor the ECG during the infusion.
   c. Never administer potassium by I.V. push or I.M.
   d. Monitor the serum potassium level (normal, 3.5 to 5.5 mEq/L).
   e. Monitor intake and output accurately. Use a urometer if necessary.
2. **Provide client and family teaching.** Teach the client to eat foods high in potassium, particularly if he is receiving steroid, diuretic, or digoxin therapy. Such foods include orange juice, bananas, cantaloupe, peaches, potatoes, dates, and apricots.
3. **Prevent client injury** by assessing the potassium level in clients receiving digoxin. Hypokalemia potentiates the action of digoxin; therefore, the client receiving digoxin must be monitored closely for digoxin toxicity (e.g., nausea, vomiting, anorexia, yellow haze).

VII. HYPERKALEMIA

A. **Description.** Hyperkalemia (i.e., potassium excess) is a serum potassium level above 5.5 mEq/L.

B. **Etiology**
1. Decreased renal excretion due to renal failure
2. Hypoaldosteronism
3. Acidosis
4. Severe tissue trauma (e.g., burns, massive infection)
5. Excessive intake of potassium supplement (rare)
6. Use of a tight tourniquet while drawing blood, hemolysis of blood sample, drawing blood above the site where the potassium is being infused, or administration of expired blood products that results in a false serum potassium level. This is referred to as factitious or *pseudohyperkalemia.*

C. **Assessment findings**
1. **Clinical manifestations**
   a. Cardiac arrhythmias
   b. Muscle weakness, paresthesias, and possibly paralysis
   c. Irritability and anxiety
   d. Abdominal cramps with diarrhea
2. **Laboratory and diagnostic study findings**
   a. Serum potassium level is above 5.5 mEq/L.
   b. Electrocardiogram (ECG) reveals tall, tented T waves; prolonged PR interval and QRS duration; absent P waves; and ST-segment depression.

D. **Nursing management**
1. **Prepare for and assist with aggressive therapy,** as prescribed. Various therapies may be implemented.
   a. Cation-exchange resins (e.g., Kayexalate), administered orally or by retention enema, draw potassium into the bowel so that it may be excreted in the feces.
   b. Calcium gluconate antagonizes the adverse cardiac conduction abnormalities.
   c. Parenteral sodium bicarbonate alkalinizes the plasma and causes a temporary shift of potassium into the cells.
   d. Parenteral regular insulin and glucose cause a temporary shift of potassium into the cells.
   e. Hemodialysis removes potassium from blood.
2. **Prevent client injury.**
   a. Assess for signs of muscular weakness, cardiac arrhythmias, parasthesias, nausea, and intestinal colic.
   b. Evaluate and verify all high serum potassium levels. To avoid false reports, do not prolong the use of a tourniquet when drawing blood, caution the client not to exercise the extremity before drawing blood, and take the blood sample to the laboratory immediately after being drawn.
   c. Monitor the ECG for abnormalities.
   d. Monitor the serum potassium level (normal, 3.5 to 5.5 mEq/L).
   e. When administering potassium I.V., always administer it with an infusion pump to prevent excessive intake.

3. **Provide client and family teaching.**
   a. Advise clients at increased risk for hyperkalemia (e.g., those with renal failure) to avoid potassium-rich foods. Foods low in potassium include butter, margarine, cranberry juice, ginger ale, gumdrops or jelly beans, hard candy, and honey. Foods high in potassium include coffee, cocoa, tea, dried fruits, dried beans, and whole grain breads.
   b. Caution the client to use salt substitutes sparingly, because most contain approximately 60 mEq of potassium per teaspoon.
   c. Assess the client who is receiving potassium-sparing diuretics for hyperkalemia.

VIII. HYPOCALCEMIA

A. Description. Hypocalcemia (i.e., calcium deficiency) is a serum calcium level below 8.5 mg/dl.

B. Etiology
   1. Primary or surgical hypoparathyroidism due to thyroidectomy
   2. Pancreatitis
   3. Inadequate vitamin D intake or synthesis
   4. Renal failure
   5. Drug therapy (e.g., aminoglycosides, corticosteroids, caffeine)
   6. Insufficient calcium intake

C. Assessment findings
   1. **Clinical manifestations**
      a. Tetany (i.e., tingling in fingers and circumoral area; muscle spasms associated with pain in extremities and face)
      b. Positive Trousseau's sign (see *Figure 3-1*) and Chvostek's sign (i.e., twitching of muscles supplied by the facial nerve when the nerve is tapped just below the ear lobe)
      c. Carpopedal spasms
      d. Hyperactive deep tendon reflexes and seizures due to neuromuscular irritability
   2. **Laboratory and diagnostic study findings**
      a. Serum calcium level is below 8.5 mg/dl.
      b. Electrocardiogram reveals a prolonged QT interval.

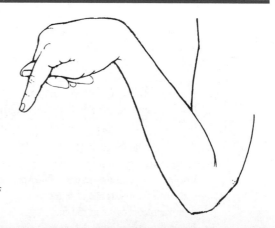

FIGURE 3–1

In hypocalcemia, Trousseau's sign results after inflating a blood pressure cuff to about 20 mm Hg over systolic pressure on the upper arm. As the blood supply to the ulnar nerve is obstructed, carpopedal spasm develops, usually within 2 to 5 minutes.

Source: Smeltzer, S.C. , and Bare, B.G. *Brunner and Suddarth's Textbook of Medical-Surgical Nursing,* 9th ed. Philadelphia: Lippincott Williams & Wilkins, 2000.

D. Nursing management

1. **Prepare for and assist with therapy, as prescribed.**
   a. Institute and maintain seizure precautions.
   b. Administer parenteral calcium. Take precautions to prevent tissue infiltration, which can lead to tissue necrosis and sloughing.
   c. Do not add calcium to parenteral solutions containing bicarbonate or phosphorus; this causes a precipitate to form.
   d. Administer calcium cautiously to a client receiving digoxin; calcium potentiates the action of digoxin, increasing the risk of cardiac arrest.
   e. Maintain a relaxed, quiet environment, and promote adequate rest.
2. **Administer vitamin D,** which increases calcium absorption from the GI tract.
3. **Provide client and family teaching.**
   a. Instruct the client to increase dietary intake of calcium to 1,000 to 1,500 mg/day (e.g., milk products, green leafy vegetables, fresh oysters); alcohol and caffeine in high doses inhibit calcium absorption.
   b. Instruct clients at risk for osteoporosis to maintain adequate dietary intake of calcium or take calcium supplements.
   c. Instruct the client on the value of regular exercise, which decreases bone loss.
4. **Monitor the serum calcium level** (normal, 8.5 to 10.5 mg/dl).

IX. HYPERCALCEMIA

A. Description. Hypercalcemia (i.e., calcium excess) is a serum calcium level above 10.5 mg/dl.

B. Etiology

1. Excessive calcium administration or intake
2. Movement of calcium from bones to serum, as occurs in prolonged immobilization and malignant neoplastic diseases
3. Decreased renal excretion due to renal failure
4. Drug therapy with thiazide diuretics
5. Hyperparathyroidism

C. Assessment findings

1. **Clinical manifestations**
   a. Anorexia, nausea, and vomiting
   b. Constipation
   c. Muscular weakness, incoordination
   d. Altered level of consciousness (e.g., slurred speech, confusion, lethargy, coma)
   e. Polyuria and polydipsia
   f. Cardiac arrhythmias
   g. Hypoactive deep tendon reflexes
2. **Laboratory and diagnostic study findings**
   a. Serum calcium level is above 10.5 mg/dl.
   b. Electrocardiogram reveals a shortened QT interval, bradycardia, and heart blocks.

D. Nursing management

1. **Prepare for and assist with therapy, as prescribed.**
   a. Administer parenteral saline solution to dilute serum calcium and inhibit tubular reabsorption of calcium.
   b. Administer parenteral phosphate to enhance deposition of calcium.

    c. Administer furosemide (Lasix) to increase calcium excretion.

    d. Monitor the serum calcium level (normal, 8.5 to 10.5 mg/dl).

    e. Treat the underlying cause, which may include calcitonin for hyperparathyroidism and mithramycin and corticosteroids for cancers.

2. Maintain normal bowel elimination pattern.

    a. Assess for dehydration, mental confusion, and psychotic behavior.

    b. Encourage 3 to 4 quarts of fluid daily (fluids containing sodium help with calcium excretion) and dietary fiber intake to help with constipation.

3. Institute injury-prevention measures for mental confusion. Keep bed side rails up, keep bed brakes locked, reposition the client often, and secure all invasive lines.

4. Provide client and family teaching on the causes and treatment of hypercalcemia.

    a. Teach the client about the importance of early ambulation to reduce calcium loss from bones during hospitalization.

    b. Encourage the client to participate in daily weight-bearing activities.

X. HYPOMAGNESEMIA

A. Description. Hypomagnesemia (i.e., magnesium deficiency) is a serum magnesium level below 1.5 mEq/L.

B. Etiology

1. Poor nutrition
2. Alcoholism
3. GI and renal losses without replacement

C. Assessment findings

1. Clinical manifestations

    a. Positive Trousseau's sign (see *Figure 3-1,* page 57) and Chvostek's sign

    b. Neuromuscular irritability

    c. Insomnia

    d. Mood changes

    e. Cardiac arrhythmias

2. Laboratory and diagnostic study findings

    a. Serum magnesium level is below 1.5 mEq/L.

    b. Electrocardiogram (ECG) reveals a flattened T wave, prominent U wave, and ST-segment depression.

D. Nursing management

1. Prepare for and assist with therapy, as prescribed.

    a. Administer parenteral magnesium replacement therapy on an infusion pump to prevent rapid administration and to prevent cardiac arrest.

    b. Monitor for signs of magnesium toxicity, including hot, flushed skin; diaphoresis; anxiety or lethargy; hypotension; and laryngeal stridor.

    c. Monitor the ECG and pulse for abnormalities.

    d. Monitor the serum magnesium level (normal, 1.5 to 2.5 mEq/L).

2. Prevent injury.

    a. Institute and maintain seizure precautions.

    b. Institute safety measures for mental confusion.

    c. Assess the client's ability to swallow before administering oral medications or feeding him; dysphagia may occur in clients with magnesium depletion.

    d. Monitor clients on digoxin closely because a magnesium deficit predisposes to digoxin toxicity.

  3. Provide client and family teaching.

    a. Discuss the misuse of diuretics and laxatives if necessary.

    b. Identify dietary sources of magnesium, including nuts, whole grains, cornmeal, spinach, bananas, and oranges, and encourage increased intake of these foods.

XI. HYPERMAGNESEMIA

A. Description. Hypermagnesemia (i.e., magnesium excess) is a serum magnesium level above 2.5 mEq/L.

B. Etiology

  1. Renal failure

  2. Overuse of magnesium-containing antacids

  3. Excessive magnesium administration

  4. Overuse of enemas or laxatives containing magnesium

  5. Severe dehydration, as occurs in diabetic ketoacidosis

C. Assessment findings

  1. Clinical manifestations

    a. Hot, flushed skin

    b. Hypoactive reflexes

    c. Hypotension, bradycardia

    d. Depressed respirations, lethargy, drowsiness, and absent deep tendon reflexes with increasing magnesium level

    e. Cardiac arrhythmias

  2. Laboratory and diagnostic study findings

    a. The serum magnesium level is above 2.5 mEq/L.

    b. Electrocardiogram reveals prolonged QT interval and atrioventricular blocks.

D. Nursing management

  1. Prepare for and assist with therapy, as prescribed.

    a. Discontinue all parenteral and oral magnesium.

    b. During respiratory or cardiac emergencies, collaborate with the respiratory therapist providing ventilatory support. Administer I.V. calcium gluconate, as prescribed, to antagonize the neuromuscular effects of magnesium.

    c. Prepare the client for hemodialysis.

    d. Administer diuretics and 0.45% normal saline, which causes excretion of magnesium.

    e. Monitor the serum magnesium level (normal, 1.5 to 2.5 mEq/L).

  2. Prevent injury.

    a. Monitor vital signs, cardiovascular status, respiratory status, patellar reflexes, and changes in level of consciousness closely.

    b. Institute safety precautions, including keeping bed side rails up, keeping bed brakes locked, and repositioning the client often.

  3. Provide client and family teaching.

    a. Teach the client about the adverse effects associated with the overuse of magnesium-containing antacids and cathartics.

    b. Instruct the client to read all over-the-counter drug labels carefully for magnesium content.

XII. HYPOPHOSPHATEMIA

A. Description. Hypophosphatemia (i.e., phosphorus deficiency) is a serum phosphorus level below 2.5 mg/dl.

B. Etiology

1. Overzealous intake or administration of carbohydrates
2. Total parenteral nutrition administration
3. Prolonged intense hyperventilation, alcohol withdrawal, and diabetic ketoacidosis
4. Excess phosphorus binding by antacids containing magnesium, calcium, or albumin
5. Severe dehydration, as occurs in diabetic ketoacidosis

C. Assessment findings

1. **Clinical manifestations**
   a. Irritability, apprehension, weakness, numbness, confusion, seizure, and coma
   b. Hypoxia leading to an increase in respiratory rate and respiratory alkalosis
   c. Muscle weakness, muscle pain and, at times, acute rhabdomyolysis (i.e., disintegration of striated muscle)
   d. Chronic loss of phosphorus possibly causing bruising and bleeding because of platelet dysfunction
   e. Increased susceptibility to infection
2. **Laboratory and diagnostic study findings**
   a. Serum phosphorus level is less than 2.5 mEq/L.
   b. The serum magnesium level may be decreased because of increased urinary excretion of magnesium.

D. Nursing management

1. **Prepare for and assist with therapy, as prescribed.**
   a. During administration of total parenteral nutrition to malnourished clients, gradually introduce the solution to avoid rapid shifts of phosphorus into the cells.
   b. Monitor the serum phosphorus level (normal, 2.5 to 4.5 mg/dl).
   c. Monitor for possible complications of I.V. phosphorus administration, which may include hypocalcemia.
2. **Prevent injury.**
   a. Assess vital signs, signs of apprehension, confusion, and changes in mental status.
   b. Institute seizure and safety precautions. Keep bed side rails up, keep bed brakes locked, and reposition the client often.
3. **Provide client and family teaching.** Discuss the importance of preventing infection because hypophosphatemia may produce changes in granulocytes.

XIII. HYPERPHOSPHATEMIA

A. Description. Hyperphosphatemia (i.e., phosphorus excess) is a serum phosphorus level above 4.5 mg/dl.

B. Etiology

1. Renal failure
2. Chemotherapy for neoplastic disease
3. High phosphorus intake
4. Profound muscle necrosis

C. Assessment findings
1. **Clinical manifestations**
    a. Soft tissue calcification
    b. Tetany (a high serum phosphorus level causes a low concentration of serum calcium)
    c. Anorexia, nausea, and vomiting
    d. Muscle weakness, hyperreflexia, and tachycardia
2. **Laboratory and diagnostic study findings**
    a. Serum phosphorus level is above 4.5 mEq/L.
    b. X-ray studies may show skeletal changes with abnormal bone development.

D. Nursing management
1. **Prevent injury.**
    a. Institute seizure precautions and monitor for seizures.
    b. Monitor the serum phosphorus level (normal, 2.5 to 4.5 mg/dl).
2. **Provide client and family teaching.**
    a. Instruct the client to avoid foods high in phosphorus, which include hard cheese, cream, nuts, whole-grain products, dried fruits, and dried vegetables.
    b. Instruct the client to avoid phosphate-containing substances, such as certain laxatives and enemas.

XIV. METABOLIC ACIDOSIS

A. Description.
Metabolic acidosis is an acid-base imbalance resulting from excessive absorption or retention of acid or excessive excretion of bicarbonate (HCO_3).

B. Etiology
1. Ketoacidosis
2. Lactic acidosis
3. Prolonged fasting
4. Salicylic poisoning
5. Oliguric renal disease
6. Abnormal HCO_3 losses, which can occur in loss of fluid from the lower GI tract from surgery, drains, or severe diarrhea

C. Assessment findings
1. **Clinical manifestations**
    a. Headache
    b. Drowsiness and confusion
    c. Weakness
    d. Increased respiratory rate and depth
    e. Nausea and vomiting
    f. Diminished cardiac output with pH below 7, which results in hypotension, cold and clammy skin, and cardiac arrhythmias
2. **Laboratory and diagnostic study findings**
    a. Arterial blood gas (ABG) studies reveal abnormal values: pH below 7.35 and HCO_3 below 22 mEq/L.
    b. Serum potassium level reveals hyperkalemia.

D. Nursing management
1. **Prepare for and assist with therapy, as prescribed.**

a. Monitor ABG values.

b. When appropriate, administer sodium bicarbonate.

c. Monitor the serum potassium level closely as acidosis is reversed.

d. Treat chronic metabolic acidosis (seen with chronic renal failure) by administering calcium to avoid tetany, use of alkalizing agents, and hemodialysis or peritoneal dialysis.

2. **Prevent injury.**

a. Monitor cardiovascular status closely, noting blood pressure, pulse rate and rhythm, capillary refill time, and temperature and color of extremities.

b. Institute safety precautions. Keep bed side rails up, keep bed brakes locked, and secure all invasive lines properly.

XV. METABOLIC ALKALOSIS

A. **Description.** Metabolic alkalosis is an acid-base imbalance characterized by excessive loss of acid or excessive gain of bicarbonate (HCO_3).

B. **Etiology**

1. Loss of hydrogen and chloride ions because of prolonged vomiting or gastric suctioning (most common cause)

2. Excessive intake of alkali (e.g., antacids, baking soda)

C. **Assessment findings**

1. **Clinical manifestations**

a. Tingling of the fingers and toes

b. Dizziness, belligerence, or confusion

c. Tetany

d. Slow, shallow respirations; possibly apnea

2. **Laboratory and diagnostic study findings**

a. Arterial blood gas (ABG) studies reveal abnormal values: pH above 7.45 and HCO_3 above 26 mEq/L.

b. Urine chloride concentrations help to differentiate between vomiting or diuretic ingestion or one of the causes of mineralocorticoid excess.

D. **Nursing management**

1. **Prepare for and assist with therapy, as prescribed.**

a. Monitor ABG values.

b. Monitor intake and output carefully; use a urometer if necessary.

c. Provide treatment to correct the underlying cause as ordered.

d. Administer sodium chloride to restore normal fluid volume (continuing volume depletion serves to maintain the alkalosis).

e. Correct electrolyte deficits, particularly of potassium and sodium.

f. Treatment of chronic metabolic alkalosis (seen in long-term diuretic therapy, chronic ingestion of milk and calcium carbonate, and external drainage of gastric fluids) is aimed at treating the underlying acid-base disorder.

2. **Prevent injury.**

a. Monitor respiratory rate and pattern and auscultate lung sounds.

b. Institute safety precautions. Keep bed side rails up, keep bed brakes locked, and secure all invasive lines.

XVI. RESPIRATORY ACIDOSIS

A. **Description.** Respiratory acidosis is an acid-base imbalance characterized by increased partial pressure of arterial carbon dioxide and decreased blood pH.

B. **Etiology**
   1. Chronic obstructive respiratory disorders, such as bronchial asthma and emphysema
   2. Acute disorders, such as chest-wall trauma, pulmonary edema, atelectasis, pneumothorax, drug overdoses, pneumonia, and Guillain-Barré syndrome
   3. Any condition that results in hypoventilation

C. **Assessment findings**
   1. **Clinical manifestations**
      a. Acute respiratory acidosis
         – Increased pulse and respiratory rate
         – Increased blood pressure
         – Mental cloudiness and feeling of fullness in head
      b. Chronic respiratory acidosis
         – Weakness
         – Dull headache
   2. **Laboratory and diagnostic study findings.** Arterial blood gas (ABG) studies reveal abnormal values: pH below 7.35 and partial pressure of carbon dioxide above 45 mm Hg.

D. **Nursing management**
   1. **Prepare for and assist with therapy, as prescribed.**
      a. Monitor ABG values.
      b. Improve ventilation with bronchodilators; postural drainage; antibiotic therapy to treat infection; regular coughing, turning, and deep breathing; and mechanical ventilation as appropriate.
      c. Treat the underlying cause.
      d. Treat chronic respiratory acidosis (e.g., the client who has chronic obstructive pulmonary disease and hypoxic stimulus for breathing) by administering low-flow oxygen therapy to prevent respiratory arrest.
   2. **Prevent injury.**
      a. Position the client in semi-Fowler's position (or another comfortable position) to ease the work of breathing.
      b. Maintain a quiet, relaxing environment; cluster activities to allow for periods of uninterrupted rest.
      c. Keep needed items within the client's reach.
      d. Monitor cardiovascular status, noting blood pressure, pulse rate and rhythm, capillary refill time, and temperature and color of extremities.
      e. Monitor respiratory status, noting respiratory rate, rhythm, difficulty, level of consciousness, and peripheral and buccal cyanosis.
      f. Maintain fluid and electrolyte balance.

XVII. RESPIRATORY ALKALOSIS

A. Description. Respiratory alkalosis is an acid-base imbalance characterized by decreased partial pressure of arterial carbon dioxide and increased blood pH.

B. Etiology

1. Most commonly, hyperventilation due to anxiety, hypoxia, or improper mechanical ventilation
2. Fever
3. Salicylate poisoning

C. Assessment findings

1. **Clinical manifestations**
   a. Lightheadedness
   b. Inability to concentrate
   c. Convulsions
   d. Positive Chvostek's sign
   e. Muscle twitching

2. **Laboratory and diagnostic study findings.** Arterial blood gas (ABG) studies reveal abnormal values: pH above 7.45 and partial pressure of carbon dioxide below 35 mm Hg.

D. Nursing management

1. **Prepare for and assist with therapy, as prescribed.**
   a. Monitor ABG values.
   b. Aim treatment at the underlying cause, such as decreasing pain, fever, and anxiety.
   c. Encourage the client to take slow, deep breaths.
   d. Treat chronic respiratory alkalosis (from chronic hypocapnia resulting in decreased serum bicarbonate) the same as acute respiratory alkalosis. Clients with chronic alkalosis are usually asymptomatic.

2. **Prevent injury.**
   a. Assess the respiratory rate and pattern.
   b. Institute and maintain seizure precautions as necessary.
   c. Assess sources of anxiety and intervene to help reduce anxiety.
   d. Assist the client with activities as necessary.

Study questions

1. When teaching a client with hypokalemia, which foods should the nurse instruct the client to increase?

1. Whole grains and nuts
2. Milk products and green, leafy vegetables
3. Pork products and canned vegetables
4. Orange juice and bananas

2. Which intervention is *most* appropriate for the client who is hyperventilating and develops respiratory alkalosis?

1. Administering low-flow oxygen therapy
2. Preparing to administer sodium bicarbonate
3. Encouraging slow, deep breaths
4. Administering sodium chloride I.V.

3. The nurse is totaling the intake and output for a client diagnosed with septicemia who is on a clear liquid diet. The client intakes 8 oz of apple juice, 850 ml of water, 2 cups of beef broth, and 900 ml of half-normal saline solution and outputs 1,500 ml of urine during the shift. How many milliliters should the nurse document as the client's intake?

_____

4. Which assessment data does the nurse document when a client diagnosed with hypocalcemia develops a carpopedal spasm after the blood-pressure cuff is inflated?
1. Positive Trousseau's sign
2. Positive Chvostek's sign
3. Paresthesia
4. Tetany

5. Which clinical manifestation would the nurse expect to assess in a client with hypernatremia?
1. Muscle weakness and paresthesia
2. Fruity breath and Kussmaul's respirations
3. Muscle twitching and tetany
4. Tented skin turgor and thirst

6. A client with a history of chronic obstructive pulmonary disease has the following arterial blood gas results: partial pressure of oxygen (Po_2), 55 mm Hg, and partial pressure of carbon dioxide (Pco_2), 60 mm Hg. When attempting to improve the client's blood gas values through improved ventilation and oxygen therapy, which is the client's primary stimulus for breathing?
1. High Pco_2
2. Low Po_2
3. Normal pH
4. Normal bicarbonate (HCO_3)

7. Which intervention should the nurse perform when caring for a client diagnosed with fluid volume deficit?
1. Assessing urinary intake and output with a urometer
2. Obtaining the client's weight weekly at different times of the day
3. Monitoring arterial blood gas (ABG) results
4. Maintaining I.V. therapy at the keep-vein-open rate

8. Which client situation requires the nurse to discuss the importance of avoiding foods high in potassium?
1. Prescribed diuretics
2. Ileostomy
3. Metabolic acidosis
4. Renal disease

9. For the client diagnosed with hypomagnesemia, which nursing intervention would be appropriate?
1. Instructing the client on the importance of preventing infection
2. Avoiding the use of a tight tourniquet when drawing blood
3. Teaching the client the importance of early ambulation
4. Instituting seizure precautions to prevent injury

10. Which electrolyte would the nurse identify as the _major_ electrolyte responsible for determining the concentration of the extracellular fluid?
1. Potassium
2. Phosphate
3. Chloride
4. Sodium

11. Which medication would the nurse anticipate administering for a client with a potassium level of 6.2 mEq/L?
1. Potassium supplements
2. Kayexalate
3. Calcium gluconate
4. Sodium tablets

12. Which clinical manifestation would lead the nurse to suspect that a client is experiencing hypermagnesemia?
1. Muscle pain and acute rhabdomyolysis
2. Soft-tissue calcification and hyperreflexia
3. Hot, flushed skin and diaphoresis
4. Increased respiratory rate and depth

13. In planning the care for a client receiving furosemide and digoxin, which laboratory data would be the *most* important to assess?
1. Sodium level
2. Magnesium level
3. Potassium level
4. Calcium level

14. A client has the following arterial blood gas (ABG) values: pH of 7.34, partial pressure of arterial oxygen of 80 mm Hg, partial pressure of arterial carbon dioxide of 49 mm Hg, and a bicarbonate level of 24 mEq/L. Based on these results, which intervention should the nurse implement?
1. Administering low-flow oxygen
2. Encouraging the client to cough and deep-breathe
3. Instructing the client to breathe slowly into a paper bag

4. Nothing, because these ABG values are within normal limits.

15. Which would the nurse expect the health care provider to order for the client diagnosed with metabolic acidosis?
1. Potassium
2. Sodium bicarbonate
3. Serum sodium level
4. Bronchodilator

16. Which electrolyte abnormality would the nurse suspect if the client's electrocardiogram (ECG) showed a shortened QT interval and bradycardia?
1. Hypercalcemia
2. Hyperkalemia
3. Hypocalcemia
4. Hypokalemia

Answer key

1. The answer is 4.
The client with hypokalemia needs to increase the intake of foods high in potassium. Orange juice and bananas are high in potassium, along with raisins, apricots, avocados, beans, and potatoes. Whole grains and nuts would be encouraged for the client with hypomagnesemia; milk products and green, leafy vegetables are good sources of calcium for the client with hypocalcemia. Pork products and canned vegetables are high in sodium and are encouraged for the client with hyponatremia.

2. The answer is 3.
The client who is hyperventilating and subsequently develops respiratory alkalosis is losing too much carbon dioxide. Measures that result in the retention of carbon dioxide are needed. Encourage slow, deep breathing to retain carbon dioxide and reverse respiratory alkalosis. Administering low-flow oxygen therapy is appropriate for chronic respiratory acidosis. Administering sodium bicarbonate is appropriate for treating meta-

bolic acidosis, and administering sodium chloride is appropriate for metabolic alkalosis.

3. The answer is 2,470.
The fluid intake includes 8 oz (240 ml) of apple juice, 850 ml of water, 2 cups (480 ml) of beef broth, and 900 ml of I.V. fluid for a total of 2,470 ml intake for the shift.

4. The answer is 1.
In a client with hypocalcemia, a positive Trousseau's sign refers to carpopedal spasm that develops usually within 2 to 5 minutes after applying and inflating a blood pressure cuff to about 20 mm Hg higher than systolic pressure on the upper arm. This spasm occurs as the blood supply to the ulnar nerve is obstructed. Chvostek's sign refers to twitching of the facial nerve when tapping below the ear lobe. Paresthesia refers to numbness or tingling. Tetany is a clinical manifestation of hypocalcemia denoted by tingling in the tips of the fingers around the mouth, and muscle spasms in the extremities and face.

5. The answer is **4.**
Hypernatremia refers to elevated serum sodium levels, usually above 145 mEq/L. Typically, the client exhibits tented skin turgor and thirst in conjunction with dry, sticky mucous membranes, lethargy, and restlessness. Muscle weakness and paresthesia are associated with hypokalemia; fruity breath and Kussmaul's respirations are associated with diabetic ketoacidosis. Muscle twitching and tetany may be seen with hypocalcemia or hyperphosphatemia.

6. The answer is **2.**
A chronically elevated Pco_2 level (above 50 mm Hg) is associated with inadequate response of the respiratory center to plasma carbon dioxide. The major stimulus to breathing then becomes hypoxia (low Po_2). High Pco_2 and normal pH and HCO_3 levels would not be the primary stimuli for breathing in this client.

7. The answer is **1.**
For the client with a fluid volume deficit, assessing the client's urine output (using a urometer if necessary) is essential to ensure an output of at least 30 ml/hour. The client should be weighed daily, not weekly, and at same time each day, usually in the morning. Monitoring ABGs is not necessary for this client. Rather, serum electrolyte levels would most likely be evaluated. The client also would have an I.V. rate of at least 75 ml/hour, if not higher, to correct the fluid volume deficit.

8. The answer is **4.**
Clients with renal disease are predisposed to hyperkalemia and should avoid foods high in potassium. Clients receiving diuretics, with ileostomies, or with metabolic acidosis may be hypokalemic and should be encouraged to eat foods high in potassium.

9. The answer is **4.**
Instituting seizure precautions is an appropriate intervention, because the client with hypomagnesemia is at risk for seizures.

Hypophosphatemia may produce changes in granulocytes, which would require the nurse to instruct the client about measures to prevent infection. Avoiding the use of a tight tourniquet when drawing blood helps prevent pseudohyperkalemia. Early ambulation is recommended to reduce calcium loss from bones during hospitalization.

10. The answer is **4.**
Sodium is the electrolyte whose level is the primary determinant of the extracellular fluid concentration. Sodium, a cation (e.g., positively charged ion), is the major electrolyte in extracellular fluid. Chloride, an anion (e.g., negatively charged ion), is also present in extracellular fluid, but to a lesser extent. Potassium (a cation) and phosphate (an anion) are the major electrolytes in the intracellular fluid.

11. The answer is **2.**
The client's potassium level is elevated; therefore, Kayexalate would be ordered to help reduce the potassium level. Kayexalate is a cation-exchange resin, which can be given orally, by nasogastric tube, or by retention enema. Potassium is drawn from the bowel and excreted through the feces. Because the client's potassium level is already elevated, potassium supplements would not be given. Neither calcium gluconate nor sodium tablets would address the client's elevated potassium level.

12. The answer is **3.**
Hypermagnesemia is manifested by hot, flushed skin and diaphoresis. The client also may exhibit hypotension, lethargy, drowsiness, and absent deep tendon reflexes. Muscle pain and acute rhabdomyolysis are indicative of hypophosphatemia. Soft-tissue calcification and hyperreflexia are indicative of hyperphosphatemia. Increased respiratory rate and depth are associated with metabolic acidosis.

13. The answer is **3.**
Diuretics such as furosemide may deplete

serum potassium, leading to hypokalemia. When the client is also taking digoxin, the subsequent hypokalemia may potentiate the action of digoxin, placing the client at risk for digoxin toxicity. Diuretic therapy may lead to the loss of other electrolytes such as sodium, but the loss of potassium in association with digoxin therapy is most important. Hypocalcemia is usually associated with inadequate vitamin D intake or synthesis, renal failure, or use of drugs, such as aminoglycosides and corticosteroids. Hypomagnesemia generally is associated with poor nutrition, alcoholism, and excessive GI or renal losses, not diuretic therapy.

14. The answer is **2.**
The ABG results indicate respiratory acidosis requiring improved ventilation and increased oxygen to the lungs. Coughing and deep breathing can accomplish this. The nurse would administer high oxygen levels because the client does not have chronic obstructive pulmonary disease. Breathing into a paper bag is appropriate for a client hyperventilating and experiencing respiratory alkalosis. Some action is necessary, because the ABG results are not within normal limits.

15. The answer is **2.**
Metabolic acidosis results from excessive absorption or retention of acid or excessive excretion of bicarbonate. A base is needed. Sodium bicarbonate is a base and is used to treat documented metabolic acidosis. Potassium, serum sodium determinations, and a bronchodilator would be inappropriate orders for this client.

16. The answer is **1.**
An ECG showing a shortened QT interval and bradycardia suggests hypercalcemia. The ECG pattern typically associated with hyperkalemia reveals tall, tented T waves, a prolonged PR interval and QRS duration, absent P waves, and ST-segment depression. The ECG associated with hypocalcemia typically shows a prolonged QT interval. With hypokalemia, the ECG reveals a flattened T wave, prominent U wave, ST-segment depression, and a prolonged PR interval.

4 *Pain*

I. STRUCTURE AND FUNCTION OF PAIN SYSTEMS

A. The **peripheral nervous system**, including spinal and cranial nerves, carries pain impulses to and from the central nervous system (CNS).

   1. Afferent nerve fibers carry impulses *to* the CNS.

     a. **Somatic afferent fibers** carry impulses from the skin, skeletal muscles, joints, and tendons to the CNS.

     b. **Visceral afferent fibers** carry impulses from the viscera to the CNS.

   2. Efferent nerve fibers carry impulses *from* the CNS.

     a. The **visceral efferent system** is responsible for responding to the CNS afferent impulses that innervate the involuntary body activities of smooth muscles, cardiac muscle, and glands.

     b. The **somatic efferent system** is responsible for responding to the CNS afferent impulses that innervate the voluntary body activities of skeletal muscles, tendons, and joints.

   3. Nociceptors are naked nerve endings found in nearly every tissue of the body. These respond to thermal, chemical, and mechanical stimulation. The two major types of receptors are the A-delta fibers and C fibers. (See *Figure 4-1*.)

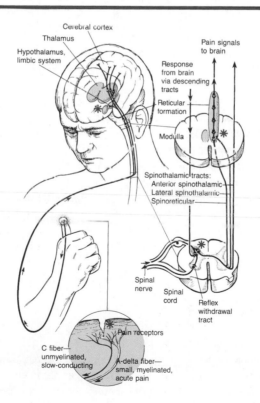

FIGURE 4–1

Neural pathways of pain and fibers transmitting pain

Source: Bullock, B.A., and Henze, R.L. *Focus on Pathophysiology.* Philadelphia: Lippincott Williams & Wilkins, 2000.

      a. The A-delta fibers conduct impulses at a very rapid rate and are responsible for transmitting acute sharp pain signals from the peripheral nerves to the spinal cord.

      b. The C fibers transmit sensory input at a much slower rate and produce slow, chronic pain.

B. The **autonomic nervous system** regulates involuntary vital functions. It comprises sympathetic and parasympathetic divisions. It also contains neurotransmitters.

  1. **Sympathetic nervous system** functions

      a. Fight, flight, or freeze response to alarm or stress (e.g., pain)

      b. Whole-person response, by which the body mobilizes defenses in response to stress

      c. Control of the adrenal medullae, sweat glands, blood vessels, and piloerector muscles in hair

  2. **Parasympathetic nervous system** functions

      a. Exhaustion or shock response with intense or prolonged stress (e.g., pain), triggered when sympathetic system no longer functions

      b. Specific organ responses

      c. Control of many body functions, such as digestion and elimination

  3. **Neurotransmitters** are chemicals that modify or enable transmission of nerve impulses between synapses.

      a. Cholinergic neurotransmitters involve acetylcholine.

      b. Adrenergic neurotransmitters include:

         – epinephrine

         – norepinephrine

         – dopamine

         – serotonin.

C. The **central nervous system** comprises the spinal cord and the brain.

  1. The **spinal cord** transmits painful stimuli to the brain and motor responses and pain perception to the periphery.

      a. Spinal cord pathways (nerve tracts)

         – Afferent tracts to the brain

         – Efferent tracts from the brain

      b. In the substantia gelatinosa, located in lamina II of the spinal cord's dorsal horn, fibers carry information about pain from the periphery. These fibers converge with larger fibers and form connections (i.e., synapses) with transmission cells (T cells) and fibers from the brain that carry inhibitory pain information.

  2. The **brain** processes and interprets transmitted pain impulses.

      a. The midbrain contains many centers for control, association, and relay of impulses, including:

         – reticular formation

         – medulla

         – hypothalamus (i.e., center for brain opiates)

         – thalamus (i.e., relay station and center for pain perception)

         – limbic system (i.e., center for emotion and environmental responses).

      b. In the sensory cortex, tactile sensory impulses from the periphery are interpreted and understood.

      c. The motor cortex initiates motor responses to data reaching the sensory cortex.

      d. The frontal lobes contain areas for:

         – attention (an essential component of the pain experience)

         – memory

- cognition
- emotion
- decision making.

II. ESSENTIAL CONCEPTS OF PAIN

A. Description
1. **Characteristics of pain**
   a. Pain is subjective and personal; it exists wherever and whenever a client says it does.
   b. Physiologic pain may sometimes broaden to encompass emotional hurt.
   c. Pain is a symptom, not a disease entity.
   d. Pain is a valuable diagnostic indicator; it usually indicates tissue damage or pathology.
   e. Pain is usually reported as severe discomfort or an uncomfortable sensation.
2. **Components of pain**
   a. A **stimulus** may be mechanical, chemical, thermal, or mental.
   b. The **sensation of hurt** relies on intact reception, transmission, perception, and interpretation.
   c. **Reaction** may involve musculoskeletal, autonomic, and psychologic responses. Reaction to pain also relies on an intact nervous system.
3. **Phases of the pain experience**
   a. **Anticipation of pain** may produce fear and anxiety, which affect a person's response to sensation and typically intensify the perception of pain.
   b. The **sensation of pain** is often affected by how anticipation was managed; pain increases anxiety, which increases pain.
   c. The **aftermath of pain** is the most neglected phase. The client's response to the pain experience may indicate fear, embarrassment, or guilt, all of which can affect future experiences with pain.
4. **Pain effects**
   a. **Beneficial effects of pain.** Pain can serve as a warning sign of injury and signal the need for treatment. Pain can also protect the body from further injury.
   b. **Detrimental effects of pain**
      - Pain poses a threat to basic needs by:
        - interfering with the ability to meet food, fluid, and sleep needs
        - affecting elimination
        - interfering with breathing and meeting oxygen needs
        - limiting mobility, leading to impaired skin integrity and altered ability for self-care.
      - Pain poses a threat to higher-level needs by:
        - interfering with relationships with significant others, communication, sexuality, social involvement, and job performance
        - causing spiritual distress and potentially leading to violence
        - delaying rehabilitation, enabling pain itself to become the disability.
5. **Types of pain**
   a. **Acute pain** can be described as:
      - rapid in onset
      - usually temporary, lasting no more than 6 months
      - subsiding spontaneously, with or without treatment.

    b. **Chronic pain** is marked by:
- gradual onset
- lengthy duration, more than 6 months
- periodic recurrence
- absence of a useful purpose
- the potential for becoming a major complication.

    c. **Cutaneous and superficial pain** involves:
- abrupt onset
- sharp, stinging quality.

    d. **Deep pain** is marked by:
- somatic pain from organs in any body cavity
- slower onset
- burning quality
- diffusion and radiation
- possibly, nausea and vomiting.

    e. **Referred pain** is pain originating at one site that is perceived in another. Referred pain follows dermatome and nerve root patterns. (See *Figure 4-2.*)

    f. **Phantom pain** may follow amputation or mastectomy; the client feels pain as if it were in the absent part.

    g. **Intractable pain** refers to moderate to severe pain that cannot be relieved by any known treatment.

B. Etiology

  1. **Physiologic factors**. Pain commonly results from an injury or disease process; other physiologic factors may contribute. Common causes include:

    a. musculoskeletal disorder caused by spasm, rupture, ischemia, or stretching

    b. visceral disorders

    c. cancer

    d. vascular disorders (caused by cold, pulling, displacement, or distention)

    e. inflammation

    f. contagious disease

    g. trauma (surgical or accidental)

    h. diagnostic tests (e.g., biopsy, venipuncture, invasive scanning)

    i. unmet basic needs (e.g., flatus after abdominal surgery)

    j. necessary nursing interventions (e.g., ambulation or coughing after surgery)

    k. pregnancy, labor, and delivery

    l. chemical irritants (e.g., release of histamine, bradykinin, prostaglandins, leukokinins)

    m. allergic responses

    n. neuralgia, such as after herpes zoster infection, resulting from scarring and degenerative changes in nerves

    o. causalgia, such as after peripheral nerve injury.

  2. **Psychological and emotional factors** may cause or augment pain.

    a. Stress of emotion may produce observable physiologic changes (e.g., chronic excessive muscle contractions).

    b. Psychological factors that can cause a person to interpret pain as more severe or less severe include:
- isolation
- anxiety
- fear
- anticipation of pain.

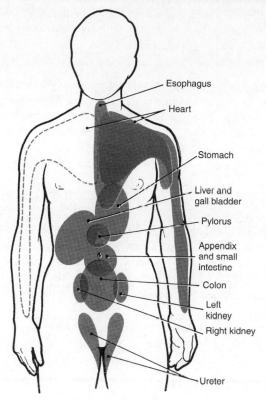

FIGURE 4–2
Typical areas of referred pain from visceral organs

Source: Bullock, B.A., and Henze, R.L. *Focus on Pathophysiology.* Philadelphia: Lippincott Williams & Wilkins, 2000.

    c. A client's past experiences with pain influence the meaning attached to the pain experience and affect his expectations of the health care team.

3. **Atypical response patterns** to pain may be demonstrated by some people. Variations in adaptation depend on factors such as:
   a. personal perception of appropriate behavior
   b. ability for self-distraction
   c. attempts to adjust to prolonged pain.

4. **Social factors** that can affect pain perception include:
   a. group status
   b. state of involvement at time of pain episode (e.g., an injury sustained during a sporting event may not be perceived as significant until after the event is over)
   c. role changes in family and social groups.

5. **Economic factors** that can contribute to pain perception include:
   a. threat to job or work role
   b. cost of treatment
   c. cost of caregiver or care for the family.

      6. Cultural factors influencing pain perception may include:

         a. whether the person's culture encourages or discourages expression of pain

         b. whether or not the culture teaches that suffering can serve some higher purpose (e.g., spiritual cleansing or a test of faith)

         c. the cultural view of health care provider and system roles.

C. Physiology. The physiology of pain is not completely understood, however, various models and theories of pain transmission and perception have been proposed. The gate-control model and the central-control theory overlap somewhat in current thought; both are useful.

    1. Gate-control model (See *Figure 4-3.*)

      a. Nerve fibers carry touch and pain impulses from receptors on the skin to the spinal cord.

      b. Nerve cells in the substantia gelatinosa (SG) of the spinal cord receive these touch and pain impulses.

      c. Impulses then proceed through transmission cells to the brain.

      d. Increased input over large fibers (A-alpha, A-beta, and A-gamma fibers) inhibits some pain impulses over smaller fibers (A-delta and type C fibers); fewer pain impulses reach transmission cells for transmission to the brain.

      e. Decreased input over large fibers allows more pain impulses to reach transmission cells.

      f. Fibers from the brain send inhibiting information to the SG, which serves as a gate for pain control.

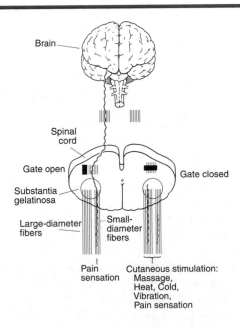

FIGURE 4–3

Gate control theory of pain

Source: Morton, P.G., et al. *Critical Care Nursing,* 8th ed. Philadelphia: Lippincott Williams & Wilkins, 2005.

2. **Central control theory of pain**
   a. Some neuropeptides (e.g., substance P) present in the SG seem to be pain-specific neurotransmitters that facilitate pain transmission.
   b. Endogenous molecular neuropeptides called brain opiates (e.g., endorphins, enkephalins) are opium-like compounds that have profound analgesic properties.
   c. Specific neuroreceptors bind with morphine and brain opiates.
   d. Certain events or situations trigger the release of brain opiates (e.g., cutaneous stimulation such as massage, electrical stimulation, pain itself, tissue injury, placebos, acupuncture, and transcutaneous electric nerve stimulation).
3. **Specificity theory**
   a. This theory proposes that pain originates in specific pain receptors, not in free nerve endings.
   b. This theory does not explain pain modulation by variables, such as social and cultural factors. It also does not account for pain syndromes, such as causalgia and phantom pain.
4. **Pattern theory**
   a. This theory relates pain intensity to the strength of the stimulus and the summation effect of continued stimulation.
   b. This theory has been proposed because of the inadequacies of the specificity theory. However, it does not explain psychological factors related to pain.
5. **Psychological theories**
   a. In many cases, pain results from emotion, hostility, guilt, or depression. It is not clearly understood why negative emotions effect pain on a physiologic level.
   b. Persons with pain-prone personalities use pain as a means to communicate.
   c. According to the psychogenic theory, pain arises from a perceived threat to self.

D. Clinical manifestations
1. **Sympathetic nervous system manifestations** occur with pain of low to moderate intensity or with severe superficial pain of short duration. These responses may include:
   a. skin pallor, coldness, and clamminess
   b. altered vital signs (i.e., elevated blood pressure, pulse rate, and respiratory rate)
   c. diaphoresis
   d. dilated pupils.
2. **Parasympathetic nervous system manifestations** occur with pain of severe intensity and long duration or deep pain. These responses may include:
   a. skin pallor
   b. altered vital signs (e.g., decreased blood pressure and pulse rate)
   c. nausea and vomiting
   d. weakness, fainting, and prostration
   e. possible loss of consciousness.
3. **Behavioral and musculoskeletal manifestations** include:
   a. postures to splint, hold, or protect painful areas
   b. muscle spasms
   c. skeletal muscle rigidity
   d. reflex abnormalities
   e. grimacing and clenching of jaws or fists
   f. rapid blinking, squinting eyes, or darting glance
   g. drawn facial expression and twitching facial muscles
   h. moaning, sighing, and crying
   i. restlessness

   j. immobility

   k. quiet and withdrawn response when touched

   l. anorexia, nausea, and vomiting.

  4. Psychologic manifestations may include:

   a. fear

   b. anxiety

   c. anger or irritation

   d. depression

   e. inability to concentrate

   f. desire for extra attention from others.

NURSING PROCESS OVERVIEW

III. THE CLIENT IN PAIN

 A. Assessment. Throughout the health history and physical examination, assess for common signs and symptoms of pain as described in section II.D. The Joint Commission on Accreditation of Healthcare Organizations has required all health care organizations to plan, support, and coordinate activities and resources to assure the pain of all clients is recognized and addressed appropriately. **Pain is now considered the fifth vital sign.** Clients have the right to appropriate assessment and management of pain. (See *Box 4-1.*)

  1. Health history

   a. Always believe the client's account and rating of pain. Keep in mind that pain assessment depends mainly on subjective data; objective signs must be confirmed by the client, except in certain cases when physiologic changes are obvious.

  b. Ask the client about the nature of the pain, including:

   – description (e.g., piercing, aching, shooting, burning, stinging, constant, intermittent, sharp, dull)

   – onset or time of occurrence (Ask the client when it began, how often it occurs, and what time of day it occurs.)

   – duration (Ask the client how long it lasts, and whether it is constant or intermittent.)

   – location (Have the client describe or point to the area or areas of pain. When documenting, use the client's words and give the correct anatomic terms.)

   – intensity or severity, such as mild, moderate, severe, or excruciating (Have the client rate the severity of pain on a scale of 1 to 10, with 1 representing the least pain and 10 the most severe, or use a color scale, with green representing the least pain and red representing the most severe.)

   – apparent or suspected cause

   – meaning of the pain to the client

   – apparent or suspected precipitating, aggravating, or alleviating factors.

  c. **Listen carefully to how the client describes the pain,** believe the client, and evaluate implied messages about the pain.

  2. Physical examination

  a. **Assess vital signs.**

  b. **Inspection.** Using all of your senses, observe:

   – nonverbal behavior

   – the painful body part or area

   – unusual odors

BOX 4-1
Special nursing care considerations

- **Assess the client's pain.** Determine intensity by using a 1 to 10 scale, with 10 being the worst pain the client has ever had and 1 being no pain. Determine the location and whether the pain radiates. Determine what the client was doing before the pain began and whether anything causes the pain to be less or more (e.g., taking deep breaths, lying in a fetal position). Ask if the pain is throbbing, dull, or sharp.
- **Rule out complications.** Make sure that the pain is related to the client's identified condition and is not a sign of developing complications. For example, a client is expected to have pain soon after abdominal or hip surgery. However, the nurse should make sure that the client's pain results from the surgery, not from a complication such as hemorrhage. In such a case, the nurse should:
  – assess the surgical dressing
  – assess bowel sounds or the neurovascular status of both legs in the case of hip surgery
  – assess vital signs, such as blood pressure and pulse rate.

- **Take action and intervene** as follows:
  – If the assessment data are within normal limits for the client's condition, administer appropriate medication as prescribed.
  – If the assessment data are abnormal for the client's condition, assess further. If indicated, notify the health care provider or perform appropriate activities, such as repositioning, ambulation, or distraction.
- **Assess risk for injury and institute safety measures after administering pain medications** that may cause drowsiness, impaired judgment, memory loss, or disorientation (e.g., raise bed side rails, lower the bed, place call signal in position for easy use).
- **Evaluate effectiveness of medication interventions** 30 minutes after administration (e.g., use a 10-point scale to measure and compare the client's comfort or discomfort level before and after medication).
- **Document pain,** related nursing interventions, and the client's responses.

- position or posture
- environment
- relationships, if others are present.
  c. **Palpation.** Palpate painful areas for:
  - heat
  - edema
  - masses.

B. **Nursing diagnoses**
  1. Acute pain
  2. Chronic pain
  3. Ineffective coping or compromised family coping

C. **Outcome identification and planning.** The major goals for the client experiencing pain include relief of pain or discomfort, a decrease in the intensity of pain and discomfort, absence of complications, and ability to verbalize knowledge of how to effectively cope with pain.

D. **Implementation**
  1. **Intervene to alter the source or progress of pain**.
     a. Prepare the client for scheduled surgery or other treatment, such as irradiation, to remove or reduce the cause of pain (e.g., tumor, infection).
     b. Explain how the treatment works to control pain.
     c. Explain alternative therapies, such as hypnosis, if the client or health care provider desires. (*Note:* Why hypnosis is effective for some clients remains unclear; it may stimulate brain opiates or produce a purely psychological effect.)
     d. Administer medication for pain or other problems causing pain (e.g., infection, postsurgical flatus) as prescribed. (See *Drug chart 4-1*, page 80.)

DRUG CHART 4-1
Pain medications

Classifications	Indications	Selected interventions
Antibiotics cefaclor penicillin G streptomycin sulfisoxazole tetracycline	Reduce discomfort, fever, edema, and inflammation associated with infection	■ Check the client's history for drug allergies before administering, and check whether culture has been obtained. ■ After multiple doses, assess the client for superinfection (thrush, yeast, diarrhea); notify the health care provider if these occur. ■ Assess the insertion site for phlebitis if antibiotics are being administered I.V. ■ To assess the effectiveness of antimicrobial therapy, monitor the client's white blood cell count and temperature. ■ Monitor peaks and troughs for aminoglycosides.
Anxiolytics diazepam hydroxyzine	Decrease stress and anxiety, thereby reducing interpretation of pain	■ Caution the client that alcohol and other drugs, such as antihistamines, potentiate the effect of tranquilizers. ■ Ensure the client's safety.
Nonopiod analgesics acetaminophen acetylsalicylic acid	Treat mild to moderate pain; blocks the generation of pain impulses through peripheral mechanism	■ Caution the client that overdose may be toxic to the liver. ■ Report tinnitus (ringing in ears), which is a sign of ASA toxicity.
Nonsteroidal antiinflammatory drugs ibuprofen idomethacin ketorolac naproxen	Reduce inflammatory process, thereby reducing pain	■ Administer with food to minimize gastric upset. ■ Inform the client that the medication may have an anticoagulant effect.
Opioid analgesics codeine meperidine morphine oxycodone pentazocine propoxyphene	Depress the central nervous system and inhibit pain impulses	■ Avoid overdosing, which can lead to tolerance and dependence. ■ Monitor the client's respiratory function. ■ Explain proper use of patient-controlled analgesia (PCA) machine if being used.
Skeletal muscle relaxants carisoprodol cyclobenzaprine dantrolene methocarbamol	Relieve pain-producing muscle spasm and spasticity	■ Caution the client that alcohol and other drugs, such as antihistamines, potentiate the effect of muscle relaxants. ■ Ensure the client's safety.

e. Relieve or prevent factors that aggravate pain (e.g., coughing, vomiting, diarrhea, constipation, bladder fullness, and infection).

f. Reduce or remove noxious stimuli (e.g., cast, elastic bandage, or weight; foreign body in eye; wrinkles in sheets; unsupported heavy bedding; excessive noise; excessively hot or cold environment; glaring lights).

g. As prescribed, provide nonpharmacologic pain-relief interventions, such as cutaneous stimulation, back rubs, biofeedback, acupuncture, transcutaneous electric

CLIENT AND FAMILY TEACHING 4-1
The client experiencing pain

■ Discuss additional nonpharmacologic pain interventions, including distraction, imagery, elevating an affected extremity, transcutaneous electric nerve stimulation, and biofeedback.
■ Discuss what the pain means to decrease the client's concerns about the cause of pain (e.g., cancer, incurable disease).
■ Encourage the client to take pain medication when the pain is just starting; this will aid in the medication's effectiveness and decrease the amount needed.
■ Encourage the client to lie in a quiet room with minimal distractions to aid the effectiveness of the medication.
■ Teach the client appropriate and safe ways to administer pain medications; also teach potential adverse effects, how often to take pain medication, and when to notify a health care provider if pain is not relieved.
■ Discuss the painful experience before and after episodes to help decrease any fear or shame associated with the perceived inability to cope with pain appropriately.
■ Discuss the client's previous experiences with pain, including how it was managed and how the client wants to manage current pain.
■ Assist the client to identify and use effective coping strategies, including those indicated by his cultural beliefs.
■ Discuss the appropriate way to store pain medications to prevent accidental overdosage or child tampering.
■ Teach the client what he needs to learn to meet any knowledge deficit related to pain or its treatment.

nerve stimulation, dorsal column stimulation, counter irritation, and contralateral stimulation.

   h. Encourage noninvasive pain management techniques, such as guided imagery, relaxation, and distraction (with music, TV, or reading) to reduce focus on pain and increase other impulses, which may help block pain impulses.

   i. Provide heat and cold application as prescribed; these methods may relieve edema and may produce anesthesia.

   j. Note any age-related effects on the client's response to pain and medication administration, and adjust interventions accordingly.

   k. Refer the client to a pain center or pain clinic, as recommended, for special treatment of pain that does not respond to therapy.

   l. Encourage activity or perform passive range-of-motion exercises. Mild activity or assisted activity, although painful, helps relieve stiffness of arthritic joints and sore muscles, eventually reducing pain; activity may also increase endorphin levels.

   m. Ensure proper body alignment and reposition regularly; although movement may hurt, repositioning and proper alignment relieves muscle strain and joint stiffness and helps relieve pain.

   n. Use behavior-modification techniques as appropriate.

   o. Involve family members to help them understand pain control, the client's response, and to enhance their ability to provide comfort and emotional support.

   p. Involve other disciplines (e.g., clergy, social worker, counselor, occupational therapist) as necessary.

   q. When performing painful procedures, work gently, swiftly, and skillfully to minimize the amount of pain generated and the time required.

   r. Provide adequate rest for the client or the painful body part.

  2. Intervene to alter psychosocial, economic, and cultural factors influencing pain. (See *Client and family teaching 4-1.*)

   a. Explain all interventions, treatments, or symptoms that may frighten or worry the client; anxiety or fear increases a client's perception of the severity of pain.

   b. Stay with the client during pain episodes, and convey empathy and concern. This can help decrease stress and anxiety and ease feelings of isolation and loneliness.

c. Establish a trusting relationship with the client by keeping promises and providing excellent physical care.

d. Promote the client's sense of control by allowing him to make choices regarding therapy as appropriate and, if applicable, by using client-controlled analgesia.

e. When talking with the client, avoid such words as *complain, attack,* and *victim,* which imply helplessness and criticism and may interfere with pain control; instead, use such neutral or positive terms as *explain, episode,* and *experience.*

f. As prescribed, administer medication to reduce stress and anxiety that may contribute to pain.

g. Discuss situational factors that may influence pain (e.g., loss of job, recent divorce, death in family, serious illness). This may help decrease anxiety and reassure the client that others are there to help, which can combat feelings of isolation and loneliness.

h. As necessary, refer the client to psychological counseling, occupational therapy, and other resources to help deal with psychosocial problems.

E. Outcome evaluation
1. The client reports reduced pain after pain-relief interventions; use the pain scale.
2. The client is able to verbalize effective coping strategies to address acute or chronic pain.
3. The client displays a change in various responses to pain, such as:
   a. sympathetic nervous system responses
   b. parasympathetic nervous system responses
   c. behavioral and musculoskeletal responses (verbal and nonverbal)
   d. psychological responses.

Study questions

1. A client who had abdominal surgery 3 days earlier complains of sharp, throbbing abdominal pain that ranks 8 on a scale of 1 (no pain) to 10 (worst pain). Which intervention should the nurse implement *first*?
1. Obtaining an order for a stronger pain medication because the client's pain has increased
2. Assessing the client to rule out possible complications secondary to surgery
3. Checking the client's chart to determine when pain medication was last administered
4. Explaining to the client that the pain should not be this severe 3 days postoperatively

2. Which term refers to pain that has a slower onset, is diffuse, radiates, and is marked by somatic pain from organs in any body activity?

1. Acute pain
2. Chronic pain
3. Superficial pain
4. Deep pain

3. Which intervention should the nurse plan for a client with arthritis who remains in bed too long because it hurts to get started?
1. Telling the client to strictly limit the amount of movement of his inflamed joints
2. Teaching the client's family how to transfer the client into a wheelchair
3. Teaching the client the proper method for massaging inflamed, sore joints
4. Encouraging gentle range-of-motion exercises after administering aspirin and before rising

4. Which intervention should the nurse include as a nonpharmacologic pain-relief intervention for chronic pain?
   1. Referring the client to a therapist for hypnosis
   2. Administering pain medication as prescribed
   3. Removing all glaring lights and excessive noise
   4. Using transcutaneous electric nerve stimulation

5. A 10-year-old boy falls off his bicycle, grabs his wrist, and cries, "Oh, my wrist! Help! The pain is so sharp, I think I broke it." Based on these data, the pain the boy is experiencing is caused by impulses traveling from receptors to the spinal cord along which type of nerve fibers?
   1. Somatic efferent fibers
   2. Type C fibers
   3. Autonomic nerve fibers
   4. Type A-delta fibers

6. Which pain theory provides information *most* useful to nurses in planning pain-reduction interventions?
   1. Central-control theory
   2. Gate-control theory
   3. Specificity theory
   4. Pattern theory

7. One day after open reduction and internal fixation of the left hip, a client is complaining of pain. Which data would cause the nurse to refrain from administering the pain medication and to notify the health care provider instead?
   1. Left hip dressing dry and intact
   2. Blood pressure of 114/78 mm Hg; pulse rate of 82 beats per minute
   3. Left leg in functional anatomic position
   4. Left foot cold to touch; no palpable pedal pulse

8. Which term would the nurse use to document pain at one site that is perceived in another site?

   1. Referred pain
   2. Phantom pain
   3. Intractable pain
   4. Aftermath of pain

9. A client who had abdominal pain 1 day earlier complains of abdominal pain that ranks 9 on a sale of 1 (no pain) to 10 (worst pain). Which interventions should the nurse implement? (Select all that apply.)
   1. Assessing the client's bowel sounds
   2. Taking the client's blood pressure and apical pulse
   3. Obtaining a pulse oximeter reading
   4. Notifying the health care provider
   5. Determining the last time the client received pain medication
   6. Encouraging the client to turn, cough, and deep-breathe.

10. Which intervention is the *most* appropriate to assist a client who is expressing concern about the possible loss of job-performance abilities and physical disfigurement 6 months after sustaining severe burn injuries?
   1. Referring the client for counseling and occupational therapy
   2. Staying with the client as much as possible and building trust
   3. Providing cutaneous stimulation and pharmacologic therapy
   4. Providing distraction and guided imagery techniques

11. A client who has chronic pain, loss of self-esteem, no job, and bodily disfigurement from severe burns over the trunk and arms is admitted to a pain center. Which evaluation criteria would indicate the client's successful rehabilitation?
   1. The client remains free of the aftermath phase of the pain experience.
   2. The client experiences decreased frequency of acute pain episodes.
   3. The client continues normal growth and development with intact support systems.

4. The client develops increased tolerance for severe pain in the future.

12. Which scientific rationale, if believed by the nurse, would indicate that she understands the concept of pain?
1. Intractable pain may be relieved by treatment.
2. Pain is an objective sign of a more serious problem.
3. Psychological factors rarely contribute to a client's pain perception.
4. Pain sensation is affected by a client's anticipation of pain.

13. After a 5-year-old boy received a small paper cut on his finger, his mother let him wash it and apply a small amount of antibacterial ointment and a bandage. Then she let him watch TV and eat an apple. This is an example of which type of pain intervention?
1. Pharmacologic therapy
2. Control and distraction
3. Environmental alteration
4. Cutaneous stimulation

14. Which statement represents the *best* rationale for using noninvasive and non-pharmacologic pain-control measures in conjunction with other measures?
1. These measures are more effective than analgesics.
2. These measures decrease input to large fibers.
3. These measures potentiate the effects of analgesics.
4. These measures block transmission of type C fiber impulses.

15. When evaluating a client's adaptation to pain, which behavior indicates appropriate adaptation?
1. The client distracts himself during pain episodes.
2. The client denies the existence of any pain.
3. The client reports no need for family support.
4. The client reports pain reduction with decreased activity.

16. One day after abdominal surgery, a client is complaining of severe, throbbing abdominal pain, described as 9 on a rating scale of 1 (no pain) to 10 (worst pain). Assessment reveals bowel sounds in all four quadrants and that the dressing is dry and intact. Which intervention would the nurse implement *first*?
1. Calling the health care provider immediately
2. Explaining to the client how to do imagery
3. Medicating the client as prescribed
4. Encouraging turning, coughing, and deep breathing

Answer key

1. The answer is **2.**
The nurse's immediate action should be to assess the client in an attempt to exclude possible complications that may be causing the client's complaints. The health care provider ordered the pain medication for routine postoperative pain that is expected after abdominal surgery, not for such complications as hemorrhage, infection, or dehiscence. The nurse should never administer pain medication without assessing the client first. Obtaining an order for a stronger medication may be appropriate after the nurse assesses the client and checks the chart to see whether the current analgesic is ineffective. Checking the client's chart is appropriate after the nurse determines that the client is not experiencing complications from surgery. Pain is subjective, and each person has his own level of pain tolerance. The nurse must always believe the client's complaints of pain.

2. The answer is **1**.

Deep pain has a slow onset, is diffuse and radiates, and is marked by somatic pain from organs in any body activity. Acute pain is rapid in onset, usually temporary (less than 6 months), and subsides spontaneously. Chronic pain is marked by gradual onset and lengthy duration (more than 6 months). Superficial pain has abrupt onset with a sharp, stinging quality.

3. The answer is **4**.

Aspirin raises the pain threshold and, although range-of-motion exercises hurt, mild exercise can relieve pain on rising. Strict limitation of motion only increases the client's pain. Having others transfer the client into a wheelchair does not increase the client's mobility and increases his feelings of dependency. Massage increases inflammation and should be avoided with this client.

4. The answer is **4**.

Nonpharmacologic pain relief interventions include cutaneous stimulation, back rubs, biofeedback, acupuncture, transcutaneous electric nerve stimulation, and more. Hypnosis is considered an alternative therapy. Medications are pharmacologic measures. Although removing glaring lights and excessive noise help to reduce or remove noxious stimuli, it is not specific to pain relief.

5. The answer is **4**.

Type A-delta fibers conduct impulses at a very rapid rate and are responsible for transmitting acute sharp pain signals from the peripheral nerves to the spinal cord. Only Type A-delta fibers transmit sharp, piercing pain. Somatic efferent fibers affect the voluntary movement of skeletal muscles and joints. Type C fibers transmit sensory input at a much slower rate and produce a slow, chronic type of pain. The autonomic system regulates involuntary vital functions and organ control such as breathing.

6. The answer is **1**.

No one theory explains all the factors underlying the pain experience, but the central-control theory discusses brain opiates with analgesic properties and how their release can be affected by actions initiated by the client and caregivers. The gate-control, specificity, and pattern theories do not address pain control to the depth included in the central-control theory.

7. The answer is **4**.

A left foot cold to touch without a palpable pedal pulse represents an abnormal finding on neurovascular assessment of the left leg. The client is most likely experiencing some complication from surgery, which requires immediate medical intervention. The nurse should notify the health care provider of these findings. A dry and intact hip dressing, blood pressure of 114/78 mm Hg, pulse rate of 82 beats per minute, and a left foot in functional anatomic position are all normal assessment findings that do not require medical intervention.

8. The answer is **1**.

Referred pain is pain occurring at one site that is perceived in another site. Referred pain follows dermatome and nerve root patterns. Phantom pain refers to pain in a part of the body that is no longer there, such as in amputation. Intractable pain refers to moderate to severe pain that cannot be relieved by any known treatment. Aftermath of pain, a phase of the pain experience and the most neglected phase, addresses the client's response to the pain experience.

9. The answers are **1, 2, 5**.

The nurse must rule out complications prior to administering a pain medication, so her interventions would include assessing to make sure the client has bowel sounds and determining if the client is hemorrhaging by checking the client's blood pressure and pulse. The nurse must also make sure the pain medication is due according to the health care provider's orders. Obtaining a pulse oximeter reading and turning, coughing, and deep breathing will not help the client's pain. There is no need to notify the health provider in this situation.

10. The answer is **1.**
Because it has been 6 months, the client needs professional help to get on with life and handle the limitations imposed by the current problems. Staying with the client, building trust, and providing methods of pain relief, such as cutaneous stimulation, medications, distraction, and guided imagery interventions, would have been more appropriate in earlier stages of postburn injury, when physical pain was most severe and fewer psychologic factors needed to be addressed.

11. The answer is **3.**
Even though the client may experience an aftermath phase, progress is still possible, as is effective rehabilitation. Aftermath reactions may occur but need not interfere with rehabilitation. Acute pain is not expected at this stage of recovery. Conditioning probably would produce less pain tolerance.

12. The answer is **4.**
Phases of the pain experience include the anticipation of pain. Fear and anxiety affect a person's response to sensation and typically intensify the pain. Intractable pain is moderate to severe pain that cannot be relieved by any known treatment. Pain is a subjective sensation that cannot be quantified by anyone except the person experiencing it. Psychologic factors contribute to a client's pain perception. In many cases, pain results from emotions, such as hostility, guilt, or depression.

13. The answer is **2.**
The mother's actions are examples of control and distraction. Involving the child in care and providing distraction took his mind off the pain. Pharmacologic agents for pain — analgesics — were not used. The home environment was not changed, and cutaneous stimulation, such as massage, vibration, or pressure, was not used.

14. The answer is **3.**
Noninvasive measures may result in release of endogenous molecular neuropeptides with analgesic properties. They potentiate the effect of analgesics. No evidence indicates that noninvasive and nonpharmacologic measures are more effective than analgesics in relieving pain. Decreased input over large fibers allows more pain impulses to reach the central nervous system. There is no connection between type C fiber impulses and noninvasive and nonpharmacologic pain-control measures.

15. The answer is **1.**
Distraction is an appropriate method of reducing pain. Denying the existence of any pain is inappropriate and not indicative of coping. Exclusion of family members and other sources of support represents a maladaptive response. Range-of-motion exercises and at least mild activity, not decreased activity, can help reduce pain and are important to prevent complications of immobility.

16. The answer is **3.**
The client should be medicated as ordered. On the first postoperative day, clients commonly complain of severe pain. Further assessment by the nurse revealing a dry dressing and bowel sounds indicate the absence of complications. The ordered analgesic therefore should be given. The client's current condition does not require immediate medical treatment. The client is in pain and must be medicated. Imagery is not appropriate, and because of the client's pain level, he probably is unable to concentrate fully enough to learn how to do the imagery. Turning, coughing, and deep breathing are important interventions in the postoperative period, but they are related to improving respiratory function, not pain. Above all else, the client must be medicated.

5 Respiratory disorders

I. STRUCTURE AND FUNCTION OF THE RESPIRATORY SYSTEM

A. Structures (See *Figure 5-1*.)

1. The **upper respiratory tract** consists of the nose and sinuses, pharynx, epiglottis, and larynx; all parts are lined with mucus-secreting cells and cilia. The uppermost structures contain olfactory sensors.

2. The **lower respiratory tract** consists of the trachea, right and left mainstem bronchi, segmental bronchi, terminal bronchioles, and alveoli. Type I alveolar cells are epithelial cells that form alveolar walls; type II alveolar cells secrete surfactant that prevents alveolar collapse; and type III alveolar cells ingest foreign matter and act as an important defense mechanism.

3. **Lungs.** Situated in the thoracic cavity on either side of heart, the lungs are bounded by the clavicles, ribs, vertebrae, and diaphragm. The right lung contains three lobes; the left lung contains two lobes. The lungs' primary lobules contain millions of alveolar sacs.

4. **Chest cavity.** This closed compartment is bounded on top by neck muscles and at the bottom by the diaphragm. The sternum, thoracic vertebrae, 12 ribs, and the intercostal muscles form its outer wall. The chest cavity includes the lungs, heart, great vessels, and esophagus.

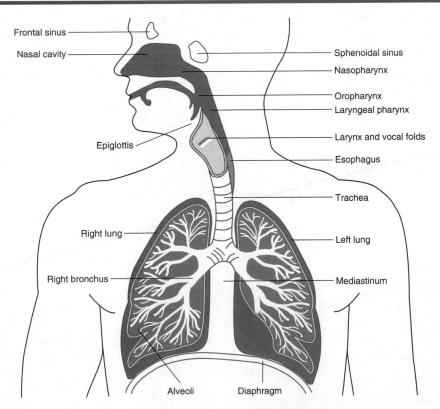

FIGURE 5-1

The respiratory system, showing respiratory structures and the structures of the thorax

5. **Pleura.** Parietal and visceral pleura surround the lungs; these two membranes are separated by the intrapleural space.
6. **Respiratory muscles**
   a. The **diaphragm**, a dome-shaped muscle separating the thoracic and abdominal cavities, is innervated by the phrenic nerve (a branch of the vagus nerve).
   b. The **external intercostal muscles** connect the adjacent ribs and slope downward and forward; the **other accessory muscles** include scalene muscles and the sternocleidomastoid muscles.
7. **Pulmonary blood supply** to the lungs is provided by the pulmonary and bronchial arteries.
8. **Neurologic control.** Ventilation is governed by the medulla oblongata, which contains inspiratory and expiratory centers. The neurologic system controls the rate and depth of respiration to meet the body's metabolic needs.

B. **Function.** The respiratory system provides gas exchange by means of ventilation, oxygen transport, and tissue perfusion; helps maintain acid-base balance; and serves as an immune defense.
   1. The **upper respiratory tract** is responsible for:
      a. air conduction to the lower respiratory tract
      b. protection of the lungs from foreign matter by clearing particulate matter from inspired air through the action of cilia and mucus-secreting cells
      c. warming and humidifying inspired air.
   2. **Lower respiratory tract**
      a. The **trachea** is a continuous tube that connects the larynx and the lungs.
      b. **Bronchi** conduct air to the alveoli.
      c. **Alveoli** receive and exchange oxygen (O_2) and carbon dioxide (CO_2) across the alveolar membrane to the pulmonary capillaries.
   3. **Lungs**
      a. **Ventilation.** During inspiration, air flows from the environment into the lungs, O_2 and CO_2 exchange takes place in the alveoli, and air flows from the lungs to the outside during expiration.
      b. **Diffusion of gases** occurs across the alveolar membrane according to pressure gradients from areas of high to low concentration. The pressure gradient of O_2 is greater in the lung than in the pulmonary capillaries, causing O_2 to diffuse across the alveolar membrane into the pulmonary capillaries. The pressure gradient of CO_2 is lower in the lung than in the pulmonary capillaries, causing CO_2 to diffuse from the pulmonary blood vessels to the lungs.
      c. **Acid-base regulation.** Changes in CO_2 concentration of the blood can cause shifts in pH levels. To maintain acid-base balance, the physiologic buffer system of the lungs responds to changes in CO_2 levels. The respiratory rate increases to blow off CO_2 and decreases to retain CO_2 formation, thereby restoring acid-base balance. (See *Table 5-1*, page 90.)
   4. **Chest cavity.** The act of breathing requires that the chest cavity is a closed compartment whose only opening to the outside is the trachea.
   5. **Pleura.** Negative pressure created by the intrapleural space helps effect elastic recoil of the lungs. A thin film of fluid allows the membranes to glide over each other and prevents separation between the lungs and the chest wall.
   6. **Respiratory muscles** assist breathing by rising on expiration and lowering on inspiration. During inspiration, the intrathoracic pressure becomes negative, and air is drawn into the lungs because the intrathoracic pressure is less than atmospheric pressure.

TABLE 5-1
Arterial blood gases

Type	Causes	Clinical manifestations	Treatment
Respiratory acidosis pH < 7.35; partial pressure of arterial carbon dioxide ($Paco_2$) > 45 mm Hg (too much carbon dioxide [CO_2] = too much acid = acidosis)	Respiratory failure, respiratory arrest, pulmonary edema, chronic obstructive pulmonary disease, pneumonia, pneumothorax, atelectasis, overdose, aspiration	*If sudden onset:* increased heart rate, decreased level of consciousness (LOC), feeling of fullness after vasodilation from CO_2 in head, dysrhythmias *If chronic:* weakness, dull headache	■ *Improve ventilation (chest physiotherapy):* turn, cough, deep-breathe; suction; oxygen (O_2) ■ Assess vital signs, breath sounds, and neurologic assessment signs. ■ Monitor arterial blood gases (ABG) and pulse oximetry readings.
Respiratory alkalosis pH > 7.45; $Paco_2$, < 35 mm Hg (too little CO_2 = too little acid = alkalosis)	Hyperventilation, pain, anxiety, hypoxemia, ventilators	Lightheadedness, unable to concentrate, numbness, tingling, tinnitus	■ Treat the cause. ■ Encourage slow breaths.
Metabolic acidosis pH < 7.35; bicarbonate (HCO_3) ≤ 22 mEq/L (too little HCO_3 = too little base = acidosis)	Diabetic ketoacidosis; starvation (ketoacidosis), lactic acidosis; renal failure; diarrhea; acetylsalicylic acid poisoning	Changes in LOC (confusion, drowsiness), headache, nausea and vomiting, Kussmaul's respirations (increased rate and increased depth), dysrhythmias	■ Administer sodium bicarbonate; monitor intake and output, ABGs, vital signs, and dysrhythmias; use seizure precautions.
Metabolic alkalosis pH > 7.45; HCO_3 > 26 mEq/L (too much HCO_3 = too much base = alkalosis)	Vomiting, nasogastric tube; diuretics; antacids, too much HCO_3; too much I.V. HCO_3 ordered by health care provider	Tingling, dizziness and bradypnea (conserve O_2), hypertonic muscles, dysrhythmias	■ Restore fluid volume and electrolytes. ■ Monitor vital signs, intake and output, ABGs, and dysrhythmias. ■ Perform a neurologic assessment.

7. **Pulmonary blood supply**
   a. The pulmonary circulation provides for the gas-exchange functions of the lungs; the bronchial circulation supplies the cells of the lungs with blood to meet their nutritional needs.
   b. Pulmonary circulation provides for tissue perfusion.
   c. In normal anatomic shunting, a small amount of blood from bronchial, pleural, and coronary circulation bypasses pulmonary circulation and therefore is not oxygenated. In abnormal physiologic shunting, a large amount of unoxygenated venous blood mixes with oxygenated blood in the left heart chambers as a result of adequate pulmonary perfusion with inadequate or absent alveolar ventilation.
8. **Neurologic control.** Many receptor sites assist in the brain's control of respiratory function. Central chemoreceptors respond to chemical changes, peripheral receptor sites respond to CO_2 levels, and baroreceptors respond to changes in arterial blood pressure.

II. **THE RESPIRATORY SYSTEM**

A. Assessment

1. **Health history**

    a. **Elicit a description of the client's present illness and chief complaint**, including onset, course, duration, location, and precipitating and alleviating factors. Cardinal signs and symptoms of respiratory dysfunction include:
       - dyspnea (i.e., labored breathing)
       - orthopnea (i.e., difficulty breathing in all positions except upright)
       - cough, which may be hacking, brassy, wheezing, productive, or nonproductive
       - increased sputum production, which may be purulent (yellow or green), rusty, bloody, or mucoid sputum
       - chest pain
       - wheezing and crackles
       - clubbing of fingers
       - hemoptysis
       - cyanosis (e.g., buccal, peripheral).

    b. **Explore the client's health history for risk factors** associated with respiratory disease, including:
       - personal or family history of lung disease
       - smoking (the most significant contributing factor in lung disease)
       - occupational or vocational exposure to allergens or environmental pollutants
       - age-related changes in lung capacity and respiratory function
       - history of upper respiratory infection
       - postoperative changes resulting in diminished respiratory excursion.

2. **Physical examination**

    a. **Inspection**
       - Observe general appearance, noting body size, age, skin quality and color, and posture.
       - Inspect configuration and movement of the thorax during respiration.
       - Assess characteristics of respiration, including rate, rhythm, depth, and muscles used for breathing. The normal resting adult breathes at 12 to 20 breaths per minute.
       - Note the presence of cough and the nature and character of sputum (e.g., clear, purulent, bloody, tenacious).
       - Note clubbing of fingers (i.e., angle of nail bed greater than 160 degrees and distal phalangeal depth greater than interphalangeal depth) and softening of nail beds.

    b. **Palpation.** Palpate the chest to detect painful areas or masses on the chest surface, and evaluate chest excursion and the presence or absence of fremitus (i.e., vibration).

    c. **Percussion.** Assess chest sounds to evaluate underlying tissues. Resonant sound indicates air-filled lung (normal), whereas dull or flat sound suggests presence of firm mass (usually abnormal).

    d. **Auscultation.** Listen to air movement in the lungs to detect normal or adventitious breath sounds.
       - Vesicular sounds are low-pitched, rustling sounds heard over most of lung field, most prominently on inspiration. They indicate normal, clear lungs.
       - Bronchial sounds are high-pitched, tubular sounds with a slight pause between inspiration and expiration. They are normal over large airways.

        – Bronchovesicular sounds are the combination of vesicular and bronchial sounds, normally heard anteriorly to the right or left of the sternum and posteriorly between the scapulae; inspiration and expiration are equal.

        – Adventitious breath sounds are crackles (i.e., fine to coarse), wheezes (i.e., sibilant or sonorous), and pleural friction rub.

   3. **Laboratory and diagnostic studies**

      a. **Radiographic and scanning studies** are done to visualize respiratory system structures. The studies include chest radiography, chest tomography, lung scan, computed tomography scan, positron-emission tomography scan, fluoroscopy, and barium swallow.

      b. **Endoscopic studies** are invasive techniques performed to visualize pulmonary structures and obtain tissue specimens. These studies include bronchoscopy, esophagoscopy, and mediastinoscopy.

      c. **Thoracentesis** involves needle aspiration of pleural fluid for diagnostic and therapeutic purposes.

      d. **Needle biopsy** is an invasive technique that involves entering the lung or pleura to obtain tissue for analysis.

      e. **Spirometry** (i.e., pulmonary function testing) is a noninvasive technique used to determine lung volumes, ventilatory function, airway resistance, and distribution of gases.

      f. **Sputum culture** determines the presence of pathogenic organisms.

      g. **Arterial blood gas (ABG) studies** determine oxygen (O_2) and carbon dioxide content and evaluate the body's acid-base balance. (See *Table 5-1,* page 90.)

      h. **Pulse oximetry** is a noninvasive method of continuously monitoring the O_2 saturation of hemoglobin, an effective tool to monitor sudden changes in O_2 saturation. Normal pulse oximetry readings are 93% to 100%; if the reading is less than 93%, respiratory comprise will occur.

B. Nursing diagnoses

   1. Ineffective breathing pattern
   2. Impaired gas exchange
   3. Ineffective tissue perfusion (peripheral)
   4. Activity intolerance
   5. Acute or chronic pain
   6. Risk for infection
   7. Anxiety
   8. Ineffective coping
   9. Deficient knowledge

C. Outcome identification and planning.

Goals for management of respiratory problems focus on improved breathing patterns, gas exchange and tissue perfusion, increased activity tolerance, pain relief, decreased anxiety, improved coping, and increased knowledge of disease process and therapeutic management.

D. Implementation

   1. **Assess respiratory status and tissue perfusion,** including respiratory rate, depth, and effort; level of consciousness; lung sounds; buccal and peripheral cyanosis; capillary refill time; color and consistency of sputum; and pulse oximetry.

   2. **Improve breathing patterns.**

      a. Encourage upright position (semi-Fowler's or high-Fowler's position) at least 30 to 45 degrees.

CLIENT AND FAMILIY TEACHING 5-1
Guidelines for a client with a respiratory disorder

- Complete all antibiotic therapy; do not save the medication for another time.
- Eat well-balanced, nutritious meals; avoid alcohol intake.
- Increase fluid intake to help thin secretions; fill a 2-L bottle with water every night and drink it before the next night.
- Alternate rest with activity; avoid fatigue and overexertion; conserve energy.
- Avoid cold winds, irritants, smoking, and second-hand smoke.

- Avoid crowds or people with infections or colds.
- Deep-breathe and cough at least every 2 hours.
- Wash hands thoroughly to help prevent infection transmission.
- Throw tissues away in a plastic bag; do not leave used tissues on counters or the floor.
- Receive influenza and streptococcal pneumonia immunizations at prescribed times.
- Make all scheduled medical visits for chest radiographs and follow-up care.

    b. Encourage the client to increase fluid intake to at least 2 to 3 L of fluid each day, unless contraindicated as in heart failure.

3. **Promote gas exchange.**
       a. Collaborate with a respiratory therapist when administering oxygen therapy. Analyze ABG values and pulse oximetry to determine the need for oxygen therapy. Assist in administering nebulizer, metered dose inhaler, or intermittent positive-pressure breathing treatment.
       b. Encourage effective coughing. Instruct the client to take three deep breaths in through the nose and out through the mouth, and on the third breath pull in the abdominal muscles and cough twice forcefully with the mouth open. Encourage the client to lie on the affected side to splint the area if there is pain when coughing.
       c. Encourage the client to eliminate or minimize exposure to all pulmonary irritants, and advise him to quit smoking.

4. **Improve activity tolerance.** Encourage the client to alternate rest with activity to prevent overexertion that may exacerbate symptoms and to increase activity gradually.

5. **Provide pain management.**
       a. Assess the client for pain, and exclude other potential complications.
       b. Instruct the client about splinting when the client has chest pain.
       c. Position the client to decrease pain, and administer pain medications as needed.

6. **Promote infection-control measures.**
       a. Instruct the client to avoid crowds or people with known colds, flu, or respiratory infection.
       b. Implement standard precautions and droplet or airborne precautions as indicated.

7. **Promote coping and minimize anxiety.**
       a. Support the client in dealing with emotional stress by discussing positive coping strategies (i.e., relaxation techniques, guided imagery, and enrollment in a pulmonary rehabilitation center).
       b. Reassure the client, provide concise explanations, and remain calm to reduce the client's anxiety, thereby decreasing his O_2 need.

8. **Provide client and family teaching.**
       a. Instruct the client to report danger signs and symptoms, including a change in color of the sputum, numbness and tingling in extremities, and difficulty with breathing.
       b. Provide additional teaching as detailed in *Client and family teaching 5-1*.

E. Outcome evaluation

1. The client demonstrates resolution of acute processes.
2. The client maintains normal vital signs.
3. The client demonstrates improved pulmonary function study results, and the ABG values are within normal ranges.
4. The client reports eased breathing effort.
5. The client's lungs are clear on auscultation.
6. The client maintains gas exchange at preillness level.
7. The client has capillary refill times of less than 3 seconds, no peripheral cyanosis, and no buccal cyanosis.
8. The client displays normal cardiopulmonary function.
9. The client can perform activities without shortness of breath.
10. The client reports relief or control of dyspnea and chest discomfort.
11. The client remains free from infection.
12. The client reports and exhibits reduced anxiety.
13. The client can identify strategies to cope effectively with illness.
14. The client verbalizes an understanding of administration and the purpose of prescribed medications.
15. The client verbalizes an understanding of the disease process and measures to prevent complications, including infection and lifestyle modifications.
16. The client reports symptom improvement with self-care strategies.
17. The client incorporates health-maintenance behaviors into his lifestyle.

III. PNEUMONIA

A. Description. Pneumonia is an inflammatory process involving the respiratory bronchioles, alveolar space and walls, and lobes, caused primarily by chemical irritants or by specific bacterial, viral, fungal, mycoplasmal, or parasitic organisms. Pneumonia is the most common cause of death from infectious disease in North America and the fourth leading cause of death among elderly persons.

B. Etiology

1. **Bacterial pneumonia** may be caused by the following organisms:
   a. *Streptococcus pneumoniae* (hemolytic type A; accounts for 90% of cases)
   b. *Staphylococcus aureus*
   c. *Haemophilus influenzae* (type B)
   d. *Klebsiella pneumoniae, Pseudomonas aeruginosa, Escherichia coli, Enterobacter,* and other gram-negative enteric bacilli.
2. **Nonbacterial pneumonia** may be caused by the following organisms:
   a. *Mycoplasma pneumoniae*
   b. Influenza viruses, parainfluenza viruses, and other viral infections
   c. *Pneumocystis carinii*
   d. *Aspergillus fumigatus.*
3. **Causes of and contributing factors** to pneumonia include:
   a. inability to move pulmonary secretions
   b. aspiration pneumonia due to an abnormal swallowing mechanism or tube feedings
   c. clients who are immunosuppressed
   d. frequent alcohol intoxication
   e. immobility

f. cigarette smoking.

C. Pathophysiology. The infecting organisms trigger inflammation of the airways. Inflammatory exudate fills the alveolar air spaces, producing lung consolidation. Impaired gas exchange in the alveoli leads to various degrees of hypoxia, depending on the amount of lung tissue affected.

D. Assessment findings

1. **Clinical manifestations**
   a. Dullness with consolidation on percussion of chest
   b. Bronchial breath sounds auscultated over consolidated lung fields; egophony "EE" to "AY"
   c. Sudden onset fever greater than 100° F (37.8° C)
   d. Shaking chills (with bacterial pneumonia)
   e. Chest pain aggravated by hacking cough
   f. Dyspnea, respiratory grunting, and nasal flaring
   g. Flushed cheeks; cyanotic lips and nail beds
   h. Purulent sputum
   i. Anxiety and confusion
   j. In elderly clients, the only signs may be mental status change and dehydration.

2. **Laboratory and diagnostic study findings**
   a. Chest radiograph shows density changes, primarily in the lower lung fields.
   b. Sputum culture and sensitivity are positive for a specific causative organism.
   c. White blood cell (WBC) count is elevated in pneumonia of bacterial origin; WBC count is depressed in pneumonia of mycoplasmal or viral origin.

E. Nursing management (See section II.D.)

1. **Administer prescribed medications,** which may include antibiotics, mucolytics, expectorants, or antitussive agents. (See *Drug chart 5-1,* pages 96 and 97.)
2. **Promote infection-control measures,** especially droplet precautions as indicated.
3. **Prevent aspiration pneumonia in a client receiving tube feedings.** Keep the client in an upright position during feedings and for 30 minutes afterward. Check for residual gastric contents; if more than double the rate of infusion, stop feeding and reevaluate.

IV. CHRONIC OBSTRUCTIVE PULMONARY DISEASE

A. Description

1. Chronic obstructive pulmonary disease (COPD), also known as *chronic airflow limitation,* is a group of disorders associated with persistent or recurrent obstruction of airflow, which include chronic bronchitis, emphysema, and asthma. These conditions frequently overlap. Most commonly, bronchitis and emphysema occur together. Asthma frequently occurs alone without the triad of bronchitis, emphysema, and asthma.
2. The most common chronic lung disease, COPD affects an estimated 17 million persons in the United States. The incidence is rising. The most common cause is smoking cigarettes.

B. Etiology

1. **Chronic bronchitis and emphysema.** Major causes of and contributing factors to these disorders, which are irreversible, include:
   a. smoking

DRUG CHART 5-1
Medications for respiratory disorders

Classifications	Indications	Selected interventions
Adrenergics (sympathomimetics) epinephrine isoetharine metaproterenol terbutaline	Dilate bronchial smooth muscles to relieve bronchospasm	■ When the client is using an inhaler, instruct him to exhale forcefully, use his lips to form a tight seal around the inhaler, press the top of inhaler and inhale deeply, and hold his breath as long as possible; instruct him to wait 3 to 5 minutes before taking a second inhalation. ■ When administering epinephrine subcutaneously in an emergency situation, always use a tuberculin needle and monitor the client closely. ■ Instruct the client that nervousness, anxiety, insomnia, tachycardia, palpitations, and headache may occur.
Antibiotics aminoglycosides (gentamicin, tobramycin) amoxicillin erythromycin penicillin tetracycline	Prevent or treat infections caused by pathogenic microorganisms	■ Before administering the first dose, assess the client for allergies and determine whether culture has been obtained. ■ After multiple doses, assess the client for superinfection (thrush, yeast infection, diarrhea); notify the health care provider if superinfection occurs. ■ Assess the insertion site for phlebitis if antibiotics are being administered I.V. ■ To assess the effectiveness of antibiotic therapy, monitor the white blood cell count. ■ Monitor peaks and troughs for aminoglycosides.
Anticoagulants I.V. heparin oral warfarin sodium	Prevent recurrence of emboli (have no effect on emboli that are already present)	■ For heparin therapy, monitor partial thromboplastin time (PTT), for which the therapeutic range should be 1.5 to 2 times the normal PTT or control. Antidote is protamine sulfate. ■ For Coumadin therapy, monitor the International Normalized Ratio (INR), the therapeutic level for which is 2 to 3. Antidote is AquaMEPHYTON (vitamin K). ■ Instruct the client to report bruising, unexplained bleeding, or dark, tarry stools; use a soft-bristle toothbrush; be cautious when using sharp objects and machinery; wear a medi-alert bracelet, and notify health care providers (dentist, pharmacist) that he is on anticoagulant. ■ If bleeding occurs, instruct the client to apply direct pressure to the wound; if bleeding does not stop after 5 minutes, get medical help.
Subcutaneous Low-dose heparin (5000 units)	Prevent deep-vein thrombosis (Heparin activates antithrombin III, which inactivates newly formed factor Xa and thrombin.)	■ Administer subcutaneously in the client's abdomen, 1″ (2.5 cm) from the umbilicus. Do not aspirate; do not massage. Not necessary to monitor PTT.
Bronchodilators (xanthine derivatives) theophylline	Relax bronchial smooth muscle	■ Monitor serum level of theophylline (therapeutic level, 10-20 µg/ml). ■ Provide medication at regular intervals before meals and with a full glass of water. ■ Instruct the client to notify the health care provider of irritability, restlessness, headache, insomnia, dizziness, tachycardia, palpitations, or seizures. ■ Do not crush sustained-release (SR or XL) capsules or tablets.

DRUG CHART 5-1

Medications for respiratory disorders *(continued)*

Classifications	Indications	Selected interventions
Corticosteroids oral—dexamethasone, hydrocortisone, methylprednisolone, prednisone inhalable—beclomethasone I.V.—Solu-Medrol, Solu-Cortef	Combat severe immune or inflammatory responses	▪ Instruct the client to take the medication exactly as directed and to taper it rather than stop it abruptly, which could cause serious withdrawal symptoms leading to adrenal insufficiency, shock, and death. ▪ Forewarn the client that the medication may cause reportable cushingoid effects (weight gain, moon face, buffalo hump, and hirsutism) and may mask signs and symptoms of infection.
Low-molecular-weight heparin enoxaparin	Prevent deep vein thrombosis by preferentially inactivating factor Xa	▪ Administer in the anterolateral abdominal wall. Do not aspirate; do not massage. Insert air bubble into syringe. Not necessary to monitor PTT.
Mast cell inhibitor cromolyn sodium	Inhibit mast cell, thereby releasing chemical mediators that result in bronchodilation and a decrease in airway inflammation	▪ Teach the client to insert the capsule in the nebulizer device, exhale completely, place the mouthpiece between his lips, inhale deeply, hold breath for 10 seconds, and then exhale. ▪ Instruct the client that the inhaler is to be used prophylactically before exercise, not for an acute asthma attack.
Mucolytic, expectorant, and antitussive agents acetylcysteine benzonatate guaifenesin	Facilitate sputum expectoration for disorders characterized by thick, resistant secretions	▪ Instruct the client to take syrups undiluted and not to eat or drink anything for at least 15 minutes after taking the medication. ▪ Instruct the client to not chew benzonatate perles, which must be swallowed whole.
Thrombolytic therapy alteplase (tissue plasminogen recombinant TPA) streptokinase urokinase	Dissolve the thrombi and emboli more quickly and restore more normal hemodynamic functioning of pulmonary circulation	▪ Be sure to follow hospital protocol when administering these medications.

   b. air pollution

   c. occupational exposure to respiratory irritants

   d. allergies

   e. autoimmunity

   f. infection

   g. genetic predisposition

   h. aging.

2. **Asthma** is a reversible diffuse airway obstruction with a possible genetic component. It may be extrinsic or intrinsic.

   a. **Extrinsic factors** include external agents or specific allergens (e.g., dust, foods, mold spores, insecticides).

   b. **Intrinsic factors** include upper respiratory infection, exercise, emotional stress, cold, or other nonspecific factors.

   c. **Status asthmaticus** is a severe and persistent asthma that lasts longer than 24 hours and does not respond to conventional therapy.

C. **Pathophysiology.** COPD disrupts airway dynamics, resulting in obstruction of airflow into or out of the lungs.

1. **Chronic bronchitis.** Hypertrophy and hypersecretion in goblet cells and bronchial mucus glands leading to increased sputum secretion, bronchial congestion, narrowing of bronchioles, and small bronchi.

2. **Emphysema.** Increased size of air spaces (i.e., "dead space") with loss of elastic recoil of lung due to hyperinflation of distal airways causing airway obstruction. Destruction of alveolar walls and diffuse airway narrowing causes resistance to airflow because of loss of supporting structure and bronchospasm further impede airflow.

3. **Asthma.** Basic pathologic changes include narrowing of the bronchial airways, bronchospasms, increased mucus, and mucosal edema secondary to inflammation.

D. **Assessment findings**

1. **Clinical manifestations**

   a. **Chronic bronchitis**
      - History of productive cough that lasts 3 months per year for 2 consecutive years
      - Persistent cough, known as *smoker's cough,* usually in the winter months
      - Persistent sputum production
      - Recurrent acute respiratory infections
      - Dusky color leading to cyanosis
      - Clubbing of fingers

   b. **Emphysema**
      - History of chronic bronchitis
      - Slow onset of symptoms (typically over several years), which can lead to right-sided heart failure (i.e., cor pulmonale)
      - Progressive dyspnea, initially only on exertion and later also at rest
      - Progressive cough and increased sputum production, especially during bouts of infection; use of accessory muscles
      - Anorexia with weight loss and profound weakness

   c. **Asthma**
      - Chest tightness and dyspnea
      - Cough
      - Wheezing
      - Expiration more strenuous and prolonged than inspiration
      - Use of accessory muscles of respiration
      - Hypoxia with restlessness, anxiety, cyanosis, weak pulse, and diaphoresis

2. **Laboratory and diagnostic study findings**

   a. **Chronic bronchitis**
      - Pulmonary function studies identify decreased forced expiratory volume (FEV), decreased forced vital capacity (FVC), increased residual volume (RV), and total lung capacity (TLC) that is normal to slightly increased.
      - Chest radiograph shows an enlarged heart with a normal or flattened diaphragm.
      - Arterial blood gas (ABG) studies during the acute phase show significantly increased partial pressure of arterial carbon dioxide ($Paco_2$) and decreased partial pressure of arterial oxygen (Pao_2).
      - Pulse oximeter reading less than 93%.
      - Sputum culture reveals secondary bacterial infection with gram-negative or gram-positive organisms, such as *Diplococcus pneumoniae* and *H. influenzae.*

    b. **Emphysema**
- Pulmonary function studies identify decreased FEV, decreased FVC, increased RV, and increased TLC.
- Chest radiograph shows a flattened diaphragm, decreased vascular markings with hyperradiolucence, and increased anteroposterior diameter (i.e., "barrel chest").
- ABG studies detect increased $Paco_2$ and decreased Pao_2.
- Pulse oximeter reading is less than 93%.
- Blood analysis reveals polycythemia (i.e., increased numbers of red blood cells in response to hypoxemia).

    c. **Asthma.** Pulmonary function studies during an acute episode identify markedly decreased FEV, increased RV, and increased TLC in response to air trapping. These study values improve after treatment.

E. Nursing management (See section II.D.)

  1. **Provide nursing care for the client with chronic bronchitis or emphysema.**

    a. **Administer prescribed medications,** which may include antibiotics, bronchodilators, mucolytic agents, and corticosteriods. (See *Drug chart 5-1,* pages 96 and 97.) Antibiotics should be administered at the first sign of infection, such as a change in sputum. Opioids, sedatives, and tranquilizers, which can further depress respirations, should be avoided.

    b. **Clear airways** with postural drainage, percussion (i.e., clapping) or vibrating, and suctioning as appropriate.

    c. **Promote infection control.** Encourage the client to obtain influenza and pneumonia vaccines at prescribed times.

    d. **Improve breathing patterns.** Demonstrate and encourage diaphragmatic and purse-lip breathing. Have the client take a deep breath and blow out against closed lips.

    e. **Administer oxygen.** A low arterial oxygen level is the client's primary drive for breathing. Oxygen flow rate should be no more than 2 to 3 L per minute. Higher levels will cause the client to quit breathing.

    f. **Discuss the importance of smoking cessation and avoiding second-hand smoke.** Discuss ways to quit smoking and make appropriate referrals. Compromise is not acceptable; the client must stop smoking.

  2. **Provide nursing care for the client with asthma.**

    a. **Administer prescribed medications,** which may include adrenergics, bronchodilators, and corticosteroids for acute attack. Encourage use of a cromolyn inhaler as prophylactic treatment. (See *Drug chart 5-1,* pages 96 and 97.)

    b. **Provide treatment during an acute asthmatic attack.**
- Stay with the client and keep him calm and in an upright position.
- Do purse-lip breathing with the client; encourage relaxation techniques.

    c. **Implement measures to prevent asthmatic attacks.** Teach the client the following skills:
- Identify and eliminate or minimize exposure to pulmonary irritants.
- Remove rugs and curtains from the home, change air filters frequently, keep the home as dust free as possible, and keep windows closed during windy and high pollen days.
- Use an inhaler and take medications as prescribed, and notify the health care provider when not gaining complete relief.
- Notify the health care provider when a respiratory infection occurs.

- Obtain influenza and pneumonia vaccines at prescribed times.
- Monitor peak expiratory flow rate.

3. **Provide referrals** to the Asthma and Allergy Foundation of America, American Lung Association, and Smokenders. (See appendix A.)

V. OCCUPATIONAL LUNG DISEASE

A. Description
1. Occupational lung disorders (i.e., pneumoconioses) are nonneoplastic alterations of the lung from exposure to organic or inorganic dusts and noxious gases in the workplace. They commonly do not produce signs or symptoms in the early stages.
2. The most common types include silicosis, asbestosis, and coal workers' pneumoconiosis (CWP), also known as *black lung*.

B. Etiology
1. **Silicosis** results from inhaling silica dust in such occupations as mineral mining, stone cutting, quarrying, abrasives manufacturing, and ceramic and pottery work.
2. **Asbestosis** results from inhaling asbestos dust and particles in occupations related to manufacture, handling, and removal of asbestos-containing materials. (*Note:* There are more than 4,000 known uses of asbestos fiber.)
3. **CWP** results from accumulation of coal dust in the lungs, most commonly from coal mining.

C. Pathophysiology. The effects of inhaling dusts, particles, or gases depend on the substance's composition, its antigenic or irritating properties, the amount inhaled, duration of exposure, and the person's overall health status.
1. **Silicosis.** Chronic inhalation of silica particles produces nodular lesions throughout the lungs. These lesions become fibrotic, enlarged, and fused, resulting in obstructive and restrictive lung changes.
2. **Asbestosis.** Inhaled asbestos fibers enter the alveoli, which eventually become obliterated by fibrous tissue surrounding the particles. Progressive pleural fibrosis and plaque formation lead to restrictive lung disease, diminished lung volume, impaired gas exchange, hypoxemia and, eventually, cor pulmonale. Asbestosis also is associated with bronchogenic cancer.
3. **CWP.** Inhaled coal dust is deposited in the alveoli and bronchioles. Eventually, the alveoli and bronchioles become clogged with dust, macrophages, and fibroblasts, leading to the formation of coal macules, the primary lesion of CWP. As these macules enlarge, bronchiolar dilation and emphysema result.

D. Assessment findings
1. **Clinical manifestations**
   a. **Silicosis.** Symptoms indicative of hypoxemia, severe airway obstruction, and right-sided heart failure (i.e., cor pulmonale) are evident. Edema may occur secondary to right-sided heart failure.
   b. **Asbestosis.** Progressive dyspnea, mild to moderate chest pain, anorexia, and weight loss are evident. With progression of asbestosis, cor pulmonale and respiratory failure may result.
   c. **CWP.** Initially, chronic cough and sputum production are evident. As CWP progresses, the client has dyspnea and coughs up large amounts of black fluid. Eventually, cor pulmonale and respiratory failure occur.

2. **Laboratory and diagnostic study findings**
    a. Chest radiograph findings vary for the specific disorder:
        - In silicosis, nodular formation to massive fibrosis and densities are identified in lung fields as the disease progresses.
        - In asbestosis, interstitial density is seen in the lower lung fields.
        - In CWP, nodular densities are seen in the upper lung fields.
    b. Pulmonary function tests reveal decreased forced vital capacity, forced expiratory volume, total lung capacity, and diffusing capacity of carbon dioxide as the disease progresses.
    c. Arterial blood gas studies show decreasing partial pressure of arterial oxygen and increasing partial pressure of arterial carbon dioxide values with disease progression.

E. Nursing management (See section II.D.)
    1. **Implement nursing care for a client experiencing acute symptoms.**
        a. Maintain a patent airway by suctioning or endotracheal intubation.
        b. Maintain cardiac output.
        c. Initiate mechanical ventilation if respiratory failure occurs.
    2. **Implement nursing care for a client with chronic disease.** There is no specific treatment for pneumoconioses. Interventions for chronic disease are aimed at managing complications and preventing infections:
        a. Administer prescribed medications, which may include medications used to treat chronic obstructive pulmonary disease (COPD).
        b. Maintain bronchial hygiene.
        c. Implement additional interventions as for COPD.
    3. **Provide a referral** to the American Lung Association. (See appendix A.)

VI. ACUTE RESPIRATORY FAILURE

A. Description. Acute respiratory failure (ARF) results when the exchange of oxygen (O_2) for carbon dioxide (CO_2) in the normal lungs cannot match the rate of O_2 consumption and CO_2 production in body cells.

B. Etiology
    1. Airway obstruction
    2. Restrictive lung disease
    3. Central nervous system disorder, such as head trauma or stroke
    4. Drug overdose
    5. Anesthesia and surgical procedures

C. Pathophysiology. ARF occurs when O_2 and CO_2 exchange in normal lungs fails to fulfill the oxygen needs of the body, causing alveolar hypoventilation. Effects include hypoxia (partial pressure of arterial oxygen [Pao_2] < 80 mm Hg) with or without hypercapnia (partial pressure of arterial carbon dioxide [$Paco_2$] > 45 mm Hg).

D. Assessment findings. Evaluation of the precipitating event is important in differentiating ARF from acute lung damage (e.g., acute respiratory distress syndrome) and chronic respiratory conditions with acute changes (e.g., chronic obstructive pulmonary disease).
    1. **Clinical manifestations**
        a. Dyspnea
        b. Tachypnea
        c. Tachycardia

   d. Headache
   e. Cyanosis
   f. Anxiety, confusion, and restlessness
   g. Decreased or absent breath sounds
   h. Adventitious breath sounds such as crackles and wheezing
2. **Laboratory and diagnostic study findings**
   a. Arterial blood gas studies reveal a Pao_2 of less than 80 mm Hg and $Paco_2$ of more than 45 mm Hg; the pH is less than 7.35 (i.e., respiratory acidosis).
   b. The electrocardiogram shows cardiac arrhythmias.
   c. Chest radiograph detects lung field changes, depending on causative factors.

E.   Nursing management (See section II.D.)
   1. **Restore and maintain a patent airway** by suctioning or performing endotracheal intubation as ordered.
   2. **Administer oxygen therapy** to maintain adequate alveolar ventilation.
   3. **Institute mechanical ventilation** if the client's condition deteriorates. (See section XIII.)
   4. **Maintain effective tracheobronchial hygiene.**
   5. **Monitor cardiac status.**

VII. PULMONARY EMBOLISM

A. Description. Pulmonary embolism is the obstruction of one or more pulmonary arteries by a thrombus or thrombi, originating somewhere in the venous system or in the right side of the heart. Pulmonary embolism affects an estimated 6 million adult Americans yearly, resulting in about 100,000 deaths.

B. Etiology
   1. **Thrombus formation**
      a. Venous stasis, which may result from prolonged immobilization, sitting, or standing
      b. Vessel-wall injury
      c. Hypercoagulability of the blood
   2. **Pulmonary embolism**
      a. Prolonged immobility
      b. Chronic lung disease
      c. Heart failure
      d. Thrombophlebitis
      e. Hematologic disorders
      f. Lower extremity fractures or surgery
      g. Pregnancy or hormonal contraceptive use

C. Pathophysiology
   1. Thrombus formation may occur in the deep veins of the legs (most common site); in pelvic, renal, or hepatic veins; in the right heart; and in the upper extremities.
   2. A dislodged thrombus may travel to the pulmonary arterial bed, where obstruction leads to an altered ventilation-perfusion ratio and an increase in alveolar dead space. The area of obstruction continues to ventilate but receives little or no blood supply, resulting in decreased pulmonary vascular blood pressure and increased pulmonary artery pressure.

3. Unrelieved obstruction may result in right ventricular heart failure and shock; total occlusion of the main pulmonary artery is rapidly fatal.

D. Assessment findings
1. Clinical manifestations
a. Chest pain, which may be sudden, sharp or mild, and substernal or pleuritic, depending on the site and extent of obstruction
b. Sense of impending doom
c. Tachycardia
d. Dyspnea
e. Anxiety and restlessness
f. Decreased breath sounds on auscultation and crackles, usually with pleural friction rub
g. Signs of circulatory collapse (e.g., weak, rapid pulse; hypotension)
2. Laboratory and diagnostic study findings
a. Arterial blood gas (ABG) studies reveal a partial pressure of arterial oxygen of less than 60 mm Hg, indicating hypoxemia.
b. Blood analysis detects elevated levels of lactate dehydrogenase, bilirubin, and fibrin split products.
c. A ventilation-perfusion lung scan shows areas of deficient ventilation and perfusion.
d. Pulmonary angiogram (most specific for diagnosis) detects intra-arterial filling defects and obstruction of the pulmonary artery branch.
e. D-dimer test is elevated (> 250 µg/L).

E. Nursing management (See section II.D.)
1. Administer prescribed medications, which may include anticoagulants (initial therapy includes I.V. heparin followed by warfarin), enoxaparin, and thrombolytics. (See *Drug chart 5-1,* pages 96 and 97.)
2. Provide nursing care for the client experiencing symptoms of acute pulmonary embolism.
a. Call for help, and stay with the client.
b. Administer nasal oxygen immediately.
c. Establish an I.V. route.
d. Prepare the client for a stat perfusion lung scan, ABG determinations, and pulmonary angiography.
e. Assist with transferring the client to the intensive care unit.
f. Prepare to administer small doses of morphine to relieve anxiety and alleviate chest discomfort.
3. Implement measures to prevent pulmonary emboli by minimizing the risk for deep vein thrombosis.
a. Perform active or passive range-of-motion exercises to prevent venous stasis. Move the legs in a "pumping" motion, and encourage early ambulation.
b. Administer low doses of heparin (enhances the activity of antithrombin III, a major plasma inhibitor of clotting factor X); prophylactic warfarin and prophylactic enoxaparin may be administered.
c. Apply antiembolism stockings or intermittent pneumatic leg-compression devices to help improve venous return.
d. Instruct the client not to do activities that increase venous stasis, such as crossing legs, sitting for long periods, and wearing constricting knee-high socks.
e. Instruct the client to elevate the legs above heart level.

f. Instruct the client to increase fluids to prevent hemoconcentration due to fluid deficit.

VIII. PLEURAL EFFUSION

A. Description. Pleural effusion is a collection of fluid in the pleural space, which is located between the visceral and parietal surfaces.

B. Etiology. Pleural effusion usually results from such diseases as neoplastic tumors (of which bronchogenic cancer is the most common malignancy), heart failure, tuberculosis, pneumonia, pulmonary infection, and connective tissue disease.

C. Pathophysiology. The pleural space contains a small amount of lubricating fluid that allows the pleural surfaces to move without friction. Excess fluid accumulates in the space until it becomes clinically evident. The effusion can be composed of a clear fluid, or it can be bloody or purulent.

D. Assessment findings. The size of the effusion determines the severity of symptoms.
1. **Clinical manifestations**
   a. **Large pleural effusion**
   - Shortness of breath
   - Minimal or no breath sounds
   - Dull, flat sound when percussed
   - Tracheal deviation away from the affected side (may occur when significant accumulation of fluid occurs)
   b. **Small to moderate pleural effusion**
   - Respiratory difficulty or comprised lung expansion may not be evident.
   - Dyspnea may not be present.
2. **Laboratory and diagnostic study findings**
   a. Chest radiograph shows fluid in the pleural space.
   b. Pleural fluid obtained by thoracentesis and treated with an acid-fast bacillus stain may reveal tuberculosis or red and white blood cells.

E. Nursing management. Specific treatment is directed at resolving the underlying cause. (See section II.D.)
1. **Prepare the client for thoracentesis,** which is performed to remove fluid, obtain a specimen for analysis, and relieve dyspnea.
2. **Assist the health care provider with administering chemically irritating agents,** which may be instilled to obliterate the pleural space and prevent further accumulation of fluid.

IX. CHEST TRAUMA

A. Description. Injury to the chest wall or lungs can interfere with inspiration, gas exchange, or expiration. Types of injuries include:
1. **hemothorax** (blood in the pleural space)
2. **tension pneumothorax** (air in the pleural space)
3. **open pneumothorax** (a sucking chest wound).

B. Etiology

1. **Hemothorax** results from penetrating or blunt chest injury.
2. **Tension pneumothorax** can result from disease or injury, most commonly from laceration of the lung parenchyma, tracheobronchial tree, or esophagus.
3. **Open pneumothorax** most commonly results from penetrating chest injury.

C. Pathophysiology

1. **Hemothorax.** The blood in the pleural cavity compresses the lungs and can produce blood loss, resulting in shock.
2. **Tension pneumothorax** is considered a medical emergency. Pressure in the pleural space compromises ventilation and can lead to lung collapse, decreased ventilation in the other lung, and decreased venous return to the heart, known as a mediastinal shift.
3. **Open pneumothorax**, an acutely life-threatening condition, involves an opening in the chest wall large enough to allow air passage into and out of the chest cavity with each attempted respiration; the rush of air produces a characteristic "sucking" sound. Tidal volume diminishes, and ventilation is compromised.

D. Assessment findings

1. **Clinical manifestations**
   a. Dyspnea
   b. Tachypnea, tachycardia
   c. Pain on breathing on affected side
   d. Rapid development of cyanosis
   e. Asymmetric chest movement
   f. Absent breath sounds on affected area
   g. Hypotension progressing to shock (hemothorax)
2. **Laboratory and diagnostic study findings**
   a. The electrocardiogram may reveal cardiac arrhythmias.
   b. Chest X-rays will reveal the size and type of injury.

E. Nursing management (See section II.D.)

1. **Provide emergency care.**
   a. Establish and maintain a patent airway by suctioning and endotracheal intubation as appropriate.
   b. Control hemorrhage. Treat damage to chest and other injured structures.
   c. Stabilize the chest wall if necessary.
   d. As ordered, assist with insertion of a chest tube, and maintain a closed drainage system. (See *Figure 5-2*, page 106.)
2. **Promote measures to maintain adequate chest tube drainage**. Assess the chest tube insertion site for crepitus and bleeding. Assess tubing for kinks, clots, or dependent loops. Assess the drainage chamber for color, consistency, and amount of drainage. Assess water-seal chamber for fluctuation "tidaling" with inspiration and expiration. Assess suction chamber for gentle bubbling.
3. **Promote coping.** Provide emotional support to reduce anxiety and fear.
4. **Prepare the client for surgery**, if appropriate, based on the nature of the injury.

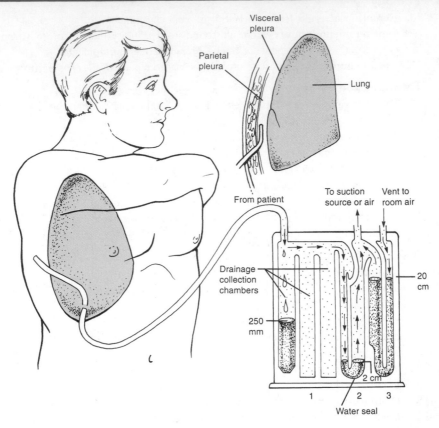

FIGURE 5-2

The Pleur-Evac system (shown above) is a common chest tube drainage-suction system used in clients with pulmonary injury, such as hemothorax or pneumothorax. It works much like the traditional bottle-suction systems.

X. ACUTE RESPIRATORY DISTRESS SYNDROME

A. **Description.** Acute respiratory distress syndrome (ARDS) is a clinical syndrome characterized by pulmonary edema and progressive decrease in arterial oxygen (O_2) content. It occurs after a serious illness or injury and accumulation of lung fluids, also known as *noncardiogenic pulmonary edema*. ARDS has been associated with a mortality rate as high as 50% to 60%. Early diagnosis and prompt treatment increase survival rate.

B. **Etiology.** ARDS results from an injury or illness. Causes may include aspiration; drug overdose; prolonged inhalation of high concentrations of O_2, smoke, or corrosive substances; shock (any cause); trauma (e.g., pulmonary contusion, multiple fractures, head injury); and systemic infection.

C. **Pathophysiology.** Injury to the alveolar capillary membrane results in leakage of blood and fluid into the alveolar interstitial spaces and alteration in the capillary bed. The fluid in the alveoli impairs gas exchange and causes extensive shunting of blood in the lungs. This leads to a ventilation-perfusion imbalance, which leads to noncardiogenic pulmonary edema.

D. Assessment findings

1. **Clinical manifestations,** usually occurring 12 to 48 hours after a serious injury or illness, may include:
   a. anxiety
   b. decreased level of consciousness
   c. dyspnea
   d. tachypnea
   e. auscultated crackles
   f. decreased functional residual capacity
   g. hypocapnia
   h. severe hypoxia
   i. marked buccal peripheral cyanosis.
2. **Laboratory and diagnostic study findings**
   a. Chest radiograph shows bilateral pulmonary infiltrates.
   b. Arterial blood gas studies reveal decreased partial pressure of arterial oxygen (≤ 60 mm Hg) despite administration of O_2 at a high flow rate (10 L/minute).

▨ E. Nursing management. Vigilant nursing management, early diagnosis, and treatment is crucial for recovery and may involve ventilatory support, medication, and supportive care. (See section II.D.)

1. **Administer prescribed medication,** which may include corticosteroids to decrease inflammation surrounding the alveoli and to stabilize the capillary membranes. Keep in mind that this therapy remains controversial because of the belief that corticosteroid use may precipitate superinfection and further impair pulmonary function. (See *Drug chart 5-1,* pages 96 and 97.)
2. **Promote measures to maintain adequate airway and ventilation.**
   a. Collaborate with the health care provider and the respiratory therapist when intubating the client and placing him on mechanical ventilation; as prescribed, institute positive end-expiratory pressure to keep alveoli distended, stretch stiff lungs, and increase O_2 and carbon dioxide (CO_2) diffusion. (See section XIII.)
   b. Maintain effective tracheobronchial hygiene.
   c. Monitor the client's hemodynamic status.
3. **Monitor fluid balance.** Assess the client for signs and symptoms of fluid volume overload, including peripheral edema and jugular vein distention.
4. **Provide adequate nutritional support** that is not high in carbohydrates, which metabolize to form excess CO_2. The diet should include 35 to 45 kcal/kg each day to meet normal requirements, with enteral or parental feeding support if necessary.

XI. AIRWAY OBSTRUCTION

A. Description. Airway obstruction refers to any mechanical impediment to oxygen delivery or absorption in the lungs.

B. Etiology. The airway may be partially obstructed or fully obstructed by aspirated food or foreign objects or from laryngospasm or edema due to inflammation, injury (e.g., blood, teeth, tongue), or anaphylaxis.

C. Assessment findings

1. A client with **complete airway obstruction** is unable to breathe or speak, becomes cyanotic, and collapses.

2. A client with **partial airway obstruction** appears anxious, uses accessory muscles to breathe, may have stridor and flared nostrils, and usually is able to speak.

D. Nursing management. Airway obstruction takes priority over any other injury or emergency problem. (See section II.D.)

1. **Implement measures to dislodge an obstructing object in a *conscious* client.**
   a. In partial obstruction, instruct the conscious client to cough forcefully; if this does not dislodge the object, perform the abdominal thrust (Heimlich) maneuver.
   b. In complete obstruction in a conscious client, immediately perform the Heimlich maneuver.

2. **Implement measures to dislodge an obstructing object in an *unconscious* client.** In partial or complete obstruction, follow these steps:
   a. Position the client on the back.
   b. Use the head-tilt–chin-lift technique to open the airway. (Use the jaw-thrust technique if a cervical spine injury is suspected.)
   c. Attempt to ventilate the client.
   d. Perform the Heimlich maneuver.
   e. Perform a finger sweep.
   f. Attempt ventilation again.
   g. Chest thrusts may be used in advanced stages of pregnancy or in a markedly obese client.
   h. Continue until the obstruction is removed.

3. **Provide a patent airway.**
   a. An oropharyngeal airway is placed by insertion of a tubelike device over the back of the tongue into the lower posterior pharynx in a spontaneously breathing but unconscious client.
   b. An esophageal obturator airway is placed by insertion of a tube through the mouth and advanced into the esophagus just below the bifurcation of the trachea in an unconscious client when endotracheal intubation is not possible; the proximal part of the tube has air holes at the level of the pharynx through which air or oxygen is delivered into the lungs.
   c. An endotracheal airway is placed by insertion of an endotracheal tube into the mouth through the vocal folds and advanced to the trachea just above the bifurcation of the trachea in an unconscious client; the endotracheal cuff at the end of the tube is inflated to secure the tube.
   d. Tracheostomy is the insertion of a tube into an opening in the trachea to bypass an upper airway obstruction, to replace an endotracheal tube, or for long-term use of a ventilator.
   e. Cricothyroidotomy is puncturing or incising into the cricothyroid membrane to establish an emergency airway when endotracheal intubation is not possible or contraindicated.

XII. NEAR-DROWNING

A. Description. Near-drowning describes the pathologic status of a person who has survived events that nearly led to drowning. Asphyxia and aspiration are the primary problems associated with drowning and near-drowning. Drowning is a leading preventable cause of accidental death in the United States. Approximately 5,500 people die of drowning every year.

B. Etiology. Alcohol ingestion is an important factor in adult drowning deaths.

C. Pathophysiology

1. **Hypoxemia occurs within 3 to 5 minutes after total immersion, and brain injury and brain death can occur within 5 to 10 minutes.**

2. **Delayed death in near-drownings result from water aspiration.**

   a. Fresh water is hypotonic and is rapidly absorbed from the alveoli, resulting in significant hypervolemia and hemodilution.

   b. Salt water is hypertonic and causes fluid to be drawn into the alveoli, resulting in hypovolemia and hemoconcentration.

3. **Immersion in very cold water and the dive reflex** — a protective mechanism that slows the heartbeat, constricts peripheral vessels, and shunts blood to the brain and heart —may prolong survival of drowning victims.

D. Assessment findings

1. **Clinical manifestations**

   a. Altered level of consciousness, restlessness, and apprehension

   b. Pulmonary edema with pink froth visible in the mouth and nose

   c. Possible hypothermia

   d. Complaints of headache or chest pain

   e. Vomiting

   f. Cyanosis

   g. Possible cardiac arrest

2. **Laboratory and diagnostic study findings.** Arterial blood gas (ABG) values show severe hypoxia and metabolic acidosis.

E. Nursing management (See section II.D.)

1. **Provide emergency care.**

   a. Initiate vigorous, purposeful cardiopulmonary resuscitation.

   b. Ventilate with 100% oxygen and positive end-expiratory pressure. (See section XIII.)

   c. Insert an I.V. line, a central venous line, an indwelling urinary catheter, or a nasogastric tube, as ordered.

   d. Initiate cardiac monitoring.

   e. Begin internal rewarming (e.g., warm peritoneal dialysis, warm aerosol inhalation) and external rewarming (e.g., hyperthermia blanket) if necessary.

2. **Provide ongoing assessment.** Monitor vital signs, level of consciousness, electrocardiogram findings, central venous pressure, intake and output, ABG values, and serum electrolyte levels.

3. **Admit the client to the intensive care unit.**

XIII. MECHANICAL VENTILATION

A. Description

1. A mechanical ventilator is a breathing device that can maintain ventilation and oxygen delivery for a prolonged period.

2. Indications for mechanical ventilation include a client experiencing a continuous decrease in oxygenation, an increase in arterial carbon dioxide, or persistent acidosis; and clients with such conditions as postoperative thoracic or abdominal surgery, drug overdose, chronic obstructive pulmonary disease, multiple trauma, shock, and multisystem failure.

B. Assessment of ventilator
1. Type of ventilator (e.g., volume-cycled, pressure-cycled, negative-pressure devices)
2. Controlling mode (e.g., control, assist/control, intermittent mandatory ventilation)
3. Tidal volume and rate settings
4. Fraction of inspired oxygen setting
5. Inspiratory pressure reached and pressure limit
6. Sigh settings if applicable
7. Presence of water in tubing, disconnection, or kinking of the tubing
8. Humidification
9. Properly functioning alarms
10. Positive-end expiratory pressure

C. Nursing management. Nursing interventions are the same whether the client is in an intensive care unit, a medical-surgical unit, or an extended-care facility. (See section II.D.)
1. **Maintain adequate airway and ventilation.**
   a. Always treat the client first then the ventilator.
   b. Maintain the endotracheal or tracheostomy tube, perform meticulous endotracheal tube care or tracheostomy care, and maintain sterility when suctioning client.
   c. Assess the lip line and ensure that end-line suction is always in the off position when not suctioning.
   d. Collaborate with the health care provider and respiratory therapist when weaning the client from the ventilator, tube, and oxygen.
2. **Prevent complications.**
   a. Frequently reposition the client to decrease complications of immobility (e.g., pulmonary, skin integrity, deep vein thrombosis).
   b. Continually monitor for and help prevent complications of ventilator use, such as:
      – increase in peak airway pressure
      – decrease in pressure or loss of volume.
   c. Continually monitor for and help prevent complications of the client's condition, such as:
      – cardiovascular compromise
      – barotrauma or pneumothorax
      – pulmonary infection.
3. **Minimize anxiety and promote family and client coping.** Provide explanations, reassurance, and support to the family and client; develop an alternative method of communication.

Study questions

1. During the nursing history, which client statement would lead the nurse to suspect pneumoconioses?
1. "I suddenly got a fever, chills, and a hacking cough."
2. "I became short of breath and started wheezing during exercise."
3. "I have worked in the coal mines for over 25 years."
4. "I am having left-sided chest pain that radiates down my left arm."

2. A client is admitted to the emergency department with an acute exacerbation of chronic obstructive pulmonary disease (COPD). Which interventions should the nurse implement while caring for this client? (Select all that apply.)

1. Administering 10 L/min of oxygen via nasal cannula
2. Placing the client in a high-Fowler's position
3. Obtaining a stat pulse oximeter reading
4. Inserting an 18-gauge needle in the anticubital space
5. Encouraging the client to breathe into a paper bag
6. Notifying the respiratory therapist

3. Which data would the nurse expect to assess in a febrile client complaining of a hacking cough and generalized malaise?
1. Conjunctivitis and nasal swelling
2. Tonsillar exudate and pain on swallowing
3. Bronchial breath sounds over lung fields with consolidation
4. Productive cough with excess mucus

4. Which nursing intervention would be important to include in the discharge teaching plan for the client diagnosed with pulmonary embolism?
1. Reducing walking to necessary activities around the house
2. Maintaining peripheral circulation with leg exercises
3. Soaking feet nightly in warm water to increase circulation
4. Avoiding bending when attempting to pick up objects

5. Which long-term goal would the nurse identify for a client diagnosed with chronic obstructive pulmonary disease (COPD)?
1. Reducing activity level to conserve functional lung tissue
2. Increasing frequency of postural drainage to every 2 hours
3. Increasing pulmonary residual volume
4. Improving pulmonary ventilation and gas exchange

6. Which intervention would the nurse implement for a client with chronic obstructive pulmonary disease who develops acute respiratory failure?
1. Beginning the initial stage of activity
2. Encouraging supine positioning
3. Managing oxygen therapy
4. Planning for home care needs

7. Which intervention would be *most* helpful in assisting the client diagnosed with chronic obstructive pulmonary disease (COPD) to develop ways to cope with the disease?
1. Encouraging the family to take increased responsibility for the client's care
2. Discouraging the client from performing activities of daily living (ADLs) if they promote fatigue
3. Teaching the client relaxation techniques and breathing retraining exercises
4. Protecting the client from knowing the prognosis of the disease

8. A client hospitalized for acute bacterial pneumonia is recovering after a course of therapy with penicillin G. Which outcome demonstrates the effectiveness of care?
1. The client has partial pressure of arterial oxygen (Pao_2) of 85 mm Hg or higher.
2. The client has partial pressure of arterial carbon dioxide ($Paco_2$) of 80 mm Hg or higher.
3. The client has decreased breath sounds.
4. The client has signs of restlessness and confusion.

9. Which nursing intervention should be included in the care plan for a client receiving mechanical ventilation?
1. Encouraging coughing to mobilize secretions
2. Ensuring that there is water in the tubing
3. Assessing the ventilator settings as prescribed by the health care provider
4. Allowing the client to vocalize feelings of powerlessness

10. Which should the nurse expect to observe in the water-seal chamber of the chest tube drainage system for a client with a hemothorax 4 hours after chest tube insertion?
1. No movement of the fluid
2. Bloody drainage
3. Vigorous bubbling
4. Fluctuation with inspiration and expiration

11. Which discharge instruction is *most* appropriate to prevent or control respiratory infections for the client diagnosed with respiratory insufficiency resulting from long-standing restrictive lung disease?
1. Taking penicillin prophylactically for life
2. Smoking low-tar (light) cigarettes
3. Receiving influenza injections
4. Having periodic studies to monitor partial pressure of oxygen (Po_2)

12. Which procedure would the nurse anticipate preparing for the client who develops a large pleural effusion?
1. Thoracentesis
2. Paracentesis
3. Bronchoscopy
4. Chest tube insertion

13. The nurse would suspect acute respiratory distress syndrome (ARDS) in a client diagnosed with hypovolemic shock secondary to multiple trauma when he exhibits which clinical manifestation?
1. Partial pressure of arterial oxygen (Pao_2) of 62 mm Hg after 2 hours of oxygen at 10 L/minute
2. Increased breath sounds with increased chest expansion
3. Partial pressure of arterial carbon dioxide ($Paco_2$) of 65 mm Hg with a Pao_2 of 85 mm Hg

4. Greenish, tenacious sputum and tachypnea

14. Which assessment findings would the nurse expect in a client with a right-sided pneumothorax?
1. Bradypnea and bronchovesicular breath sounds
2. Chronic cough and sudden onset of chills
3. Rust-colored sputum and increased temperature
4. Dyspnea and asymmetric chest expansion

15. Which nursing intervention should be included in the care plan for a client diagnosed with acute respiratory distress syndrome (ARDS)?
1. Keeping the client in prone position
2. Assessing the client for fluid volume deficit
3. Monitoring arterial blood gas (ABG) levels and cardiac status
4. Administering oxygen at a rate of 2 L/minute by nasal cannula

16. A client with a pulmonary embolism who is receiving anticoagulation therapy with warfarin has an International Normalized Ratio of 2.5, a prothrombin time of 23, and a partial thromboplastin time of 39. Based on these test results, which intervention should the nurse implement?
1. Administering the prescribed dose
2. Preparing to administer protamine sulfate
3. Withholding the dose and notifying the health care provider
4. Preparing to administer vitamin K (AquaMEPHYTON)

Answer key

1. The answer is **3.**
Pneumoconioses refers to occupational lung disease. The most common types include silicosis, asbestosis, and coal worker's pneumoconiosis (CWP). CWP results from accumulation of coal dust in the lungs, most commonly from coal mining. Sudden fever, chills, and hacking cough support the diagnosis of bacterial pneumonia. Shortness of breath and wheezing with exercise suggest the diagnosis of an acute asthmatic attack. Chest pain radiating down the left arm indicates myocardial infarction.

2. The answers are **2, 3, 6.**
The client with an acute exacerbation of COPD will be experiencing breathing difficulties, therefore sitting him in high-Fowler's position will help with breathing, a pulse oximeter reading will determine how oxygen deprived he is, and notifying the respiratory therapist would be appropriate. The client must have low oxygen (2 to 3 L/min) due to hypoxic drive for administration of 10 L/min of oxygen via nasal cannula to be appropriate; an 18-gauge needle would be used if the client is receiving blood, and then the nurse should start the I.V. therapy most distal. Having the client breathe into a paper bag is not encouraged.

3. The answer is **3.**
With pneumonia, subsequent infiltration and consolidation is evidenced by bronchial breath sounds commonly found over lung fields. Eye and nose symptoms, such as conjunctivitis and nasal swelling, are not typical in pneumonia. Tonsillar exudate and pain on swallowing are cardinal symptoms of streptococcal sore throat caused by infection of the pharynx. The cough associated with pneumonia is typically hacking and nonproductive.

4. The answer is **2.**
Pulmonary embolism is obstruction of one or more pulmonary arteries by a thrombus or thrombi, originating somewhere in the venous system or the right side of the heart. Most commonly, the thrombus originates in the deep veins of the legs. Measures to ensure adequate peripheral circulation are important. For example, leg exercises help to reduce the risk of further thrombus development by preventing venous stasis, minimizing the risk for deep vein thrombosis. Walking is encouraged rather than reduced or limited. Soaking the feet is unnecessary to increase circulation, and it is inappropriate, especially in an older person, because of its drying effect on skin and the potential for burn injury. No physiologic contraindication to bending is associated with pulmonary embolism.

5. The answer is **4.**
The underlying pathology of COPD affects the lungs' ability to ventilate and exchange oxygen and carbon dioxide. Pulmonary ventilation and gas exchange are interdependent. An effective relationship between the two parameters is necessary for successful physiologic and mental functioning. The long-term goal is to improve pulmonary ventilation and gas exchange. Decreasing the activity level does not conserve functional lung tissue. Rather, treatment should aim to increase activity while implementing work-modification and energy-conservation techniques. Postural drainage performed every 2 hours is unnecessary, because no evidence links the client's problem to retained secretions. The goal is to decrease rather than increase residual volume, which usually is high in COPD.

6. The answer is **3.**
Acute respiratory failure (ARF) results from inadequate gas exchange in the lungs. Increasing the availability of oxygen by managing oxygen therapy and assisting with secretion removal can improve ventilation. A

client experiencing ARF usually should not be started on an activity program. Energy conservation is critical at this stage. The client usually has difficulty breathing in the supine position. A semi-Fowler's or Fowler's position is encouraged to facilitate breathing. Planning for home care is important, although not at this stage. The priority need at this time is ventilation and oxygenation, and the client's level of self-care deficit is unknown at this point.

7. The answer is **3.**
Relaxation techniques and breathing retraining help a client with COPD to maximize energy supplies and use available oxygen more effectively. A client with COPD should be encouraged to be as independent as possible within his physiologic capabilities by using appropriate measures to conserve energy. Knowledge of the disease process may help the client better understand how to make the most of her life.

8. The answer is **1.**
As lung infection progresses, ventilation is interrupted. PaO_2 usually decreases, and a degree of respiratory insufficiency occurs. However, with treatment, the infection subsides, and lung function returns. PaO_2 typically rises to between 85 and 100 mm Hg. A $Paco_2$ value of 80 mm Hg indicates respiratory failure. Decreased breath sounds is an abnormal manifestation. Restlessness and confusion indicate hypoxia rather than improvement.

9. The answer is **3.**
Even though the nurse is not primarily responsible for adjusting the settings, she is responsible for the client and therefore needs to assess the ventilator settings and evaluate how the ventilator is affecting the client's overall status. When mechanical ventilation is used, the client is intubated and is unable to cough or talk. There should be no water or kinks in the tubing, and the tubing should be inspected to ensure that all connections are secure.

10. The answer is **4.**
Fluctuation with inspiration and expiration indicates that there is communication between the pleural space and the water-seal drainage system. No fluctuation typically indicates that the tubing is clotted, kinked, or the lungs have reinflated. Bloody drainage would be in the drainage chamber, not the water-seal chamber. Vigorous bubbling indicates an air leak.

11. The answer is **3.**
To aid in preventing or controlling respiratory infections, influenza injections are regularly recommended for clients with chronic respiratory problems. Broad-spectrum antibiotics are indicated only under medical supervision as a prophylactic treatment against lung infections, particularly during winter months. Penicillin is not a broad-spectrum antibiotic. Clients with lung disease should not smoke any substance in any form. PO_2 studies are indicated only if exacerbation occurs.

12. The answer is **1.**
Pleural effusion is a collection of fluid in the pleural space, which is located between the visceral and parietal surfaces. Thoracentesis is performed to remove fluid from the pleural space to obtain a specimen for analysis and to relieve dyspnea. It is the treatment of choice for pleural effusion. Paracentesis is used to treat ascites. Bronchoscopy is used for direct inspection and examination of the larynx, trachea, and bronchi. A chest tube insertion may be used for recurring pleural effusion but not for immediate treatment.

13. The answer is **1.**
One of the cardinal signs of ARDS is a low Pao_2 value after administration of a high concentration of oxygen. The oxygen cannot cross the alveoli because of the fluid in the interstitial space. Crackles, not increased breath sounds, would be heard throughout the lungs. The $Paco_2$ value (normal, 35 to 45 mm Hg) is not immediately increased because carbon dioxide can diffuse across the alveoli more

easily than can oxygen. Pao$_2$ of 85 mm Hg is within normal limits. Although the client with ARDS may be tachypneic, greenish, tenacious sputum indicates pneumonia, not ARDS.

14. The answer is **4.**
The client with a pneumothorax has dyspnea from decreased lung expansion. The breathing pattern is asymmetric because of air in pleural space. Typically, the client has tachypnea and decreased breath sounds over the pneumothorax. Bronchovesicular breath sounds are normal. Chronic cough, sudden onset of chills, rust-colored sputum, and increased temperature suggest pneumonia.

15. The answer is **3.**
For the client with ARDS, monitoring ABG levels is of paramount importance for diagnosing and evaluating the effectiveness of treatment. A decreased partial pressure of arterial oxygen (Pao$_2$) value despite a high oxygen concentration is a cardinal sign of ARDS. A rising level of Pao$_2$ reflects progress. The client should be in semi-Fowler's or high-Fowler's position to ease breathing. The nurse should assess for fluid volume overload caused by noncardiogenic pulmonary edema. Low-flow oxygen administration is indicated in treating chronic obstructive pulmonary disease. High-flow oxygen administration is indicated in cases of ARDS.

16. The answer is **1.**
Anticoagulant therapy with warfarin requires monitoring of the client's International Normalized Ratio (INR), which has a therapeutic level between 2 and 3; therefore the nurse would administer the prescribed dose. Protamine sulfate is the antidote for heparin overdose. There is no need to withhold the dose because the INR values indicate that the drug is at a therapeutic level. Vitamin K is the antidote for warfarin overdosage, but the data reflect that the drug is within normal therapeutic levels.

6 Cardiovascular disorders

I. STRUCTURE AND FUNCTION OF THE CARDIOVASCULAR SYSTEM

A. Structures of the heart. A hollow, muscular organ, the heart lies in the mediastinum (i.e., space between the two lungs) and rests on the diaphragm.

1. **Pericardium.** The heart is encased in the pericardium, a thin, membranous sac that has a visceral layer in contact with the heart and an outer parietal layer. The space between the pericardial layers contains 20 to 30 ml of serous fluid, which protects the heart from trauma and friction.

2. **Heart wall.** The heart wall is specialized muscle tissue consisting of three tissue layers:
   a. **Epicardium,** the thin, serous outer layer
   b. **Myocardium,** the thick, muscular middle layer
   c. **Endocardium,** the smooth inner layer that comes in contact with blood.

3. **Heart chambers.** A membranous muscular septum divides the heart into two distinct sides. Each side contains two chambers: an atrium and a ventricle. (See *Figure 6-1.*)
   a. The **right atrium**, a low-pressure chamber, receives systemic venous blood through the superior vena cava, inferior vena cava, and coronary sinus.
   b. The **right ventricle**, another low-pressure chamber, receives blood from the right atrium through the tricuspid valve during ventricular diastole. It then ejects deoxygenated blood through the pulmonic valve into the pulmonary artery and into pulmonary circulation during ventricular systole.
   c. The **left atrium**, a low-pressure chamber, receives oxygenated blood returning to the heart from the lung through four pulmonary veins.
   d. The **left ventricle**, a high-pressure chamber, receives blood from the left atrium through the mitral valve during ventricular diastole. It then ejects oxygenated blood through the aortic valve into the aorta and into systemic circulation during ventricular systole.

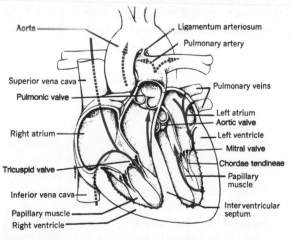

FIGURE 6-1
Structure of the heart and course of blood flow (arrows) through the chambers

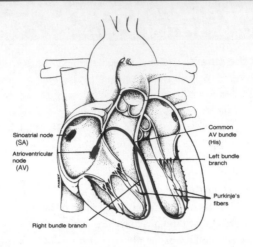

Sinoatrial node (SA)

Atrioventricular node (AV)

Common AV bundle (His)

Left bundle branch

Purkinje's fibers

Right bundle branch

FIGURE 6-2

Cardiac conduction system and landmarks, beginning with the sinoatrial node and progressing along the atrioventricular node, the common atrioventricular bundle (the bundle of His) and its branches

4. **Heart valves** connect the chambers and outflow tracts. The two types of heart valves are atrioventricular and semilunar valves. (See *Figure 6-1,* page 117.)

   a. **Atrioventricular (AV) valves** separate the atria from the ventricles.
   - The **tricuspid valve** (contains three cusps, or leaflets) is located between the right atrium and ventricle.
   - The **mitral valve** (a bicuspid valve with two cusps) is located between the left atrium and ventricle.

   b. **The semilunar valves** (each containing three cusps) are located between each ventricle and its corresponding artery.
   - The **pulmonic valve** is located between the right ventricle and pulmonary artery.
   - The **aortic valve** is located between the left ventricle and aorta.

   c. **Papillary muscles**, muscle bundles on the ventricular walls, and **chordae tendineae**, fibrous bands extending from the papillary muscles to the valve cusps, keep the valves closed during systole. This maintains unidirectional blood flow through the AV valves and prevents backflow of blood.

5. The **cardiac conduction system** consists of specialized cardiac cells that initiate or propagate electrical impulses throughout the myocardium as a precursor to cardiac muscle contraction. (See *Figure 6-2.*)

   a. **Electrical pathways**
   - The **sinoatrial (SA) node**, located at the junction of the right atrium and the superior vena cava, functions as the pacemaker for the myocardium, initiating rhythmic electrical impulses at an intrinsic rate of 60 to 100 impulses per minute.
   - The **AV node**, located in the septal wall of the right atrium, receives impulses from the SA node and relays them to the ventricles.
   - The **bundle of His,** a bundle of specialized muscle fibers in the myocardial septum, conducts impulses from the AV node. The bundle of His divides into right and left branches.
   - The **right bundle branch (RBB)** conducts impulses down the right side of the septum.

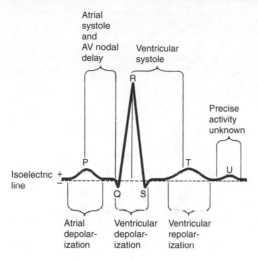

FIGURE 6-3

Correlation of mechanical and electrical activity within the heart

Source: Bullock B.L., and Henze, R.L. *Focus on Pathophysiology.* Philadelphia: Lippincott Williams & Wilkins, 2000.

- The **left bundle branch (LBB)** conducts impulses into right and left fascicles that fan out into the left ventricular muscle.
- The RBB and LBB terminate in the **Purkinje fibers,** which propagate electrical impulses into the endocardium and on to the myocardium.

b. Electrical impulse activity. Electrical impulses traveling through the cardiac conduction system can be measured and recorded by electrocardiography.

- **Phases of the electrocardiogram (ECG)** are labeled P, Q, R, S, and T. (See *Figure 6-3.*)
  - The P wave represents atrial depolarization.
  - The PR interval represents the time from the beginning of atrial depolarization to the beginning of ventricular depolarization.
  - The QRS complex represents ventricular depolarization.
  - The T wave represents ventricular repolarization.
- **Normal sinus rhythm**
  - Heart rate is 60 to 100 beats per minute.
  - P waves precede each QRS complex.
  - PR interval is 0.12 to 0.2 second.
  - QRS complex is 0.04 to 0.1 second.
  - Conduction is forward and cyclical through the conduction system.
  - Rhythm is regular with no abnormal delay.

6. The **coronary arteries** supply the heart with blood from branches that originate in the right or left sinus of Valsalva of the aortic valve cusps.

a. The **right coronary artery** supplies blood to the right heart wall.

b. The **left main coronary artery**, which divides into the left anterior descending coronary artery and the circumflex artery, supplies most of the blood to the left heart wall. (See *Figure 6-4,* page 120.)

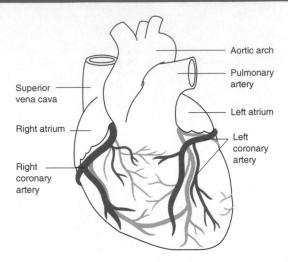

Aortic arch

Pulmonary artery

Superior vena cava

Left atrium

Right atrium

Left coronary artery

Right coronary artery

FIGURE 6-4

Diagram of the coronary arteries arising from the aorta and circulating in the heart, including some of the coronary veins

B. Functions of the heart. The heart has electrophysiologic, mechanical, and neurologic properties that coordinate to produce effective myocardial contraction and pumping of blood.

1. **Cardiac output (CO)** is defined as the volume of blood ejected by each ventricle in 1 minute; CO = SV (stroke volume) X HR (heart rate).

    a. **Stroke volume** is the amount of blood ejected by the left ventricle with each heartbeat. Several factors influence CO indirectly by affecting the SV.
    - **Preload,** the end-diastolic filling volume of the ventricle, increases by increased returning volume to ventricle.
    - **Afterload,** the resistance to left ventricular ejection, increases by increased systemic arterial pressure.

    b. **Heart rate** is the number of heartbeats per minute. Normal is 60 to 100 beats/minute.

2. **Cardiac cycle.** Each complete heartbeat, or cardiac cycle, consists of two phases in response to electrical stimulation.

    a. **Systole** is the contraction phase. It is triggered by depolarization of cardiac muscle cells, which involves a transient change in sodium and potassium ion concentration inside and outside the cell.

    b. **Diastole** is the relaxation (filling) phase. Immediately after depolarization is completed, the process reverses itself, resulting in repolarization and a return to the resting state.

3. **Heart sounds** result from vibrations caused by valve closure and ventricular filling.

    a. The **first heart sound (S1)** is associated with tricuspid and mitral valve closure.

    b. The **second heart sound (S2)** is associated with aortic and pulmonic valve closure.

    c. The **third heart sound (S3)**, known as *ventricular gallop,* is often normal in persons younger than age 30 but pathologic in older persons and occurs during the rapid ventricular filling stage of diastole.

    d. The **fourth heart sound (S4)**, or *atrial gallop,* is linked to resistance to ventricular filling, as in hypertrophy or injury of the ventricular wall.

4. **Neurologic factors regulating heart function**
   a. **Sympathetic nervous system stimulation,** with release of norepinephrine, results in arteriolar vasoconstriction, increased heart rate, and a positive inotropic effect.
   b. **Parasympathetic nervous system stimulation,** with release of acetylcholine, results in decreased heart rate and slowed AV conduction.
   c. The response of **chemoreceptors,** located in the carotid and aortic bodies, to decreased O_2 and increased CO_2 concentrations is to increase the heart rate.
   d. The response of **baroreceptors,** located in the aortic arch, carotid sinus, vena cava, pulmonary arteries, and atria, is to decrease or increase heart rate, resulting in blood pressure changes.

 ## II. CARDIOVASCULAR SYSTEM

A. **Assessment**
   1. **Health history**
      a. **Elicit a description of the client's present illness and chief complaint,** including onset, course, duration, location, and precipitating and alleviating factors. Cardinal signs and symptoms indicating altered cardiovascular function include:
         - pain over the lower sternal region and the upper abdomen characterized by heavy vicelike, "belt-squeezing" pain that may radiate to the shoulders, neck, and down the arms (Associated symptoms may include electrocardiogram [ECG] changes and arrhythmias. This pain may indicate myocardial ischemia.)
         - palpitations characterized by rapid irregular or pounding heart beat (This symptom may be associated with arrhythmias or ischemia.)
         - intermittent claudication characterized by extremity pain with exercise (This may indicate peripheral vascular disease.)
         - dyspnea characterized by difficult breathing or shortness of breath with activity (i.e., dyspnea on exertion), in the supine position (i.e., orthopnea), or sudden onset at night (i.e., paroxysmal nocturnal dyspnea) (This is commonly associated with compromised cardiac function.)
         - fatigue with or without activity (This may be associated with decreased carbon dioxide [CO].)
         - syncope with or without dizziness (This can result from a sudden decrease in CO.)
         - diaphoresis with associated clamminess and cyanosis (This reflects decreased CO and decreased peripheral perfusion.)
         - edema or weight gain greater than 3 lb in 24 hours. (This may indicate heart failure.)
      b. **Explore the client's health history for risk factors** associated with cardiovascular disease (atherosclerosis):
         - Positive family history for cardiovascular disease
         - Age (The incidence of cardiovascular disease increases after age 40.)
         - Gender (Mortality from cardiovascular disease is greater in men than in women; however, this difference decreases after menopause.)
         - Race (Mortality is greater for nonwhites than whites.)
         - Smoking (The risk of cardiovascular disease is two to four times greater for cigarette smokers than nonsmokers.)
         - Hypertension, particularly elevated systolic pressure

- Hyperlipidemia (The ratio of high-density lipoproteins [HDL] to low-density lipoproteins [LDL] is the best predictor.)
- Obesity (Contributes to the severity of other risk factors.)
- Sedentary lifestyle
- Diabetes (Uncontrolled elevated blood glucose level increases risk.)
- Stress (May contribute to developing coronary artery disease.)
- Hormonal contraceptives.

2. **Physical examination**
   a. **Vital signs.** Assess vital signs, particularly pulse rate, blood pressure, and respirations. Increased blood pressure and pulse may indicate cardiovascular disease.
   b. **Inspection**
      - Observe general appearance for signs of distress, anxiety, and altered level of consciousness.
      - Inspect the lips and buccal mucosa for central cyanosis, which reflects hypoxia.
      - Inspect the peripheral extremities for cyanosis and a capillary refill time of less than 3 seconds.
      - Assess jugular venous pressure and observe for venous distention.
   c. **Palpation**
      - Palpate all peripheral pulses including carotid, brachial, radial, femoral, popliteal, dorsalis pedis, and anterior tibial. Grade 0, no pulse; 1+, weak; 2+, normal; 3+, increased; 4+, bounding.
      - Palpate the precordium to locate the point of maximal impulse or the apical impulse.
   d. **Auscultation.** Systematically auscultate the heart for normal and abnormal heart sounds, murmurs, and friction rub, covering four main areas: aortic, pulmonary, mitral, and tricuspid. (See chapter 1.)
   e. **Perform a respiratory assessment.** (See chapter 5, section II.A.) Findings pointing to cardiovascular problems may include cough (possibly reflecting pulmonary congestion); crackles or wheezing (reflecting airway narrowing, atelectasis, or left ventricular failure); hemoptysis (possibly pointing to acute pulmonary edema); Cheyne-Stokes respiration (possibly associated with severe left ventricular failure).
   f. **Perform an abdominal assessment** (see chapter 9, section II.A), noting liver enlargement and ascites (indicating decreased venous return secondary to right ventricular failure); bladder distention (pointing to decreased CO); and bruits just above the umbilicus (reflecting abdominal aortic obstruction or aneurysm).

3. **Laboratory and diagnostic studies**
   a. **White blood cell (WBC) count** can detect signs of infection.
   b. **Lipid profile** examines cholesterol (LDL and HDL) and triglycerides.
   c. **Cardiac enzymes** examine levels of creatinine phosphokinase, troponin, and lactate dehydrogenase.
   d. **Blood coagulation studies** examine prothrombin time and partial thromboplastin time.
   e. **Chest radiograph** can determine heart size and silhouette and visualize the pulmonary system.
   f. **ECG** evaluates the heart's electrical activity.
   g. **Holter monitoring (ambulatory ECG)** allows for 24-hour continuous measurement of the heart's electrical activity.

h. **Exercise ECG (graded exercise test)** evaluates electrical activity during physical stress; a chemical-induced ECG stress test is used if the client is unable to walk or bike for a long period of time.

i. **Echocardiography** yields information about cardiac structures (especially valvular) and function.

j. **Radionuclide testing** evaluates ventricular function and myocardial blood flow and detects areas of myocardial damage. Radionuclide testing includes positron emission tomography, multiple-gated acquisition, and thallium scanning.

k. **Cardiac catheterization** enables measurement of chamber pressures and oxygen saturation.

l. **Arteriography** visualizes coronary arteries with injections of radiopaque contrast media.

m. **Ventriculography** visualizes ventricles with injection of radiopaque contrast media.

n. **Central venous pressure** reflects filling pressure of the right ventricle and helps assess cardiac function and intravascular volume status.

o. **Pulmonary artery pressure** and **pulmonary artery wedge pressure** measure left heart pressures.

p. **Arterial line** allows continuous monitoring of peripheral arterial pressures.

B. Nursing diagnoses
1. Decreased cardiac output
2. Impaired gas exchange
3. Activity intolerance
4. Acute pain
5. Risk for infection
6. Disturbed sleep pattern
7. Anxiety
8. Deficient knowledge
9. Interrupted family processes

C. Planning and outcome identification. The major goals of the client with a cardiovascular problem include enhancement of cardiopulmonary status, increased gas exchange and activity tolerance, prevention of pain and infection, improved sleep pattern, reduction of anxiety, adherence to a self-care program with an understanding of the disease process and its management, and improved family functioning.

D. Implementation
1. **Assess cardiopulmonary status.**
   a. Assess level of consciousness, heart rate and rhythm, heart sounds, blood pressure, peripheral pulses, peripheral edema, skin color and temperature, respiratory rate and lungs.
   b. Monitor arterial blood gases and pulse oximetry.
   c. Monitor ECG and telemetry.
   d. Monitor the client's intake and output; maintain 30 ml/hour urinary output, using a urometer to ensure accuracy.
2. **Enhance cardiac output.** Establish a patent I.V. line to administer fluids. An I.V. infusion control device should be used to control rate and volume to be infused.
3. **Promote gas exchange.**
   a. Collaborate with the respiratory therapist and administer oxygen to maintain oxygen saturation levels of 95% to 100% if no other disease process is present.

    b. Encourage the client to maintain semi-Fowler's position while resting in bed; keep the client on bed rest or chair rest to decrease oxygen myocardial consumption.

    c. Instruct the client to cough, deep-breathe, and turn frequently, which can decrease pooling of fluid in the lungs. Instruct the client to breathe in through the nose and out through the mouth three times and then cough forcefully on the fourth breath.

4. **Increase activity tolerance.** Balance periods of rest and exercise. Assist the client as needed with activities of daily living and self-care.

5. **Promote comfort.** Assess the client's description of chest discomfort, including location, radiation, pain duration, and what precipitated pain.

6. **Prevent infection.**

    a. Monitor skin integrity of lower extremities and incisions from cardiac surgery.

    b. Assess insertion sites from invasive procedures for signs of redness, warmth, edema, and pain.

    c. Monitor vital signs, especially for fever.

    d. Assess breath sounds for changes associated with pneumonia in clients after surgery and those requiring bed rest.

7. **Promote adequate sleep.** Attempt to cluster nursing interventions to provide the client with several hours of uninterrupted sleep.

8. **Minimize anxiety.** Offer the client opportunities to ventilate his feelings. Answer his questions truthfully, and develop a trusting and caring relationship with him and his family.

9. **Provide client and family teaching.**

    a. Teach the client and his family the basic pathophysiology of the underlying disease process.

    b. Teach the client measures to reduce modifiable risk factors, including the importance of a low-fat, low-cholesterol, low-sodium diet, smoking cessation, and adequate exercise.

    c. Teach energy conservation measures.

    d. Discuss medications, including possible adverse effects and interactions.

    e. Discuss danger signs and symptoms requiring prompt medical attention including, chest pain, increased shortness of breath, sudden onset of fever, irregular heartbeats, and weight gain of more than 2 pounds in less than 24 hours.

    f. Discuss with the client the necessity of advance directives and durable power of attorney for health care.

10. **Promote family coping.** Assist with adaptation to role changes caused by disease-related limitations and activity restrictions.

E. Outcome evaluation

1. The client demonstrates stable cardiac rhythm, vital signs, hemodynamic parameters, and urinary output.

2. The client demonstrates stabilization of cardiac rhythm with proper pacemaker pacing and sensing.

3. The client responds to cardiopulmonary resuscitation (CPR).

4. The client demonstrates clear lung sounds, capillary refill time of less than 3 seconds, and no central or peripheral cyanosis.

5. The client limits activities to a level that permits the heart to rest.

6. The client verbalizes factors and events that precipitate pain.

7. The client reports no pain during normal activities and reports relief of anginal pain with nitrate administration.

8. The client demonstrates stabilization of the inflammatory process.

9. The client is free of systemic and local infection.
10. The client sleeps at least 6 hours each night uninterrupted.
11. The client and his family display decreased anxiety.
12. The client verbalizes an understanding of the disease process and its treatment, preventive measures, and the signs and symptoms that should be reported to the health care provider.
13. Family members verbalize an understanding of CPR and the pathophysiology of the underlying disease.

III. ARRHYTHMIAS

A. **Description.** Arrhythmia (or dysrhythmia) refers to any sinus rhythm deviating from normal. (See *Figure 6-3*, page 119.)

B. **Etiology.** Arrhythmias result from altered impulse formation, altered impulse conduction, or both.

C. **Pathophysiology.** Myocardial cells that have been injured or replaced with scar tissue do not have the ability to respond to sinoatrial (SA) node impulses. Even when the SA node is functioning properly, other cardiac cells can assume the pacemaker properties when myocardial cells are injured, oxygen-deprived, or exposed to certain chemicals or drugs. When any other part of the heart except the SA node initiates the heart beat, an arrhythmia occurs.

D. **Assessment findings.** Symptoms vary from none to death.

E. **Nursing management (See section II.D.)** Administer or assist with the treatment of choice, which varies depending on the type and severity of the arrhythmia.

F. **Sinus tachycardia**
   1. **Description.** Sinus tachycardia is a heart rate greater than 100 beats per minute, originating in the sinus node. This arrhythmia has the following characteristics:
       a. **Rate** is 100 to 180 beats per minute.
       b. **P waves** precede each QRS complex.
       c. **PR interval** is normal.
       d. **QRS complex** is normal.
       e. **Conduction** is normal.
       f. **Rhythm** is regular.
   2. **Etiology.** Causes of sinus tachycardia include exercise, anxiety, fever, drugs, anemia, heart failure, hypovolemia, and shock.
   3. **Assessment findings.** Sinus tachycardia is often asymptomatic, but the clinical manifestations may include:
       a. occasional palpitations
       b. hypotension
       c. angina with cardiovascular disease.
   4. **Nursing management.** Administer the prescribed treatment. Treatment is directed at the primary cause, which usually is not cardiac related. Carotid sinus pressure or a beta-adrenergic blocker may be used to reduce the heart rate quickly. (See *Drug chart 6-1*, pages 126 to 129.)

(Text continues on page 129.)

DRUG CHART 6-1

Medications for cardiovascular disorders

Classifications	Indications	Selected interventions
Analgesic—antipyretic-nonsteroidal-antiinflammatory drugs acetaminophen acetylsalicylic acid ibuprofen	Relieve pain, fever, and inflammation	▪ Instruct the client to take the medication with a full glass of water and just after food. ▪ Warn the client that GI symptoms (nausea, vomiting, bleeding, ulceration) can occur when taking these medications on a long-term basis. ▪ The the client to report tinnitus (ringing in ears), a sign of aspirin toxicity.
Angiotensin-converting enzyme inhibitors captopril enalapril lisinopril	Prevent angiotensin I from converting to angiotensin II, a potent vasoconstrictor, thereby decreasing peripheral vascular resistance; blocks the secretion of aldosterone from adrenal gland	▪ Monitor the client's blood pressure; if less than 90/60 mm Hg, hold and question the order. ▪ Teach the client about orthostatic hypotension. ▪ Instruct the client not to discontinue abruptly.
Angiotensin II receptor antagonists losartan valsartan	Block angiotensin II at the receptor sites, thereby decreasing peripheral vascular resistance; block the secretion of aldosterone from the adrenal gland	▪ Monitor the client's blood pressure; if less than 90/60 mm Hg, hold and question the order. ▪ Teach the client about orthostatic hypotension. ▪ Instruct the client not to discontinue abruptly.
Antiarrhythmics Class IA—quinidine, procainamide Class IB—lidocaine Class IC—flecainide Class II—propranolol Class III—amiodarone Class IV—see calcium channel blockers; atypical—adenosine	Reduce automaticity, slow conduction of electrical impulses through the heart, and prolong the refractory period of myocardial cells	▪ Take apical pulse rate before administering the drug. Notify the health care provider if the rate falls below 60 beats per minute. Teach the client to monitor and record his pulse. ▪ Make sure that the client is being closely monitored on telemetry, with frequent blood pressure monitoring; when administering I.V., do not leave the client. ▪ Monitor serum drug levels to maintain therapeutic range.
Antibiotics aminoglycosides (gentamycin, tobramycin) amoxicillin erythromycin penicillin tetracycline	Prevent or treat infections caused by pathogenic microorganism	▪ Before administering the first dose, assess the client for allergies; also note whether a culture has been obtained. ▪ After multiple doses, assess the client for superinfection (thrush, yeast infection, diarrhea); notify the health care provider if these occur. ▪ Assess the insertion site for phlebitis if antibiotics are being administered I.V. ▪ To assess the effectiveness of antimicrobial therapy, monitor white blood cell count (WBC). ▪ Monitor peaks and troughs for aminoglycosides.
Anticholinergics atropine	Block effects of vagus nerve stimulation	▪ Monitor vital signs closely. ▪ Monitor telemetry. ▪ Administer at a rate of 1 mg or less over 1 minute.

DRUG CHART 6-1

Medications for cardiovascular disorders *(continued)*

Classifications	Indications	Selected interventions
Anticoagulants I.V. heparin oral warfarin sodium	Prevent recurrence of emboli but have no effect on emboli that are already present	▪ For heparin therapy, monitor partial thromboplastin time (PTT), for which therapeutic range should be 1.5 to 2 times the normal PTT or control. Antidote is protamine sulfate. ▪ For Coumadin therapy, monitor the International Normalized Ratio (INR), for which the therapeutic level is 2 to 3. Antidote is AquaMEPHYTON (vitamin K). ▪ Instruct the client to report bruising, unexplained bleeding, or dark, tarry stools; use a soft-bristle toothbrush; be cautious when using sharp objects and machinery; wear medi-alert bracelet; and notify any health care provider (dentist, pharmacist) that he is on anticoagulant therapy. ▪ If bleeding occurs, instruct the client to apply direct pressure to the wound; if bleeding does not stop after 5 minutes of direct pressure, tell him to get medical help.
Subcutaneous low-dose heparin (5,000 units)	Prophylactically prevent deep-vein thrombosis; heparin activates antithrombin III, which inactivates newly formed factor Xa and thrombin	▪ Administer subcutaneously in the abdomen, 1″ (2.5 cm) from the umbilicus. Do not aspirate; do not massage. Not necessary to monitor partial thromboplastin time (PTT).
Antilipemic agents cholestyramine clofibrate colestipol **HMG-CoA reductase inhibitors** lovastatin	Lower the serum cholesterol level by binding bile salts in the bowel and forming an insoluble complex that is excreted in the stool	▪ Mix medication with 60 ml of water or fruit juice to mask the unpleasant flavor. ▪ Instruct the client to increase his fluid intake to prevent constipation. ▪ Instruct the client to take the medication at night due to enzyme that metabolizes cholesterol. ▪ Monitor the client's cholesterol level; it should be < 200 mg/dl.
Antiplatelet agents aspirin dipyridamole ticlopidine	Inhibit the aggregation of platelets to form a plug; platelets do not initiate thrombus formation as readily when taking antiplatelets	▪ Instruct the client to take his medication with food to decrease gastric irritation. ▪ Remind the client to inform health care providers that he is taking these medications and to be careful when taking over-the-counter medications. ▪ Instruct the client to report bruising, bleeding gums, nosebleeds, or bleeding in the stools.
Beta-adrenergic blockers atenolol metoprolol nadolol propranolol	Decrease the heart rate and the force of contraction and reduce vasoconstriction by antagonizing beta-receptors in the myocardium and vasculature	▪ Monitor pulse; if apical pulse falls below 60 beats per minute, hold and question the order. ▪ Monitor blood pressure; if less than 90/60 mm Hg, hold and question the order. ▪ Teach the client about orthostatic hypotension. *(continued)*

DRUG CHART 6-1

Medications for cardiovascular disorders *(continued)*

Classifications	Indications	Selected interventions
Beta-adrenergics beta only — dobutamine beta or alpha plus beta — dopamine epinephrine metaraminol	Increase myocardial contractili- ty and heart rate, which in turn raises blood pressure; alpha plus beta-adrenergic activity	▪ Must be administered on an I.V. continuous drip; assess the I.V. site. ▪ Monitor blood pressure at least every 5 to 15 minutes. ▪ Epinephrine is administered IVP.
Calcium channel **blockers** diltiazem nifedipine verapamil	Inhibit calcium ions from cross- ing myocardial and vascular smooth muscle, thereby pro- ducing vasodilation and de- creased myocardial contractility	▪ Monitor pulse; if apical pulse falls below 60 beats per minute, hold and question the order. ▪ Monitor blood pressure; if less than 90/60 mm Hg, hold and question the order. ▪ Teach the client about orthostatic hypotension.
Cardiac glycosides digitoxin digoxin	Increase the force of myocar- dial contractions and slow heart rate and conduction through the atrioventricular node and bundle of His	▪ Monitor pulse; if apical pulse falls below 60 beats per minute, hold and question order. ▪ Monitor digoxin level (therapeutic level, 0.8 to 2). ▪ Monitor potassium level (normal, 3.5 to 5.5 mEq/L); hypokalemia potentiates digoxin toxicity (signs and symptoms include anorexia, nausea, and vomiting).
Corticosteroids oral hydrocortisone oral methyprednisolone oral prednisone	Strengthen the biologic mem- brane, which inhibits capillary permeability and prevents leak- age of fluid into the injured area and development of ede- ma (exact mechanism un- known)	▪ Instruct the client to take the medication exactly as directed and to taper the drug rather than stop it abruptly, which could cause serious withdrawal symptoms leading to adrenal insufficiency, shock, and death. ▪ Forewarn the client that the drug may cause re- portable cushingoid effects (weight gain, moon face, buffalo hump, and hirsutism) and may mask signs and symptoms of infection.

Diuretics
loop diuretic — furosemide
potassium-sparing diuretic —
  spironolactone
thiazide diuretic — chloroth-
  iazide
	Decrease blood volume, which
	decreases the workload of the
	heart
		▪ Monitor potassium level; do not administer if the
		patient is hypokalemic or hyperkalemic.
		▪ Monitor intake and output; increase fluid intake.
		▪ Monitor blood pressure; if less than 90/60 mm
		Hg, hold and the question order.
		▪ Teach the client about orthostatic hypotension.
		▪ Teach the client to weigh himself daily and re-
		port weight gain of more than 2 lb in 1 day.
		▪ Question the order if the client is dehydrated.

Low molecular-weight **heparin** enoxaparin	Prophylactically prevent deep vein thrombosis; LMW mole- cules are short and preferen- tially inactivate newly formed factor Xa	▪ Administer in the anterolateral abdominal wall. Do not aspirate; do not massage. Insert an air bub- ble into the syringe. Not necessary to monitor PTT.
Opioid analgesics codeine hydrocodone hydromorphone morphine propoxyphene	Relieve moderate to severe pain by reducing pain sensa- tion, producing sedation, and decreasing the emotional upset often associated with pain; most often schedule II drugs	▪ Assess the pain for location, type, intensity, and what increases or decreases it; rate pain on scale of 1 (no pain) to 10 (worst pain). ▪ Rule out any complications. Is this pain routine or expected? Is this pain a complication that needs immediate intervention?

DRUG CHART 6-1
Medications for cardiovascular disorders *(continued)*

Classifications	Indications	Selected interventions
Opioid analgesics *(continued)*		■ Medicate according to pain scale findings. Institute safety measures — bed in low position, side rails up, and call light within reach. Evaluate effectiveness of pain medication in 30 minutes.
Nitrates isosorbide dinitrate nitroglyc- erin sublingual, topical, patch, tablet, I.V.	Reduce myocardial oxygen de- mand by promoting vaso- dilation and by increasing oxy- gen supply to myocardial tissue	■ Inform the client that a headache is a common adverse effect. ■ Monitor blood pressure; teach client about or- thostatic hypotension. ■ For topical administration, be sure to wear gloves, remove the old patch, apply to a hairless area, and date and time the new patch. ■ For I.V. administration, dilute the drug and ad- minister by continuous infusion, with constant monitoring of blood pressure and pulse.
Stool softeners docusate calcium docusate sodium	Decrease the surface tension of the fecal mass to allow water to penetrate into the stool; pre- vents the client from straining on defecation	■ Instruct the client to increase his fluid and fiber intake. ■ Instruct that client that he does not have to have a daily bowel movement, what is normal for him, and about not getting constipated.
Thrombolytic agents alteplase streptokinase urokinase	Dissolve thrombi or emboli in the coronary arteries	■ Follow hospital protocol when administering a thrombolytic agent. ■ Monitor the client for internal bleeding every 15 to 30 minutes for the first 8 hours and then every 1 hours throughout therapy.
Vasodilators diazoxide hydralazine nitroprusside sodium	Decrease preload (venous dila- tors) and afterload (arterial dila- tors); act directly on blood ves- sels to cause dilation and de- crease peripheral vascular resistance	■ Monitor blood pressure; if less than 90/60 mm Hg, hold and question the order. ■ For I.V. administration, have the client on a car- diac monitor. ■ Keep the client on bed rest, with safety precau- tions instituted.

G. Sinus bradycardia

1. **Description.** Sinus bradycardia is a heart rate less than 60 beats per minute originat- ing in the sinus node. This arrhythmia has the following characteristics:

   a. **Rate** is less than 60 beats per minute.

   b. **P waves** precede each QRS complex.

   c. **PR interval** is normal.

   d. **QRS complex** is normal.

   e. **Conduction** is normal.

   f. **Rhythm** is regular.

2. **Etiology.** Causes of sinus bradycardia include drugs, vagal stimulation, hypoendocrine states, anorexia, and hypothermia or sinus node involvement in myocardial infarction. This arrhythmia may be normal in athletes.

3. **Assessment findings.** Sinus bradycardia is often asymptomatic, but clinical manifestations may include:

   a. fatigue

   b. lightheadedness

   c. syncope.

4. **Nursing management.** If the client is symptomatic, maintain adequate CO by treating the underlying cause and administering the anticholinergic drug atropine as prescribed. (See *Drug chart 6-1,* pages 126 to 129.) If appropriate, provide nursing care for the client who has or will receive a pacemaker. (See section XI.)

H. Paroxysmal atrial tachycardia and supraventricular tachycardia

1. **Description.** Paroxysmal atrial tachycardia (PAT) or supraventricular tachycardia (SVT) is an abrupt onset of rapid heartbeat (palpitations), originating in the atria. PAT or SVT have the following characteristics:

   a. **Rate** is 150 to 250 beats per minute.

   b. **P waves** are ectopic and may be found in preceding T waves.

   c. **PR interval** is shortened (0.12 second).

   d. **QRS complex** is normal and may be distorted because of aberrancy.

   e. **Conduction** is normal.

   f. **Rhythm** is regular.

2. **Etiology.** Causes of PAT or SVT include extreme emotions (e.g., anger, fear), drugs, alcohol, smoking, and caffeine. This arrhythmia usually is not associated with heart disease.

3. **Assessment findings**

   a. Palpitations

   b. Lightheadedness

   c. Dyspnea

   d. Anginal pain

4. **Nursing management** depends on the client's overall clinical situation and how well he tolerates the arrhythmia. Administer the prescribed treatment to decrease the heart rate and eliminate the underlying cause. The nurse may:

   a. assist with carotid sinus pressure or any vagal maneuver

   b. administer prescribed medication, which may include antiarrhythmics and cardiac glycosides (See *Drug chart 6-1,* pages 126 to 129.) (Adenosine is often the drug of choice for treatment of SVT.)

   c. assist with cardioversion. (See *Box 6-1.*)

I. Atrial fibrillation

1. **Description.** Atrial fibrillation is disorganized and uncoordinated twitching of atrial musculature caused by overly rapid production of atrial impulses. This arrhythmia has the following characteristics:

   a. **Rate.** Atrial rate is 350 to 600 beats per minute; ventricular response rate is 120 to 200 beats per minute.

   b. **P wave** is not discernible, with an irregular baseline.

   c. **PR interval** is not measurable.

   d. **QRS complex** is normal.

   e. **Conduction** is normal through the ventricle and irregular through the atrioventricular (AV) junction because of the overwhelming number of impulses from the atria.

   f. **Rhythm** is irregular and usually rapid unless controlled.

BOX 6-1
Important points for assisting with defibrillation or cardioversion

- Always shout "all clear," and make sure that no one is touching the bed or the client before discharging.
- Apply defibrillator pads as indicated.
- Make sure that the correct amount of joules is applied before defibrillating or cardioverting the client.

- Cardioversion is an elective procedure that requires informed consent. The client will be sedated during this procedure.
- Automated external defibrillation is available in many nonacute areas. Be sure to follow verbal directions.

2. **Etiology.** Causes of atrial fibrillation include atherosclerosis, rheumatic mitral valve stenosis, heart failure, congenital heart disease, chronic obstructive pulmonary disease, hypothyroidism, and thyrotoxicosis.
3. **Assessment findings.** Atrial fibrillation may be asymptomatic, but clinical manifestations may include:
   a. palpitations
   b. dyspnea
   c. pulmonary edema
   d. signs of cerebrovascular insufficiency.
4. **Nursing management.** Administer the prescribed treatment to decrease ventricular response, decrease atrial irritability, and eliminate the cause.
   a. Administer prescribed medication, which may include a cardiac glycoside or a calcium channel blocker. (See *Drug chart 6-1,* pages 126 to 129.)
   b. Assist with cardioversion. (See *Box 6-1.*)
   c. For clients with chronic atrial fibrillation, implement anticoagulant therapy, as appropriate, to prevent thromboemboli from forming in the atria. (See *Drug chart 6-1,* pages 126 to 129.)

J. Atrioventricular blocks
   1. **Description.** An AV block is a conduction defect within the AV junction that impairs conduction of atrial impulses to ventricular pathways. The three types are first degree, second degree, and third degree. This arrhythmia has the following characteristics:
      a. **Rate**
         – **First degree.** Rate is usually 60 to 100 beats per minute or the inherent ventricular rate.
         – **Second degree.** Rate is slowed; the atrial rate is 2 to 4 times faster than the ventricular rate.
         – **Third degree.** Rate is slowed, usually 40 to 60 beats per minute or the inherent ventricular rate.
      b. **P wave** is normal and present in each type of block.
      c. **PR intervals**
         – **First degree.** PR intervals are prolonged, usually 0.2 second.
         – **Second degree.** PR intervals may be progressively lengthening, as in type I (Mobitz I or Wenckebach), or fixed, as in type II (Mobitz II).
         – **Third degree.** No relationship between P waves and QRS complexes exists; PR intervals cannot be measured.
      d. **QRS complex**
         – **First and second degrees.** QRS complex is usually normal.
         – **Third degree.** QRS complex is widened (0.1 second) if originating from ventricles or is of normal duration if originating from the AV junction below the block.

        e. **Conduction**
- **First degree.** Conduction is delayed in the AV junction.
- **Second degree.** Impulses are not regularly conducted through the AV junction.
- **Third degree.** All sinus impulses are blocked; conduction through the ventricles is abnormal.

        f. **Rhythm** is regular in each type of block.

  2. **Etiology.** Causes of AV blocks include congenital and atherosclerotic heart disease (most common), certain drugs (e.g., digoxin, vagotonic agents, sympatholytic agents, beta-adrenergic blockers), and hypokalemia.

  3. **Assessment findings**

        a. **First degree** is asymptomatic.

        b. **Second degree.** Clinical manifestations include vertigo, weakness, and an irregular pulse.

        c. **Third degree.** Clinical manifestations include hypotension, angina, and heart failure.

  4. **Nursing management**

        a. **First degree.** No treatment is necessary. Discontinue the causative drug if indicated.

        b. **Second degree.** Administer atropine as prescribed to increase heart rate. (See *Drug chart 6-1,* pages 126 to 129.)

        c. **Third degree.** Administer atropine as prescribed to support ventricular escape rhythm. Prepare and assist with pacemaker insertion (see section XI), which provides repetitive electrical stimuli to the heart muscle to control the heart rate.

K. **Premature ventricular contractions**

  1. **Description.** Early or premature ventricular contractions (PVCs) are caused by increased automaticity of ventricular muscle cells. PVCs usually are not considered harmful but are of concern if more than six occur in 1 minute, if they occur in pairs or triplets, if they are multifocal, or if they occur on or near a T wave. PVCs have the following characteristics:

        a. **Rate.** Underlying rhythm is usually 60 to 100 beats per minute.

        b. **P wave.** Underlying rhythm is normal; premature beat has no P wave.

        c. **PR interval.** Underlying rhythm is normal; premature beat has no PR interval.

        d. **QRS complex.** Underlying rhythm is normal; premature beat is wide and bizarre (0.1 second) and may have one focus or a variety of foci (multifocal), resulting in many different configurations.

        e. **Conduction** is retrograde through the conduction system.

        f. **Rhythm** is usually irregular when premature beat occurs; it may be in a regular pattern, as in bigeminy.

  2. **Etiology.** Causes of PVCs include factors linked to irritability of ventricular muscle cells, including normal variance, exercise, increased catecholamines, electrolyte imbalance, digoxin toxicity, hypoxia, and myocardial damage.

  3. **Assessment findings.** PVCs may be asymptomatic, but clinical manifestations may include:

        a. palpitations

        b. weakness

        c. lightheadedness.

  4. **Nursing management.** Assess the cause (e.g., hypoxia, hypokalemia, ischemia, pain) of PVCs and treat as indicated. Treatment is indicated if the client has underlying disease because PVCs may precipitate ventricular tachycardia or fibrillation.

BOX 6-2
Ventricular fibrillation/pulseless ventricular tachycardia algorithm

- Assess airway, breathing, and cardiovascular status.
- Perform cardiopulmonary resuscitation (CPR) until the defibrillator is attached.
- Defibrillate up to three times if needed for ventricular fibrillation/ventricular tachycardia (VF/VT):
  - 200 joules
  - 200 to 300 joules
  - 360 joules.
- Check the rhythm after the first three shocks.

If your client is experiencing persistent or recurrent VF/VT:
- Continue CPR, and intubate at once.
- Obtain I.V. access.
- Epinephrine: 1 mg I.V. push, repeat every 3 to 5 minutes.
- Vasopressin: 40 units I.V.; one time only
- Defibrillate: 360 joules.
- Administer medications of probable benefit (see antiarrhythmics in *Drug chart 6-1*, pages 126 to 129).
- Defibrillate: 360 joules; 360 joules after each dose of medication.
- Pattern should be drug then shock.

    a. Assess for life-threatening PVCs (more than six PVCs per minute); multifocal PVCs; a PVC every other beat (bigeminy), every third beat (trigeminy), or every fourth beat (quadrigeminy); or PVCs that occur in a vulnerable phase of conduction cycle (R on T), and administer lidocaine immediately.

    b. Administer an antiarrhythmic medication, as prescribed. The medication of choice is lidocaine or amiodarone. For long-term therapy, procainamide or quinidine may be effective. (See *Drug chart 6-1*, pages 126 to 129.)

L. Ventricular tachycardia

  1. Description. Ventricular tachycardia is three or more consecutive PVCs. It is considered a medical emergency because CO cannot be maintained because of decreased diastolic filling. It has the following characteristics:

    a. **Rate** is 100 to 250 beats per minute.

    b. **P wave** is blurred in the QRS complex, but the QRS complex has no association with the P wave.

    c. **PR interval** is not present.

    d. **QRS complex** is wide and bizarre; **T wave** is in the opposite direction.

    e. **Conduction** is abnormal through ventricular tissue.

    f. **Rhythm** is usually regular.

  2. Etiology. The cause is linked to irritability of ventricular muscle.

  3. Assessment findings

    a. Lightheadedness

    b. Weakness

    c. Dyspnea

    d. Unconsciousness

  4. Nursing management

    a. Administer an antiarrhythmic medication, as prescribed. If the client is conscious, I.V. lidocaine may be indicated; if lidocaine is not successful, procainamide or amiodarone may be indicated. (See *Drug chart 6-1*, pages 126 to 129.)

    b. If the client is conscious or if lidocaine is unsuccessful, assist with cardioversion. (See *Box 6-1*, page 131.)

    c. If rhythm deteriorates to ventricular fibrillation or if the client is pulseless, assist with defibrillation (see *Box 6-1*, page 131) and use the Advanced Cardiac Life Support (ACLS) algorithm for resuscitation. (See *Box 6-2*.)

M. Ventricular fibrillation

1. **Description.** Ventricular fibrillation is rapid, ineffective quivering of ventricles that may be rapidly fatal. This arrhythmia has the following characteristics:

   a. **Rate** is rapid and uncoordinated, with ineffective motions.

   b. **P wave** is not seen.

   c. **PR interval** is not seen.

   d. **QRS complex** is seen as an undulation with no specific pattern.

   e. **Conduction** is unorganized, with many foci firing at once.

   f. **Rhythm** is irregular without a pattern.

2. **Etiology.** The cause of ventricular fibrillation is most commonly myocardial ischemia or infarction. It also may result from untreated ventricular tachycardia, electrolyte imbalances (e.g., hypokalemia and hypercalcemia), digoxin or quinidine toxicity, or hypothermia.

3. **Assessment findings**

   a. Loss of consciousness

   b. Pulselessness

   c. Loss of blood pressure

   d. Cessation of respirations

   e. Possible seizures

   f. Sudden death

4. **Nursing management**

   a. Assist with defibrillation (see *Box 6-1*, page 131, and *Box 6-2*, page 133) and CPR.

   b. Administer prescribed antiarrhythmic medications. (See *Drug chart 6-1*, pages 126 to 129.)

   c. Automated external devices are being placed in many stores, airlines, organizations, and nonacute care settings. These devices have defibrillator pads that are placed on the client's chest and when the device detects ventricular fibrillation it shocks the client automatically. This device is being used by many laypersons with success.

N. Ventricular asystole

1. **Description.** Ventricular asystole is described as a lack of QRS complexes, heartbeat, palpable pulse, and respiration. Without immediate intervention, ventricular asystole is fatal. This arrhythmia has the following characteristics:

   a. **Rate** is not present.

   b. **P wave** may be visible but does not conduct through the AV node and ventricles.

   c. **QRS complex** is not present.

   d. **Conduction** is possible through the atria only.

   e. **Rhythm** is not present.

2. **Etiology.** Causes of ventricular asystole may include any of the reasons for the previously described arrhythmias if medical treatment was not successful.

3. **Assessment findings**

   a. Loss of consciousness

   b. No respirations

   c. Pulselessness

   d. Sudden death

4. **Nursing management.** As indicated, assist with CPR; administer drugs, such as atropine and epinephrine (see *Drug chart 6-1*, pages 126 to 129); and provide nursing care for the insertion of a transthoracic, transvenous, or external pacemaker if necessary. (See section XI.)

IV. CORONARY ARTERY DISEASE

A. **Description.** Coronary artery disease (i.e., CAD, coronary atherosclerosis) results from focal narrowing of large and medium-sized coronary arteries due to intimal plaque formation. The most common cardiac disorder in the United States, the incidence of CAD increases progressively with age.

B. **Etiology**
   1. Causes vary and may involve a combination of such factors as genetic predisposition, metabolic disturbances, arterial hypertension, and altered platelet function that predisposes the vessel to plaque formation.
   2. Risk factors
      a. Advanced age
      b. Chronic stress
      c. Diabetes mellitus
      d. Family history
      e. Hormonal contraceptive use
      f. Hyperlipidemia
      g. Hypertension
      h. Male or postmenopausal female
      i. Obesity
      j. Sedentary lifestyle
      k. Smoking

C. **Pathophysiology.** CAD begins with the formation of fatty, fibrous plaques on the intima of coronary arteries. These plaques narrow the arterial lumen, reducing the volume of blood that can flow through the artery to the heart. Reduced coronary blood flow leads to myocardial ischemia and various degrees of cell damage. Plaque formation also predisposes the vessel to thrombus formation and subsequent embolism.

D. **Assessment findings**
   1. **Clinical manifestations**
      a. Angina. The most characteristic symptom, angina (also known as *chest pain*) is marked by mild to severe retrosternal pain (typically described as burning or squeezing) that may radiate to the arm, jaw, neck, or shoulder. It is usually precipitated by exertion, cold, heavy meals, smoking, or excitement (or may occur at rest because of vasospasm) and is relieved by rest and nitrates.
      b. Nausea and vomiting
      c. Dizziness and syncope
      d. Diaphoresis and cool, clammy skin
      e. Apprehension or a sense of impending doom
   2. **Laboratory and diagnostic study findings.** The client's electrocardiogram (ECG) may appear normal when the client is pain free; it may show ischemic changes (ST depression, T-wave inversion) during angina episodes or exercise.

E. **Nursing management (See section II.D.)**
   1. **Administer prescribed medications,** which may include nitrates, antiplatelets, antilipemics, beta-adrenergic blockers, and calcium channel blockers. (See *Drug chart 6-1,* pages 126 to 129.)

CLIENT AND FAMILY TEACHING 6-1
Guidelines for the client with coronary artery disease

- Participate in a regular exercise program.
  - Walk, swim, or perform low-impact aerobics. (Avoid activities that require sudden bursts of movement.)
  - Warm-up, perform the activity for 20 to 30 minutes, then cool down.
  - Avoid eating 2 hours before exercising.
  - Avoid extremes of cold or hot weather.
  - Avoid any activity that causes chest pain, shortness of breath, or undue fatigue.
- Modify diet.
  - Adhere to a low-fat, low-cholesterol, low-sodium diet.
  - Increase fiber to decrease the cholesterol level and prevent constipation.
  - Avoid excessive caffeine intake.
  - Eat smaller portions.
- Stop smoking to prevent vasoconstriction.
- Do not use any over-the-counter medications without consulting a pharmacist. Diet pills, nasal decongestants, and many other medications increase the heart rate.

- Keep a list of your medications that you are currently taking with you at all times; wear a medic-alert bracelet; and keep a record of all anginal attacks with the date, time, and activity that caused the pain.
- Manage anginal attacks properly.
  - Stop all activity; remain sitting upright.
  - Place a nitroglycerin (NTG) tablet under your tongue or take one NTG spray (should burn; causes headache, flushing, and dizziness).
  - Wait 5 minutes; if no relief, take another tablet or spray.
  - If no relief after an additional 5 minutes, take another tablet or spray; then seek medical attention immediately.
- Carry NTG with you at all times.
  - Keep tablets in a tightly capped, dark-colored container.
  - Replace tablets every 5 months.
  - You may take NTG before activities that cause angina (e.g., sexual activity, climbing stairs).

   2. **Provide care during an acute anginal attack.**
      a. Instruct the client to stop all activity, place one nitroglycerin (NTG) tablet (or take one NTG spray) under the tongue, and wait 5 minutes. If relief is not experienced, instruct him to take another tablet (or spray) and wait 5 minutes. If relief is still not experienced, instruct the client to take another tablet (or spray), and get medical help immediately; stay with him at all times.
      b. Request a STAT 12-lead ECG.
      c. Support and reassure the client and his family during an anginal episode.
   3. **Promote pain relief.** Encourage the client to reduce activity to a point at which pain does not occur.
   4. **Prepare the client for possible treatment.**
      a. Percutaneous transluminal coronary angioplasty (PTCA) compresses the blockage (atheroma) into the intimal lining of the artery, thereby increasing blood flow through the artery, or possibly by inserting an intravascular stent over the balloon during a PTCA.
      b. Coronary artery bypass grafting uses a blood vessel from the body to bypass the occluded vessel, thereby increasing blood flow to the myocardium.
   5. **Provide client and family teaching** to promote optimal management of the disease and to minimize anxiety.
      a. Encourage the client and his family to participate in a cardiac rehabilitation program. Also encourage support group participation.
      b. Encourage the client's family to take a CPR course.
      c. Guidelines for the client with CAD are given in *Client and family teaching 6-1.*
   6. **Provide referrals** to the American Heart Association. (See appendix A.)

V. MYOCARDIAL INFARCTION

A. **Description.** Myocardial infarction (MI) is destruction of myocardial tissue in regions of the heart abruptly deprived of adequate blood supply because of reduced coronary blood flow. In the United States, more than 1 million cases of MI are reported annually. The incidence of MI is far greater in men than women.

B. **Etiology**

1. Coronary artery narrowing due to atherosclerosis, coronary artery spasm, or complete arterial occlusion by embolism or thrombus
2. Decreased coronary blood flow due to hemorrhage or shock, causing a profound imbalance between myocardial oxygen supply and demand

C. **Pathophysiology.** In an MI, inadequate coronary blood flow rapidly results in myocardial ischemia in the affected area. The location and extent of the infarct determine the effects on cardiac function. Ischemia depresses cardiac function and triggers autonomic nervous system responses that exacerbate the imbalance between myocardial oxygen supply and demand. Persistent ischemia results in tissue necrosis and scar tissue formation, with permanent loss of myocardial contractility in the affected area. Cardiogenic shock may develop because of inadequate CO from decreased myocardial contractility and pumping capacity.

D. **Assessment findings**

1. **Clinical manifestations**
   a. Chest pain (Typically, chest pain is persistent and crushing; located substernally with radiation to the arm, neck, jaw, or back; and unrelieved by rest or nitrates. A silent MI may produce no pain.)
   b. Diaphoresis and cool, clammy, pale skin
   c. Nausea and vomiting
   d. Dyspnea with or without crackles
   e. Palpitations or syncope
   f. Restlessness and anxiety or feeling of impending doom
   g. Tachycardia or bradycardia
   h. Decreased blood pressure
   i. Altered S3 heart sound (indicates left ventricular failure)

2. **Laboratory and diagnostic study findings**
   a. Electrocardiogram. Myocardial ischemia causes the T wave to be larger and inverted; in epicardial myocardial ischemia, the ST segment is elevated; in endocardial myocardial ischemia, the ST segment is depressed.
   b. Serum enzyme studies reveal elevated levels of creatinine phosphokinase, lactate dehydrogenase, and troponin.
   c. The white blood cell count is elevated.

E. **Nursing management (See section II.D.)**

1. **Administer drug therapy.**
   a. Administer prescribed medications, which may include morphine, nitrates, antilipemics, thrombolytics, and anticoagulants in an acute situation; or stool softeners during rehabilitation. (See *Drug chart 6-1,* pages 126 to 129.)
   b. Remember MONA: morphine, oxygen, nitroglycerin, and aspirin for immediate treatment of a myocardial infarction.
2. **Provide ongoing assessment.**

     a. Monitor cardiac enzymes.

     b. Monitor hemodynamic parameters as necessary through the multilumen pulmonary artery catheter.

3. **Minimize anxiety.** Reassure the client, and explain procedures as the situation warrants.

4. **Minimize metabolic demands.** Institute a liquid diet; advance to a low-sodium, low-cholesterol, low-fat, solid diet as tolerated.

5. **Prepare the client for treatment,** such as percutaneous transluminal coronary angioplasty and coronary artery bypass grafting (See section IV.E.4.)

6. **Provide client and family teaching.**

     a. Encourage family members and significant others to take a cardiopulmonary resuscitation course.

     b. Guidelines for the client with coronary artery disease are provided in *Client and family teaching 6-1,* page 136.

7. **Provide referrals** for the American Heart Association. (See appendix A.)

VI. HEART FAILURE

A. Description

1. **Heart failure** is a syndrome of pulmonary or systemic circulatory congestion caused by decreased myocardial contractility, resulting in inadequate CO to meet oxygen requirements of tissues. The incidence of heart failure increases with aging.

2. **Heart failure classification**

     a. Left-sided (or left ventricular)

     b. Right-sided (or right ventricular)

B. Etiology.
The primary causes of heart failure are disorders producing decreased myocardial contractility (e.g., coronary artery disease [CAD], valvular heart disease, hypertension, cardiomyopathy, dysrhythmias, cor pulmonale secondary to lung disease, constrictive pericarditis, and pericardial tamponade).

C. Pathophysiology

1. **Left-sided heart failure** Congestion occurs primarily in the lungs from backup of blood into pulmonary veins and capillaries because of left ventricular pump failure. As blood backs up into the pulmonary bed, increased hydrostatic pressure causes fluid accumulation in the lungs. Blood flow is consequently decreased to the brain, kidneys, and other tissues.

2. **Right-sided heart failure.** Congestion in systemic circulation results from right ventricular pump failure. As blood backs up into systemic circulation, increased hydrostatic pressure produces peripheral and dependent pitting edema. Venous congestion in the kidneys, liver, and GI tract also develops.

D. Assessment findings

1. **Clinical manifestations**

     a. **Left-sided heart failure**

       – Dyspnea on exertion, paroxysmal nocturnal dyspnea, or orthopnea

       – Moist crackles on lung auscultation

       – Frothy blood-tinged sputum

       – Tachycardia with S3 heart sound

       – Pale, cool extremities

  - Peripheral and central cyanosis
  - Decreased peripheral pulses and capillary refill time longer than 3 seconds
  - Decreased urinary output (< 30 ml/hour)
  - Easy fatigability
  - Insomnia and restlessness
    b. **Right-sided heart failure**
      - Dependent pitting edema (peripheral and sacral)
      - Weight gain
      - Nausea and anorexia
      - Jugular vein distention (JVD)
      - Liver congestion (e.g., hepatomegaly), ascites, or weakness
  2. **Laboratory and diagnostic study findings**
     a. Chest radiograph reveals cardiomegaly and vascular congestion of lung fields.
     b. Electrocardiogram identifies hypertrophy or myocardial damage.
     c. Arterial blood gas studies reveal decreased partial pressure of arterial oxygen and increased partial pressure of arterial carbon dioxide.
     d. Pulse oximeter readings may be less than 95%, indicating decreased oxygen saturation.
     e. Multilumen pulmonary artery catheter shows elevated pulmonary artery and capillary wedge pressures in left-sided heart failure and elevated central venous pressure in right-sided heart failure.

E. Nursing management (See section II.D.)
  1. **Administer medications,** which may include cardiac glycosides, diuretics, angtiotensin-converting enzyme inhibitors, vasodilator therapy, and antilipemics. (See *Drug chart 6-1*, pages 126 to 129.)
  2. **Provide ongoing assessment.**
     a. Monitor hemodynamic parameters and heart rate and rhythm through the multilumen pulmonary artery catheter.
     b. Weigh the client daily. Notify the health care provider if the client gains 3 lb or more per day, which is a sign of fluid retention.
     c. Monitor serum electrolyte levels daily.
  3. **Prevent complications of immobility.** Instruct the client in or assist in performing range of motion exercises. Apply antiembolism stockings to prevent deep vein thrombosis.
  4. **Provide a low-sodium diet, as prescribed,** to decrease fluid retention and subsequently the workload of the heart.
  5. **Provide client and family teaching** for the client with CAD. (See *Client and family teaching 6-1*, page 136.)
  6. **Provide referrals** to the American Heart Association and home health care agencies. (See appendix A.)

VII. ACUTE PULMONARY EDEMA

A. Description. Acute pulmonary edema is a condition of rapid fluid accumulation in the extravascular (alveoli and interstitial) lung spaces. This condition is considered a medical emergency.

B. Etiology
  1. **Major causes of acute pulmonary edema**

     a. Left ventricular heart failure (most common cause), myocardial infarction, or other cardiac disorders

     b. Circulatory overload from infusions or transfusions

     c. Lung injury (e.g., smoke inhalation, pulmonary embolism)

     d. Drug hypersensitivity, allergy, poisoning, or opioid overdose

     e. Central nervous system damage (e.g., stroke, head trauma)

     f. Pulmonary infections (e.g., viral, bacterial, parasitic pneumonia)

  2. Certain procedures and treatments (e.g., cardioversion, coronary artery bypass grafting, or postanesthesia)

C. Pathophysiology. Engorged with blood, the pulmonary capillaries eventually cannot hold their contents, and fluid leaks into adjacent alveoli or interstitial spaces. Fluid accumulation causes the lungs to stiffen and impairs normal expansion, resulting in severe hypoxia.

D. Assessment findings

  1. Clinical manifestations

     a. Dyspnea and cough producing copious blood-tinged, frothy sputum

     b. Crackles and wheezes heard throughout the lung fields on auscultation

     c. Tachycardia or other arrhythmias

     d. Cyanotic, cold, clammy, diaphoretic skin

     e. Restlessness or anxiety or both

     f. Jugular vein distention

  2. Laboratory and diagnostic study findings

     a. Chest radiograph shows vascular congestion of lung fields ("butterfly" appearance).

     b. Multilumen pulmonary artery catheter shows elevated central venous, pulmonary artery, and capillary wedge pressures.

     c. Arterial blood gas studies reveal decreased partial pressure of arterial oxygen and increased partial pressure of arterial carbon dioxide.

     d. Pulse oximeter readings may be less than 93%, indicating a decrease in oxygen saturation.

E. Nursing management (See section II.D.)

  1. Administer prescribed medications, which may include morphine, diuretics, and cardiac glycosides. (See *Drug chart 6-1,* pages 126 to 129.)

  2. Position the client upright to decrease venous return and allow maximum lung expansion.

  3. Provide continuous assessment.

     a. Monitor ventilation. Assist with intubation or other measures as necessary; the client should have positive end-expiratory pressure to reduce venous return, lower pulmonary capillary pressure, and improve oxygenation.

     b. Monitor vital signs and hemodynamic parameters (by multilumen pulmonary artery catheter), assessing respiratory and cardiovascular status at least hourly.

     c. Assess renal status through output and electrolyte monitoring.

  4. Minimize anxiety. Provide reassurance and support to the client and his family members.

  5. Provide client and family teaching.

     a. Discuss the importance of daily weight measurement and intake and output monitoring to determine the need for further diuresis.

     b. Cover the need for rest periods and a gradual increase in daily activity.

     c. Review dietary guidelines, including foods low in sodium and high in potassium to replace that lost from diuretic therapy.

VIII. CARDIAC ARREST

A. **Description.** Cardiac arrest is defined as sudden, unexpected cessation of the heart's pumping action and effective circulation.

B. **Etiology**
1. **Ventricular fibrillation** is the major cause of cardiac arrest. Precipitating factors include myocardial infarction (MI), heart failure, near drowning, acute hemorrhage, hypoxia, pulmonary embolus, and ventricular irritation.
2. **Asystole** may trigger cardiac arrest. Precipitating factors include drug overdose, hemorrhage, anaphylaxis, and respiratory acidosis.
3. **Electromechanical dissociation** may cause cardiac arrest. Precipitating factors include severe MI, cardiac tamponade, and hemorrhage.
4. **Cardiac standstill** resulting from severe hypoxia is a possible cause of cardiac arrest.
5. **Circulatory collapse with acute hypotension** due to vasodilation or hypovolemia may cause cardiac arrest.

C. **Pathophysiology.** Cardiac arrest is the cessation of effective circulation because of the heart suddenly stopping; there is an immediate loss of consciousness and an absence of pulses (especially the carotid pulse); ventricular fibrillation or asystole occur.

D. **Assessment findings**
1. Immediate loss of consciousness
2. Absence of palpable pulses and heart sounds (absence of carotid pulse most reliable sign)
3. Apnea or gasping respirations
4. Ashen-gray skin

E. **Nursing management**
1. **Initiate cardiopulmonary resuscitation (CPR).** Cardiac arrest represents a medical emergency requiring immediate CPR to restore heart function and circulation. All health care team members should complete a CPR course, such as the American Heart Association Health Care Provider course or ACLS course. *Box 6-2* (page 133) shows the advanced cardiac life support (ACLS) ventricular fibrillation algorithm.
   a. Begin resuscitation measures immediately. Because of the life-threatening nature of cardiac arrest, prompt identification of arrest and initiation of CPR is essential. The nurse should not waste valuable time assessing blood pressure or listening for a heartbeat. CPR must restore circulation within approximately 4 minutes after the onset of cardiac arrest to prevent irreversible brain damage.
   b. Summon assistance, and establish a patent airway.
   c. Provide artificial ventilation by mouth-to-mouth resuscitation or with an Ambu bag; start oxygen as soon as possible.
   d. Provide artificial circulation through external cardiac compression.
   e. Assist with defibrillation using direct-current countershock for ventricular fibrillation or tachycardia. (See *Box 6-1*, page 131.)
2. **Administer a patent I.V. line if it is not already in place.**
3. **Administer emergency drugs,** as ordered. *Box 6-2*, page 133, shows the ACLS algorithm for ventricular fibrillation.
4. **Provide client and family teaching.** (See section II.D.9.) Encourage family members to complete an American Heart Association or American Red Cross CPR course.
5. **Promote family coping.**

>   *a.* Provide emotional support to the client's family as necessary.
>   *b.* Assist with the grieving process if death occurs.
> 6. **Address the possibility of organ donation** with the client's family, keeping in mind that this is a difficult time for them.

IX. ENDOCARDITIS

A. Description. Endocarditis is an infection of the endocardium or heart valves resulting from invasion of bacteria or other organisms. It may be acute, subacute, or chronic.

B. Etiology

1. **Causative organisms**
    a. Bacteria (e.g., *Streptococcus viridans, Staphylococcus aureus,* enterococci)
    b. Fungi (e.g., *Candida albicans,* Aspergillus)
    c. Rickettsiae

2. **Predisposing factors**
    a. History of valvular heart disease
    b. Prosthetic valve replacement surgery
    c. Debilitation
    d. Indwelling catheter placement
    e. Prolonged I.V. antibiotic therapy
    f. I.V. drug abuse
    g. Dental surgery

C. Pathophysiology. Ineffective organisms travel through the bloodstream and are deposited on heart valves or other portions of the endocardium. This triggers fibrin and platelet aggregation, which engulfs the organisms, forming friable verrucous vegetations. The vegetations typically form on valves but also may extend to the endocardium. Vegetations covering the valve surface can lead to ulceration and necrosis, with subsequent deformity and dysfunction of the valve leaflets.

D. Assessment findings

1. **Clinical manifestations**
    a. Weakness and fatigue
    b. Weight loss and anorexia
    c. Fever, with chills and diaphoresis
    d. Cough
    e. Arthralgia
    f. Splenomegaly
    g. Petechiae of the anterior trunk, conjunctivae, and mucosa
    h. Splinter hemorrhages in nail beds
    i. Skin changes, such as Roth's spots, Osler's nodes, or Janeway lesions
    j. New heart murmur or a change in an existing murmur, especially in the presence of fever

2. **Laboratory and diagnostic study findings**
    a. Blood analysis findings include:
       – positive blood cultures for causative organisms
       – elevated white blood cell count and erythrocyte sedimentation rate
       – anemia.
    b. Echocardiogram shows valvular damage.

    c. Electrocardiogram identifies changes indicating arrhythmias and cardiomegaly.

E. Nursing management (See section II.D.)

1. **Administer prescribed medications,** which include antibiotics. (See *Drug chart 6-1,* pages 126 to 129.)
2. **Provide ongoing assessment.**
    a. Monitor temperature at regular intervals.
    b. Draw blood for serial cultures to evaluate the effectiveness of therapy.
    c. Observe for signs and symptoms of heart failure, cerebral vascular complications, and valve stenosis or regurgitation.
3. **Prepare the client for possible valve replacement,** which greatly improves the prognosis for clients with severely damaged heart valves.
4. **Provide client and family teaching.**
    a. Discuss the need for prophylactic antibiotics before dental work; childbirth; genitourinary, GI, or gynecologic procedures; or any procedure or event that can cause transient bacteremia.
    b. Review signs and symptoms of complications to watch for and report.
    c. Discuss the need for regular temperature monitoring.

X. PERICARDITIS

A. Description. Pericarditis is inflammation of the pericardium, the fibroserous sac that surrounds the heart. It may be acute or chronic.

B. Etiology

1. Pericarditis, particularly the acute form, may be idiopathic.
2. Identified causes include:
    a. bacterial, fungal, or viral infections
    b. neoplasms
    c. connective tissue disorders
    d. hypersensitivity reactions
    e. injury to the pericardium (e.g., myocardial infarction, trauma, cardiac surgery)
    f. drugs (e.g., hydralazine, procainamide)
    g. high-dose radiation therapy to the chest
    h. uremia
    i. aortic aneurysm with pericardial leakage
    j. myxedema with cholesterol deposits in the pericardium.

C. Pathophysiology

1. **Acute pericarditis** may be fibrinous or effusive, producing serous or hemorrhage exudate.
2. **Chronic constrictive pericarditis** is marked by progressive pericardial thickening.

D. Assessment findings

1. **Clinical manifestations**
    a. Sharp, sudden pain over the precordium, radiating to the neck and left scapular region. Pain may be aggravated by breathing or movement and typically decreases when the client sits and leans forward.
    b. Dyspnea (from decreased carbon dioxide) and orthopnea
    c. Tachycardia
    d. Pericardial friction rub

    e. Distant heart sounds

    f. Increased cardiac dullness on percussion

    g. Absent apical impulse

    h. In the presence of cardiac tamponade, pallor, cool and clammy skin, hypotension, pulsus paradoxus, and jugular vein distention

2. **Laboratory and diagnostic study findings**

    a. Blood analysis reveals normal or elevated white blood cell count and erythrocyte sedimentation rate.

    b. Pericardiocentesis reveals positive pericardial fluid culture.

    c. ECG shows ST-segment elevation, T-wave inversion, and diminished QRS voltage with effusion.

    d. Echocardiography detects a free space echo between the ventricular wall and pericardium.

E. Nursing management (See section II.D.)

1. **Provide pain relief.**

    a. Administer prescribed pain medication, which may include morphine to relieve pain during the acute phase; nonsteroidal anti-inflammatory drugs; and corticosteroids. (See *Drug chart 6-1,* pages 126 to 129.)

    b. Place the client in an upright and leaning forward position, which tends to relieve pain.

    c. Place the client on bed rest until fever, chest pain, and friction rub disappear.

2. **Monitor for signs and symptoms of cardiac tamponade,** such as hypotension, muffled heart sounds, and pulsus paradoxus.

3. **Prepare the client for possible pericardiocentesis,** as ordered.

XI. PACEMAKER IMPLANTATION

A. Description. A cardiac pacemaker is a temporary or permanent electronic device that provides electrical stimuli to the heart muscle to initiate and maintain cardiac contractions when the heart's natural pacemakers are unable to do so. Pulses are generated from a battery-operated pacer unit and transmitted to the heart through electrodes placed in direct contact with the heart muscle wall.

B. Classification. Universal pacemaker classification involves a three-letter identification code.

1. The first letter identifies the **chamber paced:** A (atrium), V (ventricle), or D (dual).

2. The second letter identifies the **chamber sensed:** A (atrium), V (ventricle), or D (dual).

3. The third letter identifies the **mode of response:** T (triggered), I (inhibited), or D (both).

C. Types of pacemakers

1. **Temporary pacemakers** are used in emergencies for short-term pacing.

2. **Permanent pacemakers** are used for long-term pacing.

    a. **Demand pacemakers** (i.e., synchronous or noncompetitive pacemakers) are the most commonly used. The pacer fires only when the rate of spontaneous beats drops below the preset minimum rate. The sensing and pacing electrodes usually are placed in a ventricle.

    b. **Fixed pacemakers** (i.e., asynchronous or competitive pacemakers) are used less often. The rate and rhythm of pacer beats are unaffected by spontaneous heart beats. The pacing electrode is in a ventricle.

    c. **Atrioventricular pacemakers** are used in the A-V sequential mode, and sensing and pacing electrodes are placed in the atria and the ventricles; this pacemaker mimics the client's own intrinsic cardiac function.

D. Indications

1. **Temporary pacemakers**
   a. Diagnostic testing, such as hemodynamic assessment or antiarrhythmic drug evaluation
   b. Acute myocardial infarction
   c. Acute and chronic atrioventricular (AV) block
   d. Overdrive suppression of arrhythmia
   e. Symptomatic bradycardia or tachycardia

2. **Permanent pacemakers**
   a. Stokes-Adams syncope
   b. Sinus node dysfunction
   c. AV conduction abnormalities
   d. Chronic bundle branch block
   e. Recurrent tachyarrhythmias

E. Insertion routes

1. **Temporary pacemakers** are inserted by transvenous and transthoracic (usually emergency) routes. The catheter tip is positioned in the apex of the right ventricle.
2. **Permanent pacemakers** are inserted by transvenous and epicardial routes. Generator implantation is usually under the skin below the right or left pectoral region or below the clavicle.

F. Complications

1. **Complications within the body** include local infections at the insertion site, arrhythmias (from irritation of the ventricular wall by the electrode), perforation of the myocardium, or abrupt loss of pacing because of a high ventricular threshold.
2. **Malfunctions of the pacemaker** include battery failure, breakage or dislocation of the electrodes and electronic failure, and exposure to electromagnetic fields.

G. Nursing management (See section II.D.)

1. **Provide care for a client with a temporary pacemaker.**
   a. Monitor the peripheral insertion site (i.e., antecubital, brachial, jugular, subclavian, or femoral vein) for infection, bleeding, and placement.
   b. Assess pacemaker function, heart rate, and rhythm frequently; note deviations from settings.
   c. Ensure that all connections are secure.
   d. Monitor for ventricular dysrhythmia, the most common complication during insertion.

2. **Provide care for a client with a permanent pacemaker.**
   a. Assess pacemaker function, heart rate, and rhythm frequently; note deviations from settings.
   b. Assess the insertion site for bleeding, hematoma, or infection.
   c. Document data about model, date, and time of insertion; location of pulse generator; stimulus threshold; and pacer rate on the client's chart and at the head of the bed.
   d. Provide reassurance and emotional support.
   e. Teach the client and family to:

- carry a card specifying important pacemaker information at all times
- monitor pulse daily, and report any deviations to the health care provider
- comply with prescribed physical activity limitations
- watch for and promptly report signs and symptoms of complications
- keep scheduled appointments for regular pacemaker checkup
- avoid electromechanical devices that could interfere with pacing.

XII. HEMORRHAGE

A. **Description.** Hemorrhage is a loss of a large amount of blood internally or externally in a short period. The source may be arterial, venous, or capillary.

B. **Etiology**
   1. **External hemorrhage** may be caused by penetrating trauma and lacerations.
   2. **Internal hemorrhage** may be caused by blunt or penetrating trauma, blood dyscrasias, and ruptured aortic aneurysm.

C. **Pathophysiology.** Severe hemorrhage can lead to hypovolemic shock, which results in inadequate filling of the vascular compartment; it occurs when 15% to 20% of circulating blood volume is loss. A loss of effective circulating blood volume causes inadequate organ and tissue perfusion, resulting in cellular metabolic death. Severe hemorrhage necessitates emergency intervention.

D. **Assessment findings**
   1. **Clinical manifestations**
      a. Obvious bleeding from wound or orifices
      b. Signs of internal bleeding (e.g., ecchymoses, occult or frank blood in urine or stool)
      c. Cold, moist, pale skin
      d. Apprehension
      e. Hypotension
      f. Tachycardia
      g. Oliguria
   2. **Laboratory and diagnostic study findings**
      a. Blood studies detect decreased hematocrit and hemoglobin.
      b. Guaiac testing may detect occult blood in stool.

E. **Nursing management (See section II.D.)**
   1. **Provide emergency care.**
      a. Ensure a patent airway and start cardiopulmonary resuscitation, if necessary.
      b. Apply pressure over the bleeding area or involved artery (external bleeding); apply a tourniquet only as a last resort to stop bleeding.
      c. Apply medical antishock trousers, as indicated.
      d. Elevate and immobilize the injured body part (for external bleeding), and position the client in the supine position.
      e. Start a peripheral large-gauge I.V. line for blood replacement; administer fluids (lactated Ringer's solution) and blood products as ordered.
      f. Insert an indwelling catheter with a urometer, monitor urinary output every 15 to 30 minutes; report urinary output less than 30 ml/hour.
   2. **Provide drug therapy.**
      a. Administer prescribed medications, which may include dopamine to improve cardiovascular performance. (See *Drug chart 6-1*, pages 126 to 129.)

b. Cautiously use analgesics or opioids when relieving pain.

3. **Provide continuous assessment.** Assess the client closely, including vital signs, skin temperature, color, central venous pressure, arterial blood gases, electrocardiogram, hematocrit, and hemoglobin concentration.

4. **Prepare the client for surgery if indicated.**

XIII. VALVULAR DISORDERS OF THE HEART

A. **Description.** Two types of valvular disorders are narrowing (i.e., stenosis) of the valve opening and failure of a valve to close completely (i.e., insufficiency or regurgitation).

B. **Etiology.** Valvular heart disorders result from congenital defects, trauma, ischemic damage, degenerative changes, and inflammation. Rheumatic endocarditis is the most common cause.

C. **Pathophysiology.** The tricuspid, bicuspid (mitral), pulmonic, or aortic valve of the heart is unable to control the one-way flow of blood through the heart. The valve is unable to open and close at the appropriate times as the heart contracts and relaxes through the cardiac cycle, which results in blood leaking back through the valve and impeded blood flow.

1. **Mitral valve prolapse syndrome** prevents the mitral valve from closing completely, resulting in valvular regurgitation in which blood from the left ventricle seeps back into the left atrium.

2. **Mitral stenosis** results in progressive thickening and contracting of the mitral valve cusps, which causes narrowing and obstruction of blood flow. This leads to low carbon dioxide and pulmonary venous hypertension.

3. **Mitral insufficiency** (i.e., regurgitation) results when the chordae tendineae shorten and prevent complete closure of the leaflets, causing backflow of blood from the left ventricle into the left atrium. The left atrium must dilate to accommodate the blood flow from lungs and backflow of blood from the left ventricle.

4. **Aortic valve stenosis** results when the leaflets fuse and partially close the opening between the heart and the aorta; the obstructed flow causes left ventricular hypertrophy.

5. **Aortic insufficiency** (i.e., regurgitation) results when the leaflets do not completely seal the aortic orifice, allowing backflow of blood from the aorta into the left ventricle.

D. **Assessment findings**

1. **Mitral valve prolapse syndrome** may be asymptomatic and the first symptom may be an extra heart sound referred to as a *mitral click.*

2. **Mitral stenosis.** Clinical manifestations include progressive fatigue, hemoptysis, and dyspnea on exertion.

3. **Mitral insufficiency.** Clinical manifestations include palpitation of the heart, dyspnea on exertion, and cough due to pulmonary congestion.

4. **Aortic valve stenosis.** Clinical manifestations include dyspnea, angina pectoris, and a loud, rough systolic murmur over the aortic area.

5. **Aortic insufficiency.** Clinical manifestations include an increased force of the heartbeat, an arterial pulsation in the neck, exertional dyspnea, and breathing difficulties.

E. **Nursing management (See section II.D.)**

1. **Educate the client on the need for prophylactic antibiotics** before any invasive procedure to include dental work, genitourinary or GI procedures, and I.V. therapy. (See *Drug chart 6-1,* pages 126 to 129.)

2. **Implement nursing care for the client** undergoing valve repair or replacement, which in most instances is the treatment of choice.
   a. Teach the client and his family about valvuloplasty, the repair of the affected valve, if appropriate. The type of valvuloplasty depends on the cause and type of valve dysfunction.
      - Commissurotomy is a procedure performed to separate fused leaflets.
      - Annuloplasty is the repair of the junction of the valve leaflets and the muscular heart wall.
      - Chordoplasty is the repair of the chordae tendineae.
   b. Teach the client and his family about valve replacement, if appropriate.
      - A mechanical valve is a ball and cage or disk design.
      - Xenografts are tissue valves from pigs (porcine) or cows (bovine).
      - Homografts are human valves obtained from cadaver tissue donations.
      - Autografts are obtained by excising the client's own pulmonic valve and portion of the pulmonary artery for the use as the aortic valves.
   c. Valvuloplasty and valve replacements require the client to be admitted to critical care units for constant nursing care because of the potential complications of thromboembolism, infection, bleeding, hypertension, arrhythmias, and mechanical obstruction.
   d. Educate the client about lifelong oral anticoagulant therapy with certain types of valves replacements. (See *Drug chart 6-1*, pages 126 to 129.)
   e. Provide discharge instructions, including education on wound care, diet, activity, medication, and self-care.
3. **Perform proper nursing management if the patient develops heart failure because of his inability to have surgery to replace or repair the valves;** see section VI for nursing management.

Study questions

1. When assessing a client with angina, which assessment data is considered a common precipitating factor for pain?
1. Exposure to warmth
2. Smoking
3. Prolonged rest
4. Eating a light meal

2. After being diagnosed with an acute myocardial infarction (MI) and stabilized, a female client denies pain. Her vital signs and heart rhythm are stable but she appears agitated and uses her call light more often. Which nursing intervention would be the *initial* step in addressing the client's needs?
1. Assessing her blood pressure more frequently

2. Explaining that another episode is unlikely
3. Encouraging her to discuss her feelings about the MI
4. Telling her not to worry because she is being closely monitored

3. Which behavior indicates that a client diagnosed with heart failure is being compliant with the discharge teaching plan?
1. The client demonstrates better nutrition habits by gaining 10 lb.
2. The client returns to the hospital as an inpatient less frequently.
3. The client significantly improves the activity level.
4. The client attends all the medication teaching classes.

4. Discharge teaching for a client diagnosed with coronary artery disease should include which nursing intervention?
1. Decreasing intake of dietary fiber
2. Eating two hours before exercising
3. Decreasing cigarette smoking
4. Participating in regular exercise

5. Assessment of a client diagnosed with heart failure reveals moderate dyspnea, clammy and very pale skin, and cough producing frothy, blood-tinged sputum. Based on these findings, the nurse suspects that the client is experiencing which complication?
1. Angina
2. Myocardial infarction (MI)
3. Pulmonary edema
4. Endocarditis

6. For the client experiencing a cardiac arrest, which nursing intervention should the nurse implement *first*?
1. Assessing the client's blood pressure
2. Establishing a patent airway
3. Auscultating heart sounds
4. Assisting with defibrillation

7. While performing discharge teaching for a client with chronic heart failure, the nurse should stress which topic?
1. The need for a high-impact aerobic exercise program
2. A high-sodium, low-potassium diet
3. The signs and symptoms of pulmonary edema
4. The possibility of the need for surgical procedures

8. Four days after an acute anterior wall myocardial infarction (MI), a 63-year-old client progresses from a first-degree atrioventricular (AV) block to a second-degree Mobitz II AV block over 6 hours. Although the client is asymptomatic, the nurse should anticipate instituting which intervention?
1. Assisting with pacemaker implantation
2. Administering digoxin
3. Administering lidocaine by I.V. bolus
4. Increasing the I.V. fluid infusion to 175 ml/hour

9. A client with a prosthetic heart valve has a nursing diagnosis of "deficient knowledge." Which intervention is *most important* for the nurse to include in the client's discharge teaching plan?
1. Reporting cold or flulike symptoms promptly
2. Taking antibiotic prophylaxis for invasive procedures
3. Daily pulse rate assessment
4. Maintenance of bed rest for any chest pain

10. After assisting with insertion of a temporary transvenous pacemaker, which assessment data would be *most important* to document?
1. Cardiovascular response to the pacemaker
2. Emotional state
3. Activity level
4. Pacemaker information (e.g., type, settings)

11. A client develops symptomatic sinus bradycardia. Which medication would the nurse expect to administer?
1. Atropine
2. Lidocaine
3. Amiodarone
4. Procainamide

12. When assessing a client's radial pulses, the nurse finds them to be irregular, with the apical pulse rate about 10 beats faster than the radial pulse rate. The nurse would suspect which cardiac arrhythmia?
1. Atrial fibrillation
2. Second-degree atrioventricular (AV) block
3. Ventricular tachycardia
4. Sinus bradycardia

13. Which clinical manifestation would the nurse expect to assess in a client diagnosed with pericarditis?
1. Sharp, sudden pain over the precordium, radiating to the left scapular region
2. Weakness, fatigue, and petechiae of the anterior trunk and conjunctivae
3. Crushing chest pain radiating down the left arm plus nausea and vomiting
4. Hepatomegaly, jugular vein distention (JVD), and dependent peripheral edema

14. A middle-aged client with coronary artery disease has been hospitalized three times in the last 6 months, suggesting noncompliance with the medication regimen. When preparing the client for discharge this time, which intervention should the nurse implement?
1. Reteaching the client about the medication and dosing schedule
2. Collecting more data to help identify reasons for noncompliance
3. Teaching the client's family about the medication and need for compliance
4. Arranging for outpatient follow-up examinations to ensure compliance.

15. Before discharge, a client who is receiving cardiac rehabilitation after a myocardial infarction (MI) should be able to do which activity?
1. Bed rest with sitting up in a chair twice each day
2. Walking the length of the hallway twice each day
3. Isometric exercises three times daily
4. Walking up and down two flights of stairs daily

16. The nurse is assisting a client diagnosed with R/O myocardial infarction (MI) to ambulate to the bathroom when the client starts complaining of chest pain. Which inventions should the nurse implement? (Select all that apply.)
1. Escorting the client back to the bed
2. Administering oxygen via nasal cannula
3. Instructing the client to take slow deep breaths
4. Administering subinguinal nitroglycerin (NTG)
5. Calling a code via the telephone
6. Placing the client in Trendelenburg's position

Answer key

1. The answer is **2.**
Any activity that increases myocardial oxygen demands, such as smoking, can lead to anginal pain. Smoking also causes vasoconstriction that can precipitate anginal attacks. Exposure to cold and subsequent constriction, not exposure to warmth that causes dilation, may precipitate anginal pain. Rest typically relieves anginal pain, except with anginal pain caused by vasospasm. In this case, chest pain may occur at rest. Light meals are recommended; heavy meals should be avoided because increased oxygen is needed to digest food.

2. The answer is **3.**
Because the client's vital signs are stable, she is most likely experiencing anxiety related to the acute event. The nurse should encourage her to express her feelings about the MI to help reduce her anxiety level. Assessing her blood pressure more frequently would be appropriate if her vital signs were not stable. Plus, frequent checks would tend to increase her already heightened level of anxiety. Explaining that another episode is unlikely or telling her not to worry ignores her feelings and blocks further communication. False or empty reassurance does not meet her needs.

3. The answer is **2.**
Less frequent hospital admissions indicate that the client is experiencing better heart function and therefore must be complying with his discharge plan. Weight gain may be

a result of fluid retention from possible non-compliance with medications (e.g., diuretic therapy) or with dietary recommendations for a low sodium intake. A significant improvement in activity level usually is not possible for clients with CHF. Medication teaching classes is but one aspect of his discharge plan. Although attendance at the classes may help with compliance, it does not ensure his compliance.

4. The answer is **1.**
The client should participate in a regular exercise program, such as walking, swimming, or low-impact aerobics, for at least 20 to 30 minutes a day plus a warm-up and cool-down time. A high-fiber diet is encouraged to help decrease the cholesterol level. The client should avoid eating for 2 hours before exercise because digestion increases blood supply to the GI system and decreases supply to heart muscle. The client must quit smoking.

5. The answer is **3.**
Frothy, blood-tinged sputum appearing in conjunction with dyspnea and clammy, pale skin indicates pulmonary edema with interstitial fluid overload in the lungs because of left ventricular failure. Although dyspnea and clammy, pale skin may coexist with angina or MI, frothy, blood-tinged sputum would be absent. Weakness, fatigue, fever, diaphoresis, arthralgia, and petechiae typically are evidence of endocarditis.

6. The answer is **2.**
If a client experiences cardiac arrest, the first action is to establish a patent airway and then administer artificial ventilation and oxygen. Resuscitation measures need to be started immediately because of the life-threatening nature of a cardiac arrest. Valuable time is wasted by assessing the client's blood pressure or auscultating for heart sounds, because circulation must be restored within approximately 4 minutes after the onset of cardiac arrest to prevent irreversible brain damage. Defibrillation is used after initial resuscitation efforts have been initiated.

7. The answer is **3.**
For the client with chronic CHF, teaching topics must include the signs and symptoms of pulmonary edema. This condition is a medical emergency situation requiring prompt evaluation and treatment. Otherwise, it could progress to death. A structured exercise program involving daily low-impact aerobic exercises also would be included. However, this topic is less of a priority than the signs and symptoms of pulmonary edema. Dietary instructions should address an intake of low-sodium, high-potassium foods, especially if the client is receiving diuretic therapy. Discussion of possible surgical procedures is inappropriate for the client with chronic CHF.

8. The answer is **1.**
Progression of an AV block, a conduction defect, in the presence of an anterior wall MI is an indication for pacemaker implantation. Administering digoxin would most likely potentiate the client's AV block. Lidocaine is indicated for treatment of ventricular arrhythmias, not conduction defects. Increasing the infusion of I.V. fluids in the presence of an MI could precipitate heart failure.

9. The answer is **2.**
Because of the increased risk for endocarditis from transient bacteremia, the client needs instruction about notifying all health care providers who may perform invasive procedures that he has a prosthetic heart valve. Prophylactic antibiotics should be given before the procedure to prevent transient bacteremia. The client needs to report any unexplained fever, not cold or flulike symptoms. Daily pulse assessment and bed rest are not necessary. Pulse assessment is a teaching topic for clients with pacemakers; bed rest is a teaching topic for clients with myocardial infarction.

10. The answer is **1.**
After insertion of a temporary transvenous pacemaker, the client's telemetry, pulse, and blood pressure should be closely monitored to ensure proper pacemaker capture and

function. Pacemaker information and the client's emotional state and activity level also should be documented. However, these areas are not as critically important as is the client's cardiovascular response. The client's activity levels usually are restricted to bed rest.

11. The answer is **1.**

Atropine is used to treat sinus bradycardia in clients who are symptomatic. Lidocaine, amiodarone, and procainamide are used to treat ventricular tachycardia and ventricular fibrillation.

12. The answer is **1.**

Irregular radial pulses in conjunction with up to a 10-beat difference between the apical and radial pulse rates indicate atrial fibrillation. Second-degree AV block is a conduction defect evidenced by a slow rate (atrial rate two to four times faster than ventricular rate), progressively lengthening or fixed PR interval, and normal P wave and QRS complex. Ventricular tachycardia is evidenced by a rate of 100 to 250 beats per minute, no PR interval, wide and bizarre QRS complex, and abnormal conduction through ventricular tissue. Sinus bradycardia refers to a heart rate less than 60 beats per minute with all other electrocardiogram waveforms within normal parameters.

13. The answer is **1.**

Sharp, sudden pain over the precordium that radiates to the left scapular region is a characteristic clinical manifestation of pericarditis and inflammation of the pericardium (e.g., sac that surrounds the heart). The pain may be aggravated by breathing or movement. Weakness, fatigue, and petechiae of the anterior trunk and conjunctivae indicate endocarditis. Crushing chest pain radiating down the left arm accompanied by nausea and vomiting is associated with a myocardial infarction. Hepatomegaly, JVD, and dependent peripheral edema are manifestations of right-sided heart failure.

14. The answer is **2.**

To ensure compliance, the nurse needs more information to determine if there is a specific reason why the client is not complying with the medication regimen. The client may have a valid reason, such as financial constraints or lack of accessibility to the pharmacy, that needs to be identified and addressed. It is questionable whether or not reteaching would be effective for this client. Teaching the family and arranging for outpatient follow up may help with compliance, but these also may cause the client to feel a loss of control over his condition and its management.

15. The answer is **2.**

Before discharge, a realistic goal of cardiac rehabilitation for a client after an MI is the client's ability to walk the hallway twice daily. The client should not be on bed rest except in the initial post-MI period. Cardiac rehabilitation begins on admission. Isotonic exercises are recommended. Isometric exercises, which strain the heart (such as in Valsalva's maneuver), are to be avoided. At this time, the client would be unable to climb two flights of stairs. However, this may be a goal for later in the cardiac rehabilitation period.

16. The answers are **1, 2, 4.**

Chest pain is a sign of angina that may lead to an MI. The nurse must first prevent further exertion by the client by escorting him back to the bed. The nurse should then administer oxygen to increase perfusion to the heart muscle and subinguinal NTG to increase vasodilatation to the myocardium. Taking deep breaths will not help the chest pain, the client is not coding at this time, and placing the client with his head downward will not help relieve chest pain.

7 *Peripheral vascular disorders*

I. STRUCTURE AND FUNCTION OF PERIPHERAL CIRCULATION

A. Structures

1. **Arteries**

   a. The **aorta** is the first vessel carrying blood out of the heart. Sections of the aorta include the ascending aorta, aortic arch, thoracic aorta, and abdominal aorta.

   b. The aorta branches into **arteries** and then into **arterioles,** the smallest arteries, to distribute blood to the body. (See *Figure 7-1.*) Arterioles end in microcirculation, or capillaries.

   c. **Arteries** consist of an outer layer of connective tissue (tunica adventitia), a middle layer of muscle (tunica media), and an inner layer of endothelial cells (tunica intima).

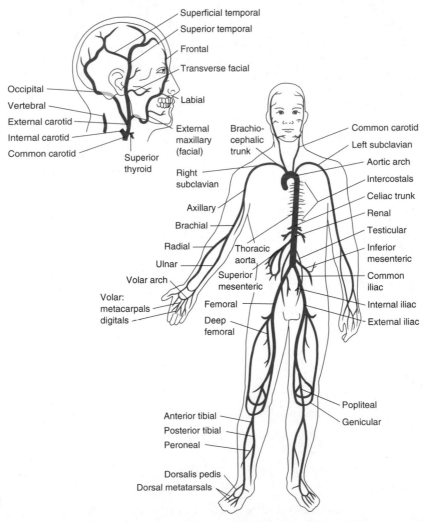

FIGURE 7-1
Principal systemic arteries

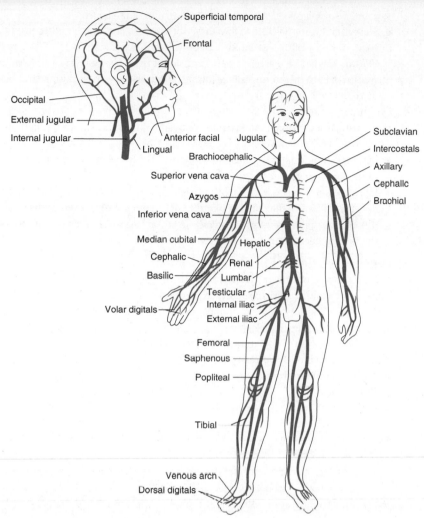

FIGURE 7-2
Principal systemic veins

The thick, elastic muscle layer of the arteries can withstand higher pressures than can veins and can dilate or constrict depending on messages sent to it.

2. **Capillaries,** thin-walled vessels through which nutrients and waste products pass, consist of a layer of endothelial cells and basement membrane surrounded by a pericapillary sheath of connective tissue.

3. **Veins**

    a. Blood travels from capillaries into a system of collecting vessels known as **veins.** (See *Figure 7-2.*)

        – **Venules,** the smallest veins, join to form progressively larger veins.

        – The **superior vena cava** receives blood from the veins of the head, neck, upper extremities, and chest. The superior vena cava drains into the right atrium of the heart.

- The **inferior vena cava** receives blood from the veins below the diaphragm. The inferior vena cava drains into the right atrium of the heart.
  b. **Superficial veins** lie close to the surface of the skin. The most important superficial veins are those of the extremities. **Deep veins** lie near arteries.
  c. **Venous tissue.** Like arteries, veins consist of three tissue layers — the tunica adventitia, tunica media, and tunica intima. Tissue in the veins is thinner and less elastic than in the arteries.
  4. **Lymphatic system**
  a. **Lymphatics** are small, thin, veinlike vessels that conduct lymph through the body. They tend to lie near veins.
  b. **Lymph nodes** are small, oval bodies connected by lymphatics. Lymph flows through these nodes on its way to the veins.
  c. **Lymph ducts.** Valves and smooth muscle contractions act to direct lymph in one direction by way of the right lymphatic duct (draining the right side of the head, neck, thorax, and upper arms) and thoracic duct (draining most of the rest of the body) to the right and left brachiocephalic veins.

B. Functions

1. **Arteries** carry blood away from the heart to supply nutrients and oxygen to tissues.
2. **Capillaries** allow for the exchange of oxygen and carbon dioxide between the blood and body tissues. They also serve to connect the arterioles and venules.
3. **Veins** carry deoxygenated blood and waste products of cellular metabolism to the heart.
4. **Lymphatic system.** The lymphatics collect lymph from tissues and return it to the blood. This system helps protect the body from infection by microorganisms.
5. **Dynamics of blood flow**
   a. **Vessel walls**
   - Vasodilation, an increase in the diameter of a blood vessel, allows for delivery of more blood to an area.
   - Vasoconstriction, a decrease in the diameter of a blood vessel, allows for delivery of less blood to an area.
   - Regulatory mechanisms from the nervous system and local tissues provide for vasodilation and vasoconstriction as needed.
   b. The **precapillary sphincter,** which encircles the entrance to the capillary, dilates as needed to increase blood flow and, as a result, tissue oxygenation.
   c. The **return of blood to the heart** is promoted through several factors:
   - Pumping action of the heart
   - Pressure exerted on the veins by skeletal muscles
   - Valves in the veins (except for the vena cava and the portal, cerebral, intraabdominal, and pulmonary veins), which break the hydrostatic column of blood into smaller units (This facilitates movement of blood in one direction and with reduced pressures.)
   - Pressure gradient between the veins and the atrium (Normal venous pressure is much lower than arterial pressure and is lower in the right atrium than in the feet. This pressure gradient enables veins to channel blood from capillaries to the heart's right side.)
   - Changes in abdominal and thoracic pressures caused by breathing (Inspiration creates an intrathoracic vacuum and facilitates blood flow to the right atrium.)
   - Venous volume and pressure, which is regulated actively by neurogenic venoconstriction caused by alpha-adrenergic nerves and passively by the elastic recoil of

the vein wall after distending pressure falls below the level necessary to hold the vein in a rounded shape.

NURSING PROCESS OVERVIEW

II. PERIPHERAL CIRCULATION

A. Assessment

1. **Health history**

   a. **Elicit a description of the client's present illness and chief complaint,** including onset, course, duration, location, and precipitating and alleviating factors. Assess exercise tolerance (especially important in arterial disorders) and for pain caused by tissue ischemia. Cardinal signs and symptoms indicating altered peripheral vascular function include arterial insufficiency (e.g., pain with exercise, rest pain, absent or diminished pulses, dependent rubor) and venous insufficiency (e.g., aching, cramping, pulses are present, peripheral edema).

   b. **Explore the client's health history for modifiable risk factors,** including smoking, hypertension, obesity, sedentary lifestyle, stress, diabetes mellitus. Also assess for **nonmodifiable risk factors,** including heredity, gender, and age.

2. **Physical examination**

   a. **Inspection.** An adequate supply of arterial blood to the extremities produces normal-appearing skin and nails and good tissue healing.

   – Assess skin color and temperature changes.
   - Coolness, possibly indicating deficient blood supply
   - Pallor, associated with diminished blood supply
   - Blanching, which may indicate diminished arterial pressure in a body part
   - Rubor, which may occur with chronic ischemia
   - Cyanosis, resulting from insufficient blood oxygen and, if localized, indicating poor circulation in that area
   - Necrosis and ulceration, which can occur in arterial and venous disorders, with symptoms depending on cause
   – Assess for muscle atrophy and loss of strength and joint mobility, which occurs in chronic ischemia.

   b. **Palpation.** Measure pulse volume using the peripheral pulse grading system: 0, absent; 1+, weak and thready; 2+, normal; 3+, full; 4+, bounding.

   c. **Auscultation**

   – Assess for bruits, which are heard most easily during systole; pitch correlates with degree of stenosis.
   – Assess capillary refill time, which indicates peripheral perfusion and cardiac output; acceptable time is less than 3 seconds.
   – Measure blood pressure, using the standard arm pressure measurement and ankle-arm index (i.e., ankle systolic pressure divided by arm systolic pressure). A normal ankle-arm index is greater than 1. An ankle-arm index of 0.5 to 0.8 indicates moderate outflow disease; an ankle-arm index of less than 0.5 indicates severe outflow disease.

3. **Laboratory and diagnostic studies**

   a. **Doppler ultrasound** is a simple, inexpensive, highly reliable procedure used to obtain qualitative and quantitative information electronically about blood flow in arteries or veins.

    b. **Plethysmography** is a procedure involving measurable changes in calf volume that correspond to changes in blood volume. This test procedure is used to assess changes in venous volume and carotid artery blood flow.

    c. The **treadmill test** is an exercise test done to evaluate total extremity blood flow after exercise and to detect pain occurring with exercise or signs of activity intolerance, such as shortness of breath.

    d. **Digital subtraction angiography** or **digital I.V. angiography** is a radiologic technique that uses an image-intensifier video system to display vessels on a television monitor.

    e. **Phlebography (venography)** is a procedure involving radiologic visualization of veins after injection of contrast medium.

    f. **Angiography** is a procedure involving radiologic visualization of arteries after injection of contrast medium.

    g. The ^{125}**I-fibrinogen uptake test** is a sensitive, expensive, and time-consuming screening test for acute calf vein thrombosis. This test involves injection of radioactive iodine.

B. Nursing diagnoses
1. Ineffective peripheral tissue perfusion
2. Activity intolerance
3. Acute pain
4. Impaired physical mobility
5. Impaired skin integrity
6. Risk for infection
7. Disturbed body image
8. Ineffective individual coping
9. Deficient knowledge
10. Noncompliance

C. Planning and outcome identification. The major goals for the client with a peripheral vascular disease include increased arterial blood supply to the extremities; decreased venous congestion; improvement of activity tolerance and ability to carry out activities of daily living; pain relief; improved mobility; maintenance of tissue integrity; absence of complications; improvement of self-image; and adherence to a self-care program with an understanding of the disease process and its management.

D. Implementation
1. **Assess the client's neurovascular status** by assessing for the six "Ps" on both extremities.

    a. **Pain.** Determine if the pain occurs with exercise (how much), with rest, or at all times; assess pain on a scale of 1 (no pain) to 10 (worst pain); and assess the type of pain.

    b. **Paresthesias.** Assess if the client can determine sharp or dull pain (use a cotton-tipped applicator) on all five toes, the bottom of the foot, and up the leg.

    c. **Polar.** Feel the client's feet to determine if they are warm or cold.

    d. **Paralysis.** Ask the client to move his toes, ankle, and knee; observe him ambulating.

    e. **Pallor.** Assess the color of the client's feet in neutral, dependent, and elevated positions.

    f. **Pulses**
- Assess lower extremity pulses (the dorsalis pedis, the popliteal, and posterior tibial pulses), rating the quality between 0 (absent) and 4+ (bounding).
- Mark the pulse with an "X," especially if the pulse is difficult to palpate.

- If unable to assess pulses, always use a Doppler ultrasound device to detect the pulse. Mark the pulse with an "X."

2. **Promote tissue perfusion.**
   a. Assess lower extremities for peripheral edema, hair distribution, and skin characteristics (e.g., dry, scaly, moist).
   b. Encourage walking on flat surfaces or in a swimming pool to promote blood flow and help develop collateral circulation.

3. **Increase activity tolerance.** Balance periods of rest and exercise. Assist as needed with activities of daily living and self-care. Maintain bed rest as ordered. Gradually resume activities as tolerated.

4. **Provide pain relief.**
   a. Administer pain medications, as prescribed.
   b. Institute nonpharmacologic pain measures, such as rest of the affected extremity and relaxation techniques.
   c. Advise the client with intermittent claudication to understand the limits in ambulation.

5. **Prevent hazards of immobility.**
   a. Instruct the client about the importance of proper turning, positioning, and deep-breathing techniques.
   b. Perform passive and active range-of-motion exercises on all extremities to promote blood flow and prevent contractures.

6. **Maintain skin integrity.**
   a. Assess wound characteristics to determine if they are arterial or venous. Perform wound care as ordered using aseptic technique.
   b. Measure circumference of extremities for changes related to an increase or decrease in edema.

7. **Prevent infection.** Monitor vital signs, especially for fever. Inspect the wound and the surrounding area for redness, edema, and pain.

8. **Enhance body image and coping.** Encourage the client to verbalize feelings related to altered appearance (i.e., wounds and ulcers), altered function of body part, or loss of body part.

9. **Provide client and family teaching to enhance compliance with treatment.**
   a. Teach the client about the importance of adhering to treatment. Provide information about possible complications, including gangrene and widespread infection.
   b. Discuss medications, including possible adverse effects and interactions.
   c. Discuss danger signs and symptoms requiring prompt medical attention, including increased edema, increased pain, foul-smelling purulent drainage from the wound, and complaints of numbness or coldness in the extremity.
   d. Discuss issues concerning an advanced directive and a durable power of attorney for health care.

E. Outcome evaluation

1. The client demonstrates increased tissue perfusion to the extremities, as evidenced by warm skin, improved skin color, decreased muscle pain with exercise, and palpable peripheral pulses.

2. The client complies with measures to promote vasodilation and prevent vasoconstriction and trauma.

3. The client increases physical mobility, gradually progressing to an optimal activity level while controlling pain-inducing activity.

4. The client is able to tolerate self-care activities and reports decreased fatigue.

5. The client reports freedom from pain and increased activity tolerance.
6. The client maintains skin integrity.
7. The client demonstrates resolution of the infectious process with the use of prescribed medications and the absence of signs and symptoms of systemic or local infection.
8. The client projects an improved self-image and acknowledges positive changes in body image.
9. The client verbalizes feelings and demonstrates appropriate coping skills in dealing with disorders of the peripheral vascular system.
10. The client verbalizes an understanding of the disease process, preventive measures, treatments, and signs and symptoms of complications that should be reported to the health care provider.
11. The client complies with the medical treatment, medication therapy, activity restrictions, and follow-up visits with the health care provider.

III. PERIPHERAL ARTERIAL OCCLUSIVE DISEASE

A. **Description.** Peripheral arterial occlusive disease is a form of arteriosclerosis involving occlusion of arteries, most commonly in the lower extremities. It may be acute or chronic.

B. **Etiology**
1. **Acute occlusion** may result from trauma, thrombosis, or embolism. About 90% of acute occlusions occur in the lower extremities.
2. **Chronic occlusion** may be caused by:
    a. atherosclerosis
    b. inflammation
    c. thrombosis
    d. embolism
    e. trauma
    f. autoimmune response.

C. **Pathophysiology**
1. **Narrowing of the arterial lumen or damage to the endothelial lining** can result from such factors as atherosclerotic buildup of lipid deposits or arteriosclerosis obliterans that cause arterial occlusion. This leads to reduced or absent peripheral blood flow and, if unchecked, tissue ischemia and eventual necrosis.
2. **Acute arterial occlusion** results in an immediate decrease in arterial blood flow distal to the occlusion, with a resultant decrease in nutrient and oxygen supply to perfused tissue.
3. In **chronic arterial occlusion**, gradual onset allows for some development of collateral circulation around areas of occlusion. Chronic nutrient and oxygen deficit causes more trophic changes than acute occlusion.
4. **Effects of arterial occlusion in the lower extremities**
    a. Aortoiliac arterial stenosis and occlusion
    b. Femoropopliteal arterial stenosis and occlusion
    c. Arterial ulcers of distal toes, anterior tibia, and lateral malleolus
    d. Distal arterial embolization of large or small vessels of the feet
5. **Effects of arterial occlusion in the upper extremities**
    a. Subclavian steal syndrome, resulting in arm ischemia from blockage of the subclavian artery with subsequent incomplete perfusion from the carotid artery

b. Thoracic outlet syndrome, resulting from pinching of the subclavian artery by muscle, the first rib, or the clavicle

D. Assessment findings

1. Clinical manifestations of acute arterial occlusion (commonly called *the six Ps*):
   a. Pain or loss of sensory nerves secondary to ischemia
   b. Paresthesias and loss of position sense
   c. Polar or coldness
   d. Paralysis
   e. Pallor due to empty superficial vessels (can progress to mottled, cyanotic, and cadaverous cold leg)
   f. Pulselessness

2. Clinical manifestations of chronic arterial occlusion
   a. Intermittent claudication, which is calf muscle pain occurring when muscle is forced to contract without adequate blood supply (e.g., after walking a certain measurable distance). The calf muscle pain is alleviated with rest.
   b. Resting pain, which is pain at rest when limited blood flow cannot meet very low tissue requirements.
   c. Trophic changes in skin and nails, such as dryness, scaling, and thinning of skin; decreased or absent hair growth; brittle and thickened nails; and gangrenous changes marking death and decay of tissues.

3. Laboratory and diagnostic study findings
   a. Doppler ultrasound flow studies reveal that extremity blood pressure measurements in the legs are lower than in the arms.
   b. Angiography may confirm the diagnosis and shows vascular obstructions or aneurysms and the presence of collateral circulation.
   c. Digital subtraction angiography visualizes vascular obstructions, aneurysms, narrowing of vessels, and atherosclerotic plaque.

E. Nursing management

1. **Administer prescribed medications,** such as vasodilators, anticoagulants, antilipemic agents, thrombolytics, and antiplatelet drugs. (See *Drug chart 7-1,* pages 162 to 164.)

2. **Provide proper positioning.**
   a. Place the client's legs in a dependent position in relation to the heart to improve peripheral blood flow
   b. Avoid raising the client's feet above heart level unless specifically prescribed by the health care provider (e.g., as part of Burger-Allen exercises).
   c. Keep the client in a neutral, flat, supine position if in doubt about the nature of his peripheral vascular problems.

3. **Promote vasodilation.**
   a. Provide insulating warmth with gloves, socks, and other outerwear as appropriate.
   b. Keep room temperatures comfortably warm.
   c. Instruct the client to warm himself with warm drinks or baths.
   d. Never apply a direct heat source to the extremities. Limited blood flow combined with possible paresthesias can lead to tissue damage from heat earlier than would occur with normal circulation.
   e. Teach the client about the vasoconstrictive effects of nicotine and caffeine, emotional stress, and chilling; discuss ways to avoid or minimize these risk factors.
   f. Teach the client to avoid constricting clothes, such as garters, knee-high stockings, and belts. *(Text continues on page 164.)*

DRUG CHART 7-1
Medications for peripheral vascular disorders

Classifications	Indications	Selected interventions
Angiotensin-converting enzyme inhibitors captopril enalapril maleate lisinopril	Prevent angiotensin I from converting to angiotensin II, a potent vasoconstrictor, thereby decreasing peripheral vascular resistance; blocks the secretion of antidiuretic hormone (ADH)	■ Monitor blood pressure; if less than 90/60 mm Hg, hold and question the order. ■ Teach the client about orthostatic hypotension. ■ Instruct the client to not discontinue abruptly and to keep a record of blood-pressure readings between visits with the health care practitioner.
Angiotensin II receptor antagonists losartan valsartan	Block angiotension II at tissue receptor sites, thereby decreasing peripheral vascular resistance; blocks the secretion of aldosterone from the adrenal gland	■ Monitor blood pressure; if less than 90/60 mm Hg, hold and question the order. ■ Teach the client about orthostatic hypotension. ■ Instruct the client to not discontinue abruptly and to keep a record of blood-pressure readings between visits with the health care practitioner.
Antibiotics aminoglycosides (gentamycin, tobramycin) amoxicillin erythromycin penicillin tetracycline	Prevent or treat infections caused by pathogenic microorganism	■ Before administering the first dose, assess the client for allergies and determine whether a culture has been obtained. ■ After multiple doses, assess the client for superinfection (thrush, yeast infection, diarrhea); notify the health care provider if these signs occur. ■ Assess the insertion site for phlebitis if antibiotics are being administered I.V. ■ To assess the effectiveness of antibiotic therapy, monitor the white blood cell count. ■ Monitor peaks and troughs for aminoglycosides.
Anticoagulants I.V. heparin oral warfarin sodium	Prevent recurrence of emboli; no effect on emboli that are already present	■ For heparin therapy, monitor partial thromboplastin time (PTT), for which the therapeutic range should be 1.5 to 2 times the normal PTT or control; antidote is protamine sulfate. ■ For Coumadin therapy, monitor the International Normalized Ratio, for which the therapeutic level is 2 to 3; antidote is AquaMEPHYTON (vitamin K). ■ Instruct the client to report bruising, unexplained bleeding, or dark, tarry stools; use a soft bristle toothbrush; be cautious when using sharp objects and machinery; and wear a medi-alert bracelet. ■ Remind the client to inform all health care providers that he is taking these medications. ■ If bleeding occurs, instruct the client to apply direct pressure to the wound; if bleeding does not stop after 5 minutes of direct pressure, get medical help.
Subcutaneous low-dose heparin (5,000 units)	Prophylactically prevent deep vein thrombosis; heparin activates antithrombin III, which inactivates newly formed factor Xa and thrombin	■ Administer subcutaneously in the abdomen 1″ (2.5 cm) from the umbilicus. ■ Do not aspirate; do not massage. ■ Not necessary to monitor PTT.

DRUG CHART 7-1

Medications for peripheral vascular disorders *(continued)*

Classifications	Indications	Selected interventions
Antilipemic agents cholestyramine clofibrate colestipol **HMG-CoA reductase inhibitor** probucol	Lower serum cholesterol level by binding bile salts in the bowel and forming an insoluble complex that is excreted in the stool	■ Mix the medication with 60 ml water or fruit juice to mask the unpleasant flavor. ■ Instruct the client to increase his fluid intake to prevent constipation. ■ Instruct the client to take at night due to an enzyme that metabolizes cholesterol. ■ Monitor the client's cholesterol level; it should be <200 mg/dl.
Antiplatelet agents aspirin dipyridamole ticlopidine	Inhibit the aggregation of platelets to form a plug; platelets do not initiate thrombus formation as readily when taking antiplatelets	■ Instruct the client to take the medication with food to decrease gastric irritation. ■ Remind the client to inform health care providers that he is taking these medications and to be careful when taking over-the-counter medications. ■ Instruct the client to notify the health care provider if bruising, bleeding gums, nosebleeds, bleeding in the stools, or tinnitis occur.
Beta-adrenergic blockers atenolol metoprolol nadolol propranolol	Decrease the heart rate and the force of contraction; reduces vasoconstriction by antagonizing beta receptors in the myocardium and vasculature	■ If apical pulse rate falls below 60 beats per minute, hold and question the order. ■ Monitor blood pressure; if less than 90/60 mm Hg, hold and question the order. ■ Teach the client about orthostatic hypotension. ■ Teach the client about possible adverse effects.
Calcium channel blockers diltiazem nifedipine verapamil	Inhibit calcium ions from crossing myocardial and vascular smooth muscle, thereby producing vasodilation and decreasing myocardial contractility	■ If apical pulse rate falls below 60 beats per minute, hold and question the order. ■ Monitor blood pressure; if less than 90/60 mm Hg, hold and question the order. ■ Teach the client about orthostatic hypotension.
Central alpha agonists clonidine methyldopa	Stimulate alpha-adrenergic receptors in the central nervous system, resulting in decreased sympathetic outflow	■ If apical pulse rate falls below 60 beats per minute, hold and question the order. ■ Monitor blood pressure; if less than 90/60 mm Hg, hold and question the order. ■ Teach the client about orthostatic hypotension.
Diuretics loop diuretic—furosemide potassium-sparing diuretic— spironolactone thiazide diuretic—chlorothiazide	Decrease blood volume, which decreases the heart's workload	■ Monitor potassium level; do not administer if the client is hypokalemic or hyperkalemic. ■ Monitor intake and output; maintain fluid intake. ■ Monitor blood pressure; if less than 90/60 mm Hg, hold and question the order. ■ Teach the client about orthostatic hypotension. ■ Teach the client to weigh himself daily and report weight gain of more than 2 lb in 1 day. ■ Encourage foods high in potassium and potassium supplements.
Low-molecular-weight heparin enoxaprin	Prophylactically prevent deep-vein thrombosis by preferentially inactivating factor Xa	■ Administer in the anterolateral abdominal wall. ■ Do not aspirate; do not massage. ■ Insert air bubbles into the syringe. ■ Not necessary to monitor PTT.

(continued)

DRUG CHART 7-1
Medications for peripheral vascular disorders *(continued)*

Classifications	Indications	Selected interventions
Opioid analgesics codeine hydrocodone hydromophone morphine propoxyphene	Relieve moderate to severe pain by reducing pain sensation, producing sedation, and decreasing the emotional upset often associated with pain; most often schedule II drugs	■ Assess the pain for location, type, intensity, what increases or decreases it; rate pain on scale of 1 (no pain) to 10 (worst pain). ■ Rule out complications. Is this pain routine or expected pain? Is this a complication that needs immediate intervention? ■ Medicate according to pain scale findings. Institute safety measures—bed in low position, side rails up, and call light within reach. ■ Evaluate effectiveness of pain medication in 30 minutes.
Thrombolytic agents alteplase streptokinase urokinase	Dissolve thrombi or emboli in the coronary arteries	■ Follow hospital protocol when administering a thrombolytic agent. ■ Monitor for internal bleeding every 15 to 30 minutes for the first 8 hours and then every 4 hours throughout therapy.
Vasodilators diazoxide hydralazine nitroprusside sodium	Decrease preload by acting directly on blood vessels to cause dilation and decrease vascular resistance	■ Monitor blood pressure; if less than 90/60 mm Hg, hold and question the order. ■ For I.V. administration, have the client on a cardiac monitor. ■ Keep the client on bed rest, with safety precautions instituted.

4. **Promote and teach skin and foot care.** (See *Client and family teaching 7-1.*)
5. **Promote activity and mobility.**
    a. Use an orthoframe, trapeze, foot cradle, or padded foot board to promote healing and protect skin.
    b. For a client with decreased arterial function but without activity-limiting tissue damage, encourage a program of balanced exercise and rest to promote development of collateral circulation.
    c. Instruct the client to recognize pain or intermittent claudication as an indication to limit activity during exercise (i.e., view onset of pain as a signal to stop and rest).
6. **Provide a referral** to the American Heart Association. (See appendix A.)
7. **Provide care for a client undergoing angiography or percutaneous transluminal angioplasty.**
    a. Before the procedure, provide information related to the procedure; validate that informed consent has been obtained; mark peripheral pulses; obtain diagnostic data as ordered; and withhold food and fluids as prescribed.
    b. After the procedure, maintain bed rest as prescribed, keeping the involved extremity extended; monitor vital signs and assess peripheral pulses and circulation every 15 minutes for 2 hours and then every hour for 4 hours; assess for bleeding, hematoma, or edema at the catheter insertion site; encourage oral fluids; and monitor urine output.
8. **Provide care for a client receiving an autogenous saphenous vein or a synthetic bypass graft.**
    a. Prepare the client for surgery, and mark the site of the peripheral pulses.

---

    b. Monitor the client carefully after the procedure (especially for the first 24 hours) for signs of graft occlusion as manifested by decreased arterial perfusion.

    c. Position the involved extremity in the position prescribed by the health care provider to prevent constricted arterial flow and edema.

    d. Monitor the client for development of compartment syndrome (i.e., edema of calf muscles), which can impede circulation and necessitate fasciotomy, an incision in the fascia to relieve pressure on vessels.

    e. Be alert for embolization with ischemia of the foot and lower leg.

    f. Anticipate and take steps to prevent complications of any surgical procedure involving general anesthesia, particularly respiratory problems and infection. (See chapter 21.)

  9. **Provide care for a client who has received an axillofemoral or axillobifemoral bypass graft or an endarterectomy (i.e., removal of atheromatous plaque).**

    a. Avoid positioning the client on the side of the graft or incision after the procedure.

    b. Warn the client not to wear tight clothing, which can lead to graft occlusion.

    c. Instruct the client on signs and symptoms of infection to report to the health care provider.

 10. **Provide care for a client undergoing a sympathectomy** (i.e., interruption of sympathetic impulses to a lower extremity that eliminates vasospasm and improves peripheral blood flow).

 11. **Provide care for client undergoing an amputation.** (See section VIII.)

IV. DEEP VEIN THROMBOSIS

  A. **Description.** Deep vein thrombosis (DVT) is a blood clot formation in the deep veins of the lower extremities or in the pelvic veins leading to venous insufficiency.

  B. **Etiology.** Thrombus formation occurs when two of three conditions of Virchow's triad are present:

    1. **Venous stasis.** Conditions contributing to venous stasis include surgery, obesity, pregnancy, heart failure, and immobility.

2. **Hypercoagulability.** Conditions associated with hypercoagulability include malignant neoplasms, dehydration, blood dyscrasias, and hormonal contraceptive use.
3. **Venous wall injury.** Constriction of the leg due to garters, straps, or trauma to lower extremities may cause injury to venous walls.

C. Pathophysiology

1. A clot forms when platelets adhere to the vein lining or endothelium, release adenosine diphosphate, and begin the process of platelet aggregation, platelet plug, and clot formation. As a clot enlarges, it may block blood flow through the vein and obstruct venous drainage from the area distal to the clot.
2. Within 24 to 48 hours after formation, the clot may dislodge and travel to the pulmonary artery (i.e., pulmonary embolism), a life-threatening emergency.
3. Postphlebotic syndrome, or chronic venous insufficiency, results from dysfunctional valves that reduce venous return, increase venous pressure, and cause venous stasis; it follows most severe cases of DVT and may take 5 to 10 years to develop.

D. Assessment findings

1. **Clinical manifestations**
   a. **DVT** may be asymptomatic or may produce some or all of the following clinical manifestations:
   – edema (usually unilateral), erythema, and calf or thigh warmth associated with inflammation of phlebitis
   – pain in calf muscle on dorsiflexion (Homans' sign) due to stretching of inflamed vein
   – tenderness in calf or thigh
   – low-grade fever.
   b. **PPS** has the following hallmark signs:
   – chronic edematous limbs
   – thick, coarse, brownish skin around the ankles
   – venous stasis ulcers.
2. **Laboratory and diagnostic study findings**
   a. Doppler ultrasonography findings are diminished or absent compared with those for the opposite leg.
   b. Impedance plethysmography shows a decrease in venous volume that normally results from blood trapped below the level of the cuff.
   c. ^{125}I-labeled fibrinogen shows increased radioactivity in the progression of the clot; the test does not reveal thrombi that have already formed.
   d. Phlebography (venography) shows an unfilled segment of the vein in an otherwise completely filled vein with its connecting collaterals; this test is generally most indicative in diagnosing venous thrombosis.

E. Nursing management (See section II.D.)

1. **Administer prescribed medications,** which include anticoagulants and may include thrombolytics, analgesics, and prophylactic anticoagulants. (See *Drug chart 7-1,* pages 162 to 164.)
2. **Provide proper positioning.**
   a. Elevate the client's legs above heart level and have the client avoid prolonged standing or sitting to promote venous return.
   b. Instruct the client to avoid activities or positions that produce pressure on leg muscles.

    c. Maintain the client in a flat, supine position (bed rest may be used to facilitate healing) if in doubt regarding positioning.

  3. Promote venous return in the unaffected leg.

    a. Instruct the client to maximize the effects of the calf muscle pump to augment venous return by walking with a heel-toe gait and doing similar exercises if confined to bed.

    b. After surgery, encourage deep-breathing exercises, early ambulation to promote venous return, use of antiembolism stockings, and use of sequential compression devices to help prevent DVT.

    c. Elevate the foot of the bed about 6″ (15.2 cm) while the client is sleeping to promote venous return.

  4. Maximize comfort.

    a. Decrease discomfort through measures that promote venous return.

    b. Apply warm packs to the legs to reduce pain.

  5. Provide care associated with medical and surgical interventions, as appropriate.

    a. Assess postoperative clients and clients with decreased activity and a history of DVT for signs of thrombophlebitis.

    b. Observe the lower extremities for skin changes.

    c. Carefully monitor venous and arterial function in the affected extremity after invasive vein procedures, which may include phlebography, thrombectomy, embolectomy, vein ligation, or interruption of the vena cava with a device to prevent emboli.

    d. Assess for hemorrhage, infection, nerve damage, and DVT after surgical removal of varicose veins.

  6. Instruct the client to avoid sources of pressure above the knees (e.g., crossing the legs, sitting in chairs that are too high, and wearing garters and knee-high stocking).

V. VENOUS STASIS ULCERS

A. Description. Venous stasis ulcers are excavations of the skin surface resulting from sloughing of inflamed necrotic tissue, usually in the lower extremities. The incidence of venous stasis ulcers is increasing, especially in elderly people.

B. Etiology

  1. Postphlebotic syndrome and venous stasis (the most common cause)

  2 Deep vein obstruction from abdominal tumor or pregnancy

  3. Valvular incompetency in the ileofemoral vein

  4. Major burns

  5. Sickle cell disease

  6. Neurogenic disorders

  7. Hereditary factors

C. Pathophysiology. Over time, incompetent valves in veins result in excessive venous pressure and subsequent rupture of small skin veins and venules. Chronic changes of subcutaneous fibrosis, cutaneous atrophy, and lymphatic obstruction associated with stasis contribute to tissue breakdown and infection in local tissues. After the skin breaks down and venous ulcers develop, healing is prolonged and difficult. The problem may be lifelong.

D. Assessment findings

  1. Common clinical manifestations

    a. Visible skin ulcers

        b. Dark pigmentation

        c. Eczema or stasis dermatitis

        d. Normal arterial pulses

        e. Pain, ranging from mild discomfort to dull aching (typically relieved by leg elevation)

    2. **Laboratory and diagnostic study findings** (See section IV.D.2.)

E. Nursing management (See section II.D.)

    1. **Administer medications,** which may include antibiotics. (See *Drug chart 7-1,* pages 162 to 164.)

    2. **Provide for ulcer debridement and healing.**

        a. Remove dead or damaged material from the wound, using wet-to-dry dressings with saline solution and coarse-mesh gauze filled with cotton.

        b. Use whirlpool therapy to debride the ulcer bed.

        c. Consider using an enzymatic debrider to aid removal of debris.

        d. Prepare for surgical debridement, if necessary.

        e. Assist in application of an Unna's boot (dressing of medicated gauze covered with elastic wrap), as ordered.

    3. **Provide additional nursing interventions** to promote venous return and healing, maximize comfort, and provide client education for measures to prevent venous stasis ulcer. (See section IV.E; see also *Client and family teaching 7-1,* page 165.)

VI. VARICOSE VEINS

A. Description. Varicose veins are abnormally dilated veins with incompetent valves occurring most commonly in the lower extremities and lower trunk, usually in the great and small saphenous veins. (See *Figure 7-3.*) Varicose veins are fairly common, affecting about 15% of the adult population. The incidence is about three times greater among women than men.

B. Etiology

    1. Congenital valve or vein wall defects

    2. Valve damage from trauma, obstruction, deep vein thrombosis (DVT), or inflammation

    3. Chronic venous distention associated with occupations requiring prolonged standing, obesity, or pregnancy

    4. Systemic conditions that interfere with venous return

    5. Loss of vein wall elasticity with aging

C. Pathophysiology. Weakened vein walls cannot withstand normal pressure and dilate with pooling of blood. Vein dilation prevents the valve cusps from meeting, resulting in increased backup pressure in lower vein segments. Increased dilation increases valve stretching and worsens the condition.

D. Assessment findings

    1. **Clinical manifestations**

        a. The most obvious manifestation is dilated, twisting, discolored veins, usually of the legs but possibly on the lower trunk.

        b. Many people experience few symptoms beyond dilated leg veins and mild leg aching after prolonged standing.

        c. Other people experience more serious effects, such as:

           – easy leg fatigue

           – cramping (especially nocturnal) and a feeling of heaviness in the legs

           – ankle edema

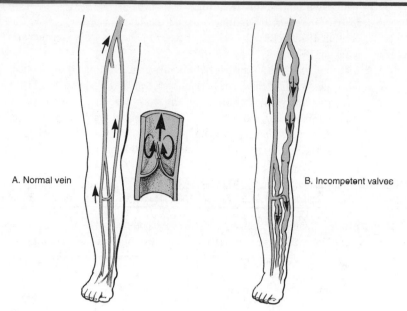

FIGURE 7-3

Varicose veins

A. Normal vein with competent valves. **B.** Incompetent valves with tortuous, dilated segments; promotes stasis of blood in lower extremities.

Source: Bullock, B.L., and Henze, R.L. *Focus on Pathophysiology*. Philadelphia: Lippincott Williams & Wilkins, 2000.

- – signs and symptoms of deep venous insufficiency
- – rarely, bleeding with abrasion of a vein surface.

  2. **Laboratory and diagnostic study findings**

  a. The Brodie-Trendelenburg test evaluates valve competency. Blood flows into the superficial veins from the deep veins if the communicating veins are incompetent.

  b. Perthes' test reveals if the deep vein system and communicating veins are competent. If the vessels do not empty but become distended on walking after a tourniquet is applied, valve obstruction is inferred.

  c. Doppler ultrasonography can detect retrograde blood flow in superficial veins with incompetent valves.

  d. Plethysmography reveals a change in venous blood volume.

  e. Phlebography (venography) shows abnormalities in vein anatomy during various leg disorders.

E. Nursing management (See section II.D.)

  1. **Promote venous return in the unaffected leg.** Discuss the importance of changing positions frequently and elevating legs above the heart.

  2. **Provide care associated with medical and surgical interventions, as appropriate.**

  a. Prepare the client for surgery, if scheduled. (See chapter 21.)

  b. Postoperatively, observe for skin changes, monitor venous and arterial function carefully, and assess for hemorrhage, infection, nerve damage, and DVT.

3. **Provide client and family teaching.**
   a. Instruct the client to avoid anything that can increase pressure above the knees (e.g., crossing the legs, sitting in chairs that are too high, wearing garters and knee-high stockings).
   b. Instruct the client on the use of antiembolism stockings, support hose, or elastic stockings. Instruct the client to put on stockings while lying down with legs in the air to promote venous return. Apply the stockings to clean, dry legs. The stockings may be removed once or twice daily and should be washed and air dried regularly. (See *Client and family teaching 7-1*, page 165.)
   c. Discuss the importance of losing weight if the client is obese.

VII. LYMPHEDEMA

A. Description. Lymphedema is tissue edema caused by obstructed lymph flow in an extremity. It may be primary or secondary. Primary lymphedema may be congenital (i.e., present at birth), praecox (i.e., developing early in life), or tardia (i.e., developing late in life). Lymphedema praecox is the most common type, with peak incidence occurring in the second decade of life and most commonly affecting females.

B. Etiology
1. **Primary lymphedema,** also known as *lymphedema of unknown origin* or *idiopathic lymphedema,* may be associated with:
   a. aplasia (no lymph vessels)
   b. hypoplasia (smaller or fewer lymph vessels than normal)
   c. hyperplasia (larger or more numerous lymph vessels).
2. **Secondary lymphedema** results from damage or obstruction of the lymph system by disease or procedure, such as:
   a. trauma
   b. neoplasms
   c. mosquito-transmitted filariasis
   d. inflammation
   e. surgical excision of axillary, inguinal, or iliac lymph nodes
   f. high-dose radiation therapy.

C. Pathophysiology
1. Collection of lymph distal to a blocked lymphatic results in increased intralymphatic pressures, causing lymphatic wall dilation and valve incompetency. Resultant backward lymph flow produces lymphatic dilation and valve incompetency in distal lymphatics and, if unchecked, eventually in even the smallest peripheral lymphatics. Increased intralymphatic pressure leads to protein accumulation in the interstitial spaces. Protein accumulation increases colloid osmotic pressures in the tissues, resulting in fluid retention and edema.
2. Chronic lymph congestion leads to fibrosis, formation of dense connective tissue in subcutaneous tissue.

D. Assessment findings
1. **Clinical manifestations**
   a. **Primary lymphedema**
      – Nonpitting edema
      – Dull, heavy sensation

- Absence of pain
- Roughened skin without ulceration of skin or cellulitis
- Marked limb enlargement

b. **Secondary lymphedema**
- Secondary lymphedema related to filariasis may produce:
  - intermittent episodes of high fever with chills
  - malaise and fatigue
  - tender regional lymphadenopathy
  - severe muscle pain
  - areas of erythema with increased edema and elephantiasis (i.e., severe edema).
- Secondary lymphedema related to neoplasms commonly causes nonpainful lymph node enlargement or edema.

2. **Laboratory and diagnostic study findings**
   a. **Lymphangiography** injects a contrast medium into lymphatic vessels, which can be visualized on the radiograph. The lymphomatous lymph nodes retain the contrast agent for up to 1 year.
   b. **Lymphoscintigraphy** injects a radioactive colloid subcutaneously, which uptakes into the lymph system. Serial images visualize abnormal lymph nodes.

E. Nursing management (See section II.D.)
   1. **Administer prescribed medications,** which may include diuretics and anticoagulants. (See *Drug chart 7-1,* pages 162 to 164.)
   2. **Assess the client's neurovascular status.**
   3. **Assess for lymphedema.**
      a. Measure and compare extremities for enlargement in all clients at risk.
      b. Assess for coexisting symptoms of lymphedema (initially pitting then brawny and nonpitting edema, no pain, and absence of infection) to rule out venous disorder as the cause of edema.
   4. **Promote lymphatic drainage**
      a. Collaborate with physical therapy for arm or leg lymphedema, which includes mechanical or manual squeezing of tissue followed by specific active and passive exercises to press stagnant lymphatic fluid into the blood stream.
      b. Elevate the affected extremity (e.g., elevate the arm on a pillow with the elbow higher than the shoulder and the hand higher than the elbow).
      c. Apply an elastic sleeve or stocking if prescribed for chronic lymphedema.
      d. Measure the circumference of the affected extremity with a tape measure to assess the client's progress.
      e. Prepare the client for excisional removal of edematous subcutaneous tissue, if planned.
   5. **Provide client and family teaching.** Instruct the client and his family to observe for and report red streaks on the affected extremity, fever and chills, penetrating wounds, and enlarged and tender lymph nodes.
   6. **Provide emotional support.**
      a. Assist the client with a diagnosis of neoplastic disease in coping with associated problems.
      b. Encourage the client to express fears and concerns, such as about altered body image; listen actively.
      c. Assist the client experiencing altered body image to select concealing clothing and take other measures to emphasize positive aspects of body image.

VIII. EXTREMITY AMPUTATION

A. **Description.** Extremity amputation is surgical resection of a limb or a part of a limb. Peripheral vascular disease accounts for most lower extremity amputations.

B. **Indications**
   1. **Life-threatening situations**
      a. Severe toxicity due to gangrene, usually caused by chronic arterial occlusion
      b. Malignant tumors
      c. Severe osteomyelitis
   2. **Intractable limb pain** from:
      a. Chronic infections
      b. Trophic ulcers
   3. **Chronic and severe functional impairment due to a damaged extremity** from:
      a. injury, including crushing wounds
      b. congenital deformities
      c. chronic ischemia from extensive peripheral vascular disease.

C. **Types**
   1. **Open or guillotine amputation** is usually performed on an infected limb because it allows the wound to drain freely. A second surgery for residual limb revision and closure is done after infection has been eradicated. (See *Figure 7-4.*)
   2. **Closed or flap amputation** is performed when there is no evidence of infection and no need for draining. (See *Figure 7-4.*)

D. **Prostheses**
   1. **Types of prostheses**
      a. A **total-contact rigid dressing** sometimes is applied in the operating room (immediate prosthetic fitting) to protect the residual limb from injury and prevent residual limb edema by gently compressing tissue.
      b. A **permanent leg prosthesis** is a rigid dressing that connects to an adjustable pylon and foot-ankle assembly to permit walking. This prosthesis must be changed three to four times before application of a permanent prosthesis, because the residual limb shrinks with healing.
      c. A **soft dressing** may be used when frequent inspection of the residual limb is required. A wound drainage device may be necessary.
   2. **Level of amputation.** The two factors that determine the level of amputation are adequate circulation to the limb and prosthetic requirements. The most distal site that can heal successfully is used. (See *Figure 7-4.*)

E. **Complications.** Infection, bleeding, skin breakdown, and pain are common complications of amputation. Immediate prosthetic fitting is thought to reduce problems of infection and bleeding.

F. **Nursing management (See section II.D.)**
   1. **Administer prescribed medications,** which may include opioid analgesics and antibiotics. (See *Drug chart 7-1,* pages 162 to 164.)
   2. **Provide proper positioning, and take measures to prevent contractures.**
      a. After 48 hours, avoid elevating the residual limb to prevent the formation of contractures.

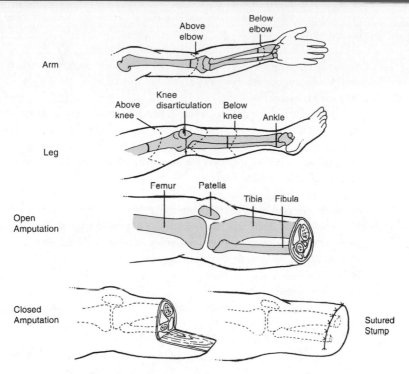

FIGURE 7-4

The most common amputations of the extremities occur in landmarks and are known generally as below the elbow, above the elbow, at the ankle (also called *Syme's operation*), below the knee, and above the knee. The operations are usually called open amputation, indicating that the wound remains open for drainage until infection resolves and the wound can be closed, or closed or flap amputation, indicating that there is no infection to contraindicate closing the wound immediately after the operation.

       b. Avoid positioning the residual limb in an externally rotated, abducted position to prevent contractures.

       c. Prevent abduction contractures by adducting the residual limb on a regular schedule.

       d. Initiate exercises to prevent contractures as soon as possible (ideally, on the first or second postoperative day), including active range-of-motion exercises for the remaining leg, strengthening exercises for the arms, and hyperextension of the residual limb.

       e. Have the client who received a prosthesis immediately walk as early as the first postoperative day to help prevent contractures (using a rigid cast prevents hip and joint contractures).

       f. Position the client prone for several hours each day.

   3. Maintain skin integrity.

       a. Inspect the residual limb and all bony prominences daily for evidence of skin breakdown or infection.

       b. Provide a high-protein diet with vitamin and mineral supplements.

       c. Keep the client well hydrated with oral or I.V. fluids.

4. **Minimize phantom limb pain.** Phantom limb sensation occurs in 1% to 10% of all clients with amputations, especially in above-the-knee amputations, for some time after the amputation.

   a. Keep the client active to help decrease phantom limb pain.

   b. Believe the client who reports phantom pain. The pain phenomenon is real to the client. Medicate for pain as ordered.

5. **Monitor for excessive bleeding.**

   a. Outline blood stains on dressings with a pen and observe every 10 minutes for 24 hours for an increase in size. Report excessive bleeding at once.

   b. Keep a large tourniquet at the bedside in case of massive hemorrhage.

6. **Assess and intervene as indicated for hematoma formation,** which delays wound healing and provides a culture medium for bacterial growth. Assist the surgeon with hematoma aspiration as necessary.

7. **Take steps to prevent residual limb edema.**

   a. Elevate the residual limb on a pillow for 24 to 48 hours to improve venous return, prevent edema, and promote comfort. Do not elevate the residual limb for more than 48 hours, which could lead to hip contracture.

   b. Apply a plaster cast sock or elastic compression stocking to the residual limb immediately after surgery.

8. **Provide support to the client and family.** Amputation may affect self-image and may be difficult to accept, particularly by a young person. Keep in mind, however, that a person suffering chronic pain may welcome amputation.

   a. Encourage self-care and independent mobility, and promote a positive self-concept. Observe carefully for signs of depression or despondency.

   b. Assess the client's and family's adaptation to the amputation and provide support as needed.

9. **Assess for and intervene as necessary to prevent or control general postoperative complications** that prolong healing and delay a return to self-care. (See chapter 21.)

10. **Provide client and family teaching for residual limb care.**

   a. Instruct the client to wash the residual limb with mild soap, rinse carefully, and dry thoroughly and to perform careful daily inspection with a mirror for redness, blistering, or abrasions.

   b. Instruct the client to avoid putting adhesive bandages or tape on the residual limb. They may irritate the skin and cause sores and infection when pulled off.

   c. Advise the client to avoid applying creams or lotions (softens skin excessively) or alcohol (dries the skin, leading to cracking) to the residual limb.

   d. Discuss wearing a woolen residual limb sock without holes or darned areas and washing clothing in cool water with mild soap to prevent shrinkage.

11. **Provide client and family teaching for proper prosthesis use and care.**

   a. Instruct the client to put the prosthesis on immediately after arising and keep it on all day to prevent residual limb edema.

   b. Advise the client to clean the prosthesis socket daily with a damp cloth. Also advise the client to avoid pouring water into the socket, which may damage leather parts and cause metal parts to rust. Instruct him to dry the prostheses thoroughly to prevent skin irritation.

   c. Stress the importance of never adjusting or mechanically altering the prosthesis without professional help.

   d. Urge the client to schedule a yearly appointment for follow-up evaluation of the prosthesis and necessary adjustments.

  e. Instruct the client to inspect and care for the remaining foot. (See *Client and family teaching 7-1*, page 165.)

12. **Provide a referral** to the National Amputee Foundation and Amputee Shoe and Glove Exchange. (See appendix A.)

IX. HYPERTENSIVE VASCULAR DISEASE

A. **Description.** Hypertensive vascular disease is an intermittent or sustained elevation in systolic or diastolic blood pressure. It occurs as two major types, which include primary (essential) hypertension and secondary hypertension. About 20% of the adult population develops hypertension. More than 90% of these cases are primary hypertension, and about 10% are secondary hypertension.

B. **Etiology**
1. **Primary hypertension** has no identifiable medical cause.
   a. **Nonmodifiable risk factors** include:
   - family history
   - gender (Men are at greater risk than women.)
   - race (In the United States, blacks have twice the risk of whites.)
   - age.
   b. **Modifiable risk factors** include:
   - stress
   - obesity
   - high dietary intake of sodium or saturated fats
   - excessive caffeine, alcohol, or tobacco use
   - hormonal contraceptive use
   - sedentary lifestyle.
2. **Secondary hypertension.** Conditions associated with secondary hypertension include:
   a. renal vascular disease
   b. primary hyperaldosteronism
   c. pheochromocytoma
   d. coarctation of the aorta
   e. thyroid, parathyroid, or pituitary dysfunction
   f. pregnancy-induced hypertension.

C. **Pathophysiology.** Increased peripheral resistance controlled at the arteriolar level is the basic pathophysiologic cause for elevated blood pressure. The cause of increased peripheral resistance is poorly understood, but the following factors tend to perpetuate the hypertensive state:
1. Stimulation of the vasomotor center (located in the medulla of the brain) sends impulses through the sympathetic nervous system to the sympathetic ganglia. Acetylcholine released by the preganglionic neurons cause the postganglionic nerve fibers to release norepinephrine, which causes the constriction of the blood vessels, thereby increasing blood pressure.
2. The adrenal medulla secretes epinephrine, which results in vasoconstriction of the peripheral vessels.
3. Vasoconstriction of the blood vessels causes the release of renin; renin leads to the formation of angiotensin I, which converts to angiotensin II, a potent vasoconstrictor.
4. Secretion of aldosterone by the adrenal cortex causes sodium and water to be retained, which leads to an increase in intravascular volume.

5. Uncontrolled hypertension increases the risk of various complications, including stroke, coronary artery disease, heart failure, renal failure, and eye changes.

D. Assessment findings

1. **Clinical manifestations**
   a. Hypertension usually produces no symptoms until vascular changes occur in the heart, brain, or kidneys.
   b. Physical examination may reveal no abnormalities, but changes may be seen in the retina.
   c. The client may exhibit epistaxis, occipital headache, or a flushed face if symptomatic.

2. **Laboratory and diagnostic study findings**
   a. Serial blood pressure readings. The following results are diagnostic of hypertensive disorders: a minimum of three readings on separate occasions measuring above 135/85 mm Hg in persons younger than age 60 or 160/85 mm Hg in persons older than age 60.
   b. Urinalysis detects an increased protein level and the inability to concentrate urine.
   c. I.V. pyelography and a renogram show renovascular disease.
   d. Blood urea nitrogen and creatinine levels are increased because of renal involvement.
   e. Electrocardiogram shows left ventricular hypertrophy.
   f. Chest radiograph shows left ventricular hypertrophy.

E. Nursing management (See section II.D.)

1. **Administer medications,** as prescribed. (See *Drug chart 7-1,* pages 162 to 164.)
   a. Medications may include thiazide, loop, and potassium-sparing diuretics; calcium channel blockers; beta-adrenergic blockers; angiotensin-converting enzyme inhibitors; angiotensin II receptor antagonists, central-alpha agonists, vasodilators, and antilipemic agents (HMG-CoA reductase inhibitors). The "stepped-care" approach for primary hypertension progresses through the preceding medications, used alone or in combination. Prepare the client for a possible "trial and error" approach to determining the right medication regimen.
   b. Instruct the client to continue medication even if such adverse effects as dizziness, lightheadedness, or impotency occur. Advise the client to notify his health care provider of adverse effects so the medication can be changed.
   c. Not all persons with primary hypertension need medication to achieve and maintain blood-pressure control. A nonpharmacologic approach is helpful for individuals with mild hypertension and is an effective adjunctive therapy for those receiving medications. A nonpharmacologic approach consists primarily of teaching, and its success depends on the client's compliance with necessary lifestyle modifications.

2. **Monitor blood pressure.** Because many people experience transient blood pressure elevations during examination, remeasurement after about 10 minutes is recommended to obtain a more accurate reading.

3. **Provide client and family teaching.**
   a. Advise the client to reduce his weight by restricting his caloric intake (especially cholesterol and fats).
   b. Instruct the client to restrict sodium intake (collaborate with a dietitian) and reduce or avoid alcohol and caffeine intake (caffeine stimulates the sympathetic nervous system).
   c. Urge the client to stop smoking, if applicable. This is a lifestyle modification that must be addressed.

      d. Encourage the client to conduct a regular physical activity and exercise program. Exercise enhances the sense of well-being, provides an outlet for emotional tension, raises serum levels of high-density lipoproteins, and aids in weight control. Recommend a gradually progressive program of aerobic activity, such as walking, jogging, or swimming; discourage isometric exercises such as weight lifting.

      e. Promote relaxation techniques (i.e., progressive relaxation, meditation, autogenic training, biofeedback, and yoga).

      f. Discuss the importance of regular blood-pressure monitoring. Teach the client how to take blood-pressure measurements and keep a record of the readings. Instruct him to take the record to future medical appointments.

      g. Discuss the importance of lifelong medical follow-up examinations. Remind the client that the disease is known as the "silent killer" because severe organ damage can occur even if the client is asymptomatic.

      h. Teach the client and his family about the disease process, factors contributing to symptoms and risks, and the importance of effective management. Evaluate the client's compliance.

   4. Intervene in a hypertensive crisis (blood pressure needs to be lowered immediately).

      a. Monitor I.V. antihypertensive medication administration; assess blood pressure and heart rate every 5 to 15 minutes; stay with the client, and maintain bed rest with the side rails up and the call light within reach.

      b. Assess for target organ damage as manifested by:
- restlessness, confusion, somnolence, coma, seizures, blurred vision, headache, nausea, and vomiting (i.e., signs of hypertensive encephalopathy)
- signs of left ventricular failure and myocardial ischemia
- azotemia, oliguria, protein, sediment, and red blood cells in urine in cases of renal damage.

   5. Provide a referral to the American Heart Association. (See appendix A.)

X. HYPOTHERMIA AND FROSTBITE

A. Description. Hypothermia refers to an abnormally low core body temperature (below 94° F [34.4° C]) resulting from exposure to cold environmental temperatures. Frostbite involves damage to tissue and blood vessels from exposure to extreme cold.

B. Etiology. Hypothermia is caused by extreme exposure to cold. It has a high mortality rate for elderly people, infants, people with chronic health problems, and people who are homeless. Frostbite occurs mostly in the feet, hands, nose, and ears after extreme exposure to cold.

C. Pathophysiology. Vasoconstriction of blood vessels secondary to extreme exposure to cold results in a decreased blood supply to the peripheral circulation. The decreased blood supply causes damage and possible necrosis of affected areas.

D. Assessment findings
   1. Hypothermia
      a. Subnormal body temperature
      b. Altered level of consciousness, including apathy, drowsiness, and coma
      c. Weak or undetectable peripheral pulses
      d. Cardiac arrhythmias, possibly cardiac arrest
      e. Signs and symptoms of hypoxia and acidosis

2. Frostbite
   a. Cold tissue
   b. Hard tissue
   c. White to bluish-white skin
   d. Numbness or pain
   e. Blisters
   f. Edema

E. Nursing management (See section II.D.)

1. Initiate cardiopulmonary resuscitation, if indicated.
2. Implement measures to rewarm the client.
   a. Use a hyperthermia blanket (external), warmed humidified oxygen, and warmed I.V. fluids (internal).
   b. Monitor the client's body temperature with an esophageal or rectal thermistor probe.
   c. Monitor vital signs, central venous pressure, electrocardiogram, arterial blood gases, and intake and output.
3. Administer I.V. fluids and sodium bicarbonate, as ordered.
4. Implement appropriate measures for the client with frostbite.
   a. Protect the affected area from injury, handle it gently, use a protective cradle if indicated, and maintain strict aseptic technique.
   b. Rewarm the body part (e.g., in a warm whirlpool).
   c. Elevate the body part.
   d. Do not massage the affected area.

XI. AORTIC ANEURYSMS

A. Description

1. An aneurysm is a dilation involving an artery formed at a weak point in the vessel wall; the aneurysm may be saccular (i.e., on one side of vessel only) or fusiform (i.e., entire arterial segment becomes dilated).
2. The three types of aortic aneurysms are abdominal aortic aneurysm (AAA), thoracic aortic aneurysm, and dissecting aneurysm of the aorta.
3. Aortic aneurysms occur primarily in men older than age 50.
4. The mortality rate for clients with ruptured aneurysm is very high.

B. Etiology. Most aneurysms are caused by atherosclerosis.

C. Pathophysiology. All aneurysms involve a damaged media layer of the vessel caused by congenital weakness, trauma, or disease. Large and medium-sized arteries are affected when lipids, calcium, blood components, carbohydrates, and fibrous tissue accumulate on the artery's intimal layer. This plaque weakens the artery, making it more susceptible to aneurysms. In some situations, the aorta may develop a tear in the intima or the media layer, resulting in a dissection.

D. Assessment findings

1. **Associated findings.** Risk factors include genetic predisposition, smoking, and hypertension.
2. **Clinical manifestations**
   a. **AAA.** Approximately two thirds of clients with AAA are asymptomatic, but clients may complain of feeling the "heart beating" in the abdomen or an abdominal mass, presence of a pulsatile mass in the middle and upper abdomen, or a systolic bruit.

b. **Thoracic aortic aneurysms.** Clinical manifestations may include constant, boring chest pain when lying in the supine position, brassy cough, hoarseness, and dysphagia.

c. **Dissecting aneurysm of the aorta.** Clinical manifestations may include the sudden onset of severe and persistent "tearing" or "ripping" in the anterior chest or back that extends to the shoulders, epigastric area, and abdomen and include cardiovascular, neurologic, and GI symptoms, depending on the location of the dissection.

3. **Laboratory and diagnostic study findings**

   a. Computed tomography determines the size of the aneurysm.

   b. Ultrasound determines the size of the aneurysm.

   c. Routine chest radiographs often detect aneurysms.

E. Nursing management (See section II.D.)

1. **Administer medications,** which may include antihypertensive medications. (See *Drug chart 7-1*, pages 162 to 164.)

2. **Prepare the client for serial ultrasonography,** which is conducted every 6 months to assess size of the aneurysm.

3. **Ensure that no additional pressure is exerted in the abdominal cavity,** such as by enemas, belts, or trauma.

4. **Implement nursing care for the client undergoing surgery to repair an aneurysm.** When the aneurysm is larger than 2" (5 cm) or there is a possibility of rupture, it will be surgically removed. (See chapter 21.)

5. After surgery, instruct the client to modify his lifestyle as if he had been diagnosed with hypertension because atherosclerosis is the primary cause of aneurysm. (See section IX.E.)

Study questions

1. After right femoral angiography that occurred 4 hours earlier, the nurse notices that the client's right leg and foot are cool and pale and that she is unable to palpate any pulses in the foot. Which nursing intervention would the nurse implement *first*?

1. Reassuring the client that this is a common complication
2. Notifying the client's health care provider immediately with the findings
3. Elevating the leg and administering an analgesic as ordered
4. Ambulating the client to restore circulation to the foot

2. A 24-year-old female client has been admitted for evaluation of severe right leg lymphedema of idiopathic origin. Which statement describes the rationale for addressing the client's reaction to the problem in the care plan?

1. Lymphedema signals cancer.
2. The infection results from inadequate bathing.
3. Leg edema can cause severe limb disfigurement.
4. Altered circulation may necessitate leg amputation.

3. Which nursing intervention should be included when caring for a client who has undergone a closed below-the-knee amputation of the right leg because of gangrene of the right foot?

1. Monitoring for bleeding and wound healing
2. Explaining about a second surgery in preparation for prosthesis fitting
3. Placing the residual limb in a dependent position immediately after surgery
4. Positioning the residual limb in an externally rotated, abducted position

4. At a blood pressure screening clinic, an elderly client exhibits a reading of 169/94 mm Hg. Which statement by the nurse would be most appropriate?
1. "Your blood pressure is normal. Please come back in a year and have it checked again."
2. "Your blood pressure is slightly elevated. Please have it checked again in the next 6 months."
3. "Your blood pressure is slightly elevated. Make an appointment to see your doctor in the next few weeks."
4. "Your blood pressure is dangerously elevated. Please have it evaluated immediately at the emergency department."

5. During an assessment of a client with intermittent claudication associated with exercise, which data would be *most important* for the nurse to assess?
1. Leg color, temperature, pulses, and pain description
2. Smoking history, deep vein thrombosis (DVT) history, and presence of edema
3. Allergy and medication history, and usual activity pattern
4. Menopausal state, occupation, and socioeconomic status

6. During a local health fair, a 45-year-old client presents with blood pressure of 140/92 mm Hg. Which interventions should the nurse implement? (Select all that apply.)
1. Explaining that this is a normal blood pressure
2. Instructing the client to see his health care provider as soon as possible
3. Instructing the client go to the nearest emergency department immediately
4. Discussing the importance of a low-fat, low-cholesterol, low-salt diet
5. Explaining the proper way to perform Burger-Allen exercises
6. Instructing the client to quit smoking, if appropriate.

7. Which rationale is *most* appropriate for placing a client's legs in a dependent position in relation to the heart for a client with chronic arterial occlusive disease of the lower extremities?
1. Improve activity tolerance
2. Decrease pain
3. Reduce risk for disuse syndrome
4. Improve peripheral blood flow

8. Which assessment data indicates that a client admitted for abdominal surgery under general anesthesia is at increased risk for developing postoperative deep vein thrombosis?
1. The client is 5'7" and 125 lb.
2. The client walks 2 miles daily for exercise.
3. The client has a history of three uneventful pregnancies.
4. The client requires bed rest for a short time after the surgery.

9. Which nursing intervention should be included for a client diagnosed with peripheral arterial occlusive disease?
1. Teaching about proper foot care
2. Warning against alcohol ingestion
3. Promoting a low-residue diet
4. Encouraging the use of heavy, tight, support stockings

10. Approximately 12 hours after a heparin infusion is started for a client diagnosed with deep vein thrombosis of the right leg, the client reports gum bleeding when brushing his teeth. Which intervention should the nurse implement?
1. Discontinuing the heparin infusion immediately
2. Notifying the health care provider of the client's symptoms
3. Administering a coumarin derivative as an antidote
4. Reassuring the client that this is normal

11. Three days after a foot amputation, a client complaining of severe pain in the foot cannot understand why the missing foot hurts so much. Which intervention should the nurse implement?
1. Assessing the residual limb site for signs and symptoms of bleeding and administer anticoagulants
2. Reassuring the client that phantom pain commonly occurs and eventually should subside, then administering an analgesic
3. Reassuring the client that phantom pain is rare and will soon disappear, and then administering a sedative
4. Monitoring the client carefully for infection in the residual limb and elevating the limb for 72 hours

12. A client is being discharged to a rehabilitation unit after a below-the-knee amputation resulting from peripheral vascular disease. Which goal would provide the *best* measure to evaluate the expected outcome of absence of wound infection?
1. The client demonstrates urinary output within normal limits.
2. The client reports pain relief from pain medication.
3. The client demonstrates a respiratory rate within normal limits.
4. The client maintains body temperature within normal range.

13. A woman with essential hypertension whose blood pressure remains elevated reports that she never eats salt but does not like to take her pills because they "make me dizzy and I go to the bathroom all night." Based on this information, which nursing diagnosis would be most appropriate for this client?
1. Noncompliance with the self-care program related to negative effects of prescribed therapy
2. Deficient knowledge related to the relation between the treatment regimen and disease control

3. Noncompliance with the self-care program related to recent short-term memory loss
4. Deficient knowledge related to the relationship between the medication's adverse effects and its therapeutic effects

14. The client diagnosed with essential hypertension has a blood pressure of 224/118 mm Hg, pulse rate of 74 beats per minute, and a respiration rate of 22. Which additional assessment data would be *essential* to collect to determine the possibility of complications associated with hypertension?
1. Last blood glucose level
2. Most recent bowel movement
3. Complaints of chest pain
4. Presence of leg cramps

15. Which statement indicates that a client with essential hypertension understands and can comply with the therapeutic regimen to achieve long-term control of hypertension?
1. "I know that if I take my antihypertensive medications, I do not need to worry about my diet."
2. "I must never discontinue a prescribed medication without my doctor's permission."
3. "I can adjust the dosage of my antihypertensive medication based on my home blood pressure readings."
4. "I need to continue taking my antihypertensive medication even if adverse effects develop."

16. Which clinical manifestation would the nurse expect to find when assessing a client with varicose veins?
1. Dilated, twisting, discolored veins and nocturnal cramping
2. Intermittent claudication and nonpalpable pedal pulses
3. A positive Homans' sign and an edematous, reddened calf
4. Marked limb enlargement and nonpitting edema

Answer key

1. The answer is **2.**

The nurse's assessment findings indicate an acute occlusion of arterial circulation, possibly by an embolus or thrombus after angiography. This necessitates immediate intervention by the health care provider to restore circulation to the leg. Because the assessment findings are not normal, reassuring the client would be inappropriate. Although pain medication would be appropriate, elevating the leg would further impede arterial circulation to the foot. Ambulation and calf muscle exercises would cause further tissue ischemia.

2. The answer is **3.**

The client is experiencing lymphedema praecox, the most common type of idiopathic lymphedema, with a peak incidence in the second decade of life. This disorder results in nonpitting edema with mild to severe enlargement of the limb. Because of the client's age and developmental level, the client may be at risk for disturbed body image because of the limb enlargement. The nurse must address this area in the client's care plan. Cancer is not a cause of idiopathic lymphedema; however, lymphedema can be associated with neoplasms. Lymphedema is not an infection, but it may result from one. Extremity amputation would not be indicated in this case.

3. The answer is **1.**

In the immediate postoperative period, bleeding and infection are the most common postoperative complications after amputation. Careful monitoring of the residual limb for signs and symptoms of bleeding and wound healing is crucial. A second surgery is done for open or guillotine amputations, not for closed amputations. The residual limb should be elevated for 24 to 48 hours postoperatively to control edema. Positioning the residual limb in an externally rotated, abducted position can cause contractures.

4. The answer is **3.**

Although the reading is slightly elevated, it is not dangerously high. The client should be instructed to have his blood pressure evaluated within the next few weeks by his health care provider. Waiting 6 months or 1 year is too long to wait for a follow-up evaluation. Because the blood pressure reading is only slightly elevated, there is no need for immediate evaluation in the emergency department.

5. The answer is **1.**

Intermittent claudication, calf leg pain associated with exercise, is symptomatic of ischemia caused by arterial occlusive disorders of the legs. Leg color, temperature, pulses, and pain can be used to ascertain clinical symptoms of arterial problems. Nicotine can cause vasoconstriction, but edema and DVT typically do not cause intermittent claudication. Allergy and medication history, usual activity pattern, menopausal state, occupation, and socioeconomic status are areas assessed for any client. They are not the priority focus areas for a client experiencing claudication.

6. The answers are **2, 4, 6.**

A blood pressure reading over 135/85 mm Hg is considered high by the American Heart Association. The nurse should instruct the client to see his health care provider as soon as possible. Explaining the importance of a proper diet and the importance smoking cessation (if the client smokes) is priority. This blood pressure reading is not normal, but it does not warrant a visit to the emergency department. Burger-Allen exercises are leg exercises for a client with arterial occlusive disease.

7. The answer is **4.**

The client with chronic arterial occlusive disease of the lower extremities experiences an alteration in tissue perfusion to this area. As a result, placing the legs in a dependent position in relation to the heart helps to improve peripheral blood flow. This position does nothing to improve activity tolerance. Improved peripheral blood flow and subsequently improved tissue perfusion may lead to a decrease in pain, but this is not the primary reason for this position. Disuse syndrome is not typically associated with chronic arterial occlusive disease.

8. The answer is 4.
The immobility associated with the required bed rest for a short time postoperatively and resultant venous stasis represent one of the three conditions necessary for thrombus formation. Although obesity and pregnancy are associated with hypercoagulability (another of the three conditions), the client who is 5′7″ and weighs 125 lb is not obese. A history of uneventful pregnancies is not considered a risk factor for thrombus formation. Engaging in a regular exercise program is not associated as a risk factor for thrombus formation from surgery.

9. The answer is 1.
The hallmark of peripheral vascular nursing, proper foot care, is necessary to prevent further tissue injury and possible amputation. Alcohol, a vasodilator, is not specifically prohibited in arterial occlusive disease. A controlled-calorie, low-fat diet, not a low-residue diet, is appropriate. Tight garments can inhibit arterial circulation. Support stockings are indicated for venous, not arterial, insufficiency.

10. The answer is 2.
Bleeding from body orifices, such as the gums, is an adverse effect of heparin that could indicate excessive anticoagulation. In this case, notification of the health care provider and further evaluation, including laboratory tests such as activated partial thromboplastin time, are necessary. Based on the laboratory test results, the prescribed dose of heparin may

be therapeutic, and therefore no changes to the infusion rate need to be made. However, if the laboratory results reveal excessive anticoagulation, the dose of heparin may need to be decreased. The infusion would only be discontinued with a health care provider's order. A coumarin derivative would be started after the client had achieved adequate anticoagulation. Protamine sulfate, not a coumarin derivative, is the antidote for a heparin overdose. Further evaluation and assessment of other potential sites of bleeding are needed before concluding that the client's complaints are not serious.

11. The answer is 2.
Phantom pain, which is real pain, occurs in up to 10% of clients who have undergone amputation. It may persist for 2 to 3 months. After explaining phantom limb to the client, analgesic medication is needed for pain control. Bleeding is not considered the cause for the pain, and if bleeding were present, anticoagulants would only exacerbate the bleeding. Sedation is inappropriate because a sedative cannot alleviate the pain and may interfere with mobility and rehabilitation. Infection is not considered a cause for phantom pain, and elevation is contraindicated postoperatively because it can promote development of contractures.

12. The answer is 4.
Body temperature combined with improving wound pain and absence of wound drainage or induration support the expected outcome of absence of wound infection. Urinary output and respiratory rate within normal limits are not specific indicators pointing to absence of wound infection. The pain medication requirement, although important for evaluating pain relief, is not the most specific indicator for evaluating the wound status.

13. The answer is 1.
Based on the client's statements, the effects of the medication are interfering with the client's taking the medication. As a result,

the client's blood pressure is not controlled. More information is needed to determine if the client also has a lack of knowledge of the treatment regimen or a short-term memory loss problem. A knowledge deficit associated with the relation between the medication's adverse effects and therapeutic effects implies a need to tolerate adverse effects to achieve therapeutic effects, which is not considered necessary in most cases.

14. The answer is **3.**
Because of possible cardiac complications, including angina associated with hypertension, the nurse should obtain additional information about complaints of chest pain. Blood glucose elevations, bowel movements, and leg cramps are not complications associated with hypertension. However, these findings may affect the level of blood pressure elevation.

15. The answer is **2.**
Clients need to know that they should never discontinue a prescribed antihypertensive medication unless directed to do so by their health care provider, because life-threatening hypertensive crisis can result from sudden withdrawal from medication in an unsupervised setting. Although antihypertensive agents constitute a cornerstone of intervention, some clients achieve control with other means. Often, a combination of diet therapy, medications, and lifestyle modifications is effective. Independent adjustment of antihypertensive medications is not a recognized self-care principle. The available antihypertensive agents and blood pressure management regimens are so varied that individualized treatment regimens can be devised to minimize or eliminate uncomfortable adverse effects.

16. The answer is **1.**
The most obvious manifestations of varicose veins are cramps at night and dilated, twisting, discolored veins, usually of the legs but possibly on the lower trunk. Intermittent claudication and nonpalpable pedal pulses are signs of arterial occlusive disease. A positive Homans' sign and an edematous reddened calf are typical signs deep venous thrombosis. Marked limb enlargement and nonpitting edema are associated signs of lymphedema.

8 Gastrointestinal disorders

I. STRUCTURE AND FUNCTION OF THE GI SYSTEM

A. **Structure.** The GI system consists of the oral structures, esophagus, stomach, small intestine, large intestine, and associated structures. (See *Figure 8-1.*)

1. **Oral structures** include the lips, teeth, gingivae and oral mucosa, tongue, hard palate, soft palate, pharynx, and salivary glands.

2. The **esophagus** is a muscular tube extending from the pharynx to the stomach. **Esophageal openings include:**

    a. the **upper esophageal sphincter** at the cricopharyngeal muscle

    b. the **lower esophageal sphincter (LES)**, or *cardiac sphincter,* which normally remains closed and opens only to pass food into the stomach.

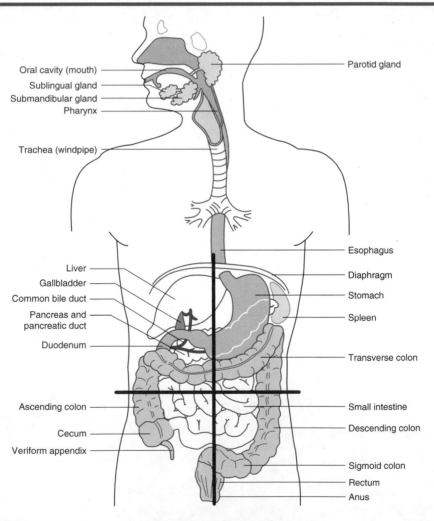

FIGURE 8-1

Organs of the digestive system and associated structures

3. The **stomach** is a muscular pouch situated in the upper abdomen under the liver and diaphragm. The stomach consists of three anatomic areas: the fundus, body (i.e., corpus), and antrum (i.e., pylorus).

4. **Sphincters.** The LES allows food to enter the stomach and prevents reflux into the esophagus. The pyloric sphincter regulates flow of stomach contents (chyme) into the duodenum.

5. The **small intestine,** a coiled tube, extends from the pyloric sphincter to the ileocecal valve at the large intestine. Sections of the small intestine include the duodenum, jejunum, and ileum.

6. The **large intestine** is a shorter, wider tube beginning at the ileocecal valve and ending at the anus. The large intestine consists of three sections:
   a. The cecum is a blind pouch that extends from the ileocecal valve to the vermiform appendix.
   b. The colon, which is the main portion of the large intestine, is divided into four anatomic sections: ascending, transverse, descending, and sigmoid.
   c. The rectum extends from the sigmoid colon to the anus.

7. The **ileocecal valve** prevents the return of feces from the cecum into the small intestine and lies at the upper border of the cecum.

8. The **appendix,** which collects lymphoid tissues, arises from the cecum.

9. The **GI tract** is composed of five layers.
   a. An inner mucosal layer lubricates and protects the inner surface of the alimentary canal.
   b. A submucosal layer is responsible for secreting digestive enzymes.
   c. A layer of circular smooth muscle fibers is responsible for movement of the GI tract.
   d. A layer of longitudinal smooth muscle fibers also facilitates movement of the GI tract.
   e. The peritoneum, an outer serosal layer, covers the entire abdomen and is composed of the parietal and viscera layers.

B. **Function.** The GI system performs two major body functions: digestion and elimination.

1. **Digestion** of food and fluid, with absorption of nutrients into the bloodstream, occurs in the upper GI tract, stomach, and small intestines.
   a. Digestion begins in the mouth with chewing and the action of ptyalin, an enzyme contained in saliva that breaks down starch.
   b. Swallowed food passes through the esophagus to the stomach, where digestion continues by several processes.
      – Secretion of gastric juice, containing hydrochloric acid and the enzymes pepsin and lipase (and renin in infants)
      – Mixing and churning through peristaltic action
   c. From the pylorus, the mixed stomach contents (i.e., chyme) pass into the duodenum through the pyloric valve.
   d. In the small intestine, food digestion is completed, and most nutrient absorption occurs. Digestion results from the action of numerous pancreatic and intestinal enzymes (e.g., trypsin, lipase, amylase, lactase, maltase, sucrase) and bile.

2. **Elimination** of waste products through defecation occurs in the large intestines and rectum. In the large intestine, the cecum and ascending colon absorb water and electrolytes from the now completely digested material. The rectum stores feces for elimination.

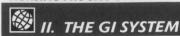

II. THE GI SYSTEM

A. Assessment

1. **Health history**

   a. **Elicit a description of the client's present illness and chief complaint,** including onset, course, duration, location, and precipitating and alleviating factors. This can provide sufficient information for diagnosis in about 80% of clients. Symptoms indicating altered GI function include:
   - lack of appetite and food intolerance, based on a recall of usual food intake within 24 hours
   - pain, including character, location, timing (e.g., before meals or after meals), and alleviating measures (The type and location of pain depends on the type of GI disease [e.g., stabbing pain, crampy pain.])
   - altered bowel-elimination patterns (See *Table 8-1.*)
   - presence of dark urine, jaundice, weight loss, nausea, or vomiting
   - previous GI tract surgery.

   b. **Explore the client's health history for risk factors** associated with GI disease, including low fiber intake; tobacco use; inadequate nutritional intake; ingestion of hot, spicy foods; and inadequate fluid intake.

2. **Physical examination**

   a. **Inspection**
   - Inspect oral structures for smooth, pink, moist oral mucosa and symmetric movement of all structures.
   - Inspect teeth and gingivae for the presence of natural teeth with filled dental caries or well-fitting dentures and no gingival redness or edema.
   - Observe the tongue for a pink and velvety appearance.
   - Observe the throat for a lack of redness or edema.
   - Inspect the client's abdomen for contour, color, scars, and striae.
   - Observe the abdominal wall for surface motion, masses, or nodules.

   b. **Auscultation**
   - Bowel sounds are present, hypoactive, hyperactive, or absent; auscultate for frequency and character of bowel sounds for a least 5 minutes before concluding that bowel sounds are absent.
   - Auscultate the right lower quadrant (RLQ), right upper quadrant (RUQ), left lower quadrant (LLQ), and left upper quadrant (LUQ) with the diaphragm of the stethoscope because bowel sounds are high pitched.

   c. **Percussion**
   - Percuss all four quadrants systemically, noting tympany (i.e., predominant sound from air in the stomach and small intestines) and dullness, which is considered abnormal.
   - Percuss the liver span, liver descent, spleen, and stomach.

   d. **Palpation**
   - Always palpate the abdomen last so that sounds from palpation are not auscultated.
   - Palpate lightly for changes in skin temperature, tenderness, or large masses.

TABLE 8-1
Altered bowel elimination patterns

Description	Signs and symptoms	Nursing interventions
Constipation Elimination pattern characterized by hard, dry stools that result from delayed passage of food residue	■ Decreased frequency of defecation ■ Hard, formed stool ■ Reported sensation of rectal fullness ■ Straining at stool ■ Painful defecation ■ Abdominal distention	■ Urge the client to increase his intake of dietary fiber. ■ Encourage increased oral fluid intake. ■ Recommend regular exercise. ■ Advise the client to establish a regular time for bowel movement. ■ Administer laxatives judiciously.
Diarrhea Frequent passage of loose, fluid, unformed stools	■ Loose, fluid stools ■ Increased frequency of defecation ■ Additional bowel sounds ■ Increased stool volume ■ Reported abdominal discomfort and cramping	■ Provide instruction on proper and safe preparation and storage of food products, such as fruits, vegetables, dairy products, and meat. ■ Teach the client how to clean cooking utensils and food containers properly to prevent epidemic diarrhea. ■ Assess the client for dehydration. ■ Encourage increased oral fluid intake. ■ Administer antidiarrheal medications as prescribed. ■ Advise the client to avoid foods that exacerbate diarrhea. Instruct him to avoid cold foods and smoking because they increase intestinal motility. ■ Provide an easily accessible bedpan or commode. ■ Provide additional perianal skin care for the client with severe diarrhea.

- Palpate deeply over the RLQ, RUQ, LLQ, and LUQ for any masses and note location, size, shape, and pulsation; always palpate tender areas last. Remember what organs are located under each of the four quadrants. (See *Figure 8-1*, page 186.)
- Palpate the liver, spleen, kidneys, and aorta for enlargement.
3. **Laboratory and diagnostic studies**
   a. **Blood and serum studies**
   - **Albumin-globulin ratio and total protein** are responsible for oncotic pressure.
   - **Alkaline phosphatase** level measures enzyme activity in bone, intestine, liver, and biliary systems.
   - **Miscellaneous tests** evaluate the absorptive activity of GI tract. These tests include iron, calcium, cholesterol, prothrombin time, carotenes, and vitamin A.
   b. **Fecal fat studies**
   - **Qualitative evaluation** measures fat content as neutral (e.g., ingested mineral oil) or fatty acid (e.g., lipids).
   - **Quantitative evaluation** measures fat content after the client eats a diet with a prescribed amount of fat, and stool is collected for 72 hours.
   - **Stool guaiac** detects occult blood in stool, indicating GI bleeding.
   c. **Radiographic studies of the GI system**
   - **Upper GI or barium swallow** involves visualization by fluoroscopy of the esophagus and stomach after the client swallows barium. Serial radiographs show outlines of the structures.

- **Lower GI or barium enema** involves instillation of barium into the large intestine, with fluoroscopy and filming used to visualize structures and determine the efficiency of emptying.

  d. **Motility studies** use manometric catheters to measure intraluminal pressure in GI structures.
  - **Esophageal manometry** evaluates peristaltic contractions and sphincter integrity.
  - **Rectal manometry** measures internal and external sphincter pressures.

  e. **Endoscopic studies** provide direct visualization of internal GI structures (and a means to obtain biopsy samples) using a long, flexible tube containing a fiberoptic light source. Endoscopic studies include esophagoscopy, gastroscopy, colonoscopy, sigmoidoscopy, and esophagogastroduodenoscopy.

  f. **Ultrasonography** produces an image of the abdominal organs and structures on the oscilloscope by using sound waves.

  g. **Computed tomography (CT)** provides cross-sectional images to allow the abdominal organs and structures to be more directly observed.

  h. **Magnetic resonance imaging** provides a supplement to ultrasonography and CT scanning but does not replace it.

  i. **Scintigraphy** detects bleeding in the abdominal cavity when endoscopy is not possible.

  j. **Gastric analysis** determines the nature of gastric secretions.

B. Nursing diagnoses
1. Diarrhea or constipation
2. Risk for deficient fluid volume
3. Imbalanced nutrition: less than body requirements
4. Risk for infection
5. Impaired oral mucous membrane
6. Risk for impaired skin integrity
7. Acute pain
8. Deficient knowledge
9. Ineffective individual coping

C. Planning and outcome identification.
The major goals for the client include attainment and maintenance of normal elimination, maintenance of adequate intake of food and fluids, absence of infection, improvement of the oral mucosa membrane and skin integrity, pain relief, increased knowledge about the disease process and its therapeutic management, and improved coping.

D. Implementation
1. **Assess GI function.**

   a. Assess the GI system, including assessing bowel sounds and the abdomen for firmness, tenderness, and edema, Measure abdominal girth, and assess for dehydration (e.g., oral mucosa, skin turgor).

   b. Ask the client the following questions:
   - Have you experienced any nausea or vomiting? What caused the nausea? What did the vomitus look like?
   - When was your last bowel movement? Is this normal for you?
   - Have there been any changes in bowel habits or stool characteristics?
   - Where is the pain, and what is its character, duration, and pattern? Does food or defecation affect the pain?

- Have you lost or gained weight in the last 6 months?
- Have you experienced belching or flatulence?

c. Assess all vomitus for content, and note undigested food and blood (i.e., coffee-ground or bright red appearance).

d. Assess all stools for consistency, odor, contents, and blood (i.e., occult or bright red).

2. **Assess nutritional and fluid balance.**
   a. Weigh the client daily in the same clothes and at the same time.
   b. Monitor strict intake and output; use a urometer as needed.

3. **Implement measures to treat diarrhea or constipation** as described in *Table 8-1*, page 189.

4. **Protect the client from infection.**
   a. Monitor vital signs.
   b. Assess perfuse watery diarrhea, which indicates infection.

5. **Maintain integrity of the oral mucosa and skin.**
   a. Instruct the client to brush his teeth daily and after meals, floss daily, and have regular dental checkups.
   b. Instruct the client to avoid any tobacco products, including smokeless tobacco.
   c. Provide meticulous perianal skin care. Advise the client to clean and dry his skin thoroughly after each episode of diarrhea.

6. **Minimize pain.** Instruct the client to avoid irritants, such as spicy or acidic foods, alcohol, caffeine, and tobacco, because they increase gastric acid production.

7. **Provide client and family teaching.**
   a. Teach the client to minimize symptoms while maintaining a well-balanced diet that follows the food guide pyramid.
   b. Teach lifestyle modifications as appropriate, such as avoidance of exacerbating foods and substances, increased fiber intake, adequate fluid intake, and stress-management techniques.
   c. Instruct the client to report danger signs and symptoms, including prolonged vomiting or diarrhea, blood in stool, and change in bowel habits.

8. **Promote client and family coping.** Allow the client and his family to ventilate their feelings about body-image changes, anxiety, and fears and concerns.

E. Outcome evaluation

1. The client returns to a normal elimination pattern as evidenced by no abdominal cramping and passage of soft, formed stool.

2. The client exhibits adequate hydration as evidenced by elastic skin turgor, moist mucous membranes, and intake equal to output.

3. The client maintains a nutritionally balanced diet and verbalizes appropriate diet modifications.

4. The client remains free from local and systemic infection.

5. The client displays intact oral mucosa with no evidence of inflammation.

6. The client demonstrates appropriate oral hygiene.

7. The client maintains intact skin integrity, including the perianal area.

8. The client is free from pain and discomfort.

9. The client verbalizes factors that precipitate or exacerbate GI conditions, as well as means of avoiding or minimizing these factors.

10. The client demonstrates compliance with the prescribed medication regimen.

11. The client is able to verbalize feelings and effective coping mechanisms that assist in his and his family's quality of life.

III. STOMATITIS

A. **Description.** Stomatitis is the inflammation of the oral mucosa.

B. **Etiology.** Stomatitis may be caused by infection, trauma, excessive dryness, irritants, toxic agents, or hypersensitivity.
   1. **Infectious agents** that can produce stomatitis include:
      a. viruses (e.g., the herpes simplex virus, which causes acute herpetic stomatitis)
      b. fungi (e.g., *Candida albicans,* which causes candidiasis or thrush).
   2. **Damage from mechanical trauma,** such as irritation from jagged teeth, cheek biting, mouth breathing, or use of a stiff toothbrush, can cause characteristic lesions.
   3. **Excessive dryness of the mouth** (i.e., xerostomia) is a common sequela of oral cancer in clients receiving psychopharmacologic agents, clients with human immunodeficiency virus infection, and clients who are predominantly mouth breathers.
   4. **Irritants and toxic agents** that can produce stomatitis include strong mouthwashes or toothpastes, tobacco, and chemotherapeutic agents.
   5. **Hypersensitivity.** Causes of aphthous ulcers (e.g., canker sores) remain unclear. Suspected predisposing factors include stress, allergies, vitamin deficiencies, and viral infection.

C. **Pathophysiology.** Destruction of the inner mucosal layer of the oral cavity results in decreased lubrication of the mucosa and disruption of the protective layers. Any fluid or food in the oral cavity further irritates the mucosa and causes inflammation, resulting in pain.

D. **Assessment findings** vary with the type of stomatitis.
   1. **Acute herpetic stomatitis** is marked by small, clear vesicles in single or multiple eruptions, commonly preceded by sore throat, headache, nausea, vomiting, and malaise. It usually lasts about 1 week.
   2. **Candidiasis** produces characteristic raised, white patches and ulcers. The infection may spread to other areas of the GI tract, the skin, or the respiratory system.
   3. **Mechanical trauma** produces various manifestations. Small lacerations or abrasions with bleeding or exudate are common.
   4. **Xerostomia** is marked by cracked and parched lips, tongue, and oral mucosa. The oral mucosa may bleed, have ulcerations, or retract.
   5. **Chemical irritation** typically produces generalized redness and edema. Chemotherapy may cause edematous, easily bruised mucosa and possibly produces ulcerations with exudate.
   6. **Aphthous ulcers** appear as well-circumscribed lesions with white centers and reddish rings around the periphery.

E. **Nursing management**
   1. **Administer medications,** which may include an antifungal agent or topical or systemic analgesics. (See *Drug chart 8-1.*)
   2. **Maintain integrity** of the oral mucosa. (See section II.D.5.)
      a. Instruct the client to brush and floss his teeth and massage his gums several times daily.
      b. Advise the client to use gauze or a sponge toothette to clean the oral mucosa when pain prevents the use of a toothbrush.
      c. Recommend the use of water, saline, or a dilute solution of hydrogen peroxide instead of toothpaste or mouthwash.
   3. **Promote adequate food and fluid intake.**

DRUG CHART 8-1
Medications for GI disorders

Classifications	Indications	Selected interventions
Antacids aluminum hydroxide calcium carbonate dihydroxyaluminum sodium carbonate magaldrate magnesium hydroxide	Neutralize the hydrochloric acid secreted by the stomach	■ Instruct the client to take 1 and 3 hours after meals and at bedtime; instruct him to avoid taking them with other medications. ■ Instruct the client to chew antacid tablets (not swallow them whole), and shake liquids before taking them.
Antibiotics aminoglycosides (gentamicin, tobramycin) amoxicillin erythromycin penicillin sulfasalazine tetracycline	Prevent or treat infections caused by pathogenic microorganisms	■ Before administering the first dose, assess the client for allergies and determine whether a culture has been obtained. ■ After multiple doses, assess the client for superinfection (thrush, yeast infection, diarrhea); notify the health care provider if these occur. ■ Assess the insertion site for phlebitis if antibiotics are being administered I.V. ■ To assess the effectiveness of antibiotic therapy, monitor the white blood cell count. ■ Monitor peaks and troughs for aminoglycosides.
Anticholinergics atropine sulfate glycopyrrolate propantheline scopolamine	Inhibit the actions of acetylcholine at cholinergic receptor sites, thereby decreasing gastric secretions	■ Advise the client that adverse effects include drowsiness and dry mouth. ■ Encourage increased fluid intake. ■ Caution the client to avoid activities, such as driving, that require alertness and concentration until the effects of the drug are known.
Antidiarrheals attapulgite diphenoxylate and atropine loperamide bismuth subsalicylate	Absorb excess water from stool	■ To assess the effectiveness of the medication, record the number and consistency of stools. ■ Monitor intake and output, daily weight, and serum electrolyte levels.
Antiemetics benzquinamide hydroxyzine metoclopramide promethazine trimethobenzamide hydrochloride	Relieve nausea and vomiting by inhibiting medullary chemoreceptor triggers; drug choice depends on the cause of vomiting	■ Advise the client that this medication may cause drowsiness. ■ Because the medication may cause chemical irritation, administer by deep I.M. injection into a large muscle mass. ■ Measure emesis and maintain accurate intake and output; monitor for dehydration.
Antifungals nystatin suspension	Treat infections caused by fungi; fungal infections are resistant to antibiotics	■ Instruct the client to rinse his mouth with water to cleanse it, "swish and swallow" to coat the oral mucosa, and hold the suspension in his mouth for at least 2 minutes.
Antispasmotics dicyclomine hydrochloride	Relax the smooth muscle of the GI tract without anticholinergic effects	■ Instruct the client to take doses before meals and at bedtime unless a timed-release form is used.

(continued)

DRUG CHART 8-1
Medications for GI disorders *(continued)*

Classifications	Indications	Selected interventions
Corticosteroids oral — dexamethasone, hydrocortisone, methylprednisolone, prednisone I.V. — Solu-Cortef, Solu-Medrol	Combat severe immune or inflammatory responses	■ Instruct the client to take the medication exactly as directed and to taper it rather than stop it abruptly, which could cause serious withdrawal symptoms (adrenal insufficiency, shock, death). ■ Forewarn the client that the medication may cause reportable cushingoid effects (weight gain, moon face, buffalo hump, and hirsutism) and may mask signs and symptoms of infection.
Histamine receptor antagonists cimetidine famotidine ranitidine	Block receptors that control the secretion of hydrochloric acid by the parietal cells	■ Instruct the client to continue taking the medication regularly, even after pain subsides. ■ When administering I.V., dilute the medication and monitor the client closely. ■ Emphasize the importance of adhering to all aspects of therapy.
Laxatives **Bulk laxatives** psyllium **Stimulant laxatives** bisacodyl senna **Stool softeners** docusate calcium docusate sodium **Saline (osmotic) laxatives** magnesium citrate magnesium hydroxide	Absorb water and increase fecal bulk; stimulate peristalsis through mucosal irritation; ease stool passage by facilitating the mixing of water with fecal mass; retain and increase water in the feces	■ Administer a bulk laxative with fluid and give immediately before it congeals. ■ Avoid overuse, which causes laxative dependence. ■ Inform the client that a daily bowel movement is not necessary for normal bowel elimination.
Mucosal protective agents misoprostol sucralfate	Protect the ulcer from the destructive action of the digestive enzyme pepsin by changing stomach acid into viscous material that binds to proteins in ulcerated tissue	■ Instruct the client to take the medication 30 to 60 minutes before meals and at bedtime. ■ Advise the client to take the medication 1 hour before or after taking an antacid. ■ Tablets may be difficult to chew; liquid preparations are available.
Opioid analgesics codeine hydrocodone hydromorphone morphine propoxyphene	Relieve moderate to severe pain by reducing pain sensation, producing sedation, and decreasing the emotional upset often associated with pain; most often schedule II drugs	■ Assess the pain for location, type, intensity, what increases or decreases it; rate pain on scale of 1 (no pain) to 10 (worst pain). ■ Rule out any complications. Is this pain routine or expected? Is it a complication that needs immediate intervention? ■ Medicate according to pain-scale findings. ■ Institute safety measures — bed in low position, side rails up, and call light within reach. ■ Evaluate the effectiveness of the pain medication in 30 minutes.
Proton pump inhibitor omeprazole pantoprazole	Prevent the final transport of hydrogen into the gastric lumen by binding an enzyme on gastric parietal cells	■ Instruct the client to take the medication regularly as prescribed by the health care provider. ■ Instruct the client to avoid any products that may cause GI irritation. ■ Administer I.V. pantoprazole with a filter.

> > *a.* Advise the client to eat a bland diet.
> >
> > *b.* Suggest that the client consume lukewarm or cold food and fluids, which may minimize discomfort and result in increased intake.
>
> **4. Minimize pain.** (See section II.D.6.)
> **5. Promote client and family coping.** (See section II.D.8.)

IV. ESOPHAGITIS

A. Description. Esophagitis is the inflammation of the esophageal mucosa. It may be acute or chronic.

B. Etiology. Esophagitis most commonly results from recurrent reflux of gastric contents into the distal esophagus. Reflux may result from:

1. incompetent lower esophageal sphincter
2. gastric or duodenal ulcers
3. prolonged nasogastric intubation.

C. Pathophysiology. Gastric hydrochloric acid from reflux of gastric juices alters the pH of the esophageal mucosa, permitting mucosal protein to be denatured; proteolytic properties of pepsin in gastric secretions are enhanced in altered pH, leading to further damage.

D. Assessment findings

1. **Clinical manifestations**
   a. Heartburn, acid regurgitation, and belching
   b. Dysphagia
   c. Esophageal pain, possibly radiating to the arms, neck, back, jaw, and substernal area (Pain may be precipitated by increased abdominal pressure, as can occur from bending, straining, obesity, or pregnancy.)
2. **Laboratory and diagnostic study findings**
   a. Esophagogastroduodenoscopy may reveal irritated, inflamed areas with possible eroded areas. Brushing and biopsy results can exclude cancer of the esophagus.
   b. Twenty-four–hour pH monitoring detects decreased pH of gastric contents.
   c. Esophagoscopy and barium swallow detect anatomic or functional derangements of esophagus secondary to acid erosion.

E. Nursing management

1. **Promote adequate nutritional intake.** Instruct the client to:
   a. eat small, frequent meals of mostly bland foods
   b. chew food thoroughly before swallowing
   c. drink fluids to aid swallowing and food passage down the esophagus
   d. refrain from laying down after eating
   e. avoid eating within 3 hours of bedtime.
2. **Assess all vomitus** for content; note undigested food and blood (i.e., coffee-ground or bright red appearance).
3. **Maintain integrity of the oral mucosa.** (See section II.D.5.)
4. **Minimize pain.** Instruct the client to avoid irritants. (See section II.D.6.) Advise the client to elevate the head of his bed with blocks to help minimize reflux.

V. GASTROESOPHAGEAL REFLUX DISEASE

A. **Description.** Gastroesophageal reflux disease (GERD) is excessive reflux of hydrochloric acid into the esophagus. The occurrence of GERD increases with age.

B. **Etiology.** GERD usually results from an incompetent lower esophageal sphincter (LES), pyloric stenosis, or a motility disorder.

C. **Pathophysiology.** A weak or incompetent LES allows backward movement of gastric contents into the esophagus; decreased esophageal peristalsis and salivary function impair clearance of the refluxed acid, resulting in mucosal injury to the esophagus.

D. **Assessment findings**
   1. **Clinical manifestations**
      a. Pyrosis (i.e., burning sensation in the esophagus)
      b. Regurgitation of sour-tasting secretions
      c. Dysphagia (i.e., difficulty swallowing) and odynophagia (i.e., pain on swallowing)
      d. Symptoms mimicking those of a heart attack
   2. **Laboratory and diagnostic study findings** (See section IV.D.2.)

E. **Nursing management (See section II.D.)**
   1. **Administer medications,** which may include antacids, histamine-receptor antagonists, and proton pump inhibitors. (See *Drug chart 8-1,* pages 193 and 194.)
   2. **Teach the client to avoid factors that increase lower esophageal irritation:**
      a. Eat a low-fat, high-fiber diet.
      b. Avoid irritants, such as spicy or acidic foods, alcohol, caffeine, and tobacco, because they increase gastric acid production.
      c. Avoid food or drink 2 hours before bedtime or lying down after eating.
      d. Elevate the head of the bed on 6″ to 8″ blocks.
      e. Lose weight if necessary.
   3. **If symptoms persist, prepare the client for surgical repair,** which includes a fundoplication (i.e., wrapping a portion of the gastric fundus around the sphincter area of the esophagus). (See *Client and Family Teaching 8-1.*)
   4. **Provide a referral** to the National Institute of Diabetic & Digestive & Kidney Diseases. (See appendix A.)

VI. PEPTIC ULCER DISEASE

A. **Description**
   1. Peptic ulcer disease involves ulcers — circumscribed breaks in the mucosa — occurring in the duodenum (duodenal ulcers), the stomach (gastric ulcers), and less commonly, the distal esophagus and the jejunum.
   2. Peptic ulcer disease occurs in 5% to 10% of the population, but only about 50% of the cases are diagnosed. Duodenal ulcers are three times more common than gastric ulcers. The peak incidence for duodenal ulcers is between ages 25 and 50. The peak incidence for gastric ulcers occurs in people older than age 50. The incidence of peptic ulcer disease is about equal among men and women.

B. **Etiology.** Peptic ulcer disease is thought to result from *Helicobacter pylori* infection. Contributing factors are related to gastric acid secretion and include:

1. altered gastric acid and serum gastrin levels
2. tobacco smoking and alcohol use
3. use of aspirin, other nonsteroidal antiinflammatory drugs, and steroids
4. genetic predisposition
5. psychosomatic or psychological factors (e.g., chronic anxiety, type A personality).

C. **Pathophysiology.** Normally, tightly packed epithelial cells protect the gastric mucosa from irritation. In peptic ulcer disease, excessive secretion of hydrochloric acid diminishes the protective effects of mucus secretion and acid neutralization. (See *Figure 8-2*, page 198.)

  1. **Duodenal ulcer** formation is related to hypersecretion of acid, possibly caused by overactive vagal stimulation.
  2. **Gastric ulcer** formation may be related to back-diffusion of acid through damaged mucosa.
  3. **Possible complications** of peptic ulcer disease include perforation, hemorrhage, and pyloric obstruction.

D. **Assessment findings**

  1. **Clinical manifestations.** Peptic ulcer disease may be asymptomatic in up to 50% of persons affected.
     a. **Duodenal ulcers**
        – Burning, aching, or gnawing pain in the right epigastrium occurring 2 to 3 hours after meals, possibly causing the client to awaken at night; relieved by eating
        – Pyrosis (i.e., heartburn), nausea, and vomiting
        – GI bleeding, a slow oozing manifested by melena or a sudden, rapid loss of large amounts of blood through hematemesis
        – Epigastric tenderness
     b. **Gastric ulcers**
        – Burning, aching, or gnawing pain in the upper epigastrium occurring 30 minutes to 1 hour after meals (rarely at night); unrelieved by eating
        – Epigastric tenderness
  2. **Laboratory and diagnostic study findings**
     a. Barium swallow shows an ulcerated area.
     b. Endoscopy identifies inflammation of gastric mucosa, ulcers, and lesions; biopsy can determine the presence of *H. pylori*.

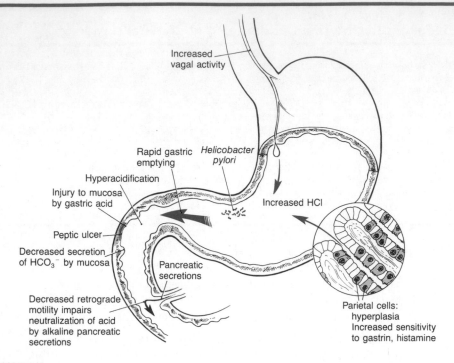

FIGURE 8-2
Pathogenesis of peptic ulcers

Source: Bullock, B.L., and Henze, R.L. *Focus on Pathophysiology.* Philadelphia: Lippincott Williams & Wilkins, 2000.

E.   Nursing management (See section II.D.)
   1. **Administer prescribed medications.**
      a. Medications may include antacids, anticholinergics, histamine-receptor antagonists, proton pump inhibitors, and mucosal protective agents. (See *Drug chart 8-1,* pages 193 and 194.)
      b. Medication for ulcers caused by *H. pylori* include bismuth subsalicylate, metronidazole, and tetracycline. These medications administered together eradicate *H. pylori* bacteria in the gastric mucosa.
   2. **Provide client and family teaching.**
      a. Teach the client methods to minimize symptoms while maintaining adequate nutrition.
         – Avoid foods that previously have caused pain. Specific dietary restrictions vary from client to client.
         – Eat three regular meals a day; small, frequent meals are unnecessary as long as the medication is taken before meals.
         – Avoid a diet rich in milk and creams, which are acid stimulants.
      b. Instruct the client to quit smoking, which decreases the secretion of bicarbonate from the pancreas into the duodenum, resulting in increased acidity in the duodenum.

    c. Teach the client about necessary lifestyle modifications aimed at decreasing stress and maximizing effective coping. Biofeedback, hypnosis, or behavior modification may be suggested.

3. **Prepare the client for diagnostic procedures, and provide postprocedure care.**

    a. Preparation for barium swallow includes no oral intake after midnight and possible laxatives to clean the GI tract. After a barium swallow, administer a laxative if indicated to prevent constipation. Stools are monitored until all barium has been eliminated.

    b. For the client undergoing gastroscopy, obtain informed consent, and instruct the client not to eat nor drink anything for 8 hours before the procedure. After the procedure, assess the gag reflex before the client consumes foods and fluids. Monitor for signs of perforation (e.g., pain, bleeding, abdominal distention).

4. **Prepare the client for surgery** if indicated (e.g., ulcers that have not responded to treatment after 12 to 16 weeks, life-threatening hemorrhage or perforation). Possible procedures include vagotomy, pyloroplasty, or distal subtotal gastrectomy, which includes Billroth I (gastroduodenostomy) or Billroth II (gastrojejunostomy).

    a. **Preoperative care**
   - Obtain informed consent.
   - Clear and empty the GI tract by administering enemas and allowing nothing by mouth.

    b. **Postoperative care**
   - Ensure that the nasogastric tube (surgically placed) is not manipulated.
   - Observe nasogastric tube aspirate.
   - Assess the surgical dressing.
   - Provide routine postoperative care. (See chapter 21.)
   - Provide discharge teaching as described in *Client and family teaching 8-1,* page 197.

5. **Provide a referral** to the National Institute of Diabetic & Digestive & Kidney Disorders. (See appendix A.)

VII. APPENDICITIS

A. Description. Appendicitis is inflammation of the vermiform appendix. It occurs in about 7% of the population and affects males more often than females. The peak incidence is between ages 10 and 30.

B. Etiology. The precipitating event in appendicitis is obstruction of the appendix lumen, which can result from a fecalith, kinking of the appendix, inflammation, or a neoplasm.

C. Pathophysiology. Obstruction of the appendix lumen causes increased intraluminal pressure and triggers an inflammatory process that can lead to infection, necrosis, and perforation. Perforation and rupture can cause peritonitis, a life-threatening complication.

D. Assessment findings

1. **Clinical manifestations**

    a. Acute abdominal pain, usually in the right lower quadrant (i.e., McBurney's point), rebound tenderness, or both

    b. Nausea and vomiting

    c. Low-grade fever

2. **Laboratory and diagnostic study findings.** White blood cell count may reveal leukocytosis.

E. Nursing management (See section II.D.)
   1. **Provide general preoperative and postoperative care.** Prompt surgery is indicated to prevent perforation. (See chapter 21.)
   2. **Provide discharge teaching** as described in *Client and family teaching 8-1*, page 197.

VIII. DIVERTICULITIS AND DIVERTICULOSIS

A. Description

   1. **Diverticulitis** is a condition involving inflammation of diverticula, small saccular herniations in the colonic wall. **Diverticulosis** exists when multiple diverticula are present without inflammation or symptoms.
   2. **Diverticulosis** develops in about 50% of persons older than age 60 in the United States. The incidence is greatest among men. **Diverticulitis** occurs in about 25% of persons with diverticulosis.

B. Etiology.
Formation of diverticula is associated with increased intraluminal pressure from such factors as a low-fiber diet, chronic constipation, and obesity. Diverticulitis occurs when food or bacteria become trapped in the diverticula, resulting in inflammation and infection. The sigmoid colon is the most common site for diverticulitis because of fecal masses that irritate and increase pressure in the colon.

C. Pathophysiology

   1. **Diverticula form** as the colonic mucosa pushes through the muscular coat at weak points. Increased intraluminal pressure is the apparent precipitating factor. The diverticula gradually fill with undigested food matter and bacteria. As they enlarge, they become more susceptible to irritation and inflammation.
   2. **Potential complications**
      a. Even a minute perforation of an inflamed diverticulum can lead to bacterial or fecal contamination of pericolic tissues.
      b. Inflamed bowel tissue may adhere to the bladder or another pelvic organ. Fistulas may form.
      c. Repeated inflammation causes the colonic wall to thicken, narrowing the lumen and possibly causing acute obstruction.
      d. Other dangerous complications include peritonitis and hemorrhage.

D. Assessment findings

   1. **Clinical manifestations**
      a. **Diverticulosis.** The client with diverticulosis is asymptomatic; multiple diverticula are present without inflammation.
      b. **Diverticulitis**
         – Change in bowel habits
         – Dull, steady, or episodic pain in the abdominal left lower quadrant or the epigastrium (depending on location of the diverticulitis)
         – Rectal bleeding
         – Anorexia
         – Low-grade fever
   2. **Laboratory and diagnostic study findings**
      a. Complete blood count evaluation may reveal an elevated white blood cell count and elevated sedimentation rate.
      b. Colonoscopy can visualize diverticula and exclude other possible causes.

    c. Barium enema shows narrowing of the colon and thickened muscle masses; this test is contraindicated in cases of acute inflammation because of the possibility of bowel perforation.

E. Nursing management (See section II.D.)

  1. Administer medications, which may include antibiotics, opioid analgesics, and antispasmodics. (See *Drug chart 8-1,* pages 193 and 194.)

  2. Teach the client about nursing care. Inform him that all nursing interventions for diverticulitis are aimed at moving the stool through the colon as easily and with as little irritation as possible.

  3. Provide measures to rest the colon during an acute exacerbation, which results when food or bacteria in the diverticula cause inflammation.

    a. Administer nothing by mouth.

    b. Administer I.V. fluids.

    c. Institute nasogastric suctioning.

    d. Keep the client on bed rest.

  4. Promote return to normal bowel elimination patterns as symptoms subside.

    a. Slowly increase oral intake until the client is drinking six to eight glasses of water daily.

    b. Offer a low-fiber diet until signs of infection decrease; then gradually increase fiber until the client is eating a high-fiber diet. If a high-fiber diet alone prevents constipation, encourage medication with caution, especially in elderly clients.

    c. Help restore the client's normal bowel elimination pattern by administering one or more of the following: bulk laxatives; stimulant laxatives; stool softeners, typically used for elderly clients because they are gentle and less likely to cause laxative dependence; saline laxatives; and at least 8 oz of water with any agent. (See *Drug chart 8-1,* pages 193 and 194.)

  5. Help prevent constipation. Encourage daily exercise, such as walking, which increases bowel peristalsis.

  6. If surgical bowel resection or colostomy is indicated, provide appropriate preoperative and postoperative care. (See chapter 21.) Provide discharge teaching as described in *Client and family teaching 8-1,* page 197.

  7. Provide referrals to the National Institute of Diabetic & Digestive & Kidney Diseases. (See appendix A.)

IX. PERITONITIS

A. Description. Peritonitis is the acute or chronic inflammation of the peritoneum, the membrane lining the abdominal cavity and covering the viscera.

B. Etiology

  1. Peritonitis usually results from bacterial (commonly, *Escherichia coli* or *Streptococcus faecalis*) invasion of the peritoneum. (See *Figure 8-3,* page 202.)

  2. Other possible causes include:

    a. chemical irritation, as can result from a ruptured bladder, ovary, or fallopian tube

    b. bile spillage into the peritoneal cavity, as can result from a ruptured gallbladder or gangrenous cholecystitis

    c. contamination of the peritoneal cavity with surgical glove powder, talc, particles of suture material, or lint from surgical drapes

    d. penetrating abdominal wound or bowel strangulation.

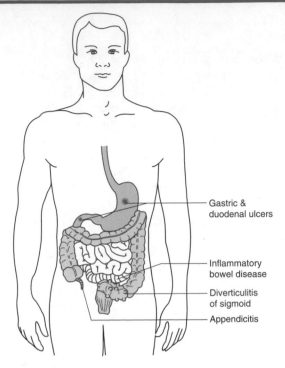

FIGURE 8-3
Common GI causes of peritonitis

C. Pathophysiology

1. Peritoneal contamination may be localized in an abscess or diffused throughout the peritoneum, depending on its origin and on the effectiveness of the client's defenses. The infectious process shunts blood to the inflamed area, leading to fluid shifts. Paralytic ileus develops in early stages. As ileus and fluid shifting progress, dehydration and, possibly, acidosis occur.

2. Life-threatening complications of peritonitis include bowel obstruction, renal failure, respiratory insufficiency, shock and, in some cases, liver failure.

D. Assessment findings

1. **Clinical manifestations**
   a. Onset of peritonitis typically is marked by severe localized or diffuse abdominal pain, with or without guarding and rebound tenderness; the abdomen is rigid and board-like.
   b. Paralytic ileus produces abdominal distention, usually with nausea and vomiting and possibly with diarrhea. Bowel sounds are decreased or absent.
   c. Fever, tachycardia, and chills point to sepsis.
   d. Shallow, guarded respirations suggest diaphragmatic involvement.
   e. Signs of dehydration and acidosis are late manifestations.

2. **Laboratory and diagnostic study findings**
   a. White blood cell count may reveal leukocytosis and possibly show leukopenia in severe cases.
   b. Paracentesis identifies the causative organism.

      c. Radiograph shows abnormal findings, which may reveal the location of the perforation.

⬛ **E.** **Nursing management (See section II.D.)**

    1. **Administer medications,** which may include antibiotics, antiemetics, and opioid analgesics. (See *Drug chart 8-1,* pages 193 and 194.)

    2. **Monitor respiratory status closely.**

    3. **Minimize pain.** Position the client to maximize comfort. Assess pain frequently.

    4. **Take steps to reduce and prevent the spread of infection.**

    5. **Provide general preoperative and postoperative care** if surgery is indicated. (See chapter 21.) Provide discharge teaching as described in *Client and family teaching 8-1,* page 197.

X. GASTROENTERITIS

A. **Description.** Gastroenteritis is the inflammation of the stomach and small intestine.

B. **Etiology.** Gastroenteritis is a generic term for various common specific and nonspecific intestinal disorders. Among the many possible causes of gastroenteritis are:

    1. bacterial food poisoning (e.g., *Staphylococcus aureus,* Salmonella, Shigella)

    2. amoebae (e.g., *Entamoeba histolytica*)

    3. adenoviruses, enteroviruses, and coxsackieviruses

    4. parasites (e.g., Ascaris, Enterobius)

    5. nonbacterial food poisoning from toxins in plants (e.g., mushrooms), seafood, or contaminated food

    6. certain drugs (e.g., antibiotics).

C. **Pathophysiology**

    1. Gastroenteritis irritates and inflames the gastric mucosa, resulting in vomiting, which is a protective mechanism that empties the contents of the stomach and portions of the small intestines when noxious or irritating substances affect the GI tract. Diarrhea is produced by toxins that stimulate secretion of water and electrolytes, destruction of the intestinal epithelial cells, and local inflammation by the organism.

    2. In healthy adults, gastroenteritis usually is a self-limited problem producing minor GI symptoms that are more inconvenient than dangerous.

    3. In young children, elderly adults, and debilitated persons, however, these GI symptoms can produce serious, possibly life-threatening fluid and electrolyte losses.

D. **Assessment findings**

    1. **Clinical manifestations** vary with the cause and the level of the GI tract involved. Possible signs and symptoms include:

       a. abdominal cramping

       b. nausea and vomiting

       c. diarrhea

       d. fever and malaise

       e. borborygmi (rumbling, gurgling, tinkling sounds heard on auscultation).

    2. **Laboratory and diagnostic study findings**

       a. Stool specimen shows leukocytes, blood, mucus, or parasite ova.

       b. Hemoglobin and hematocrit values are elevated because of dehydration from vomiting and diarrhea.

       c. Creatinine and blood urea nitrogen levels are elevated with acute diarrhea.

E.   Nursing management (See section II.D.)
1.   **Administer medications,** which may include antidiarrheals and antiemetics. (See *Drug chart 8-1,* pages 193 and 194.)
2.   **Provide measures designed to allow the GI tract to rest** (e.g., administer nothing by mouth, maintain bed rest).
3.   **Promote return to a regular diet.** As acute symptoms subside, gradually provide clear liquids (fluid electrolyte replacement provides oral replacement therapy), followed by bland diet resuming to the client's regular diet.
4.   **Provide ongoing assessment and intervene as necessary.** Closely monitor intake, output, and fluid and electrolyte status. Monitor for dehydration. Increase fluid intake with I.V. infusion if necessary.
5.   **Implement measures to treat diarrhea.** (See *Table 8-1,* page 189.)

XI. MALABSORPTION SYNDROMES

A.   Description. Malabsorption is the failure to transport dietary ingredients such as fat, carbohydrates, proteins, vitamins, and minerals, from the lumen of the GI tract into the body to meet nutritional needs.

B.   Etiology. The many possible causes of malabsorption can be divided into two categories: impaired digestion and impaired absorption.
1.   **Impaired digestion** can result from:
a. postgastrectomy, especially with gastrojejunostomy (Causes decreased pancreatic stimulation because of bypass of the duodenum, decreased mixing of food with digestive enzymes, and decreased intrinsic factor along with stagnation of contents in the proximal small bowel. This leads to bacterial overgrowth, which breaks down bile salts and impairs fat absorption.)
b. impaired function of the liver and biliary tract or pancreas, resulting in lack of digestive enzymes.
2.   **Impaired absorption** can result from:
a. tropical sprue
b. gluten-induced celiac disease
c. lactase deficiency
d. massive intestinal resection after vascular insult or short bowel syndrome
e. jejunal bypass for morbid obesity
f. inflammatory bowel disease
g. radiation enteritis.

C.   Pathophysiology. The GI tract is unable to break down food particles into molecular form for digestion, decreasing the absorption of nutrient molecules into the bloodstream. *Table 8-2* provides the specific nutrient absorption sites.

D.   Assessment findings
1.   **Clinical manifestations** depend on the cause. (See *Table 8-2.*) Common symptoms in many malabsorption syndromes include:
a. diarrhea
b. steatorrhea (i.e., pale, soft, bulky, malodorous stools)
c. abdominal distention and cramping
d. weakness

TABLE 8-2
Comparison of normal absorption with malabsorption states

Normal absorption			Malabsorption	
Small bowel	**Nutrient**	**Also requires**	**Cause**	**Signs and symptoms**
Duodenum	Iron	Gastric acid	▪ Lack of gastric acid	Pallor, anemia
	Calcium	Vitamin D parathyroid	▪ Reduced amount of vitamin D ▪ Reduced fat digestion	Chvostek's sign, Trousseau's sign, tetany, bone pain, pathologic fracture
Jejunum	Protein	Pancreatic secretions	▪ Reduced amount of pancreatic secretions or inadequate absorptive surface	Weakness, fatigue, edema, cachexia
	Carbohydrate	Pancreatic secretions	▪ Reduced amount of pancreatic secretions	Diarrhea, flatulence, abdominal distention
	Fat	Pancreatic lipase bile	▪ Reduced amount of pancreatic secretions	Steatorrhea, diarrhea, weight loss
			▪ Reduced amount of bile acid ▪ Reduced synthesis — liver ▪ Reduced amount to duodenum ▪ Reduced amount of ileal absorption	Jaundice, pruritus
	Vitamin A	Bile salts	▪ Lack of bile salts	Night blindness, dry skin and conjunctiva
	Vitamin D	Bile salts	▪ Lack of bile salts	Osteomalacia, bone pain
	Vitamin E	Bile salts	▪ Lack of bile salts	Rare to have signs or symptoms
	Vitamin K	Bile salts	▪ Lack of bile salts	Bruises easily, bleeding
	Folic acid	—	▪ Impaired mucosal absorption	Diarrhea, weight loss, irritability, forgetfulness
Ileum	Vitamin B_{12}	Intrinsic factor	▪ Gastric reaction ▪ Reduced amount of pancreatic secretion ▪ Ileal resection	Neuropathy, glossitis, anorexia
Colon	Water	—	▪ Reduced length of colon ▪ Decreased absorption ▪ Increased excretion	Watery diarrhea

   e. dry skin and hair
   f. weight loss.
2. **Laboratory and diagnostic study findings vary.**
   a. Serum albumin and protein levels are decreased because of malabsorption of protein.

     b. Hemoglobin and red blood cell counts are decreased because of malabsorption of iron or folic acid.

     c. Serum carotene level is decreased because of malabsorption of vitamin A.

     d. Fecal fat analysis reveals increased levels because of malabsorption of fat.

     e. Colonoscopy of the small intestine allows for biopsy of the mucosa, which can help diagnose tropical sprue or celiac sprue.

     f. Barium swallow with small bowel follow-through visualizes thickened intestinal mucosa.

E. Nursing management (See section II.D.)

    1. Administer medications, which may include antibiotics and antidiarrheal agents. (See *Drug chart 8-1,* pages 193 and 194.) Common supplements are water-soluble vitamins, fat-soluble vitamins, and minerals.

    2. Enhance nutritional status.

      a. Assist with initiation and maintenance of total parenteral nutrition, if indicated. (See chapter 21.)

      b. Monitor for fluid and electrolyte imbalances.

      c. Instruct the client about general nutritional concepts, including:
- basic groups in the food pyramid
- foods to be avoided, depending on the cause of malabsorption (e.g., grain products in gluten intolerance, lactose in lactase deficiency).

    3. Provide a referral to the National Institute of Diabetic & Digestive & Kidney Disorders. (See appendix A.)

XII. CHRONIC INFLAMMATORY BOWEL DISEASE

A. Description. The term inflammatory bowel disease (IBD) is used to identify two chronic inflammatory GI disorders: regional enteritis (i.e., Crohn's disease) and ulcerative colitis.

B. Etiology. Regional enteritis and ulcerative colitis are separate entities with similar causes. Both are characterized by exacerbations and remissions. Exacerbations may be triggered by pesticides, food additives, tobacco, radiation exposure, and immunologic influences. A hereditary predisposition exists in IBD.

C. Pathophysiology

    1. Regional enteritis is a subacute and chronic inflammation that extends through all layers of the bowel wall from the intestinal mucosa. Fistulas, fissures, and abscesses extend into the peritoneum, but segments of normal intestinal tissue occur between the inflammation.

    2. Ulcerative colitis is an inflammatory disease of the submucosal layer of the colon and rectum characterized by continuously occurring ulcerations and shedding of intestinal epithelium. Fat deposits and muscular hypertrophy result in a narrow, short, and thickened bowel.

D. Assessment findings

    1. Clinical manifestations

      a. Regional enteritis
- Abdominal tenderness and pain, typically colicky and increased after meals
- Diarrhea, flatulence, and steatorrhea
- Fever, malaise, and anorexia
- Signs of nutritional deficits

    - Perianal fistulas and abscesses
    - Usually occurs in ileum and ascending colon
  b. Ulcerative colitis
    - Severe diarrhea containing pus, blood, and mucosa
    - Abdominal cramping and tenderness, fever
    - Anorexia and weight loss
    - Usually occurs in the descending colon and rectum
2. **Laboratory and diagnostic study findings**
  a. Regional enteritis
    - Barium study of the upper GI tract, the most conclusive diagnostic test, reveals the classic "string sign" on an X-ray study of the terminal ileum, indicating constriction of a segment of intestine.
    - Barium enema shows ulceration and "cobblestone" appearance because of fissures surrounded by submucosal edema.
    - Colonoscopy visualizes distinct ulcerations separated by relatively normal mucosa in the ileum and ascending colon.
    - Computed tomography scan shows bowel wall thickening and fistula tracts.
  b. Ulcerative colitis
    - Barium enema shows mucosal irregularities, shortening of the bowel, and dilation of bowel loops.
    - Colonoscopy shows friable mucosa with pseudopolyps or ulcers in the descending colon and sigmoid colon.
    - Stool analysis is positive for blood. *Entamoeba histolytica,* which causes dysentery, must be ruled out.

E. Nursing management (See section II.D.)
1. **Administer medications,** which include antidiarrheals, corticosteroids (controversial), antibiotics, antispasmodics, and anticholinergic and opioid analgesics. (See *Drug chart 8-1,* pages 193 and 194.) Salicylate compounds, such as oral mesalamine (an anti-inflammatory) are prescribed during the acute phase of the illness.
2. **Enhance nutritional status.**
  a. Promote nursing care for the client who is receiving nothing by mouth, receiving oral fluids, or on total parenteral nutrition during an acute exacerbation. (See chapter 21.)
  b. Assess for fluid and electrolyte imbalance. Administer I.V. fluids and electrolytes, as indicated.
  c. Encourage a low-residue, high-protein, high-calorie diet with supplemental vitamin therapy and iron replacement.
  d. Implement measures to treat diarrhea or constipation. (See *Table 8-1,* page 189.)
3. **Minimize pain.** Address and medicate the client's pain. Promote intermittent rest periods and bed rest when the client has acute exacerbations.
4. **Promote client and family coping.** Encourage the client to seek psychotherapy to determine the factors that distress the client and how to deal with these factors to prevent exacerbations.
5. **Provide client teaching covering:**
  a. the importance of good nutrition and adequate fluid intake
  b. stress-management techniques
  c. perianal skin care
  d. the need for follow-up visits to the health care provider.

6. **Provide appropriate preoperative and postoperative care, if surgery is indicated.** (See chapters 20 and 21.) Surgery may include total colectomy with ileostomy, segmental colectomy with anastomosis, subtotal colectomy, total colectomy with continent ileostomy, and total colectomy with ileoanal anastomosis. Provide discharge teaching as described in *Client and family teaching 8-1,* page 197.

7. **Provide referrals** to the Crohn's and Colitis Foundation of America, United Ostomy Foundation, and the International Foundation for Functional Gastric Disorders. (See appendix A.)

XIII. IRRITABLE BOWEL SYNDROME

A. **Description.** Irritable bowel syndrome (IBS) is a common functional disorder of GI motility not associated with anatomic changes. It is also known as *spastic colon* or *irritable colon.* It accounts for approximately 50% of all cases of GI illness in the United States; incidence is greater among women than men.

B. **Etiology.** IBS is generally associated with such factors as:
   1. psychological stress
   2. prediverticular disease with changes in the bowel wall
   3. low-residue diet or a diet high in rich and stimulating or irritating foods
   4. alcohol consumption and smoking.

C. **Pathophysiology.** IBS develops in the absence of organic disease or anatomic abnormality. Emotional stress may disturb autonomic nervous system function, leading to disrupted intestinal motility and transit time.

D. **Assessment findings**
   1. **Clinical manifestations.** The typical triad of findings in IBS includes:
      a. abdominal pain with tenderness on palpation (Abdominal pain may be localized in the left lower quadrant, be constant or intermittent, and be relieved by passing flatulence or stool.)
      b. altered bowel habits, such as diarrhea or constipation (Diarrhea often alternates with constipation. Stools may contain increased mucus but seldom contain blood.)
      c. absence of detectable disease. (Symptoms often mimic those of other conditions, hindering the differential diagnosis. The diagnosis must first exclude any organic GI disease or abnormality.)
   2. **Laboratory and diagnostic study findings**
      a. Barium enema and colonoscopy reveal spasms, distention, or mucus accumulation in the intestine.
      b. Complete blood count shows normal findings.
      c. Stool analysis shows normal findings.

E. **Nursing management (See section II.D.)**
   1. **Administer medications,** which may include anticholinergics, antispasmodics, antidiarrheals, and bulk laxatives. (See *Drug chart 8-1,* pages 193 and 194.)
   2. **Teach the client measures to reduce symptoms by:**
      a. eating a well balanced, high-fiber diet; avoiding gas-forming foods; and avoiding fluid intake with meals because it causes abdominal distention
      b. adhering to a schedule of regular work and rest periods
      c. participating in regular exercise, which reduces anxiety and increases intestinal motility

        d. avoiding or minimizing stress-producing situations

        e. drinking six to eight glasses of water daily (not at meals) to prevent constipation

        f. adhering to a regular eating schedule and chewing food slowly and thoroughly.

  3. Promote client and family coping. Provide the client with reassurance and emotional support to help decrease anxiety and increase his sense of control over the situation and its management.

  4. Provide referrals to the International Foundation for Bowel Dysfunction. (See appendix A.)

XIV. POISONING WITH INGESTED AGENTS

A. Description. Poisoning with ingested agents is a condition resulting from accidental or deliberate ingestion of poisonous substances.

B. Etiology. Ingested agents that cause poisoning are alkaline agents or acidic agents. Alkaline agents include lye, bleach, and drain and oven cleaners. Acidic substances include toilet bowl cleaners, battery acid, and rust removers.

C. Pathophysiology. Any agents swallowed may irritate, inflame, or erode any portion of the GI tract. Any of the ingested agent may be absorbed into the systemic circulation and affect the neurologic, cardiovascular, or respiratory system.

D. Assessment findings

  1. Clinical manifestations. Depending on the agent ingested, the client may experience:

        a. burning pain in the mouth and throat

        b. dysphagia

        c. vomiting

        d. drooling

        e. respiratory distress

        f. altered level of consciousness.

  2. Laboratory and diagnostic study findings

        a. Arterial blood gases may reveal metabolic acidosis, metabolic alkalosis, or hypoxia.

        b. Blood specimen shows an increased concentration of the agent.

        c. Blood urea nitrogen and creatinine levels are increased if renal damage has occurred.

E. Nursing management (See section II.D.)

  1. Provide emergency care.

        a. Open the airway, and provide ventilation and oxygenation if needed.

        b. Position the client on his side with his head down.

        c. Suction as needed to prevent aspiration of gastric contents into the respiratory tract.

        d. When calling the poison control center to determine the correct procedure in neutralizing a poisonous agent, the type of agent, amount of agent, length of time since ingestion, and the client's age, weight, and vital signs must be provided.

        e. Remove or inactivate the poison before absorption occurs with:

          – syrup of ipecac for an alert client who has ingested a noncorrosive substance

          – gastric lavage

          – specific antidote to neutralize poisonous substance

          – milk or water for dilution if the client can swallow.

  2. Provide ongoing assessment.

        a. Obtain a blood sample for analysis as ordered.

b. Monitor neurologic status, noting seizure activity, mentation, and central nervous system depression.

3. **Insert an indwelling urinary catheter** as ordered.

4. **Provide client and family teaching.**

   a. Before discharge, provide the client with poisoning prevention guidelines.

   b. Provide the client and his family with the telephone number of the local poison contron center and instruct the client about proper storage of poisoning agents.

5. **Refer the client for psychiatric consultation if the poisoning was a suicide attempt.**

XV. ABDOMINAL TRAUMA

A. **Description.** Abdominal trauma is injury to the abdominal area caused by an external blunt or penetrating force causing damage to one or more of the organs located in the abdominal cavity.

B. **Etiology.** Abdominal injuries result from intra-abdominal trauma (e.g., gunshot wounds, stab wounds) or blunt trauma (e.g., motor vehicle crashes, falls, blows to abdominal area).

C. **Pathophysiology**

   1. The severity of intra-abdominal wounds depends on the velocity with which the missile enters the abdominal cavity. High-velocity force causes more tissue and organ damage.

   2. Blunt trauma occurs when any force hits the abdominal wall, and there is no protective covering (e.g., ribs protecting the thoracic area). The organs and tissues may become edematous, rupture, or bleed because of the trauma. Clients with blunt abdominal wounds require careful and complete assessment because hidden injuries often are not easily detected.

D. **Assessment findings**

   1. **Clinical manifestations**

      a. Visible bruises, lacerations, and penetrating wounds

      b. Abdominal distention, rebound, and maximal point tenderness (may indicate peritoneal irritation from blood or GI fluid)

      c. Pain, especially on movement, and muscle guarding

      d. Absent or diminished bowel sounds

      e. Hypotension and other signs of impending shock

   2. **Laboratory and diagnostic study findings**

      a. Guaiac testing detects occult blood in stool.

      b. Urinalysis identifies hematuria, which may indicate kidney or bladder trauma.

      c. Computed tomography may show abnormal abdominal contents or retroperitoneal damage.

      d. Abdominal and chest radiographs may reveal free air beneath the diaphragm, indicating a ruptured large internal hollow organ.

E. **Nursing management (See section II.D.)**

   1. **Provide emergency care.**

      a. Perform cardiopulmonary resuscitation if necessary, and assess the client simultaneously.

      b. Instruct the client to lie still; explain that movement may dislodge the clot, causing hemorrhage.

c. Apply pressure to external bleeding wounds.

🖐 *d.* Do not remove any penetrating object; removal could cause further internal damage.

e. Insert a nasogastric tube, an I.V. catheter, or an indwelling urinary catheter as indicated.

f. Cover exposed viscera with sterile, normal saline solution dressings.

g. Administer nothing by mouth.

2. **Provide drug therapy.**

a. Administer medications, which may include antimicrobials, opioid analgesics, and tetanus toxoid. (See *Drug chart 8-1,* pages 193 and 194.)

b. Avoid opioid administration until a definite diagnosis is made, because it may mask the clinical picture.

3. **Prepare the client for peritoneal lavage or surgery,** if indicated. (See chapter 21.)

4. **Provide discharge teaching** as described in *Client and family teaching 8-1,* page 197.

Study questions

1. The nurse would expect to assess steatorrhea in which disease process?
1. Malabsorption syndrome
2. Gastritis
3. Irritable bowel syndrome (IBS)
4. Duodenal ulcer

2. Which nursing intervention would be included in the care plan for a client with acute diverticulitis?
1. Administering bulk laxatives and increasing fluid intake
2. Encouraging a high-fiber diet and inserting a rectal tube
3. Administering nothing by mouth and initiating nasogastric suctioning
4. Administering antidiarrheal medications and encouraging a low-fiber diet

3. Which signs and symptoms would the nurse expect to find when assessing a client with esophagitis?
1. Mid-epigastric pain and tenderness
2. Abdominal distention and fever
3. Abdominal cramping and vomiting
4. Heartburn and dysphagia

4. When assessing a client admitted with a bleeding gastric ulcer, the nurse would expect to assess which type of stool?

1. Coffee-ground color
2. Clay colored
3. Black, tarry
4. Bright red

5. When developing a teaching plan for a client with gastroesophageal reflux disease (GERD), the nurse should include which discharge instruction?
1. "Elevate the foot of the bed by 6" to 8"."
2. "Lie down immediately after a meal."
3. "Take antidiarrheal medication after each loose stool."
4. "Avoid caffeine, tobacco, and peppermint."

6. A 17-year-old client with a temperature of 100.4° F (38° C) comes into the emergency department complaining of severe abdominal pain in the right lower quadrant (RLQ) and has had nausea and vomiting in the last 6 hours. Which condition would the nurse suspect?
1. Diverticulitis
2. Appendicitis
3. Gastroenteritis
4. Irritable bowel syndrome (IBS)

7. A client who has developed a malabsorption problem after receiving radiation therapy to the head, neck, and abdomen 6 months earlier is at greatest risk for nutritional problems related to which body area?
1. Teeth and tongue
2. Sigmoid and rectum
3. Small intestine
4. Large intestine

8. Which would be an appropriate outcome for the client experiencing constipation?
1. The client eats a high-fiber diet.
2. The client avoids physical exercise.
3. The client drinks one to two glasses of water daily.
4. The client maintains a sedentary lifestyle.

9. When assisting a client diagnosed with malabsorption syndrome to develop criteria for reporting stool characteristics, which stool characteristic would be *most* valuable in identifying diarrhea?
1. Quantity
2. Constituents
3. Color
4. Consistency

10. Which statement by a client with stomatitis receiving nystatin suspension indicates that the nurse's teaching has been effective?
1. "I will chew the tablet thoroughly before swallowing."
2. "I will hold the medication in my mouth for 2 minutes, swish, and then swallow."
3. "I will take the medication with food to decrease gastric irritation."
4. "I will not drink milk or any milk products at least 1 hour before taking medication."

11. Which nursing intervention would be included for the client diagnosed with irritable bowel syndrome (IBS)?
1. Instructing the client to eat a low-fiber diet

2. Administering a histamine-receptor antagonist
3. Encouraging the client to avoid fluids with meals
4. Elevating the head of the bed on 6" to 8" (5.1 to 20.3 cm) blocks

12. Which priority nursing intervention should be included when caring for a client diagnosed with gastroenteritis?
1. Encouraging optimal nutritional intake
2. Alleviating abdominal pain and cramping
3. Administering an oral antiemetic every 2 hours
4. Monitoring intake and output and electrolyte levels

13. Two days after emergency appendectomy for a ruptured appendix, a 58-year-old client has a hard, rigid abdomen and is complaining of abdominal pain that he describes as 7 on a scale of 1 (no pain) to 10 (worst pain). Which interventions should the nurse implement when caring for the client? (Select all that apply.)
1. Encouraging the client to use patient-controlled anesthesia more frequently
2. Notifying the client's health care provider immediately
3. Assessing to determine if client has bowel sounds
4. Encouraging the client to turn, cough, and deep-breathe
5. Administering an opioid analgesic I.V.
6. Determining the client's last white blood cell (WBC) count

14. Which nursing action *best* demonstrates the nurse's understanding of one of the primary complications of peritonitis?
1. Providing small, frequent meals
2. Performing frequent respiratory assessments
3. Assessing skin integrity regularly
4. Evaluating stools for color and consistency

15. Which medications are used in eradicating *Helicobacter pylori* in clients diagnosed with peptic ulcer disease?
1. Bismuth subsalicylate, metronidazole, and tetracycline
2. Antacids, proton pump inhibitors, and antiemetics
3. Antibiotics, analgesics, and corticosteroids
4. Mucosal protective agents, histamine-receptor antagonists, and antidiarrheals

16. Which client teaching instruction should be included for a client receiving corticosteroids?
1. "Avoid going out in the sun without using a sunblock."
2. "Stop taking the medication if moon face or buffalo hump occur."
3. "Take the medication on an empty stomach."
4. "Discontinue the medication gradually by tapering the dose."

Answer key

1. The answer is **1.**
Steatorrhea refers to the formation and passage of bulky, fatty stools, indicating decreased fat absorption. Steatorrhea is associated with malabsorption syndromes. This manifestation is not associated with gastritis, IBS, or duodenal ulcer.

2. The answer is **3.**
During an episode of acute diverticulitis, the bowel must be put totally at rest. The client must receive nothing by mouth, and nasogastric suctioning helps decompress the bowel. After the episode resolves and the pain subsides, the client should resume eating a low residue diet. Bulk laxatives and increased fluid intake help prevent an exacerbation of diverticulosis. A high-fiber diet would further irritate the bowel. A rectal tube is not required for diverticulitis. Diarrhea usually does not accompany diverticulitis.

3. The answer is **4.**
Common clinical manifestations of esophagitis include heartburn, acid regurgitation, belching, dysphagia, and esophageal pain radiating to the arms, neck, and jaw. Mid-epigastric pain and tenderness suggest peptic ulcer disease. Abdominal distention and fever are associated with peritonitis. Abdominal cramping and vomiting are commonly seen with gastroenteritis.

4. The answer is **3.**
For the client with a bleeding ulcer, bleeding is occurring high in the GI tract. Melena, or black, tarry stools, is a sign of bleeding high in the GI tract. The action of the digestive enzymes turns the bright red blood black and tarry before defecation occurs. Coffee-ground color is commonly used to describe emesis, indicative of digested blood from a slow bleeding gastric or duodenal lesion. Clay-colored stools would be expected with biliary obstruction. Bright red bloody stools indicate bleeding low in the GI tract.

5. The answer is **4.**
For the client with GERD, anything that can increase gastric acid production should be avoided, including caffeine, tobacco, peppermint, chocolate, onions, and fatty or fried foods. The head of the bed, not the foot of the bed, should be elevated. After eating, the client should sit up or remain upright for at least 1 hour. Diarrhea usually is not associated with GERD. Antidiarrheal medications are not indicated.

6. The answer is **2.**
Severe RLQ pain (i.e., McBurney's point), nausea, vomiting, and a low-grade fever are common clinical manifestations of appendicitis. A client with diverticulitis typically complains of pain in the left lower quadrant (LLQ) or epigastrium. Gastroenteritis is often mani-

fested by abdominal cramping, nausea, vomiting, and diarrhea. A client with IBS typically complains of altered bowel habits and pain usually localized in the LLQ that is relieved by passing flatus or stool.

7. The answer is **3.**
The small bowel (i.e., duodenum, jejunum, and ileum) is responsible for the absorption of most of the major nutrients, and a malabsorption problem would place the client at greatest risk for nutritional problems. Although an abnormality of the large bowel, including the sigmoid and rectum, could affect water reabsorption, and abnormalities of the teeth and tongue could alter the ability to ingest food, it is the small intestine that supports nutrient absorption.

8. The answer is **1.**
A high-fiber diet induces rapid movement through the colon and a large, soft stool. Lack of physical activity, inadequate fluid intake, and a sedentary lifestyle are predisposing factors for constipation. Regular physical exercise, a high-fiber diet, and plenty of water contribute to regular elimination.

9. The answer is **4.**
The consistency of the stool, which reflects the water content, is most valuable in identifying diarrhea, because an increase in fecal fluid content is most descriptive for diarrhea. It is also important to assess stool color and the presence of mucus, but these characteristics are not specific indicators of diarrhea. The quantity becomes important only when it represents a change from the person's usual elimination pattern.

10. The answer is **2.**
Nystatin suspension is prescribed for an oral fungal infection. Effective teaching is indicated by the client's statement about holding the medication in the mouth for 2 minutes, swishing, and then swallowing the medication. Chewing the tablet thoroughly would be appropriate for antacid tablets or other chewable forms of medications. Nystatin suspension is not taken with food. The client's mouth should be free of debris. Avoiding milk or milk products would be appropriate when tetracycline is prescribed.

11. The answer is **3.**
IBS is a functional disorder of motility. The client should not drink fluids with meals, because this increases abdominal distention. A high-fiber diet, not a low-fiber diet, is recommended. Histamine-receptor antagonists are used to treat peptic ulcer disease. Elevating the head of the bed is appropriate for clients with gastroesophageal reflux disease.

12. The answer is **4.**
With gastroenteritis, the client typically experiences vomiting and diarrhea, which put the client at risk for fluid volume deficit and electrolyte imbalance. Close monitoring of intake and output along with serum electrolyte levels is important to prevent any imbalances and ensure prompt treatment if an imbalance occurs. Usually, the GI tract is allowed to rest by omitting all oral intake. Flatulence and pyrosis are not common symptoms of gastroenteritis.

13. The answers are **2, 3, 6.**
Pain that rates 7 on a scale of 1 to 10 and a hard, rigid abdomen indicate peritonitis and, possibly, a ruptured appendix. This is a medical emergency; the client's health care provider should be notified. Further assessment, which would include assessing bowel sounds and determining if the client's WBC count is elevated, is needed. The nurse should always rule out complications prior to administering pain medication, and encouraging the client to turn, cough, and deep-breathe will not help peritonitis.

14. The answer is **2.**
Because of the proximity of the diaphragm to the abdominal cavity, the client is at high risk for respiratory complications. The severe

pain associated with peritonitis interferes with maximal lung expansion, further increasing the client's risk for respiratory complications. Frequent assessments of the client's respiratory status are essential. Because paralytic ileus commonly occurs, feeding a client with peritonitis and assuming that diarrhea will occur are inappropriate. Impaired skin integrity is not a primary potential complication specific to this disease. Rather, it can occur in any client on bed rest.

15. The answer is **1.**
Bismuth subsalicylate, metronidazole, and tetracycline exert a bacteriostatic effect to eradicate *H. pylori* bacteria in the gastric mucosa. Antacids, anticholinergics, histamine-receptor antagonists, proton pump inhibitors, and mucosal protectants may be used to treat peptic ulcers. However, these medications do not eradicate *H. pylori* bacteria.

16. The answer is **4.**
Corticosteroids suppress adrenal gland function. When these medications are to be discontinued, the dose must be tapered so that the adrenal gland will resume adequate functioning. Otherwise, adrenal insufficiency may occur. Because corticosteroids do not cause photosensitivity, a sunblock is unnecessary. Moon face and buffalo hump are signs of overdose (i.e., Cushing's syndrome), but the client should not stop taking the medication. Corticosteroids should be taken with food to minimize the risk of gastric upset.

9 *Endocrine and metabolic disorders*

I. STRUCTURE AND FUNCTION OF THE ENDOCRINE AND METABOLIC SYSTEMS

A. **Hormones.** Hormones are chemical substances secreted by endocrine glands directly into the blood stream to act on specific target cells. Hormones regulate growth and development, fluid and electrolyte balance, reproduction, adaptation to stress, and metabolism.

1. **Types of hormones**

   a. **Protein** or **peptide hormones** act on cell membranes by binding to receptors. Examples include insulin, vasopressin, growth hormone (GH), and adrenocorticotropic hormone (ACTH).

   b. **Amine hormones** or **amino acids** act on cell membranes. Examples include derivatives, epinephrine, and norepinephrine.

   c. **Steroids** act intracellularly to modify protein synthesis. Examples include cortisol, estrogen, and testosterone.

2. **Hormone regulation.** Hormone secretion is regulated through feedback mechanisms (i.e., for increased levels of a specific hormone, its cations or metabolites inhibit secretion; decreased levels stimulate secretion).

B. **Pituitary gland.** Located at the inferior aspect of the brain within the sella turcica (i.e., small recess in the sphenoid bone), the pituitary gland consists of anterior and posterior lobes. (See *Figure 9-1*, page 218.)

1. The **anterior lobe** synthesizes and releases hormones. Release of these hormones is regulated by the hypothalamus, which secretes releasing and inhibiting hormones. (See *Figure 9-2*, page 219.)

   a. **GH** affects growth of bones and muscles. It also influences protein, lipid, carbohydrate, and calcium metabolism.

   b. **Prolactin** affects mammary glands to stimulate milk production.

   c. **Thyroid stimulating hormone** (TSH) stimulates thyroid hormone production.

   d. **ACTH** stimulates the adrenal cortex to produce steroids (primarily cortisol).

   e. **Follicle-stimulating hormone** stimulates ovaries to develop follicles and secrete estrogen or stimulates testes to develop seminiferous tubules and perform spermatogenesis.

   f. **Luteinizing hormone**, also called *interstitial cell-stimulating hormone*, stimulates ovaries to form a corpus luteum, initiate ovulation, and produce progesterone or stimulates testes to secrete testosterone.

2. The **posterior lobe** stores and releases hormones synthesized in the hypothalamus. (See *Figure 9-2*, page 219.)

   a. **Oxytocin** stimulates uterine and mammary gland contractions.

   b. **Antidiuretic hormone** (ADH), also called *vasopressin*, acts on the distal renal tubule to increase water reabsorption. The release rate of ADH is regulated by plasma osmolality.

C. **Thyroid gland.** A butterfly-shaped gland located in the neck behind the trachea, the thyroid produces three hormones. (See *Figure 9-1*, page 218.)

1. **Thyroxine** (T_4) and **triiodothyronine** (T_3) regulate cellular metabolic activity. T_3 is produced predominantly from peripheral conversion of T_4. Secretion of T_4 and T_3 is under the control of TSH.

2. **Thyrocalcitonin** is secreted in response to high blood calcium levels. It lowers blood calcium levels by inhibiting bone resorption.

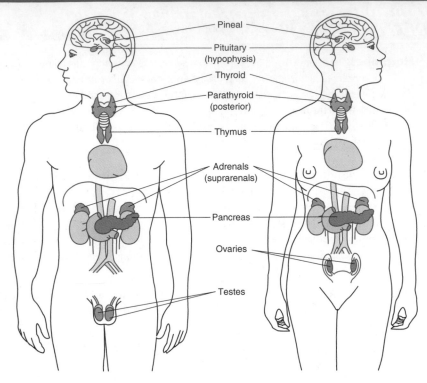

FIGURE 9-1
Major hormone-secreting glands of the endocrine system

D. Parathyroid glands
1. These small glands, usually four, surround the posterior thyroid tissue; they are often difficult to locate and may be removed accidentally during thyroid or other neck surgery. (See *Figure 9-1.*)
2. In response to a low blood calcium level, the parathyroids produce parathormone, which raises blood calcium levels by increasing calcium resorption from kidneys, intestines, and bones.

E. Adrenal glands. Located at the upper poles of both kidneys, the adrenals contain two distinct types of endocrine tissue. (See *Figure 9-1.*)
1. The **adrenal medulla,** in the center of the gland, reacts to autonomic nervous system signals to release catecholamines.
   a. **Epinephrine (adrenalin),** which accounts for approximately 90% of adrenal medulla secretions, prepares the body for the fight-or-flight response by converting glycogen, stored in the liver, to glucose and increasing cardiac output.
   b. **Norepinephrine** produces effects similar to epinephrine and produces extensive vasoconstriction.
2. The **adrenal cortex,** the outer portion of the gland, is stimulated by ACTH to produce corticosteroids.
   a. **Mineralocorticoids** (primarily aldosterone), which are released in response to angiotensin II and ACTH, increase sodium reabsorption and potassium loss primarily through the renal tubules.

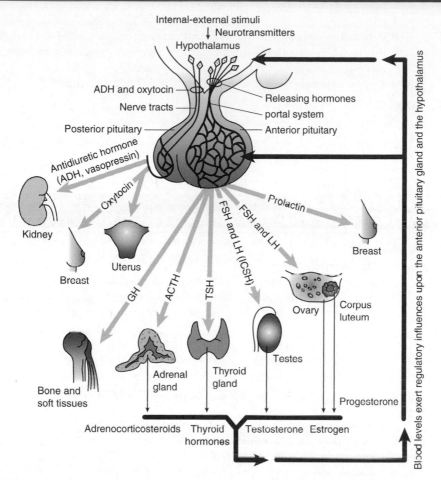

FIGURE 9-2

The pituitary gland, the relationship of the brain to pituitary action, and the hormones secreted by the anterior pituitary and the posterior pituitary

b. **Glucocorticoids** (primarily cortisol), which are released in response to ACTH, increase blood glucose by stimulating gluconeogenesis and lipolysis and decrease protein synthesis, suppress the inflammatory response, and promote sodium retention and potassium loss.

c. **Adrenal sex hormones** (i.e., androgens and estrogen) govern development of certain secondary sex characteristics. Secretion of adrenal androgens is controlled by ACTH.

F. Pancreas. A slender, elongated organ lying horizontally in the posterior abdomen behind the stomach, the pancreas functions as an exocrine and an endocrine gland. (See *Figure 9-1*.)

  1. **Exocrine functions** involve secretion of pancreatic digestive enzymes by specialized cells. (See chapter 16.)

  2. **Endocrine functions** are controlled by the alpha, beta, and delta cells of the islets of Langerhans.

     a. **Alpha cells** secrete glucagon, which increases blood glucose through gluconeogenesis.

     b. **Beta cells** secrete insulin, which regulates protein, carbohydrate, and fat metabolism by facilitating glucose, amino acid, and fatty acid transport; insulin also promotes glycogen, protein, and triglyceride synthesis.

     c. **Delta cells** secrete somatostatin (inhibitory hormone) and gastrin.

G. Gonads

1. The gonads consist of the ovaries and testes. (See *Figure 9-1,* page 218.)
2. Although the gonads exert some systemic metabolic effects, their primary function is in reproduction. (See chapter 10.)

NURSING PROCESS OVERVIEW

 ## II. ENDOCRINE AND METABOLIC SYSTEMS

A. Assessment

1. **Health history**

   a. **Elicit a description of the client's present illness and chief complaint,** including onset, course, duration, location, and precipitating and alleviating factors. Cardinal signs and symptoms indicating altered endocrine and metabolic function include:
   - unexplained weight loss or gain
   - labile mood swings and change in mental status
   - sleep-pattern disturbances
   - alteration in metabolic rate (e.g., tachycardia or bradycardia, diarrhea or constipation)
   - alteration in sexual performance (e.g., alteration in menstrual cycle, impotence).

   b. **Explore the client's health history for risk factors** associated with endocrine and metabolic disorders, including family history of endocrine disorders, radiation therapy, and trauma.

2. **Physical examination**

   a. **Assess** vital signs and measure body weight.

   b. **Inspection**
   - Observe stature, fat distribution, and shape of the face.
   - Note the color, texture, and turgor of the skin; surgical scars; and unusual bruising.
   - Note protruding or sunken eyes and lid lag or retraction.
   - Inspect hair distribution.
   - Assess for the presence of a goiter.

   c. **Palpation.** Palpate the thyroid for size, shape, consistency, symmetry, and tenderness.

   d. **Auscultation**
   - If the thyroid gland is enlarged, auscultate the thyroid to identify the localized audible vibration of a bruit.
   - Auscultate heart, lung, and bowel sounds.

3. **Laboratory and diagnostic studies.** Measurement of hormones in blood and urine reflects production and activity of hormones related to specific endocrine and metabolic disorders. Specific tests are discussed under the appropriate disorders in this chapter; broader types of testing are discussed subsequently.

    a. **Static (present time) measurement,** which is diagnostic for certain disorders, detects elevated or depressed hormone levels.

    b. **Dynamic testing** involves administration of a stimulating or suppressing agent, followed by measurement of hormone response. It requires close collaboration with laboratory personnel to ensure the correct sequence of timed specimens.

    c. **Imaging tests** assist in identifying causative factors. Studies include scans, computed tomography, magnetic resonance imaging, and bone mineral densitometry.

    d. **Selective venous sampling** can differentiate between pituitary and ectopic production of adrenocorticotropic hormone (ACTH). In this procedure, catheters are inserted into each petrosal sinus, draining the pituitary gland and peripheral vein, and ACTH levels are measured after administration of a corticotropin-releasing hormone.

    e. **Water (fluid) deprivation test** demonstrates the inability of the kidneys to concentrate urine.

    f. **Vasopressin test** demonstrates that the kidneys can concentrate urine after administration of antidiuretic hormone.

B. Nursing diagnoses
1. Deficient or excess fluid volume
2. Imbalanced nutrition: less than body requirements
3. Risk for injury
4. Risk for infection
5. Activity intolerance
6. Disturbed body image
7. Sexual dysfunction
8. Ineffective coping
9. Hyperthermia or hypothermia
10. Deficient knowledge

C. Planning and outcome identification. The goals for the client diagnosed with an endocrine or metabolic disorder include improved fluid and nutritional status; a decreased risk for injury and infection; increased activity tolerance; improved body image, sexual functioning, and coping; maintenance of normal body temperature; and an understanding of the disease process and treatments.

D. Implementation
1. **Promote fluid and nutritional balance.**
    a. Assess intake and output accurately, using a urometer if necessary.
    b. Assess for fluid-volume deficit and fluid-volume overload.
    c. Administer I.V. fluids to correct fluid deficiency as indicated.
    d. Monitor appropriate electrolyte levels.
    e. Weigh the client daily at the same time and in the same clothes.
    f. Provide client and family teaching regarding nutritional modifications as indicated.
2. **Protect the client from injury and infection.**
    a. Modify the client's environment as necessary to reduce the risk for injury.
    b. Implement measures to prevent infection. Assess surgical sites for signs of infection.
    c. Instruct the client to always wear an identification bracelet or necklace.
3. **Enhance activity tolerance.** Assist the client with activities of daily living, alternating rest periods with activity.

4. **Enhance the client's body image, sexual functioning, and coping.** Encourage the client to verbalize feelings about the disorder and its effects on his body and sexual functioning. Refer the client to a professional sex counselor, if indicated.

5. **Maintain normothermia.** Assess the client's vital signs frequently. Report a temperature higher than 104° F (38.3° C). Inspect skin color.

6. **Provide client and family teaching.**
   a. Emphasize the importance of regular follow-up evaluation and care.
   b. Teach the client danger signs and symptoms to report, including sudden changes in weight; numbness, paraesthesia, and tetany; extreme thirst; fever; and palpitations.

E. Outcome evaluation

1. The client maintains a normal fluid and electrolyte balance.
2. The client maintains a nutritionally balanced diet and verbalizes appropriate dietary modifications.
3. The client remains injury free, has no signs or symptoms of infection, and displays normal surgical wound healing, if applicable.
4. The client reports adequate energy to perform activities of daily living.
5. The client openly discusses feelings about the disorder's effects on body image.
6. The client resumes usual sexual practices.
7. The client and his family verbalize appropriate coping mechanisms to deal with the endocrine or metabolic disorder and actions to take during periods of stress.
8. The client reports stable vital signs, including temperature.
9. The client verbalizes the importance of complying with the prescribed medication regimen and plans for follow-up care.
10. The client and his family verbalize understanding of the prescribed medication regimen and of health care follow-up plans.

III. ANTERIOR PITUITARY DYSFUNCTION

A. Description. Anterior pituitary dysfunction involves undersecretion or oversecretion of anterior pituitary hormones (e.g., adrenocorticotropic hormone [ACTH], thyroid-stimulating hormone, growth hormone [GH], luteinizing hormone, prolactin [PRL]).

B. Etiology

1. **Hypopituitarism** (i.e., undersecretion)
   a. Pituitary gland infarction
   b. Surgical removal of the pituitary
   c. Genetic disorders or replacement with tumor tissue

2. **Hyperpituitarism** (i.e., oversecretion) commonly results from a secretory adenoma, which stimulates the target gland (i.e., adrenal or thyroid) or tissue.

C. Pathophysiology

1. **Hypopituitarism** affects thyroid, adrenal, and gonadal function. (See sections VI and X.)
2. **Hyperpituitarism** commonly results in altered ACTH or GH secretion, leading to Cushing's syndrome or acromegaly. (See section IX.)

D. Assessment findings

1. **Clinical manifestations**
   a. Hypopituitarism
      – Extreme weight loss

- Atrophy of all endocrine glands and organs
- Hair loss
- Impotence
- Amenorrhea
- Hypoglycemia

  b. **Hyperpituitarism**
- **Excessive GH secretion** (acromegaly in adults)
  - Coarse features (e.g., broad skull, protruding jaw, prognathism, broadening of hands and feet)
  - Thickened heel pads
  - Thick tongue
  - Change in ring and shoe size

  Excessive PRL secretion
  - Decreased libido
  - Amenorrhea
  - Impotence

2. **Laboratory and diagnostic study findings**

   a. **Hypopituitarism**
   - Computed tomography (CT) and magnetic resonance imaging (MRI) may reveal the presence and extent of pituitary tumors.
   - Serum levels of pituitary hormones may be decreased.

   b. **Hyperpituitarism**
   - Visual field examination reveals diminished visual fields.
   - CT scan and MRI may detect a tumor.
   - Serum levels of pituitary hormones may be elevated.

E.   Nursing management (See section II.D.)

1. **Administer prescribed medications,** which may include replacement of missing hormones such as GH. (See *Drug chart 9-1,* pages 224 to 226.)
2. **Prepare the client for indicated procedures or surgery.**
   a. Prepare the client for pituitary irradiation, if indicated.
   b. Prepare the client for surgical removal of a pituitary tumor (i.e., hypophysectomy), if indicated. Approaches may include transfrontal, subcranial, or oronasal-transsphenoidal. (See chapter 21.)
3. **Monitor a postsurgical client for signs of complications.**
   a. Hemorrhage
   b. Transient diabetes insipidus
   c. Rhinorrhea, which may indicate cerebrospinal leak
   d. Adrenal insufficiency (see section X) and thyroid insufficiency (see section VI)
   e. Infection, particularly meningitis (marked by fever, nuchal rigidity, headache)
   f. Visual disturbances, particularly decreased visual fields

IV. POSTERIOR PITUITARY DYSFUNCTION

A.   Description. **Posterior pituitary dysfunction** includes specific disorders involving oversecretion or undersecretion of antidiuretic hormone (ADH).

1. **Diabetes insipidus,** caused by undersecretion of ADH, results in excessive dilute urine production.

(Text continues on page 226.)

DRUG CHART 9-1
Medications for endocrine and metabolic disorders

Classifications	Indications	Selected interventions
Adrenocortical steroid inhibitors aminoglutethimide ketoconazole mitotane	Decrease cortisol production; used to reduce hyperadrenalism caused by ectopic adrenocorticotropic hormone secretion by a tumor that cannot be totally eradicated	■ Administer in divided doses to reduce nausea and vomiting, and instruct the client to continue taking the medication despite discomfort. ■ Inform the client to take safety precautions because medication may cause drowsiness and orthostatic hypotension.
Alpha-glucosidase inhibitors acarbose	Slow the digestion of some carbohydrates; aftermeal blood glucose peaks are not as high	■ Instruct the client to take the medication daily and to continue other measures (diet, exercise) to decrease blood glucose levels. ■ Advise the client that insulin may be needed during times of increased stress. ■ Forewarn the client that possible adverse effects may include hypoglycemia.
Antidiuretic hormone replacement agents desmopressin vasopressin	Conserve renal water by increasing urine osmolality and decreasing urine flow rate	■ May be administered intranasally; instruct the client to notify the health care provider if nasal stuffiness occurs. ■ I.M. injection must be administered deep I.M.; be sure to warm oil-based medications. ■ Instruct the client to report signs of water intoxication (drowsiness, lethargy, headache, sudden weight gain, severe nasal congestion); caution against adjusting dosage without consulting his health care provider.
Antithyroid agents methimazole propylthiouracil	Interfere with conversion of iodine into thyroglobulin, thereby inhibiting thyroid hormone synthesis	■ Advise the client to report flulike symptoms and fever immediately; they may be drug-induced. ■ Tell the client to report signs and symptoms of hyperthyroidism or hypothyroidism. ■ Caution the client not to use or eat products containing iodine, such as cough medicines, iodized salt, or shellfish; tell him to notify his health care providers if he is taking products containing these substances.
Biguanides metformin	Keep the liver from releasing too much glucose	■ Instruct the client to take the medication daily and to continue other measures (diet, exercise) to decrease blood glucose levels. ■ Advise the client that insulin may be needed during times of increased stress. ■ Forewarn the client that possible adverse effects may include hypoglycemia.
D-phenylalanine derivatives nateglinide	Stimulate the release of insulin from beta cells	■ Instruct the client to administer at least 1 to 30 minutes before meals. ■ Instruct the client to omit when skipping a meal.
Electrolyte replacement calcium gluconate	Maintain capillary integrity and normal functioning of the nervous, muscular, and skeletal systems	■ Administer the amount prescribed slowly through a large vein to avoid infiltration, which may cause severe necrosis and sloughing of tissue. ■ Keep the client on bed rest at least 1 hour after drug administration to prevent orthostatic hypotension.

DRUG CHART 9-1

Medications for endocrine and metabolic disorders *(continued)*

Classifications	Indications	Selected interventions
Electrolyte replacement (continued)		▪ Keep the medication at the bedside with the necessary I.V. equipment.
Growth hormone medications bromocriptine	Suppress the release of growth hormone and prolactin	▪ Administer with meals to minimize GI distress. ▪ Instruct the client to report vision problems, severe nausea or vomiting, and acute headaches. ▪ Advise the client to limit his use of alcohol.

Insulin rapid acting
  Humulin R, regular insulin
intermediate acting —Humulin N, NPH
long-acting —
  Humulin L, ultralente
insulin—
  70/30 (70% NPH and 30% R), 60/40, 50/50
	Replace endogenous insulin and maintain blood glucose levels by regulating protein, carbohydrate, and fat metabolism	▪ Answer five questions before administering insulin:
		1) When does insulin peak? Rapid-acting peaks in 2 to 4 hours; intermediate-acting in 6 to 8 hours; long-acting in 16 to 24 hours; humalog acts within 15 minutes; this is the time that hypoglycemic reaction may occur.
		2) What meal covers the peak time? Glucose or food is the antidote for insulin (e.g., 7 a.m. regular insulin is covered by breakfast).
		3) Is the client receiving nothing by mouth? If so, question the insulin order.
		4) What is the client's blood glucose level? If below 90 mg/dl, question the insulin order.
		5) Where will the shot be injected? Absorption is best in the abdomen.
		▪ Teach and demonstrate preparation; administration techniques; injection sites and rotation; insulin and equipment care, storage, and disposal.

Iodine-containing agents Lugol's solution potassium iodide	Inhibit release of stored thyroid hormone and retard hormone synthesis	▪ Administer for short term before thyroidectomy; medication has a short half-life. ▪ Dilute oral iodine solution in juice or beverage of choice; administer through straw with fluids to prevent staining of teeth.
Mineralocorticoids fludrocortisone	Replace hormones; major effect: sodium-retaining activity associated with potassium loss	▪ Explain that additional doses may be needed in times of stress. ▪ Instruct the client to report weight gain and severe headache.
Sulfonylureas acetohexamide chlorpropamide glipizide glyburide tolbutamide	Reduce blood glucose levels by stimulating pancreatic insulin production and make cell receptor sites more receptive to circulating insulin	▪ Instruct the client to take the medication daily and to continue other measures (diet, exercise) to decrease blood glucose levels. ▪ Advise the client that insulin may be needed during times of increased stress. ▪ Forewarn the client that possible adverse effects may include hypoglycemia.
Synthetic glucocorticoids cortisone dexamethasone hydrocortisone sodium succinate methylprednisolone prednisone	Replace adrenocortical; major activities are metabolic effects on carbohydrate, protein, and fat metabolism and anti-inflammatory and immunosuppressive activity	▪ Inform the client that the medication cannot be stopped abruptly but should be discontinued gradually to prevent withdrawal symptoms and, possibly, shock or death. ▪ Identify signs and symptoms of cushingoid effects to report, including weight gain, moon face, buffalo hump, and hirsutism.

(continued)

DRUG CHART 9-1

Medications for endocrine and metabolic disorders *(continued)*

Classifications	Indications	Selected interventions
Synthetic glucocorticoids *(continued)*		▪ Explain that dosage may need to be increased during times of increased stress; instruct the client to carry medication or medical identification.
Thiazolidinediones pioglitazone rosiglitazone maleate	Make muscle cells more sensitive to insulin, decreasing blood glucose levels	▪ Instruct the client to take the medication daily and to continue other measures (diet, exercise) to decrease blood glucose levels. ▪ Advise the client that insulin may be needed during times of increased stress. ▪ Forewarn the client that possible adverse effects may include hypoglycemia.
Thyroid hormone levothyroxine	Raise metabolic rate, promote gluconeogenesis, increase use of stored glycogen, stimulate protein synthesis, and affect protein and carbohydrate metabolism and cell growth	▪ Administer in the morning to avoid bedtime insomnia. ▪ Instruct the client to notify his health care provider of signs and symptoms of hypothyroidism and hyperthyroidism. ▪ Monitor cardiac response to increased metabolic rate and oxygen requirements.
Vitamins and minerals oral calcium vitamin D	Replace therapy for deficit	▪ Observe the client for symptoms of hypercalcemia (eg, nausea, vomiting, headache, mental confusion, anorexia).

---

2. **Syndrome of inappropriate ADH (SIADH),** involving oversecretion of ADH, results in excessive water conservation.

B. Etiology

1. **Diabetes insipidus**

   a. Posterior pituitary destruction from tumors

   b. Vascular accidents

   c. Surgery or hypothalamic damage

   d. Certain drugs that can interfere with ADH secretion or action (e.g., phenytoin, alcohol, lithium carbonate)

   e. Nephrogenic diabetes insipidus, familial or arising from various renal disorders

2. **SIADH**

   a. Central nervous system disorders

   b. Stimulation due to hypoxia or decreased left atrial filling pressure

   c. Pharmacologic agents (e.g., chemotherapy, chlorpropamide)

   d. Overuse of vasopressin therapy

   e. Ectopic ADH production associated with some cancers

   f. Nausea or opioid use, which can stimulate ADH secretion

C. Pathophysiology

1. **Diabetes insipidus** occurs when injury to the posterior pituitary gland causes a decrease in vasopressin secretion or an inability of the kidney tubules to respond to ADH.

2. In **SIADH,** the basic pathologic disturbances are excessive ADH activity, with water retention and dilutional hyponatremia, and inappropriate urinary excretion of sodium in the presence of hyponatremia.

D. Assessment findings

1. **Clinical manifestations**

   a. **Diabetes insipidus**
   - Profoundly increased output (5 to 20 L/day) of dilute urine
   - Nocturia
   - Extreme thirst
   - Weight loss
   - Possible tachycardia, hypotension, and weakness

   b. **SIADH**
   - Decreased urine output
   - Weight gain
   - Altered mental status (e.g., headache, confusion, lethargy, seizures, and coma in severe hyponatremia)
   - Delayed deep tendon reflexes

2. **Laboratory and diagnostic study findings**

   a. **Diabetes insipidus**
   - Plasma osmolality and serum sodium levels are elevated.
   - Water (fluid) deprivation test demonstrates inability of the kidneys to concentrate urine despite increased plasma osmolality and low plasma vasopressin level.
   - Vasopressin test demonstrates that the kidneys can concentrate urine after administration of ADH; this differentiates central (pituitary or hypothalamic) from nephrogenic diabetes insipidus.

   b. **SIADH**
   - Plasma osmolality and serum sodium levels are decreased.
   - Urinalysis detects elevated urine sodium and osmolality.
   - Serum ADH level is elevated.

E. Nursing management (See section II.D.)

1. **Provide general nursing care for diabetes insipidus and SIADH.**
   a. Assess dehydration, skin turgor, and mucous membranes.
   b. Provide meticulous skin and mouth care.
   c. Monitor serum electrolyte levels, including sodium and potassium.

2. **Provide specific nursing care for diabetes insipidus.**
   a. Administer prescribed medications, which may include ADH replacements. (See Drug chart 9-1.)
   b. Replace fluids as indicated. Assess for and report any illness, injury, or other problem that could prevent adequate fluid intake.
   c. Encourage the client to drink fluids in response to thirst. For some unknown reason, the client craves ice cold water.

3. **Provide specific nursing care for SIADH.**
   a. Administer prescribed medications, which may include furosemide (Lasix) to prevent concentration of urine; isotonic urine is excreted, achieving a change in water balance diuretics. Drugs that render the kidneys less sensitive to ADH may be prescribed; demeclocycline is preferred, but lithium may be prescribed.
   b. Restrict fluid intake as indicated.
   c. Regularly assess mental status.

V. HYPERTHYROIDISM

A. **Description.** Hyperthyroidism is a metabolic imbalance resulting from excessive thyroid hormone production. Graves' disease is the most common form. The incidence of Graves' disease is greatest between ages 30 and 40 and is higher among women than men.

B. **Etiology**
    1. Autoimmune dysfunction is the most common cause of Graves' disease; autoantibodies apparently mimic thyroid-stimulating hormone (TSH), leading to hypersecretion of thyroid hormones.
    2. Genetic factors seem to play a role.
    3. Other possible causes include:
        a. toxic nodular goiter
        b. exposure to iodine
        c. TSH-secreting pituitary tumor (rare)
        d. thyroiditis, which may be acute, subacute, or chronic.

C. **Pathophysiology**
    1. Excessive secretion of thyroid hormone leads to an increased metabolic rate, excessive heat production, and increased responsiveness to catecholamines. These actions lead to profound changes in many organ systems.
    2. Severe, acute exacerbation (i.e., thyroid storm) may be a life-threatening, emergent complication.

D. **Assessment findings**
    1. **Clinical manifestations**
        a. **Hyperthyroidism**
            - Nervousness, irritability, hyperactivity, emotional lability, and decreased attention span
            - Weakness, easy fatigability, and exercise intolerance
            - Heat intolerance
            - Weight loss and increased appetite
            - Insomnia and interrupted sleep
            - Frequent stools and diarrhea
            - Menstrual irregularities and decreased libido
            - Warm, sweaty, flushed skin with a velvety-smooth texture and spider telangiectasias
            - Tremor, hyperkinesia, and hyperreflexia
            - Exophthalmos, retracted eyelids, and staring gaze
            - Hair loss
            - Goiter
            - Bruits over the thyroid gland
            - Elevated systolic blood pressure, widened pulse pressure, and S_3 heart sound
            - In elderly clients, heart failure, atrial fibrillation, and few or none of the classic symptoms listed previously
        b. **Thyroid storm**
            - Hyperthermia
            - Hypertension
            - Delirium

  – Vomiting and abdominal pain
  – Tachyarrhythmias
 2. **Laboratory and diagnostic study findings**
    a. Serum thyroid function tests reveal increased T_4 and T_3 levels.
    b. Radioactive iodine uptake test shows an increased uptake.
    c. Serum TSH assay reveals a nondetectable TSH level.
    d. Thyroid scan reveals increased function (i.e., hot areas) in the thyroid gland.

E. Nursing management (see section II.D)
 1. **Assist the client and his family in exploring treatment options**. Include family members because the client's attention span deficit may impair his retention of information. Options include:
    a. pharmacotherapy with drugs that interfere with thyroid hormone synthesis or release. (See *Drug chart 9-1*, pages 224 to 226.)
    b. radioactive iodine therapy, which permanently limits thyroid hormone secretion by destroying thyroid tissue. (Hypothyroidism, requiring lifelong replacement therapy, usually develops at some point after this treatment.)
    c. subtotal or total thyroidectomy. (The thyroid levels must be lowered preoperatively to prevent thyroid storm; lifelong replacement therapy may be necessary.)
 2. **Promote adequate rest.** Encourage a calm environment conducive to rest and relaxation. Minimize the client's energy expenditure by assisting with activities as necessary and encouraging the client to alternate periods of activity with rest.
 3. **Promote adequate nutrition.** Monitor nutritional status. Provide increased calories and other nutritional support as needed.
 4. **Prevent injury.**
    a. Assess the client's mental status and decision-making ability; intervene as needed to ensure safety.
    b. Provide eye protection for a client with exophthalmos: patches, drops, and artificial tears. Instruct the client regarding the use of these items.
 5. **Maintain normothermia.**
    a. Reduce the client's body temperature with a cooling mattress and acetaminophen. Avoid aspirin, which may displace thyroid hormone from its carrier protein and increase hormone levels.
    b. Supply sufficient fluids to offset losses from diaphoresis
    c. Provide appropriate comfort measures for the febrile client.
 6. **Provide client and family teaching.**
    a. Reassure the client's family that any abrupt changes in the client's behavior probably are disease-related and should subside with antithyroid therapy.
    b. Encourage the client to comply with long-term medical follow-up therapy.
 7. **Provide postoperative care,** if appropriate .(See chapter 21.)
    a. Support the head and avoid tension on sutures.
    b. Monitor for complications and intervene as indicated.
    – Thyroid storm (i.e., tachycardia, hyperthermia, exaggerated symptoms of hyperthyroidism) is treated by decreasing temperature, providing supportive care, and monitoring vital signs and hemodynamic parameters for signs of heart failure.
    – Hemorrhage requires the nurse to assess surgical dressing sites and the sides and back of the neck for bleeding.
    – Injury to the recurrent laryngeal requires the nurse to notify the health care provider of any voice changes and advise the client to talk as little as possible.

- Tetany (i.e., spasms of the hands and feet and muscular twitching) occurring after accidental removal of parathyroid glands is treated by I.V. administration of calcium gluconate.
- Edema of the glottis requires the nurse to intervene if breathing difficulty occurs and to keep a tracheostomy tray at bedside at all times.

8. **Provide referrals** to the National Graves' Disease Foundation. (See appendix A.)

VI. HYPOTHYROIDISM

A. **Description.** Hypothyroidism is a state of insufficient serum thyroid hormone. Hypothyroidism is most prevalent in people between ages 40 and 50 and affects more women than men.

B. **Etiology**
   1. **Primary hypothyroidism** results from pathologic changes in the thyroid gland caused by:
      a. autoimmune thyroiditis (i.e., Hashimoto's disease)
      b. thyroidectomy
      c. radioactive iodine therapy
      d. antithyroid medication therapy.
   2. **Secondary hypothyroidism** results from failure of the pituitary gland to secrete adequate thyroid-stimulating hormone (TSH), possibly because of a tumor, surgical removal, or irradiation.

C. **Pathophysiology**
   1. Inability of the thyroid gland to secrete sufficient amounts of thyroid hormone leads to decreased cellular metabolic activities, decreased oxygen consumption, and decreased heat production. These actions produce mild to marked effects in all organ systems.
   2. A person with hypothyroidism is at risk for life-threatening myxedema coma, which can develop gradually over years or acutely in response to such precipitating factors as infection, cold exposure, or sedative use.

D. **Assessment findings**
   1. **Clinical manifestations**
      a. **Hypothyroidism**
         - Sluggishness, lethargy, depression, apathy, fatigue, and exercise intolerance
         - Memory impairment
         - Muscle aches, numbness and tingling in hands
         - Cold intolerance
         - Constipation
         - Weight gain and decreased appetite
         - Menstrual irregularities, infertility, and decreased libido
         - Dry skin, brittle nails, and dry hair
         - Nonpitting and periorbital edema
         - Husky voice and hoarseness
         - Possible goiter
         - Possible neck scar from previous thyroid surgery
         - Delay in muscle contraction and relaxation of tendon reflexes
         - Diastolic hypotension

- Bradycardia
- In elderly clients, few or no symptoms
b. **Myxedema coma**
- Hypotension
- Hypoventilation
- Hypothermia
- Stupor, possibly progressing to coma
2. **Laboratory and diagnostic study findings**
a. Thyroid function tests reveal decreased triiodothyronine and thyroxine levels.
b. Serum TSH test reveals increased TSH (primary).
c. Serum antibody tests detect presence of antithyroid antibodies (autoimmune).
d. Blood studies reveal elevated cholesterol and creatine phosphokinase.

E. Nursing management (See section II.D.)
1. **Provide pharmacotherapy.**
a. Administer prescribed medications, which will include a thyroid hormone .(See *Drug chart 9-1*, pages 224 to 226.)
b. Keep in mind that a client with hypothyroidism is very sensitive to opioids, anesthetics, and sedatives; drug degradation is delayed, and respiratory depression can develop.
c. Instruct the client and his family in the prescribed medication regimen, including purpose, dosage schedule, and signs of overreplacement and underreplacement.
2. **Administer fluids cautiously,** because the client may not be able to excrete a heavy water load. If the client has hypoglycemia, infuse a concentrated source of glucose.
3. **Provide relief of constipation,** as indicated.
4. **Prevent vascular collapse** in a client who is hypothermic. Refrain from aggressive re-warming.
5. **Institute respiratory assistance when necessary.**
6. **Implement infection prevention measures.**

VII. HYPERPARATHYROIDISM

A. Description. Hyperparathyroidism is overproduction of parathyroid hormone (PTH), resulting in high blood calcium levels and bone demineralization. Hyperparathyroidism may be primary or secondary. Primary hyperparathyroidism is a common condition, usually occurring in people older than age 60 and affecting women more often than men.

B. Etiology
1. **Primary hyperparathyroidism.** About 80% of cases are linked to a single adenoma of the parathyroid gland; the remaining cases are caused by parathyroid hyperplasia.
2. **Secondary hyperparathyroidism** results from an adaptive increase in PTH secretion associated with problems involving chronic hypocalcemia.

C. Pathophysiology
1. PTH is critical to normal calcium homeostasis. An insufficient circulating calcium level stimulates PTH production, which raises the calcium level; when the calcium level rises to normal, PTH secretion is inhibited.
2. A parathyroid adenoma or other problem can produce excessive PTH despite normal serum calcium, causing the abnormalities of primary hyperparathyroidism.

D. Assessment findings

1. **Clinical manifestations.** Although hyperparathyroidism may be asymptomatic, it may produce:
   a. fatigue, muscular weakness, and listlessness
   b. height loss and frequent fractures
   c. renal calculi
   d. anorexia, nausea, abdominal discomfort, and constipation
   e. memory impairment
   f. polyuria and polydipsia
   g. back and joint pain
   h. hypertension.

2. **Laboratory and diagnostic study findings**
   a. Total and ionized serum calcium levels are elevated.
   b. Serum phosphate levels are decreased.
   c. Urinalysis identifies hypercalciuria and hyperphosphaturia.
   d. Radiograph or bone mineral densitometry detects bone demineralization.
   e. Parathyroid hormone levels are elevated.
   f. Parathyroid scan possibly detects abnormal findings.

E. Nursing management (See section II.D.)

1. **Provide preoperative care.**
   a. Prepare the client for surgical treatment of primary hyperparathyroidism, which may include adenoma removal and hyperplastic gland resection.
   b. Force fluids to prevent dehydration, constipation, and kidney stone formation.
   c. Reduce added calcium by eliminating over-the-counter antacids, which may contain calcium; thiazide diuretics, which interfere with renal calcium excretion; and excessive intake of dairy products.

2. **Provide postoperative care,** which is similar to that for thyroidectomy. (See chapter 21.)
   a. As indicated, provide aggressive calcium supplementation after surgery to compensate for "hungry bone" syndrome. Observe the client for symptoms of hypercalcemia (e.g., nausea, vomiting, headache, mental confusion, anorexia).
   b. Assess for renal calculi; report hematuria or flank pain as necessary.
   c. Take measures to protect the client from injury.
      – Assist with activities of daily living and ambulation as necessary.
      – Encourage weight bearing to reduce calcium loss from bones.
      – Teach strategies to minimize falls, which may lead to fractures.
   d. Provide relief of constipation as indicated; prune juice, stool softeners, physical activity, and increased fluid help prevent constipation.
   e. Monitor nutritional status, and intervene as necessary. Advise the client to avoid a diet with restricted or excess calcium.
   f. Reinforce the health care follow-up schedule.

VIII. HYPOPARATHYROIDISM

A. Description. Hypoparathyroidism is parathyroid hormone (PTH) deficiency characterized by hypocalcemia, hyperphosphatemia, and neuromuscular hyperexcitablity.

B. Etiology

1. Hypoparathyroidism may be iatrogenic, caused by accidental removal of or trauma to parathyroid glands during thyroidectomy, parathyroidectomy, or radical head or neck surgery.
2. It also can result from an autoimmune genetic dysfunction (affects more women than men).
3. A reversible form may be associated with hypomagnesemia, which interferes with PTH secretion.

C. Pathophysiology

1. Reduced PTH production slows bone reabsorption, increases neuromuscular irritability, decreases serum calcium level, and increases serum phosphate level.
2. In chronic hypoparathyroidism, calcification can occur in some organs (e.g., eyes, causing cataracts; basal ganglia, possibly causing permanent brain damage).

D. Assessment findings

1. **Clinical manifestations**
   a. Anxiety and irritability
   b. Numbness, tingling, and cramps in extremities
   c. Dysphagia
   d. Photophobia
   e. Evidence of neuromuscular hyperexcitability, such as positive Chvostek's and Trousseau's signs, carpopedal spasms, bronchospasms, laryngeal spasms, arrhythmias, and convulsion
   f. Paradoxical calcification in eyes
2. **Laboratory and diagnostic study findings**
   a. Total and ionized serum calcium levels are low.
   b. Serum phosphate level is elevated.
   c. Serum parathyroid hormone level is low.

E. Nursing management (See section II.D.)

1. **Administer prescribed medications,** which include calcium and vitamin D supplements. (See *Drug chart 9-1,* pages 224 to 226.)
2. **Intervene for life-threatening tetany as indicated.**
   a. Administer I.V. calcium gluconate to prevent calcium depletion.
   b. Be alert for possible laryngeal spasm and resulting respiratory obstruction; keep a tracheostomy set available.
   c. Institute seizure precautions as per hospital protocol (padded side rails and bite blocks are controversial).
   d. Minimize environmental stimuli.
   e. After the crisis resolves, closely monitor calcium levels. Keep I.V. calcium gluconate in the client's room.
3. **Provide care for chronic hypoparathyroidism.**
   a. Encourage a diet high in calcium and low in phosphorus. Milk, milk products, and egg yolks must be avoided because they are high in phosphorus.
   b. Administer vitamin D and magnesium supplementation, as indicated. In clients receiving magnesium, observe for symptoms of hypermagnesemia (i.e., hypotension, respiratory depression, muscle weakness, and confusion).
   c. Administer oral calcium preparations, such as calcium gluconate, to supplement the diet. (See *Drug chart 9-1,* pages 224 to 226.)

4. **Provide client and family teaching** about the medication regimen, including purpose, dosage schedule, and signs and symptoms of hypocalcemia and hypercalcemia. Inform the client that dosage will be adjusted periodically based on the laboratory findings.

IX. ADRENAL HYPERFUNCTION

A. **Description.** Adrenal hyperfunction, also known as *Cushing's syndrome*, involves excessive production of adrenocortical hormones, primarily cortisol but also androgens and mineralocorticoids. The incidence is higher among women than men.

B. **Etiology**
  1. The most common cause of adrenal hyperfunction is bilateral adrenal hyperplasia (i.e., Cushing's disease).
  2. Other causes include:
    a. adrenal adenomas and carcinomas
    b. ectopic adrenocorticotropic hormone (ACTH) production by tumors in other organs, such as the lungs and pancreas
    c. glucocorticoid therapy.

C. **Pathophysiology.** Regardless of cause, impaired regulation of adrenocortical hormones results in excessive hormone levels. Manifestations of adrenal hyperfunction result from the effects of excessive adrenocortical hormone levels on various body systems and functions.

D. **Assessment findings**
  1. **Clinical manifestations** depend on the adrenocortical hormones involved and may include:
    a. weight gain and altered fat distribution (e.g., central obesity with round [moon] face and buffalo hump)
    b. muscle weakness, proximal muscle wasting, and fatigue
    c. frequent infections and poor wound healing
    d. symptoms of hyperglycemia
    e. mental status changes and mood swings
    f. menstrual disturbances such as amenorrhea
    g. diminished libido
    h. skin changes, such as striae, bruises, acne, and thinning of scalp hair
    i. hypertension
    j. hirsutism
    k. susceptibility to compression fractures
    l. edema.
  2. **Laboratory and diagnostic study findings**
    a. Serum potassium level is decreased.
    b. Serum glucose level is elevated.
    c. White blood cell count reveals depressed eosinophil and lymphocyte counts.
    d. Diurnal variation plasma levels reveal elevated plasma cortisol and 24-hour urine cortisol results.
    e. Dexamethasone suppression test results are abnormal (morning cortisol level above 5 g/dl after administration of 1 mg of dexamethasone the night before).
    f. The corticotropin-releasing hormone stimulation test reveals an elevated level of ACTH (indicative of ACTH-mediated adrenal hyperfunction).

g. Results for the 24-hour urinary free cortisol level and 24-hour urine collection for 17-hydroxycorticosteroids and 17-ketosteroids are elevated.

h. Selected radiographic and axial computed tomography studies may determine the site of ectopic ACTH production (e.g., bronchogenic oat cell carcinoma).

E. Nursing management (See section II.D.)

1. **Administer prescribed medications,** which may include adrenocortical steroid inhibitors. (See *Drug chart 9-1,* pages 224 to 226.)

2. **Take measures to protect the client from injury and infection.**
   a. Assess skin integrity regularly.
   b. Avoid agents that can damage skin (e.g., tape, strong soaps).
   c. Promote good hygiene.
   d. Modify the environment to remove or minimize hazards.

3. **Prepare the client for surgery, if indicated.** Keep in mind that any treatment modality can cause temporary (permanent with bilateral adrenalectomy) adrenal insufficiency. (See section X.) Procedures may include:
   a. adrenalectomy, if the cause is adrenal adenoma
   b. transsphenoidal hypophysectomy, if the cause is pituitary adenoma
   c. tumor resection.

4. **Encourage the client and his family to ask questions and verbalize concerns** about disease pathology, body image, treatment, and mental status.

X. ADRENAL HYPOFUNCTION

A. Description. Adrenal hypofunction is a deficiency of adrenocortical hormones. It may be primary (i.e., Addison's disease) or secondary to another problem. Adrenal hypofunction occurs in all age groups and affects both sexes about equally.

B. Etiology

1. **Addison's disease** can result from:
   a. an autoimmune process
   b. hemorrhage into the adrenal gland
   c. adrenalectomy
   d. neoplasm
   e. fungal infection
   f. tuberculosis.

2. **Secondary adrenal insufficiency** is associated with:
   a. suppression of the hypothalamic-pituitary axis from exogenous steroid use
   b. pituitary destruction or removal
   c. inadequate cortisol replacement, especially during times of stress.

C. Pathophysiology. Any problem causing adrenal cortex hypofunction results in deficiencies of adrenocortical hormones. Hormone deficiency produces various fluid, electrolyte, and metabolic disturbances.

D. Assessment findings

1. **Clinical manifestations**
   a. **Addison's disease**
      - GI complaints, such as anorexia, nausea, vomiting, abdominal pain, and diarrhea
      - Fatigue, muscle weakness, and arthralgias
      - Decreased alertness and confusion

  – Weight loss
  – Dry skin, decreased body hair, and possible increased pigmentation with excessive adrenocorticotropic hormone (ACTH) stimulation
  b. **Addisonian (adrenal) crisis**
   – Hypotension
   – Rapid, weak pulse
   – Rapid respiratory rate
   – Pallor and extreme weakness
   – Hyperthermia
 2. **Laboratory and diagnostic study findings**
  a. **Suggestive findings**
   – Serum blood glucose is decreased.
   – Serum sodium level is decreased.
   – Serum potassium level is increased.
   – White blood cell count is increased.
  b. **Definitive findings**
   – Serum cortisol levels are decreased.
   – ACTH stimulation test reveals a low to normal cortisol response.

E. Nursing management (See section II.D.)
 1. **Administer prescribed medications,** which may include synthetic glucocorticosteroids and mineralocorticosteroids. (See *Drug chart 9-1,* pages 224 to 226.)
 2. **Provide immediate treatment for an addisonian crisis.** Treatment includes I.V. fluid, glucose, and electrolytes. Corticosteroid replacement and vasopressors may be administered. The client must avoid exertion.
 3. **Help prevent adrenal crisis.**
  a. Instruct the client to take precautions to avoid unnecessary activity and events that may be stressful.
  b. Ensure that hospitalized, acutely ill clients on long-term glucocorticoid therapy receive additional doses to compensate for stress.
 4. **Provide client and family teaching.**
  a. Discuss hormone therapy, including its purpose, adverse effects, duration, symptoms of abnormalities to report to the health care provider, and the need to inform all health care providers about the steroid replacement therapy.
  b. If overreplacement of glucocorticoids is indicated, inform the client about the purpose of therapy and possible adverse effects, such as cushingoid appearance, weight gain, acne, hirsutism, peptic ulcer, diabetes mellitus, osteoporosis, infection, muscular weakness, mood swings, cataracts, and hypertension.

XI. DIABETES MELLITUS

 A. Description. Diabetes mellitus is a disorder of carbohydrate metabolism resulting from deficiency of or resistance to available insulin and is characterized by hyperglycemia. Diabetes mellitus is the third-leading cause of death from disease.
 1. **Type 1** insulin-dependent diabetes mellitus accounts for 5% to 10% of cases and typically occurs in people younger than age 25. Insulin deficiency and risk of ketosis characterize it.
 2. **Type 2** noninsulin-dependent diabetes mellitus accounts for 90% of cases and most commonly affects people older than age 40. Defects in insulin release and use, insulin

resistance, and little risk of ketosis characterize it. Due to childhood obesity, type 2 is now being diagnosed in children.

3. **Gestational diabetes** is a transitory glucose intolerance during pregnancy that resolves after delivery. It is associated with an increased risk of developing overt diabetes later in life. Gestational diabetes occurs in about 2% to 5% of all pregnancies.

4. **Diabetes associated with other conditions** is described as glucose intolerance caused by other diseases, drugs, or agents.

B. Etiology

1. **Type 1.** The exact cause is unknown, but type 1 may result from an autoimmune process possibly triggered by a virus, with genetic factors playing a part.

2. **Type 2.** Causative factors of type 2 include obesity and genetic susceptibility.

3. **Gestational diabetes.** This is related to anti-insulin effects of progesterone, cortisol, and human placenta lactogen, which increase the amount of insulin needed to maintain glycemic control.

4. **Diabetes associated with other conditions** may result from pancreatic diseases, hormonal abnormalities, or such drugs as glucocorticoids and estrogen-containing preparations.

C. Pathophysiology

1. In diabetes mellitus, insulin secretion is disproportionate to blood glucose levels as a result of deficient insulin production by beta cells; lack of adequate insulin secretion in response to high blood glucose levels; and inactivation of insulin in the circulation. Defective regulation of alpha- and beta- cell hormone release causes gluconeogenesis, resulting in mobilization rather than storage of proteins and fats. The lack of an adequate number of insulin receptors on cell surfaces impairs glucose absorption by cells, resulting in an excessive blood glucose level.

2. **Acute complications** may include diabetic ketoacidosis (DKA), hyperglycemic hyperosmolar nonketotic coma, and hypoglycemia.

   a. **DKA,** occurring in clients diagnosed with type 1 diabetes, is a severe hyperglycemia and acidosis resulting from a combination of insulin deficiency (relative or absolute) and increased levels of insulin antagonistic hormones (e.g., glucagon, cortisol, growth hormone, epinephrine). DKA is associated with failure to take insulin as prescribed, increased physical stress (e.g., infection, surgery), and psychological stress.

   b. **Hyperglycemic hyperosmolar nonketotic coma** (HHNK), occurring in clients with type 2 diabetes, is a combination of severe hyperglycemia and hyperosmolality with little or no acidosis. HHNK occurs most often in older adults and is associated with stress (e.g., infection, surgery, hyperalimentation) or ingestion of certain drugs (e.g., thiazide diuretics, glucocorticoids, phenytoin, sympathomimetics).

   c. **Hypoglycemia** is an excessive insulin-to-blood glucose ratio linked to excessive use of hypoglycemic agents (e.g., insulin, oral agents), decreased food intake, increased physical activity, excessive alcohol consumption, or renal failure (secondary to decreased insulin degradation). It can occur in clients with type 1 or type 2 diabetes.

3. **Chronic complications** include microangiopathy, macroangiopathy, neuropathy, and increased susceptibility to infection.

   a. **Microangiopathy** is the thickening of the capillary basement membrane, most prominently in the retina and glomerulus.

   b. **Macroangiopathy** is atherosclerotic changes accelerated by lipid abnormalities exacerbated by elevated blood glucose level.

c. **Neuropathy** is abnormal nerve function, possibly caused by alteration in enzyme systems and affecting nerve sheaths or neural cell function.

d. **Increased susceptibility to infection** results from an impaired ability of granulocytes to respond to infectious agents.

D. Assessment findings

1. **Clinical manifestations**

   a. **Diabetes mellitus**
   - Polyuria, polydipsia, and polyphagia
   - Weight loss
   - Fatigue and weakness
   - Visual disturbances
   - Recurrent skin, vulva, and urinary tract infections

   b. **DKA**
   - Dehydration
   - Tachycardia
   - Kussmaul's respirations
   - Acetone breath
   - Decreased level of consciousness
   - GI disturbances (e.g., nausea, vomiting, abdominal pain)

   c. **HHNK**
   - Dehydration
   - Decreased level of consciousness
   - Tachycardia
   - Hypotension

   d. **Hypoglycemia**
   - Cool, moist skin or pallor
   - Tachycardia
   - Tremor, paresthesias, confusion
   - Headache progressing to loss of consciousness or seizures
   - Clients who consistently have high blood glucose levels (> 200 mg/dl) show signs or symptoms of hypoglycemia as blood glucose levels are decreasing because of treatment, even though the client's blood glucose levels are elevated above normally accepted parameters (i.e., 160 to 180 mg/dl).

2. **Laboratory and diagnostic study findings**

   a. **Diabetes mellitus**
   - Fasting blood glucose level above 140 mg/dl or postprandial blood glucose level above 200 mg/dl measured on more than one occasion is diagnostic.
   - Glycosylated hemoglobin reveals an elevated blood glucose level over the previous 2 to 4 months.
   - Glucose tolerance test reveals blood glucose over 200 mg/dl at the 2-hour sample.

   b. **DKA**
   - Serum glucose and potassium levels are elevated.
   - Arterial blood gas values indicate metabolic acidosis.

   c. **HHNK**
   - Serum blood glucose is higher than 700 mg/dl.
   - Serum blood osmolality is higher than 330 mOsm/kg.
   - Urine specimen reveals an absence of ketosis.

– Arterial blood gas studies reveal possible mild lactic acidosis.

– Renal function test detects azotemia.

– Serum electrolyte levels reveal hypernatremia and hypokalemia.

d. **Hypoglycemia.** Serum blood glucose level is less than 70 mg/dl.

E. Nursing management (See section II.D.)

1. **Administer prescribed medications,** which may include:

   a. insulin for type 1 diabetes. (See *Drug chart 9-1,* pages 224 to 226.)

   b. sulfonylureas, thiazolidinediones, biguanides, alpha-glucosidase inhibitors, and D-phenylalanine derivatives for type 2 diabetes. (See *Drug chart 9-1,* pages 224 to 226.)

2. **Intervene as indicated for a client exhibiting signs and symptoms of DKA.** Treatment is aimed at preventing dehydration, electrolyte loss, and acidosis.

   a. Administer 0.9% normal saline I.V. at high rate, followed by hypotonic normal saline (0.45%).

   b. Monitor and administer electrolytes as prescribed. The major electrolyte of concern is potassium. Monitor the serum potassium level and electrocardiogram.

   c. Infuse regular insulin I.V. at a slow, continuous rate to decrease blood glucose, which reverses acidosis. Monitor hourly blood glucose values.

   d. Assess vital signs, lungs, intake and output, and monitor ketones.

   e. Assess for precipitating factors.

3. **Intervene as indicated to manage HHNK.**

   a. Provide treatment similar to that for DKA. Manage fluids, electrolytes, and insulin. Insulin is not as crucial because it is not needed for reversal of acidosis as in DKA.

   b. Because clients are usually older, monitor for heart failure and cardiac arrhythmias.

4. **Provide care for a client experiencing hypoglycemia.**

   a. Monitor blood glucose levels.

   b. Administer glucose. Sources include:

   – oral glucose (15 g of carbohydrate) found in a 4- to 6-oz fruit juice or regular cola, 2 to 3 tsp of sugar or honey, 2 to 4 commercially prepared glucose tablets, or 6 to 10 hard sugar candies. (Do not force oral fluids in a client with impaired consciousness.)

   – I.V. glucose (50% dextrose)

   – glucagon (I.M. or subcutaneous delivery).

   c. Administer a source of long-acting carbohydrate to prevent subsequent episodes

   d. Advise the client to carry simple sugar at all times in case of hypoglycemia.

   e. Protect the client from injury.

   f. Keep in mind that a person with long-standing diabetes may develop a defect in counterregulatory hormones, which impairs awareness of hypoglycemic symptoms and puts the person at increased risk for brain damage because of prolonged, untreated hypoglycemia.

5. **Provide teaching** as described in *Client and family teaching 9-1,* page 240.

6. **Provide referrals** to the American Diabetes Association, American Association of Diabetes Educators, and MedicAlert. (See appendix A.)

CLIENT AND FAMILY TEACHING 9-1

Guidelines for the client diagnosed with diabetes mellitus

- Discuss self-monitoring methods such as glucometers. Discuss frequency of monitoring, care and disposal of equipment, record keeping, and reporting of results.
- Instruct the client in techniques for drawing up and administering insulin and disposing of subcutaneous needles. Teach the client to use all available injection sites within one area rather than randomly rotating sites from area to area (the abdomen is the best site).
- Encourage the client to adhere to prescribed dietary modifications. Typically, the client is prescribed a low-fat, low-cholesterol, low-sodium, and high-fiber diet developed by the American Diabetes Association. Encourage the client to follow consistent meal schedules and food amounts. Discuss carbohydrate counting, which is being recommended by many dieticians.
- Encourage the client to follow an appropriate exercise program.
- Teach foot care and protection. Instruct the client to properly bathe, dry, and lubricate his feet; inspect his feet daily for redness, blisters, and ulcerations; use a mirror to check the bottoms of his feet; and wear well-fitting, closed-toe shoes.
- Instruct the client in the care of minor wounds. Instruct him to clean wounds with soap and water, apply antibiotic ointment, and notify his health care provider if signs of infection occur.
- Advise the client to avoid noxious substances (e.g., alcohol, smoking).
- Teach the client to avoid nephrotoxic substances; prevent or treat urinary tract infections immediately; and adjust medications as renal function changes.
- Encourage the client to attend annual ophthalmologic examinations, which allows for early detection and treatment of complications.
- Teach the client sick-day rules, such as continuing insulin or oral hypoglycemics as prescribed, increasing self-monitoring frequency, testing urine ketones, notifying the health care provider, and maintaining adequate fluid and caloric intake (e.g., jello, broth, regular cola, orange juice).

Study questions

1. Which assessment data would help diagnose diabetes insipidus in a client who underwent transsphenoidal surgery?
   1. Polyuria, polydipsia, and polyphagia
   2. Urine output, tented skin turgor, and urine specific gravity
   3. Nervousness, weakness, and warm, sweaty, flushed skin
   4. Constipation, cold intolerance, and sluggishness

2. Which nursing intervention would be included in fluid management for a client diagnosed with syndrome of inappropriate antidiuretic hormone (SIADH)?
   1. Rapid I.V. fluid infusion
   2. Fluid restriction
   3. Increased oral fluid intake
   4. Administration of dextrose fluids I.V.

3. A client receiving propylthiouracil should be instructed to stop the medication immediately and call the health care provider if which sign occurs?
   1. Diarrhea
   2. Palpitations
   3. Fever
   4. Weight gain

4. Which statement about analgesic therapy for a client with hypothyroidism would be appropriate to use as a basis for developing the client's care plan?
   1. Increased dosages will be needed because the client is overweight.
   2. Analgesics are not needed because the client already is lethargic.
   3. Decreased dosages are needed because of prolonged drug degradation rates.
   4. Increased dosages will be needed because of the hypermetabolic state.

nursing intervention should be
:d in the discharge teaching for the
eceiving levothyroxine?
:king serum glucose level twice daily
ng the medication at night to avoid
mnia
fying the heath care provider if diar-
, nervousness, or increased heart
occur
ng a blood test to monitor glycosy-
l hemoglobin every 3 months

outcome represents the *best* indica-
good overall diabetes control?
client reports urine glucose levels
:ating no glucosuria.
client displays a glycosylated hemo-
in level within control range.
client reports urine ketone levels re-
ing no ketonuria.
client records home glucose test re-
daily.

instruction represents the *best* rec-
idation to give a client with diabetes
ye examinations?
minations should be scheduled an-
ly."
minations should be scheduled
y 2 years."
minations are scheduled according
sion changes."
minations should be performed by
ptometrist."

client behavior would support the
g diagnosis deficient knowledge for
ent with insulin-dependent diabetes
is?
ent weight gain of 15 lb
ire to monitor blood glucose level
ping insulin doses when feeling ill
ng whenever diabetes is mentioned

sults of blood glucose monitoring for
: with diabetes who takes regular and

NPH insulin in the morning and evening reveals that the client is hyperglycemic before breakfast. Which dose of insulin would the nurse expect to be increased?
1. Morning dose of regular insulin
2. Evening dose of NPH insulin
3. Morning dose of NPH insulin
4. Evening dose of regular insulin

14. The nurse would assess for which signs and symptoms for a client diagnosed with addisonian crisis?
   1. Polyuria, polydipsia, and polyphagia
   2. Tremors, tachycardia, and headache
   3. Hypotension, rapid respirations, and pallor
   4. Positive Chvostek's sign, photophobia, and numbness

15. The nursing assessment data reveal that the client has thickened heel pads, a thick tongue, and a change in ring and shoe size.

Which scientific rationale would the nurse expect as the probable explanation for the client's symptoms?
1. Excessive growth hormone (GH) secretion
2. Undersecretion of antidiuretic hormone (ADH)
3. Excessive adrenocorticosteroid production
4. Undersecretion of the pancreatic beta cells

16. Altered level of consciousness commonly accompanies hyperglycemic hyperosmolar nonketotic coma. Which condition is the underlying pathophysiologic process accounting for this complication?
   1. Inadequate nutrition
   2. Diminished tissue perfusion
   3. Serum hyperosmolality
   4. Fluid volume excess

Answer key

1. The answer is 2.
   Diabetes insipidus is caused by an undersecretion of antidiuretic hormone, resulting in excessive dilute urine production. Assessments involving urine output, tented skin turgor indicating dehydration, and urine specific gravity values can aid in identifying diabetes insipidus. Polyuria, polydipsia, and polyphagia are characteristic manifestations of diabetes mellitus. Nervousness, weakness, and warm, sweaty, flushed skin suggest hyperthyroidism. Constipation, cold intolerance, and sluggishness suggest hypothyroidism.

2. The answer is 2.
   SIADH involves the oversecretion of antidiuretic hormone, resulting in excessive water conservation. Fluid management involves fluid restriction, because the client already has an excess amount of fluid in the body. Rapid administration of I.V. fluids, increased

oral fluid intake, and administration of dextrose-containing I.V. fluids would only exacerbate the client's water-intoxicated state.

3. The answer is 3.
   Propylthiouracil, used to treat hyperthyroidism, may cause agranulocytosis, increasing the client's risk for infection. Fever, possibly indicating infection related to agranulocytosis, must be reported promptly. Diarrhea and palpitations are signs of hyperthyroidism. Weight gain is a common consequence of decreasing thyroid hormone levels.

4. The answer is 3.
   A client with hypothyroidism has increased sensitivity to all drugs because of altered metabolism and excretion, depressed metabolic rate, and depressed respiratory status. Weight is not a factor to be considered for this client's analgesic therapy. Failure to ad-

minister analgesics when appropriate may cause unnecessary suffering. Increased dosages may lead to overdose.

5. The answer is **1.**
In hungry bone syndrome, the bones take up calcium at an accelerated rate, leading to hypocalcemia. Carpopedal spasms, caused by neuromuscular irritability, are symptomatic of hypocalcemia. Weakness and back pain are unrelated to calcium balance. Polyuria is a symptom of hypercalcemia.

6. The answer is **3.**
The client with hypoparathyroidism experiences a decrease in serum calcium levels, and calcium supplementation is necessary. Diuretic use is not necessarily discouraged; thiazide diuretics promote calcium resorption. Vitamin D is necessary for calcium absorption, but special prescription preparations may be needed. There is no contraindication to exercise, because osteoporosis is rare in this group.

7. The answer is **2.**
During periods of stress such as surgery, glucocorticoid dosages must be increased. Decreased or usual doses may lead to adrenal insufficiency.

8. The answers are **1, 5, 6.**
The client is probably having a hypoglycemic reaction. The 70/30 insulin has short-acting insulin included (30 units) that peaks in 2 to 4 hours, so the nurse should obtain the client's glucose level, determine if the client had breakfast, and provide a fast-acting glucose such as orange juice. Taking the client's vital signs will not help the client's symptoms. Because the client is alert, the nurse would not need to administer I.V. dextrose. There is no reason to immediately notify the health care provider; the nurse can treat the client and notify the health care provider later on rounds.

9. The answer is **3.**
Levothyroxine is used to treat hypothyroidism. Diarrhea, nervousness, and increased heart rate are signs of hyperthyroidism, indicating an overdose of medication and the need to notify the health care provider. Checking serum glucose levels and blood tests to monitor glycosylated hemoglobin would be appropriate for a client with diabetes mellitus. Levothyroxine should be taken in the morning to prevent insomnia.

10. The answer is **2.**
Glycosylated hemoglobin values reflect the average blood glucose level over a 2-month period and therefore provide the best evidence of how well controlled the client's blood glucose is. Urine tests for glucose and ketones reflect blood glucose control over only the past few hours. Reports of home blood glucose tests may be helpful, but studies have shown that they often are fabricated or not done as required.

11. The answer is **1.**
Current standards of care published by the American Diabetes Association recommend annual eye examinations by an ophthalmologist. The standards also recommend immediate evaluation of vision changes. Any vision change merits immediate evaluation, and an ophthalmologist, not an optometrist, is the appropriate health care professional for this eye examination.

12. The answer is **3.**
During periods of illness, insulin injections should be continued even if food intake is decreased because physical stress increases blood glucose levels. Weight gain and failure to monitor blood glucose levels represent noncompliant behavior. Crying demonstrates ineffective coping.

13. The answer is **2.**
The NPH insulin taken at supper exerts its greatest effect during the night and at breakfast. The peak action of regular insulin oc-

curs at 3 to 4 hours, so the morning or evening dose could not affect the breakfast-time blood glucose level. The morning dose of NPH dissipates long before breakfast the next morning.

14. The answer is **3.**
The signs and symptoms of an addisonian (adrenal) crisis are the clinical manifestations of shock, such as hypotension, rapid respirations, and pallor. Polyuria, polydipsia, and polyphagia are signs and symptoms of diabetes mellitus. Tremors, tachycardia, and headache are associated with hypoglycemia. A positive Chvostek's sign, photophobia, and numbness are signs of hypoparathyroidism.

15. The answer is **1.**
Thickened heel pads, thick tongue, and a change in ring and shoe size are all signs of excessive GH secretion. Undersecretion of ADH results in syndrome in inappropriate diuretic hormone. Excessive adrenocorticosteroid production leads to Cushing's disease. Undersecretion by the pancreatic beta cells results in diabetes mellitus.

16. The answer is **3.**
Hyperglycemic hyperosmolar nonketotic coma is an acute complication of diabetes mellitus involving a combination of severe hyperglycemia and hyperosmolality with little or no acidosis. The severely elevated glucose level leads to large amounts of fluid loss, resulting in dehydration and serum hyperosmolality, which lead to an altered level of consciousness (LOC). Inadequate nutrition and diminished tissue perfusion, although not linked directly to changes in the LOC, may be involved in the progression of this condition. Fluid volume excess does not occur in hyperglycemic hyperosmolar nonketotic coma.

10 *Reproductive and sexual disorders*

I. STRUCTURE, FUNCTION, AND PHYSIOLOGIC PROCESSES OF THE REPRODUCTIVE SYSTEM

A. Structures of the female reproductive system

1. **External genitalia,** also called the *vulva* (See *Figure 10-1.*)

   a. The **mons pubis,** located over the symphysis pubis, is a subcutaneous pad of adipose tissue covered after puberty with coarse pubic hair.

   b. The **clitoris,** positioned at the forward junction of the labia minora, is a small circular organ of erectile tissue covered by the prepuce (i.e., folded skin).

   c. The **labia majora,** positioned lateral to the labia minora, are two folds of adipose tissue covered by loose connective tissue and epithelium.

   d. The **labia minora,** positioned just posterior to the labia majora, are two hairless folds of connective tissue. The internal surface of this organ is covered with mucus membrane. The external surface is covered with skin.

   e. **Bartholin's glands,** located just lateral to the vaginal orifice, open into the distal vagina.

   f. **Skene's glands,** positioned just lateral to the urinary meatus, open into the urethra.

   g. The **urethral meatus,** located between the labia minora and below and posterior to the clitoris, is the external opening of the urethra.

   h. The **perineum** is an area of muscle, fascia, and ligaments between the vulva and rectum.

   i. The **fourchette** is the tissue located between the external genitalia and the anus.

   j. The **hymen,** located at the distal end of the vagina, is a thin vascular fold that tends to bleed during the first sexual encounter and may be torn during sports activities, tampon insertion, and pelvic examinations.

2. **Internal genitalia** (See *Figure 10-1.*)

   a. The **vagina** is a muscular tube located posterior to the bladder and anterior to the rectum; it extends from the cervix to the external vulva.

   b. The **uterus** is a pear-shaped organ separated from the vagina by the cervix and usually lies at a 90-degree angle to the vagina. Endometrium lines the uterus. The myometrium is the muscular uterine layer.

   c. The **ovaries** are two almond-shaped glands.

   d. The **fallopian tubes** terminate in fimbriae that surround the ovaries. This smooth, hollow tunnel is lined with mucus-secreting and ciliated cells. Beneath this mucous lining is a layer of connective tissue and muscle.

3. **The pelvis**

   a. The **pelvis** is a bony ring formed by four united bones: the two innominate bones (which include the ilium, ischium, and pubis), the coccyx, and the sacrum.

   b. For obstetric purposes, the pelvis is further divided into the **false pelvis** (i.e., superior half) and the **true pelvis** (i.e., inferior half).

   c. The pelvic types include gynecoid, anthropoid, platypelloid, and android.

4. The **breasts,** located anterior to the pectoral muscle, contain mammary glands organized into lobules with collecting ducts that terminate in the nipples.

B. Functions of the female reproductive system

1. **External genitalia**

   a. The **mons pubis** protects the pubic bone from trauma.

   b. The **clitoris** provides for sexual arousal and orgasm.

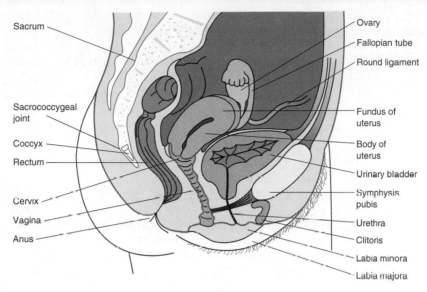

FIGURE 10-1
Female reproductive organs

    c. The **labia majora and minora** protect the external genitalia, urethra, and distal vagina.

    d. Secretions from **Bartholin's glands** lubricate the external vulva during coitus and improve sperm survival.

    e. Secretions from **Skene's glands** lubricate the external genitalia during coitus.

    f. The **urethral meatus** is the external opening of the female urethra.

    g. The **perineal muscle** expands during childbirth to enlarge the vagina, allowing for passage of the fetal head.

  2. **Internal genitalia**

    a. The **vagina** aids in conception by conveying sperm to the cervix and helps in childbirth by serving as a passageway for the fetus.

    b. The **uterus** receives the fertilized egg, provides for implantation, nourishes and protects the growing fetus, and contracts to expel the fetus during childbirth.

    c. The **ovaries** produce and release mature ova and regulate the menstrual cycle through the production of estrogen and progesterone.

    d. The **fallopian tubes** move the sperm toward the ova and the ova toward the uterus, thereby aiding in fertilization.

  3. The **pelvis** supports and protects the reproductive and other pelvic organs. During the late months of pregnancy, the false pelvis supports the uterus and helps direct the fetus into the true pelvis for birth.

  4. The **breasts** serve to produce and secrete (lactate) milk for the infant.

C. Physiologic processes of the female reproductive cycle

  1. **Menstruation,** periodic uterine bleeding, is the process that enables ovulation, fertilization, and implantation. The two cycles of menstruation include the ovarian cycle and the menstrual cycle, which are related to one another and are under hormonal influences.

a. **The ovarian cycle**
 – Under the influence of follicle-stimulating hormone (FSH), a primary follicle develops and matures on the surface of one of the ovaries.
 – Midway through the cycle, under the influence of luteinizing hormone (LH), a mature follicle ruptures and releases a mature ovum into the fallopian tube. This is referred to as **ovulation.**
 – After discharge of the ovum, the ruptured follicle becomes filled with large cells containing a special yellow matter (i.e., corpus luteum). If pregnancy does not occur, the corpus luteum degenerates. If pregnancy does occur, it persists throughout gestation and secretes progesterone.
b. The **menstrual cycle,** which is hormonally controlled, generally ranges from 22 to 34 days (average, 28 days).
 – The **menstrual phase** comprises the first 5 days of the cycle. During this phase, the thick endometrial lining of the uterus is sloughing off from the uterine wall. The detached tissues and blood pass through the vagina as the menstrual flow. The average blood loss during this period is 50 to 150 ml.
 – The **proliferative phase** comprises days 6 to 14 of the cycle. During this phase, the endometrium is repaired, glands are formed in it, and the endometrial blood supply is increased. Ovulation occurs in the ovary at the end of this stage.
 – The **secretory phase** comprises days 15 to 28 in the cycle. During this phase, rising progesterone levels cause the endometrial glands to increase in size and begin secreting nutrients, which sustain a developing embryo (if present) until it is implanted. When conception does not occur, the corpus luteum degenerates, hormone levels decrease, and the cycle begins again.
c. **Female reproductive hormones throughout menstruation**
 – **Gonadotropin-releasing hormone,** secreted by the hypothalamus, stimulates anterior pituitary secretion of FSH and LH.
 – **FSH,** secreted by the anterior pituitary, acts on an ovarian follicle causing it to mature.
 – **LH,** secreted by the anterior pituitary, acts on ovaries to secrete estrogen. LH surges at midcycle to facilitate ovulation and control the secretion of estrogen and progesterone by the corpus luteum.
 – **Estrogen,** secreted by the ovary (follicle and then corpus luteum), causes proliferation of the endometrium. It is responsible for developing and maintaining the female reproductive organs and the secondary sexual characteristics associated with the adult female.
 – **Progesterone,** secreted by the corpus luteum, is the most important hormone for conditioning and maintaining the endometrium. It causes the endometrium to become thick and secretory, allowing for implantation of a fertilized ovum.

2. Gestation and lactation
a. Fertilization of the ovum by a sperm usually occurs in the distal third of the fallopian tube. About 5 days later, the zygote implants into the uterine endometrium.
b. Human chorionic gonadotropin, secreted by chorionic villi in the endometrium of a pregnant female, stimulates the corpus luteum to secrete estrogen and progesterone until the placenta takes over.
c. From the third to the eighth week of gestation, all essential structures of the fetus form. During the remaining weeks these existing structures grow and mature. Throughout pregnancy, the placenta continues to produce progesterone and estrogen. These hormones stimulate growth of the uterus and uterine blood supply, affect contrac-

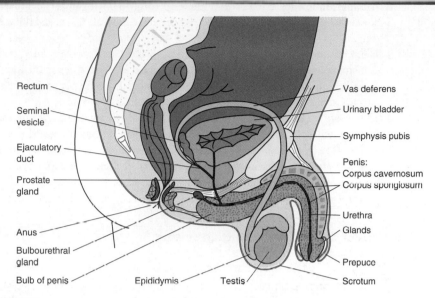

FIGURE 10-2
Male reproductive organs

tile activity, stimulate growth of mammary tissue, and affect the woman's metabolism. Normally, around the 40th week of gestation, the fetus and placenta are expelled from the body. Estrogen and progesterone play a role in initiating parturition. Under the influence of oxytocin, regular contractions increase in frequency and intensity to aid in this process of childbirth.

    d. The breasts produce and release milk for the nourishment of the neonate. The production and release of milk is influenced by prolactin, oxytocin, and suckling of the neonate. This process is referred to as lactation.

3. **Menopause** occurs when menses cease (for at least 1 year), in most women between ages 40 and 55. After menopause, the ovaries atrophy, estrogen levels fall, and changes occur in the vagina, cardiovascular system, skeletal system, and integumentary system.

D. Structures of the male reproductive system

1. **External genitalia** (See *Figure 10-2.*)

    a. The **penis** contains three columns of erectile tissue and the urethra, which terminates at the glans.

    b. The **scrotum** is divided by a septum. Each scrotal sac contains a testis, epididymis, and vas deferens.

    c. The **testes** are two ovoid glands that contain seminiferous tubules, in which spermatogenesis occurs, and interstitial cells, which produce testosterone.

2. **Internal genitalia** (See *Figure 10-2.*)

    a. The **epididymis** extends from the seminiferous tubules of each testis.

    b. The **vas deferens** extends from the epididymis and enters the ejaculatory duct in the prostate gland. This uncoiled, fibromuscular tube is surrounded by arteries, veins, and a thick, fibrous coating.

    c. The **spermatic cord** extends from the testis through the inguinal canal to the abdominal cavity. It is a bundle of blood vessels, nerves, muscle fibers, and the vas deferens.

    d. The **seminal vesicles,** positioned behind the bladder, are two convoluted pouches that empty into the ejaculatory ducts and are lined with secretory epithelium.

    e. The **ejaculatory ducts** join the seminal vesicles and urethra. They pass through the prostate gland and terminate in the prostatic urethra.

    f. The **prostate gland,** located under the bladder and surrounding the urethra, is a walnut-sized gland divided into five lobules by the urethra and ejaculatory ducts.

    g. The **urethra** leads from the base of the bladder through the prostate gland to the shaft and glans of the penis and is divided into three sections: the prostatic, membranous, and penile urethra.

    h. **Bulbourethral glands,** or **Cowper's glands,** are two pea-sized glands located beside the prostate. They drain into the urethra.

E. Functions of the male reproductive system

  1. **External genitalia**

    a. The **penis** serves as the male organ of copulation and the passageway for urine. Sexual excitement leads to venous congestion, which causes distention and erection.

    b. The **scrotum** protects and supports the testes and sperm.

    c. The **testes** produce mature, functional spermatozoa. This is referred to as spermatogenesis, which begins at puberty and continues throughout life. It occurs in several stages:

       – Spermatogonia grow and develop into primary spermatocytes, each containing 44 autosomes and 2 sex chromosomes, X and Y.

       – Primary spermatocytes divide to become secondary spermatocytes, each containing 22 autosomes and 1 sex chromosome, an X or Y.

       – Secondary spermatocytes divide to form spermatids, each retaining 23 chromosomes.

       – Spermatids mature into spermatozoa.

  2. **Internal genitalia**

    a. The **epididymis** stores sperm as it develops the power of motility and the capability to fertilize the female ovum.

    b. The **vas deferens** stores most sperm. During this time sperm continues to mature.

    c. The **seminal vesicles** produce a yellowish, alkaline fluid rich in basic sugar and protein. This fluid enhances sperm motility by nourishing the sperm and improving pH.

    d. The **ejaculatory duct** is the passage through which semen enters the urethra.

    e. The **prostate gland** secretes fluid during sexual activity to add volume to semen, enhance sperm motility, and neutralize male urethral and vaginal acidity to enhance fertility.

    f. The **urethra** serves as passageway for semen during ejaculation and as a canal for urine during voiding.

    g. The **bulbourethral glands** secrete an alkaline fluid that also neutralizes the acid secretions found in the urethra to ensure the safe passage of sperm.

  3. **Testosterone,** secreted by testicular interstitial cells (Leydig's cells), is essential for the development and maintenance of male sex organs and secondary sex characteristics. Testosterone secretion begins in utero and increases at puberty. It is controlled by LH and FSH secreted by the anterior pituitary.

F. Sexual development and identity

1. **Sexual development begins at conception.** Sex is determined by the male's XY chromosomes and female's XX chromosomes; XX chromosomes in combination with XY chromosomes can equal:
   a. girl (X from each parent)
   b. boy (X from mother and Y from father).
2. **Puberty** is the point at which sexual maturity is achieved. The events of puberty are caused by hormonal influences and controlled by the anterior pituitary in response to a stimulus from the hypothalamus. Primary sex characteristics are the external and internal organs that carry out reproductive functions (e.g., penis), and secondary sex characteristics are changes that occur throughout the body as a result of hormonal changes (e.g., voice alterations, development of facial and pubertal hair).

G. Sexual response patterns

1. According to sex researchers Masters and Johnson, **male and female sexual responses** are characterized by vasocongestion and myotonia.
2. **Sexual desire** is controlled by the limbic system of the brain and is mediated by the ratio of testosterone to estrogen.
3. **Four phases of sexual response**
   a. **Excitement,** during which physical and psychological stimulation leads to parasympathetic nerve stimulation
   b. **Plateau,** during which vasocongestion occurs
   c. **Orgasm,** during which continued stimulation leads to discharge of fluids
   d. **Resolution,** during which the genitalia return to the unstimulated state

NURSING PROCESS OVERVIEW

II. THE REPRODUCTIVE SYSTEM

A. Assessment

1. **The female**
   a. **Health history**
      – **Elicit a description of the client's present illness and chief complaint,** including onset, course, duration, location, and precipitating and alleviating factors. Cardinal signs and symptoms indicating altered female reproductive function include irregular or excessive vaginal bleeding, any bleeding after menopause or after intercourse, persistent painful menstruation, abnormal discharge, painful intercourse, urinary tract infection, and bladder dysfunction.
      – **Explore the client's health history for risk factors** associated with female reproductive disease, including noncompliance with routine gynecologic examinations (e.g., Papanicolaou [Pap] smears, mammograms, noncompliance with breast self-examinations), multiple sexual partners, multiple births, and use of hormonal contraceptives.
   b. **Physical examination**
      – **Inspection.** First, inspect the breasts then the external genitalia before performing the internal gynecologic exam.
        - Inspect breasts, noting any asymmetry, skin dimpling, or nipple discharge.
        - The vagina should appear pink with plentiful rugae in the premenopausal woman.
        - The cervix should be pink to red, firm, nontender, with a round or slitlike orifice and possibly with a watery or mucoid discharge.

- Discharge and lesions should be identified on external and internal examinations.
- **Palpation**
  - Palpate the breasts noting tenderness or masses. Client teaching for self-examination should be done during assessment.
  - Bimanually palpate the uterus and adnexa, noting masses, enlargement, or tenderness.

c. **Laboratory and diagnostic studies**
  - The **Pap test** involves cytologic analysis of a sample scraped from the cervix and other tissues to detect infections and malignant changes.
  - **Endocervical curettage** is performed to determine whether abnormal changes have occurred in the cervical canal.
  - **Endometrial smears and biopsies** are an accurate method of diagnosing cellular changes in the endometrium.
  - **Dilatation and curettage** secures endometrial or endocervical tissue for cytologic examination, controls abnormal uterine bleeding, and is a therapeutic measure for incomplete abortion.
  - **Laparoscopy** allows visualization of the pelvic structures.
  - **Hysteroscopy** allows direct visualization of all parts of the uterine cavity.
  - **Hysterosalpingography** is an X-ray view of the uterus and the fallopian tubes to evaluate infertility or tubal patency and to detect any abnormal condition in the uterine cavity.
  - **Blood tests and cultures** identify causative organisms of sexually transmitted diseases (STDs). Cultures may be obtained from the vaginal or cervical tracts or vaginal discharges. Specific studies to detect STDs include:
    - culture and sensitivity
    - Gram stain
    - rapid plasma reagin test
    - serologic testing for syphilis
    - special enzyme or antibody tests.
  - **Ovulation determination tests,** which include basal body temperature and cervical mucus assessment, evaluate fertility by checking if ovulation occurs.
  - **Hormone level studies** evaluate female fertility by checking if hormone levels are appropriate for ovulation, implantation and maintenance of pregnancy.
  - **Postcoital tests** combine ovulation detection and semen analysis to identify how sperm interacts with the vaginal and cervical environment.
  - **Mammography** is a breast imaging technique that can detect nonpalpable lesions.

2. **The male**
  a. **Health history**
    - **Elicit a description of the client's current illness and chief complaint,** including onset, course, duration, location, and precipitating and alleviating factors. Cardinal signs and symptoms indicating altered male reproductive function include pain, discharge, lesions of the genitalia, any difficulty with erection or ejaculation, and any urinary dysfunction.
    - **Explore the client's health history for risk factors** associated with male reproductive disease, including noncompliance with routine male examinations (e.g., digital rectal examinations), noncompliance with testicular self-examination, his-

tory of chronic illness (e.g., diabetes mellitus, cardiovascular disorders), certain medication therapy (e.g., antihypertensives), and multiple sexual partners.

b. **Physical examination.** Preparation for the physical examination of the male client involves asking the client to empty his bladder (unless a urine sample or urethral discharge specimen will be needed) and to disrobe and drape from the waist down. It also involves explanation, reassurance, and glove donning by the nurse.

– **Inspection.** Observe the penis, scrotum, and inguinal area.
  - Skin color and integrity, noting any discoloration and areas of redness
  - Presence of lesions
  - Discharge from the urethral meatus
  - Inability to retract the foreskin in an uncircumcised male; any irritation or inflammation of penis
  - Sparse pubic hair distribution
  - Edematous lymph nodes
  - Bulges that may indicate hernias

– **Palpation**
  - Palpate the testes, noting any masses or abnormalities.
  - Palpate the superficial inguinal area to detect enlarged or tender lymph nodes.
  - Invaginate the finger through the scrotum into the external inguinal ring to check for a hernia while the client bears down.
  - Palpate the prostate during a rectal examination. It should be firm and nontender and not protrude into the rectum. The digital rectal examination is recommended for every man older than age 40.

c. **Laboratory and diagnostic studies**
  – **Prostate-specific antigen** is used to detect prostate cancer.
  – **Prostate fluid culture** (i.e., tissue analysis) reveals disease or inflammation of the prostate gland.
  – **Nocturnal penile tumescence tests** help to determine the cause of erectile impotence.
  – **Blood tests and cultures** obtained from penile discharges evaluate causative organisms. Specific studies to detect STDs are described in section XII.
  – **Semen analysis** evaluates male fertility by checking sperm motility and quantity.

B. Nursing diagnoses
  1. Acute or chronic pain
  2. Impaired urinary elimination
  3. Risk of infection
  4. Sexual dysfunction
  5. Anxiety
  6. Situational low self-esteem
  7. Ineffective coping
  8. Deficient knowledge

C. Planning and outcome identification. The major goals for the client may include relief of pain and discomfort; return to normal elimination patterns; prevention of infection and reinfection; improvement of sexual functioning; reduction of anxiety; improvement of self-esteem and coping; and knowledge of and adherence to the treatment regimen.

D. Implementation

1. **Provide pain relief.**
   a. Believe the client's complaints of pain.
   b. Assess the pain and rule out complications that require immediate medical intervention.
   c. Treat the pain appropriately and evaluate the effectiveness of medical and nursing interventions.

2. **Promote normal elimination patterns.**
   a. Assess the client's bladder function, including occurrences of urinary burning, urgency, or retention.
   b. Assess the client's bowel function, including any change in bowel habits.
   c. Keep in mind that bowel and urinary symptoms may indicate underlying problems.
   d. Encourage the client to drink 3 to 4 qts of fluids daily.
   e. Provide nursing interventions as detailed in *Table 8-1,* page 189 to prevent and alleviate diarrhea or constipation.

3. **Minimize the risk of infection.**
   a. Assess the client for signs of infection, including vaginal or penile drainage and odor or irritation.
   b. Obtain and monitor urine specimens, vaginal or penile cultures and sensitivities, and applicable blood work.
   c. Promote safer sex practices and treatment of sex partners, as indicated.
   d. Teach the client the signs and symptoms of male or female reproductive infections, including STDs. Instruct the client to report signs and symptoms of infection to the health care provider.
   e. Encourage adequate hydration to ensure adequate diffusion of antibiotics.
   f. Instruct the client to wash his hands before and after applying topical medications.

4. **Enhance sexual functioning.**
   a. While maintaining a nonjudgmental attitude, allow the client to verbalize sexual concerns or problems.
   b. Teach the client about normal sexual and reproductive function and clarify any misconceptions.
   c. Refer the client to a specially trained therapist or counselor.

5. **Minimize anxiety and enhance self-esteem by treating the client with respect and dignity.** When caring for a client with a reproductive or sexual disorder, the nurse should:
   a. provide a therapeutic environment
   b. maintain confidentiality and privacy
   c. consider the client's sensitivity to sexual matters
   d. maintain a nonjudgmental attitude to encourage more complete disclosure
   e. offer reassurance and support to the client and his family.

E. Outcome evaluation

1. The client reports adequate pain control and no discharge.
2. The client reports relief of discomfort, urinary incontinence, urinary retention, and bowel incontinence.
3. The client remains free from urinary tract infection and incisional infection.
4. The client remains free from bleeding or infection postoperatively.
5. The client expresses concerns about sexual activity and sexuality, exhibits a positive outlook about sexuality, and seeks counseling as necessary.
6. The client demonstrates and reports reduced anxiety.

7. The client demonstrates an increase in self-esteem and voices fewer self-deprecating remarks.
8. The client verbalizes effective coping techniques when addressing issues concerning sexuality, sexual reproduction, and sexual issues.
9. The client can verbalize an understanding, preventive measures, and treatment of the disease process and the signs or symptoms that should be reported to the health care provider.

III. MENSTRUAL DISORDERS

A. **Description.** Menstrual disorders include premenstrual syndrome (PMS), dysmenorrhea, amenorrhea, and abnormal uterine bleeding.
   1. **PMS** is a cluster of symptoms occurring before onset of menstruation in the menstrual cycle.
   2. **Dysmenorrhea** is painful menstruation.
   3. **Amenorrhea** is absence of menstruation. It is primary (i.e., delayed menarche) or secondary (i.e., occurring after menarche).
   4. **Abnormal uterine bleeding** involves:
      a. menorrhagia, which is excessive bleeding at the usual time of menstrual flow
      b. metrorrhagia, which is bleeding between periods or after menopause.

B. **Etiology**
   1. **Possible causes of PMS**
      a. Estrogen excess or progesterone deficit in the luteal phase of the menstrual cycle
      b. Unidentified hormones that cause symptoms at the time of menstrual changes
      c. Possibly, beta-endorphin activity, serotonin deficiency, elevated prolactin levels, and disturbance of the hypothalamic-pituitary-ovarian axis
   2. **Dysmenorrhea**
      a. Primary dysmenorrhea is unrelated to an identifiable physical cause.
      h. Secondary dysmenorrhea is caused by a pelvic condition that leads to pain.
   3. **Amenorrhea**
      a. Primary amenorrhea may result from minor variations in body build, heredity, environmental factors, or physical, mental, and emotional development.
      b. Secondary amenorrhea may be caused by minor emotional upset, pregnancy, nutritional disturbances (i.e., obesity or anorexia), and pituitary or thyroid dysfunction. Serious, competitive athletes may also experience amenorrhea.
   4. **Abnormal uterine bleeding**
      a. Menorrhagia may be related to endocrine disturbances in early life, whereas it results from inflammatory disturbances, tumors of the uterus, or hormonal imbalance in later life.
      b. Metrorrhagia may be related to adolescence, hormonal contraceptive use, vaginal irritation from infection, cancer, a lowered level of progesterone and endometrial sloughing toward the end of the reproductive years, and psychogenic factors.

C. **Pathophysiology**
   1. **A disruption in the feedback system** between the ovarian, adrenal, thyroid, and pituitary hormonal secretions often occurs.
   2. **Pelvic pathology,** such as a uterine tumor or endometriosis, may cause abnormal menstruation.

3. In **PMS,** the estrogen-progesterone ratio is increased during the luteal phase, causing characteristic estrogen-dependent symptoms.

4. In **dysmenorrhea,** excessive prostaglandin secretion causes uterine hypercontractility and arteriolar spasm.

5. **Amenorrhea** is not a disease entity; it may be abnormal or completely normal, as in pregnancy.

6. **Abnormal uterine bleeding** is usually a symptom of some underlying disease process rather than a disease entity itself.

D. Assessment findings

1. **Associated findings.** In menstrual conditions, the client often describes abnormal menstruation in terms of how often, how long, how heavy, or how painful the menstruation is. Weight loss, inadequate nutrition, or anorexia or bulimia may also be reported.

2. **Clinical manifestations**

   a. **PMS.** Signs and symptoms include headache; fatigue; low back pain; mood swings; irritability; fear of losing control; binge eating; crying spells; and tender breasts approximately 10 days before menses each cycle.

   b. **Dysmenorrhea.** Signs and symptoms include crampy pain that begins before or shortly after onset of menstrual flow and that continues for 48 to 72 hours.

   c. **Amenorrhea.** Primary amenorrhea occurs in women older than age 16 who have not started to menstruate; secondary amenorrhea is an absence of menses for 3 cycles or 6 months after a normal menarche in an adolescent.

   d. **Abnormal uterine bleeding.** Menorrhagia is characterized by prolonged or excessive bleeding at the time of the regular menstrual flow. Metrorrhagia is characterized by vaginal bleeding between regular menstrual periods.

3. **Laboratory and diagnostic study findings**

   a. Diagnostic tests, such as pelvic ultrasonography, hysterosalpingography, and laparoscopy may reveal pelvic pathology contributing to the menstrual problem.

   b. Complete blood cell count commonly reveals decreased hemoglobin concentration and hematocrit with menorrhagia.

E. Nursing management

1. **Administer hormonal contraceptives,** if prescribed, to regulate hormonal balance. (See *Drug chart 10-1.*)

2. **Provide pain relief.** Administer prescribed pain medication. (See *Drug chart 10-1.*) Instruct the client to take analgesics before cramps start, in anticipation of discomfort. (See section II.D.1.)

3. **Promote client and family coping.** Encourage the client to include his familiy in planning working time and activities around symptomatic times.

4. **Provide client teaching.**

   a. Advise the client to maintain a well-balanced diet, eat small meals, and avoid alcohol, caffeine, and nicotine; vitamin supplements may be needed.

   b. Advise the client to keep a diary of her menstrual cycle, including occurrence and heaviness of flow and occurrence of pain and other symptoms; tell her to describe the amount of bleeding by pad count and saturation and to bring a diary to follow-up visits.

   c. Advise the client to use relaxation techniques, an exercise program, and imagery to promote comfort and relieve tension.

DRUG CHART 10-1

Medications for reproductive disorders

Classifications	Indications	Selected interventions
Androgenic steroid danazol	Inhibits gonadotropin release and depresses follicle-stimulating hormone (FSH) and luteinizing hormone; also used to treat endometriosis	▪ Instruct the client to keep an accurate record of the menstrual cycle and to report possible pregnancy immediately. ▪ Assess for weight gain; inspect for acne, edema of dependent area, and hirsutism.
Antibiotics aminoglycosides (gentamicin, tobramycin) amoxicillin erythromycin penicillin tetracycline	Prevent or treat infections caused by pathogenic microorganisms	▪ Before administering the first dose, assess client for allergies and determine whether a culture has been obtained. ▪ After multiple doses, assess the client for super infection (thrush, yeast infection, diarrhea); notify the health care provider if these occur. ▪ Assess the insertion site for phlebitis if antibiotics are being administered I.V. ▪ To assess the effectiveness of antibiotic therapy, monitor the client's white blood cell count. ▪ Monitor peaks and troughs for aminoglycosides.
Anti-infectives and antiprotozoals metronidazole	Attack amebas at intestinal and other tissue sites; also used to treat trichomoniasis	▪ Advise the client that sexual partners must be treated also. ▪ Caution the client that alcohol causes adverse effects, such as nausea, vomiting, and headache.
Antivirals acyclovir	Inhibit viral replication; used to treat herpes simplex virus types 1 and 2	▪ Inform the client that medication can decrease severity and duration of disorder but does not cure and may exacerbate it. ▪ Instruct the client to increase his fluid intake to 3,000 ml/day. ▪ When applying topical agents, always use gloves to prevent contamination, and wash hands before and after administration. ▪ Teach self-administration of vaginal creams, suppositories, and irrigants; advise the client to lie down for 30 minutes after insertion and to wear a perineal pad to prevent soiling clothes. ▪ For I.V. administration, dilute medication and administer over 1 hour on a pump.
Fertility agents bromocriptine chorionic gonadotropin clomiphene metrodin pergonal	Induce ovulation	▪ Inform the client that medication increases the likelihood of multiple pregnancies. ▪ Teach the client to keep a record of basal body temperature and consistency of vaginal mucus.
Hormonal contraceptives and other hormonal agents **Oral contraceptives** ethinyl estradiol and norethindrone	Prevent conception by inhibiting FSH secretion and thereby preventing ovulation or managing menstrual irregularities	▪ Urge the client to stop smoking to prevent possible thromboemboli. ▪ Administer injectable preparations deep I.M., and rotate injection sites. ▪ Instruct the client to take as directed and to not skip pills; caution the client that she is still at risk for sexually transmitted diseases.

(continued)

DRUG CHART 10-1
Medications for reproductive disorders (continued)

Classifications	Indications	Selected interventions
Hormonal contraceptives and other hormonal agents (continued) **Estrogens** chlorotrianisene conjugated estrogen dienestrol estradiol **Progestins** medroxyprogesterone progesterone		
Nonopioid analgesics acetaminophen	Treat mild to moderate pain; blocks the generation blocks impulse through peripheral mechanism	▪ Caution the client that overdose may be toxic to the liver.
Nonsteroidal anti-inflammatory drugs ibuprofen idomethacin ketorolac naproxen salicylates	Reduce inflammatory process-es, thereby reducing pain	▪ Administer with food to minimize gastric upset. ▪ Inform the client that medication may have anti-coagulant effect. ▪ Report tinnitus (ringing in ears), which is a sign of aspirin toxicity.
Opioid analgesics codeine morphine hydrocodone (Codone) hydromorphone (Dilaudid) propoxyphene (Darvon)	Prevent pain sensation and de-crease emotional upset often associated with pain	▪ Assess the pain for location, type, intensity, what increases or decreases it; rate pain on a scale of 1 (no pain) to 10 (worst pain). ▪ Rule out any complications. Is this pain routine or expected? Is this a complication that needs im-mediate intervention? ▪ Medicate according to pain scale findings. ▪ Institute safety measures—bed in low position, side rails up, and call light within reach. ▪ Evaluate the effectiveness of pain medication in 30 minutes.

5. **Assess client for suicidal and uncontrollable or violent behavior.** Refer the client for counseling as needed.

6. **Minimize anxiety and enhance self-esteem** by treating the client with respect and dignity. (See section II.D.5.)

IV. STRUCTURAL DISORDERS OF THE VAGINA AND UTERUS

A. Description

1. **Structural disorders of the vagina**

    a. Vesicovaginal fistula

    b. Rectovaginal fistula

    c. Cystocele

    d. Rectocele

    2. **Structural disorders of the uterus,** also known as *pelvic relaxation disorders*

      a. Uterine displacement (i.e., retroversion, retroflexion, anteversion, and anteflexion)

      b. Uterine prolapse

B. **Etiology.** Structural disorders occur congenitally or as a result of factors that lead to weakened supporting tissues of the vagina or uterus. Such factors include pregnancy, delivery, surgery, radiation therapy, and aging.

C. **Pathophysiology**

    1. **Structural disorders of the vagina**

      a. With **vaginal fistulas,** an abnormal opening is formed through impaired tissue between the bladder or rectum and the vagina, allowing a trickle of urine or feces to flow through the vagina, causing irritation and infection.

      b. **Cystocele** and **rectocele** develop as the pelvic floor muscles atrophy or weaken, allowing the bladder or rectum to bulge onto the anterior or posterior vaginal walls, interfering with urination and bowel elimination.

    2. **Structural disorders of the uterus**

      a. **Uterine displacement.** Normally, the uterus lies at a right angle to the vagina, inclined slightly forward. However, in backward displacement (i.e., retroversion and retroflexion) or forward displacement (i.e., anteversion and anteflexion), the uterus has weakened supporting structures and tilts or is flexed backward.

      b. **Uterine prolapse.** Weakened supporting ligaments allow the uterus to work its way down the vaginal canal (i.e., prolapse) or outside the vaginal orifice (i.e., procidentia).

D. **Assessment findings**

    1. **Associated findings.** The client with a vaginal fistula commonly has a history of tissue damage resulting from delivery, trauma, radiation therapy, or cancer. The client with pelvic relaxation disorder commonly has a history of childbirth, pelvic surgery, or perineal or pelvic trauma.

    2. **Clinical manifestations**

      a. **Vaginal fistulas.** Signs and symptoms include urine trickling continuously into the vagina (i.e., vesicovaginal fistula) and fecal incontinence and flatus discharged through the vagina (i.e., rectovaginal fistula). Leukorrhea along with discharge causes a foul odor.

      b. **Cystocele.** Signs and symptoms include a sense of pelvic pressure, fatigue and such urinary problems as incontinence, frequency, and urgency. Back pain and pelvic pain may also occur.

      c. **Rectocele.** Signs and symptoms include rectal pressure, constipation, uncontrollable flatus, and fecal incontinence.

      d. **Uterine displacements.** Signs and symptoms may include backache, pelvic pressure, and fertility problems, or clients may be asymptomatic.

      e. **Uterine prolapse.** Signs and symptoms include pressure and urinary incontinence or retention. Coughing or heavy lifting may aggravate symptoms. The uterine prolapse may be visible.

    3. **Laboratory and diagnostic study findings.** Instillation of methylene blue dye into the bladder helps identify the course of the vaginal fistula.

E. **Nursing management (See section II.D.)**

    1. **Provide reassurance** that structural disorders are not "normal" changes caused by aging and that treatment can alleviate symptoms.

2. **Teach Kegel exercises to strengthen perineal muscles.** Instruct the client to tighten and relax gluteal and perineal floor muscles (like starting and stopping urinary flow).

3. **Provide and teach proper perineal hygiene** to prevent infection, with perineal irrigations, douches, and sitz baths.

4. **Teach the proper use and care of a pessary,** which may be prescribed for cystocele or rectocele that cannot be corrected surgically.

5. **Explain surgical options,** including possible postoperative complications (e.g., incisional infection and urinary retention). (See chapter 21.)

   a. Vaginal fistulas may or may not require surgery. If surgery is required, a vaginal approach, abdominal approach, or a surgical repair with a urinary or fecal diversion may be done.

   b. A cystocele may require an anterior colporrhaphy. Repair of a rectocele may require a posterior colporrhaphy.

   c. Uterine displacements may require surgery to reposition the uterus.

   d. Uterine prolapse requires surgery to suture the uterus back in place or a hysterectomy.

6. **Provide postoperative care.**

   a. Monitor urine output. Insert a Foley catheter if necessary.

   b. Provide prescribed pain medications and ice packs.

   c. Encourage a well-balanced diet, heat application, and adequate rest to enhance postoperative healing.

   d. Explain the care of sutures; several methods are used.

V. GYNECOLOGIC INFECTIONS

A. Description. Gynecologic infections may or may not be sexually transmitted. (See section XII.)

1. Vulvovaginitis, a common infection in women of all ages
2. Cervicitis
3. Pelvic inflammatory disease (PID)
4. Bartholinitis and bartholinian abscess
5. Toxic shock syndrome (TSS)

B. Etiology. Gynecologic infections are caused by microorganisms, such as bacteria and fungi.

1. **Vulvovaginitis**

   a. Candida albicans (a fungus) causes candidiasis or yeast vaginitis.

   b. Gardnerella vaginalis (a bacterium) causes Gardnerella vaginitis or nonspecific vaginitis.

   c. Vulvovaginitis may be sexually transmitted.

   d. Causative organisms include *Trichomonas vaginalis* (trichomoniasis), a protozoan, and *Sarcoptes scabiei* (scabies) and *Phthirus pubis* (pubic lice), two ectoparasites.

   e. Atrophic vaginitis, an inflammatory condition caused by low estrogen levels in a postmenopausal woman, makes the vagina prone to infection by any organism.

2. **Cervicitis and PID**

   a. Chlamydia trachomatis and *Neisseria gonorrhoeae* are sexually transmitted organisms that may lead to cervicitis or PID.

    b. Escherichia coli, streptococci, and staphylococci are nonsexually transmitted organisms that may cause cervicitis or PID.

  3. **Bartholinitis and bartholinian abscess** formation are caused by *N. gonorrhoeae*, which is sexually transmitted, and by nonsexually transmitted bacteria surrounding the vulva (e.g., *E. coli*, streptococci, staphylococci).

  4. **TSS** is caused by the toxins released by *Staphylococcus aureus*. This infection may be transmitted by chronic vaginal infections, surgical wound infection, and superabsorbent tampons.

C. Pathophysiology

  1. Microorganisms invade the vulva and vaginal mucosa and may colonize and ascend the reproductive tract.

  2. Altered vaginal mucosal conditions (e.g., altered pH, disrupted normal vaginal flora, low estrogen levels) lower resistance to infection.

  3. Childbirth, abortion, and some intrauterine procedures allow bacteria to gain intrauterine access by direct invasion and possibly by spreading through the blood and lymphatics.

  4. Menstruation provides a growth media for bacteria that may ascend upward to cause salpingitis and parametritis.

  5. In TSS, magnesium absorbing fibers of tampons cause decreased magnesium levels, contributing to toxin production by bacteria in the lower reproductive tract.

D. Assessment findings

  1. Associated findings

    a. **Vulvovaginitis.** The client with nonsexually transmitted vulvovaginitis may report recent antibiotic use, hormonal contraceptive use, diabetes mellitus, menopause, pregnancy, poor hygiene, synthetic or tight-fitting undergarments and clothing, frequent douching, or use of vulvovaginal products. Clients with sexually transmitted vulvovaginitis may reveal a history of unprotected sexual activity with a new partner or one who has not been monogamous.

    b. **Cervicitis and PID.** The client may report a history of sexual activity with an infected partner; past episodes of infection; or recent childbirth, abortion, or intrauterine procedure.

    c. **Bartholinitis and bartholinian abscess.** The client may report a history of sexual activity with an infected partner.

    d. **TSS.** The client may report recent menses and tampon use.

  2. Clinical manifestations

    a. **Vulvovaginitis** typically produces complaints of discharge and possibly irritation, itching, or dysuria. On physical examination, the discharge may vary.

      – **Trichomoniasis** may produce a yellow and frothy discharge, with a red, excoriated vulva and vagina. Males are usually asymptomatic.

      – **Scabies and pubic lice** may produce itching, excoriation, burrows, papules, or visible nits or lice.

      – **Gonorrheal infection** may produce a purulent, yellow discharge.

      – **Chlamydial infection** may produce a watery to mucoid to purulent discharge.

    b. **Cervicitis**

      – Cervicitis often produces no symptoms.

      – Cervical discharge, dyspareunia, dysuria, and bleeding may occur.

    c. **PID**

      – Complaints of lower abdominal pain, fever, nausea, and vaginal discharge

– Unilateral or bilateral lower abdominal tenderness, cervical discharge, cervical motion tenderness, and adnexal tenderness on examination

d. **Bartholinitis and bartholinian abscess**
  – Acute, unilateral pain between the labia
  – Possible fever
  – Red, edematous vulva unilaterally, possibly with drainage or visible abscess

e. **TSS**
  – Sudden high fever, headache, vomiting, diarrhea, and myalgias
  – Hypotension and possibly shock
  – A red, macular rash that desquamates in 7 to 10 days
  – Possibly decreased urine output and respiratory distress

3. **Laboratory and diagnostic study findings**
  a. In **vulvovaginitis,** the culture results may be positive for *Candida, Gardnerella,* or *T. vaginalis.*
  b. In **cervicitis,** the culture results may be positive for *Chlamydia, N. gonorrhoeae,* or *Streptococcus.*
  c. In **bartholinitis,** the culture results may be positive for *E. coli, T. vaginalis, Staphylococcus,* or *Streptococcus.*
  d. In **PID,** white blood cell (WBC) count is elevated, and culture results may be positive for *Chlamydia* or *N. gonorrhoeae.*
  e. In **TSS,** WBC, blood urea nitrogen, bilirubin, and creatine phosphokinase levels are elevated.

E. Nursing management

1. **Administer prescribed medications to treat infection,** which may include antibiotics. (See *Drug chart 10-1,* pages 257 and 258.)

2. **Provide pain relief.** (See section II.D.1.)
  a. Administer opioid or nonopioid analgesics. (See *Drug chart 10-1,* pages 257 and 258.)
  b. Encourage sitz baths, warm soaks, or warm perineal irrigations as needed.

3. **Minimize the risk of infection.** (See section II.D.3.)

4. **Encourage adequate rest with activity.**

5. **Provide client teaching.**
  a. Instruct the client to abstain from sexual intercourse or use a condom during sexual activity.
  b. Instruct the client to avoid tub baths.
  c. Explain to the client that douching is unnecessary; daily showers and proper cleaning of the perineal area is sufficient.
  d. Instruct the client that adequate cleaning after voiding and defecation is important.
  e. Encourage the client not to wear tight clothing or scratch this area. Recommend loose-fitting cotton underwear.
  f. Instruct the client not to wear damp swim suits for long periods.
  g. Explain the need to recline for 30 minutes after inserting medication into the vagina (i.e., prevents medication from escaping).
  h. Advise the client to avoid superabsorbent tampons (cause of TSS).

6. **Minimize anxiety and enhance self-esteem** by treating the client with respect and dignity. (See section II.D.5.)

7. **Provide nursing care for the client with TSS.**
  a. Administer antiemetics and antidiarrheal agents for vomiting and diarrhea.
  b. Maintain hydration with I.V. fluids for clients with nausea and vomiting, fever, and shock.

   c. Assess the client's intake and output.

   d. Assess the client for signs and symptoms of dehydration.

8. **Prepare the client with a bartholinian abscess for surgical drainage as indicated.**

VI. GYNECOLOGIC BENIGN TUMORS

A. **Description.** Benign gynecologic tumors include ovarian cysts, uterine leiomyomas, and endometriosis. Most benign conditions usually do not predispose to malignancy.

  1. About 98% of ovarian cysts in women age 29 or younger are benign, but that rate decreases to 50% after age 30.

  2. Leiomyomas (i.e., fibroid tumors) occur in 20% of white women and 40% to 50% of black women.

  3. The incidence of endometriosis is increasing, possibly because of delayed childbearing. Endometriosis is common in nulliparous 25- to 35-year-old women.

B. **Etiology.** The exact cause of most gynecologic tumors is unknown.

C. **Pathophysiology**

  1. **Ovarian cysts** may be simple enlargements of the ovarian corpus luteal and follicular cysts, or they may arise from abnormal growth of the ovarian epithelium.

  2. **Leiomyomas** result from abnormal growths of new tissue that arise in the smooth muscles of the uterine wall. Characteristically, they are firm, well circumscribed, round, and gray white.

  3. In **endometriosis**, retrograde menstruation or retained remnants of embryonic epithelial tissue cause aberrant proliferation of the endometrium, which bleeds and causes adhesions during menstruation.

D. **Assessment findings**

  1. **Clinical manifestations**

    a. **Ovarian cyst.** The client may be asymptomatic or may experience signs and symptoms such as:

      – lower abdominal and back pain

      – dyspareunia (i.e., difficult or painful intercourse)

      – abnormal uterine bleeding

      – palpable ovarian mass

      – acute abdominal pain, guarding, and rebound tenderness with rupture.

    b. **Leiomyoma.** The client may be asymptomatic or may exhibit:

      – pelvic pain or backache or both

      – constipation

      – urinary retention or urgency

      – dysmenorrhea or menorrhagia or both

      – palpable enlarged or irregular uterus.

    c. **Endometriosis.** Common signs and symptoms include:

      – dysmenorrhea starting 1 or 2 days before menstruation and persisting for 2 to 3 days

      – abnormal uterine bleeding

      – dyspareunia

      – infertility

      – tender palpable masses.

  2. **Laboratory and diagnostic study findings**

     a. Endometrial biopsy, a common method of obtaining endometrial tissue, histologically reveals a pattern of whorls.

     b. Hysteroscopy may reveal abnormal growths.

E. **Nursing management (See section II.D.)**

  1. **Administer prescribed medications,** which may include androgenic steroids, hormonal contraceptives, and pain medication. (See *Drug chart 10-1,* pages 257 and 258.)

  2. **Prepare the client for surgery** by offering information and reassurance and performing routine preoperative care. (See chapter 21.) Operations may include vaginal hysterectomy, abdominal hysterectomy, and laparoscopic hysterectomy.

  3. **Provide appropriate postoperative care,** monitoring for such complications as infection, urinary retention, paralytic ileus, fluid and electrolyte imbalance, and thromboembolism. (See chapter 21.)

  4. **Monitor hemoglobin and hematocrit levels, and transfuse blood products for a client with menorrhagia.**

  5. **Provide emotional support, and encourage the client to express concerns** about body image, sexual function, and pain control. Include significant others in all teaching.

  6. **Provide a referral** to the Endometriosis Association. (See appendix A.)

VII. FIBROCYSTIC BREAST CHANGES

A. **Description.** Fibrocystic breast changes refer to a variety of nonneoplastic tissue changes within the breast that produce lumps. This condition occurs most commonly in women between ages 30 and 50. Fibrocystic breast changes may be nonproliferative or proliferative.

B. **Etiology.** The exact cause is unknown, although it is theorized that fibrocystic breast changes arise from exaggerated response of breast tissue to cyclic hormonal stimulation.

C. **Pathophysiology**

  1. **Nonproliferative changes** lead to various degrees of connective tissue fibrosis, cyst formation, and inflammation. Some ductal metaplasia or mild hyperplasia of ductal or lobular cells may result. These changes are not associated with increased risk for breast cancer, although they may make it difficult to diagnose accompanying cancerous masses.

  2. **Proliferative changes** lead to a greater degree of hyperplastic cell growth, especially in the epithelial gland components comprising the acini, ducts, and lobules. Cell changes range from mild to atypical hyperplasia. The greatest risk for malignancy is associated with atypical changes.

D. **Assessment findings**

  1. **Clinical manifestations.** Fibrocystic breast changes may be asymptomatic, or symptoms may include:

     a. palpable cysts (single or multiple, round, soft to firm, usually elastic, and mobile)

     b. tenderness

     c. dull, heavy pain and a sense of fullness, which tends to increase just before menstruation

     d. nipple discharge

     e. noticeable large, dominant cyst.

  2. **Laboratory and diagnostic study findings.** Biopsy may reveal cystic tissue.

E. Nursing management (See section II.D.)
1. **Administer prescribed medications,** which include contraceptives, diuretics, and pain medication. (See *Drug chart 10-1,* pages 257 and 258.)
2. **Provide client and family teaching.**
   a. Recommend that the client wear a supportive bra day and night for a week.
   b. Advise the client to reduce salt and caffeine intake.
   c. Instruct the client to seek primary health care if pain is not relieved after menses begins.
   d. Encourage routine mammograms and breast self-examinations.
3. **Promote coping.** Reassure the client that breast pain is rarely indicative of cancer in its early stages.

VIII. ERECTILE DYSFUNCTION (IMPOTENCE)

A. Description. Impotence refers to the inability to achieve or maintain an erection sufficient to accomplish intercourse. It may be classified as erectile or ejaculatory, and primary or secondary. The incidence of impotence increases with age.

B. Etiology
1. **Psychogenic causes**
   a. Anxiety
   b. Fatigue
   c. Depression
   d. Undue pressure to perform sexually
2. **Possible organic causes**
   a. Occlusive vascular disease
   b. Endocrine conditions (e.g., diabetes, pituitary tumors, hypogonadism)
   c. Genitourinary conditions (e.g., prostatectomy)
   d. Hematologic disorders (e.g., Hodgkin's disease, leukemia)
   e. Neurologic disorders (e.g., neuropathy, parkinsonism)
   f. Genital trauma
   g. Alcohol and drug abuse
   h Medication use (e.g., antipsychotics, anticholinergics, antihypertensives)

C. Pathophysiology
1. Pathologic processes are diverse but commonly involve decreased blood flow to the penis, altered nerve conduction, or decreased hormonal secretion.
2. Impotence may be partial or full, intermittent or constant, transient, selective for partners, and of sudden or gradual onset.

D. Assessment findings
1. **Associated findings.** The client history may reveal a chronic disease or condition, emotional or psychological problem, or use of a prescribed medication.
2. **Clinical manifestations.** Client reports difficulty with attaining or maintaining erection during sexual intercourse.
3. **Laboratory and diagnostic study findings**
   a. Nocturnal penile tumescence monitoring reveals inadequate sleep-related erections that correspond to their waking performance.
   b. Doppler studies of penile blood flow and nerve-conduction studies may be abnormal or normal.

E. Nursing management

1. **Enhance sexual functioning.** Encourage professional sex counseling, especially if impotence is of apparent psychogenic origin. (See section II.D.4.)

2. **Minimize anxiety and enhance self-esteem** by treating the client with respect and dignity. (See section II.D.5.)

3. **Help prevent impotence as a complication of chronic disease or medication use.** Encourage clients with chronic disease or who are on medications to follow up regularly and follow the health care provider's orders. Encourage them to discuss any erectile dysfunction with their health care provider; medications may be changed or treatment adjusted to promote sexual function.

4. **Provide care for the client with a penile prosthesis.** Instruct the client on its use, and monitor for bleeding, infection, pain, or displacement after surgery.

5. **Provide client teaching regarding potential drug therapy for impotence.** Explain that medications can be used to help with impotence, but certain medical conditions prohibit the use of these medications. Instruct the client to take these medications only under strict supervision by a health care provider.

IX. PENILE DISORDERS

A. Description. Conditions of the penis include phimosis, paraphimosis, and priapism.

1. **Phimosis** is a condition in which the foreskin is constricted and cannot be retracted.

2. **Paraphimosis** is a condition in which the foreskin is retracted behind the glans and cannot be replaced.

3. **Priapism** is uncontrolled, persistent erection of the penis. This is a urologic emergency.

B. Etiology

1. **Phimosis.** Poor hygiene of the uncircumcised penis plays a role in the development of phimosis.

2. **Paraphimosis** is caused by a narrow or inflamed foreskin.

3. **Priapism** results from neural or vascular pathophysiology, such as sickle cell thrombosis, spinal cord tumors, or tumor invasion of the penis and its blood vessels.

C. Pathophysiology

1. In **phimosis,** normal secretions of the prepuce accumulate and cause balanitis, with subsequent scarring and calcification preventing foreskin retraction.

2. In **paraphimosis,** after the foreskin is retracted, edema prevents reduction.

3. In **priapism,** the corpora cavernosa become engorged with blood, and venous drainage is impaired. Ischemia, fibrosis, gangrene, and impotence may result.

D. Assessment findings

1. **Phimosis** is marked by a constricted, fixed foreskin over the glans.

2. **Paraphimosis** typically involves sudden restriction of the foreskin behind the glans with edema of the penis distally.

3. **Priapism** is characterized by persistent, painful erection in the absence of sexual desire.

E. Nursing management

1. **Provide pain relief.** (See section II.D.1.)

   a. Administer opioids as prescribed. (See *Drug chart 10-1,* pages 257 and 258.)

   b. Encourage bed rest, elevation of the penis, and ice application to reduce pain and edema.

2. **Prepare the client for medical treatment.**
   a. Prepare the client with phimosis and paraphimosis for a possible circumcision.
   b. Prepare the client with priapism for a possible blood-shunting procedure.
3. **Provide postoperative care.** Monitor bleeding, administer analgesics, and change the petroleum gauze or pressure dressing as indicated. (See chapter 21.)
4. **Teach uncircumcised clients proper cleaning of the glans and prepuce.**

X. MALE REPRODUCTIVE INFECTIONS

A. **Description.** Male reproductive infections include prostatitis, orchitis, and epididymitis. These may be sexually (see section XII) or nonsexually transmitted.
   1. **Prostatitis** is inflammation of the prostate. Prostatitis may be acute or chronic.
   2. **Orchitis** is inflammation of the testes.
   3. **Epididymitis** is inflammation of the epididymis.

B. **Etiology**
   1. Microorganisms, such as bacteria, viruses, fungi, or parasites, cause genitourinary infections. The most common bacterial offenders are gram-negative organisms.
   2. Sexually transmitted organisms also can cause these infections. *Chlamydia trachomatis* is usually the cause of epididymitis in men younger than age 35. (See section XII.)
   3. Not all inflammation of the prostate, epididymis, and testes are caused by infections; some may result from trauma or chemical irritation.

C. **Pathophysiology**
   1. Microorganisms may be carried up the urethra to infect the prostate, epididymis, and testes, or they may be spread through the bloodstream.
   2. Chemical irritation and inflammation of these organs results from extravasation of urine, possibly secondary to urethral stricture or prostatic hyperplasia.
   3. Poor diffusion of antimicrobial medications into the prostate gland may cause relapsing infection in chronic prostatitis.

D. **Assessment findings**
   1. **Prostatitis**
      a. **Clinical manifestations**
         – Sudden onset of fever and chills (e.g., acute prostatitis)
         – Dysuria, urinary urgency, and urinary frequency
         – Perineal pain or low back pain
         – Tender, edematous, warm indurated prostate on palpation
      b. **Laboratory and diagnostic study findings.** Urine culture is positive for bacteria and white blood cells (WBCs).
   2. **Epididymitis**
      a. **Clinical manifestations**
         – Inguinal and scrotal pain
         – Fever
         – Tender, edematous epididymis
         – Edematous, warm scrotum
      b. **Laboratory and diagnostic study findings**
         – Urine culture may reveal bacteria and WBCs.
         – Culture of secretions may reveal *Chlamydia*.
   3. **Orchitis**

a. **Clinical manifestations** commonly include pain and edema of the testes.

b. **Laboratory and diagnostic study findings.** Specimen culture results may be positive for bacteria.

E. **Nursing management**

1. **Administer prescribed medications to treat infection,** which may include antibiotics. (See *Drug chart 10-1,* pages 257 and 258.)

2. **Provide pain relief.** (See section II.D.1.)

a. Administer prescribed pain medications, including anti-inflammatory medications.

b. Encourage bed rest, sitz baths, ice, and scrotal elevation with scrotal bridge.

3. **Minimize the risk of infection.** (See section II.D.3.)

4. **Provide client teaching.**

a. Encourage the avoidance of foods or liquids that have diuretic action or increase prostatic secretions (e.g., alcohol, coffee, tea, chocolate, cola, spices).

b. Advise the client to avoid sitting for long periods, straining, and lifting.

c. Discourage sexual activity until the infection resolves. (However, sex may be beneficial for men with chronic prostatitis.) Encourage treatment for the client's sexual partners, if indicated.

XI. PROSTATE DISORDER

A. **Description.** Benign prostatic hyperplasia (BPH) is a benign enlargement of the prostate gland.

B. **Etiology.** Although the cause is unknown, the condition is hormone dependent.

C. **Pathophysiology.** Male sex hormones stimulate growth and enlargement of the prostate. Prostatic gland enlargement or the enlarging tumor obstructs urine outflow, leading to urinary retention, stasis, and infection.

1. **Clinical manifestations**

a. Symptoms of urinary obstruction include urgency, frequency, hesitancy, decreased urine stream, and dribbling.

b. Hematuria (cancer)

c. Palpation reveals an enlarged, firm prostate (BPH) or a hard, fixed nodule (cancer).

2. **Laboratory and diagnostic study findings**

a. Acid phosphatase level is elevated, indicating cancer.

b. Renal function tests are advanced, indicating advanced BPH.

D. **Nursing management (See section II.D.)**

1. **Explain treatment options.**

a. Transurethral resection of the prostate is performed by endoscopy through the urethra. The prostate gland is removed in small chips with an electrical loop.

b. Hormonal therapy with antiandrogen agents (e.g., finasteride [Proscar]), suppresses glandular cell activity and decreases the size of the prostate.

c. Medications such as $alpha_1$-adrenergic receptor blockers (e.g., terazosin) relax the smooth muscle of the bladder neck and prostate, helping to reduce symptoms; however, long-term efficacy of these agents is unknown.

2. **Provide preoperative and postoperative care.** (See chapter 21.)

a. Teach the client about such possible complications as bleeding, infection, and thrombosis.

b. Maintain urinary catheter drainage to prevent urinary retention and infection.

🖐 *c.* Postoperatively, maintain three-way bladder irrigation to prevent hemorrhage. Be sure to obtain accurate urinary output by subtracting total Foley catheter output from bladder irrigation infused.

d. Monitor intake and output, bleeding, and vital signs.

e. Monitor and take measures to prevent infection, thrombosis, and obstructed catheter.

3. **Teach the client perineal muscle exercises** to help regain urinary control. Warn him to avoid Valsalva's maneuver until healing is complete.

XII. SEXUALLY TRANSMITTED DISEASES

A. Description

1. Sexually transmitted diseases (STDs) are infections of the genitalia and reproductive organs and other body tissues. They are transmitted by sexual activity. Acquired immunodeficiency syndrome, caused by the human immunodeficiency virus (HIV), also can be transmitted sexually, but this disorder of the immune system is discussed in chapter 11, section X.

2. **Classifications**

   a. Vulvovaginitis (see section)

   b. Cervicitis and urethritis (see section V)

   c. Pelvic inflammatory disease (see section V)

   d. Epididymitis (see section X)

   e. Genital lesions

   f. Systemic infections

3. **STDs** are the most prevalent form of infection in the United States; *Chlamydia* is the most common STD. Incidence of all STDs is rising because of increased sexual activity, greater use of nonbarrier contraceptives, and the increasingly high cost of finding and treating partners.

B. Etiology

1. **Genital lesions.** Causative organisms include herpes simplex virus (i.e., genital herpes); human papillomavirus (i.e., genital warts and condyloma acuminatum); molluscum contagiosum; *Haemophilus ducreyi* (i.e., chancroid); and *C. trachomatis* (i.e., lymphogranuloma venereum).

2. **Systemic infection.** Causative organisms include *Treponema pallidum* (i.e., syphilis) and human T-lymphotropic viruses.

C. Pathophysiology

1. **Infectious organisms** enter through the skin and mucous membrane of the genital, oral, or anal regions. They produce inflammation in surrounding tissue and in some cases ascend the reproductive tract, causing scarring and infertility (i.e., gonorrheal and chlamydial infections).

2. The **syphilis** organism travels through the bloodstream and, over many years, damages tissues such as the heart and nervous system.

3. In **genital herpes,** the virus ascends the peripheral nerve to the dorsal root ganglia, where it remains latent until such factors as fever, menses, stress, or pregnancy precipitate recurrent outbreaks.

4. Some **STDs can be transmitted to the fetus** through the placenta or the birth canal, causing spontaneous abortion or congenital infection of the neonate.

CLIENT AND FAMILY TEACHING 10-1
Health education for sexually transmitted disease

- Educate the client regarding the prevention of sexually transmitted disease (STD) through healthy sexual habits, such as abstinence and monogamy.
- Educate the client regarding early clinical manifestations of STDs that require treatment from a health care provider and the importance of follow-up evaluations to ensure the effectiveness of treatment.
- Provide a confidential setting for the treatment of STDs and follow-up evaluations.

- Emphasize the importance of adhering to pharmacologic regimens, because noncompliance may lead to resistant strains and complications.
- Reinforce the importance of having sexual partners treated.
- Explain to the client that all STD cases must be reported to the appropriate public health agency.
- Instruct the client to avoid sexual activity until cured.
- Encourage the client to use latex condoms to prevent future infections.

D. Assessment findings

1. **Associated findings.** Clients may reveal a history of unprotected sexual activity with a new partner or one who has not been monogamous.

2. **Clinical manifestations**

   a. **Genital lesions** may be apparent on inspection of the skin and mucous membranes of the genital, oral, and anal regions. Other symptoms may or may not be present.
   - Genital herpesvirus produces painful vesicles that erode to form ulcers with inguinal lymphadenopathy, possible headache, and milder recurrent outbreaks.
   - Genital warts are nonpainful, soft, fleshy papillary or sessile masses.

   b. **Systemic infections.** A nonpainful chancre with mild inguinal lymphadenopathy may be present in primary syphilis. Generalized rash, fever, and lymphadenopathy may be present in secondary syphilis.

3. **Laboratory and diagnostic study findings**

   a. In syphilis, the rapid plasma reagin test or other serologic test results are positive.
   b. With *N. gonorrhoeae,* the Gram stain, culture, and sensitivity results are positive.
   c. With herpes simplex virus, the tissue culture or antibody test is positive.
   d. With *C. trachomatis,* the tissue culture or antibody test is positive.
   e. With HIV, the antibody test is positive.

E. Nursing management

1. **Administer prescribed medications,** which may include antibiotics (penicillin for *Treponema pallidum;* ampicillin for *N. gonorrhoeae;* azithromycin for *C. trachomatis);* antiprotozoal, anti-infective, and antiviral medications; and pain medications. (See *Drug chart 10-1,* pages 257 and 258.)

2. **Minimize risk of infection.** (See section II.D.3.)

3. **Minimize anxiety and enhance self-esteem** by treating the client with respect and dignity. (See section II.D.5.)

4. **Provide client and family teaching.** (See *Client and family teaching 10-1.*)

   a. Teach the client about the disorder and its treatment, principles of transmission, possible complications, and safer sex practices (encourage use of condoms).
   b. Teach comfort and hygiene measures, such as sitz baths and saline soaks.
   c. Advise sexual abstinence until follow-up testing indicates cure or control.

5. **Encourage treatment of sexual partners.**

XIII. INFERTILITY

A. **Description.** Infertility refers to a couple's failure to achieve pregnancy within 1 to 2 years of unprotected intercourse. It may be classified as primary (i.e., never conceived a child) or secondary (i.e., at least one conception has occurred, but they currently cannot achieve a pregnancy).

B. **Etiology**
   1. Causes of female infertility may include problems with the ovary, fallopian tubes, cervix, or uterine conditions.
   2. Causes of male infertility include seminal conditions.
   3. Often, more than one factor may be responsible for the problem.

C. **Pathophysiology**
   1. **The female**
      a. **Anovulation.** The ovaries may not produce and release ova regularly or secrete sufficient progesterone to produce an endometrium sufficient for implantation.
      b. **Tubal transport problems.** Inflammation or structural abnormalities of the fallopian tubes or uterus can prevent the transportation of ovum and sperm or implantation of a fertilized ovum.
      c. **Uterine problems.** The uterus is unable to maintain the placenta formation during pregnancy.
      d. **Cervical problems.** The pH of semen or vaginal secretions or conditions of cervical mucus may alter reception to sperm and prevent fertilization.
   2. **The male.** Sperm quantity, motility, or morphology may be inadequate for fertilization.

D. **Assessment findings**
   1. **Associated findings**
      a. **The female.** The health history may include sexually transmitted diseases (STDs), reproductive tract surgery, abortions, pelvic inflammatory disease, endometriosis, adhesions, displaced uterus, or an endocrine disorder.
      b. **The male.** History findings may include STDs, genital trauma, tuberculosis, mumps, orchitis, or cryptorchidism.
   2. **Clinical manifestations**
      a. **The female**
         - Structural disorders such as uterine displacement
         - Inflammation such as salpingitis
      b. **The male**
         - Structural disorders such as cryptorchidism
         - Inflammation such as epididymitis or orchitis
   3. **Laboratory and diagnostic study findings**
      a. **The female**
         - Tubal insufflation may reveal poor tubal patency.
         - Hysterosalpingography, an X-ray study, may reveal uterine or tubal abnormalities.
         - Laparoscopy may reveal conditions that may interfere with fertility, such as endometriosis, fibroids, polyps, or congenital malformations.
      b. **The male.** Sperm count (< 20 million) or motility may be abnormal.
      c. **Combined.** Postcoital cervical mucus test result may be abnormal.

E. **Nursing management**
   1. **Promote client and family coping.**

    a. Allay anxiety or stress by providing information about the cause of infertility, diagnostic tests, and possible treatments.

    b. Encourage both partners to express feelings related to loss and disappointment, altered roles, and sexual identity.

    c. Encourage the couple to explore other options such as adoption.

2. **Aid the client undergoing assisted reproductive therapy, if indicated.**

    a. **Ovulation** may be induced with medications such as fertility medications. (See *Drug chart 10-1,* pages 257 and 258.)

    b. **Artificial insemination** is used to introduce the partner's or donor's semen into the female genital tract by artificial means. The woman must lie flat for 30 minutes after the procedure.

    c. **In vitro fertilization** is a method of fertilizing human ova outside the body by collecting the mature ova and placing them in a dish with a sample of spermatozoa. The fertilized ova then are injected into the uterus through the cervix. Discuss the possibility of multiple pregnancies with clients.

3. **Minimize anxiety and enhance self-esteem** by treating the client with respect and dignity. (See section II.D.5.)

4. **Provide ongoing reassurance.** Most clients require repeated procedures; the success rate for curing infertility is only 25% to 50%.

Study questions

1. Which intervention would be included in the teaching plan for a client diagnosed with a pelvic relaxation disorder?
1. Instructing the client to perform Kegel exercises daily
2. Advising the client to keep diary of menstrual cycle events
3. Instructing the client on the correct way to administer vaginal cream
4. Encouraging frequent sexual intercourse until treatment is completed

2. Which nursing intervention would be *most* appropriate when teaching a client with phimosis how to prevent a recurrence?
1. Discussing ways to prevent a sickle cell crisis
2. Instructing the client to apply an ice pack to the penis
3. Encouraging the client to elevate the scrotum
4. Teaching proper care of an uncircumcised penis

3. A client is 1-day postoperative transurethral resection of the prostrate and has a three-way bladder irrigation. At the end of shift, he has a urinary drainage output of 4,000 ml and has had 2,800 ml of bladder irrigant infused. How many milliliters is the client's urinary output?

_____

4. Which client statement indicates that the nurse's teaching about sexually transmitted diseases (STDs) has been successful?
1. "I will douche after each time that I have sexual intercourse."
2. "I have to take my birth control pill every day so I will not get an STD."
3. "I will make sure a condom is used every time I have sexual intercourse."
4. "STDs can be treated with medication, so I do not have to worry."

5. A three-way bladder irrigation is used after transurethral resection of the prostate (TURP) to prevent which complication?

1. Infection
2. Hemorrhage
3. Urinary retention
4. Thrombosis

6. Which signs and symptoms would the nurse assess in a client diagnosed with leiomyomas?
1. Pelvic pain and dysmenorrhea
2. Fatigue and mood swings
3. Painful vesicles and inguinal lymphadenopathy
4. Lower abdominal pain and fever

7. Which should be included when instructing a client about applying a vaginal cream?
1. Instructing the client to apply the medication when the symptoms first start
2. Warning the client not to wear a perineal pad after application of cream
3. Instructing the client to wash her hands before and after applying cream
4. Encouraging the client to douche before each application of cream

8. Which sexually transmitted disease would the nurse expect not to respond to antibiotic therapy?
1. Trichomoniasis and gonorrhea
2. Lymphogranuloma venereum and chlamydial cervicitis
3. Genital warts and molluscum contagiosum
4. Syphilis and chancroid

9. Which clinical manifestation would lead the nurse to suspect endometriosis?
1. Premenstrual and postmenstrual dysmenorrhea and abnormal uterine bleeding
2. Foul-smelling vaginal discharge accompanied by a vulvar mass or ulceration
3. Yellow and frothy discharge with a red, excoriated vulva and vagina
4. Abnormal Papanicolaou (Pap) smear findings and chronic erosions of the cervix

10. Which instruction would be included in the discharge teaching plan for a female client diagnosed with trichomoniasis and being treated with metronidazole?
1. "Drink at least 8 oz of water with each dose and take the medication before meals on an empty stomach."
2. "Avoid any alcohol intake while taking the medication and make sure the sexual partner is being treated."
3. "Stop taking the medication as soon as pain or itching subsides and store it in the refrigerator."
4. "Lie down 30 minutes after taking the medication and elevate your lower extremities."

11. For a client diagnosed with pelvic relaxation disorder who is unable to undergo a surgical repair, which is the medical treatment of choice?
1. Radiation therapy
2. Intrauterine device
3. Bed rest
4. Pessary

12. When taking the history of a 62-year-old client complaining of impotence, which statement would alert the nurse to a possible underlying cause?
1. "I have had diabetes for the last 12 years."
2. "I have never had a rectal digital examination."
3. "I have been taking a baby aspirin daily for the last 2 years."
4. "I have urinary frequency and terminal dribbling."

13. Which signs and symptoms would the nurse assess in a client diagnosed with acute prostatitis?
1. Pain and edema of the testicles
2. Inguinal and scrotal pain and edema
3. Hematuria and a firm, enlarged prostate
4. Sudden onset of fever and dysuria

14. Which information would be appropriate to discuss with a couple who are unable to conceive and taking fertility drugs?
1. Fertility drugs may cause multiple pregnancies.
2. After artificial insemination, the client should lie flat for 4 hours.
3. Exploration of other options, such as adoption, should be avoided unless it is a last resort.
4. The success rate for treating infertility is 90% to 100%.

15. Which nursing intervention would be appropriate for a client with epididymitis?
1. Applying ice and elevating the scrotum to relieve pain
2. Administering antiviral medications to fight the infection

3. Encouraging sexual activity to relieve pressure
4. Discouraging testing of sexual partners for sexually transmitted diseases

16. The nurse knows a 16-year old client diagnosed with gonorrhea understands the discharge teaching when he makes which statement?
1. "I'm not going to tell my girlfriend about this disease. It's none of her business."
2. "I'm glad that you don't have to tell anybody about this disease. I'm embarrassed."
3. "I shouldn't have any sexual activity until I've taken all my medication."
4. "Because I had this once and been treated for it, I'll never have it again."

Answer key

1. The answer is **1.**
Pelvic relaxation disorders are structural disorders resulting in a weakening of the support tissues. The goal is to strengthen the surrounding muscles. Kegel exercises (i.e., perineal exercises) help strengthen the muscles in the perineal area. The client is instructed to tighten and relax gluteal and perineal floor muscles (e.g., starting and stopping the urinary stream). Keeping a diary of menstrual cycle events, administering vaginal cream, or engaging in frequent intercourse would have no effect on the perineal muscle tone.

2. The answer is **4.**
In phimosis, the foreskin is constricted and cannot be retracted. Poor hygiene of the uncircumcised penis plays a role in development of the condition. Teaching about proper care of the uncircumcised penis is most appropriate to prevent a recurrence. Discussing ways to prevent a sickle cell crisis would be appropriate for a client with priapism (i.e., uncontrolled persistent erection). Applying ice to the penis or elevating the

scrotum would be appropriate for the client diagnosed with male reproductive infection or scrotal edema.

3. The answer is **1,200.**
The nurse must subtract the bladder irrigant infused from the total urinary drainage output to obtain the specific urinary output.

4. The answer is **3.**
The best way to prevent sexually transmitted diseases (STDs) is to use a condom every time there is sexual intercourse. Abstinence is the foolproof way. Douching and birth control pills do not prevent STDs. Some STDs do respond to antibiotics, but acquired immunodeficiency syndrome (caused by human immunodeficiency virus) does not.

5. The answer is **2.**
After TURP, three-way bladder irrigation provides continuous normal saline in the bladder to prevent hemorrhaging and occlusion of the urethreal catheter. Typically, the urine output should be light pink. Infection, urinary retention, and thrombosis are compli-

cations after a TURP, but bladder irrigation cannot prevent them.

6. The answer is **1**.
A client with a leiomyoma (i.e., fibroid tumor) may be asymptomatic or complain of pelvic pain, backache, and dysmenorrhea (i.e., painful menstruation). Fatigue and mood swings indicate premenstrual syndrome. Painful vesicles and inguinal lymphadenopathy indicate syphilis. Lower abdominal pain and fever are associated with pelvic inflammatory disease.

7. The answer is **3**.
When a vaginal cream application is prescribed, the client should be taught to wash the perineal area, apply cream with gloves, and wash her hands before and after applying the cream. The cream should be applied as prescribed, usually two to three times each day. Wearing a perineal pad helps to prevent staining of under garments. Douching is unnecessary before each application.

8. The answer is **3**.
The human papillomavirus is the organism responsible for genital warts and condyloma acuminatum. A virus also causes genital herpes. In each case, antibiotics are ineffective. Protozoa cause trichomoniasis. Bacteria cause gonorrhea, lymphogranuloma venereum, chlamydial cervicitis, syphilis, and chancroid.

9. The answer is **1**.
Common clinical manifestations associated with endometriosis include dysmenorrhea starting 1 to 2 days before menstruation and persisting for 2 to 3 days, abnormal uterine bleeding, dyspareunia, tender palpable masses, and infertility. Foul-smelling vaginal discharge accompanied by a vulvar mass or ulceration is indicative of cancer of the vulva. Yellow and frothy discharge with a red, excoriated vulva and vagina is commonly seen with trichomoniasis. An abnormal Pap smear and chronic cervical erosions are associated with cervical cancer.

10. The answer is **2**.
When a client is taking metronidazole, any intake of alcohol should be avoided because a mild to severe reaction leading to unconsciousness, convulsions, and death may occur. Even if the client is asymptomatic, the sexual partner must be treated. Abstinence should be observed until trichomoniasis is resolved. Metronidazole should be taken with food and continued until the medication is finished, even if symptoms subside. Lying down is appropriate after administering vaginal creams or suppositories.

11. The answer is **4**.
Pelvic relaxation disorders are structural disorders resulting in a weakening of the support tissues. If they cannot be corrected surgically, the medical treatment of choice is a pessary, which can provide support to the uterus and vagina. Radiation, insertion of an intrauterine device, and bed rest are not appropriate therapies for structural disorders.

12. The answer is **1**.
Impotence may result from psychogenic and organic causes. Endocrine conditions such as diabetes, pituitary tumors, and hypogonadism are possible organic causes of impotence. A rectal digital examination is important for diagnosing rectal or prostate cancer. Use of baby aspirin is expected if the client was diagnosed with coronary artery disease. Urinary frequency and terminal dribbling are signs and symptoms of benign prostatic hyperplasia.

13. The answer is **4**.
Signs and symptoms of acute prostatitis include sudden onset of fever and chills; dysuria, urgency, and frequency; perineal or low back pain; and a tender, swollen, warm, indurated prostate on palpation. Testicular pain and edema are associated with orchitis. Inguinal and scrotal pain and edema are associated with epididymitis. Hematuria and a firm, enlarged prostate suggest benign prostatic hyperplasia.

14. The answer is **1.**

Prescribed fertility drugs increase the likelihood of multiple pregnancies. After artificial insemination, the woman should like flat for 30 minutes, not 4 hours, to prevent semen from leaking out of the vagina. All options, including adoption, should be explored with the couple. The success rate for treating infertility is only 25% to 50%.

15. The answer is **1.**

For the client with epididymitis, applying ice and elevating the scrotum help to decrease pain and edema in the scrotal area. Because bacterial infection is the underlying cause, antibiotics, not antivirals, should be administered. Although encouraging sexual activity may be helpful for clients with chronic prostatitis, it cannot relieve pressure and is not appropriate for epididymitis. Sexual partners should be tested for sexually transmitted diseases, because an infection such as *Chlamydia* may have contributed to epididymitis.

16. The answer is **3.**

The client should not have sexual activity until the infection is cured, which should be after all the medication is taken. The client should tell the partner about the infection, and the nurse must make a report to the appropriate public health department. Gonorrhea can be contracted again following successful treatment.

11 *Immunologic disorders*

I. STRUCTURE AND FUNCTION OF THE IMMUNE SYSTEM

A. **Functions of the immune system**
   1. **Defense** against physical injury and infection
   2. **Maintenance of homeostasis,** a state of equilibrium of the internal environment

B. **Organs and tissues of the immune system** include the bone marrow and lymphoid tissue, which comprise the thymus gland, lymph nodes, spleen, tonsils, and adenoids.
   1. **Bone marrow** is specialized soft tissue filling the spaces in cancellous bone of the epiphyses. It is responsible for:
      a. releasing mature B lymphocytes into the blood circulation
      b. moving T lymphocytes from bone marrow to the thymus.
   2. The **thymus** is a single unpaired gland that is located in the mediastinum and is the primary central gland of the lymphatic system. Its primary function is allowing the T lymphocytes to develop before migrating to the lymph nodes and the spleen.
   3. **Lymph nodes** and vessels perform several important functions, such as:
      a. transporting lymph
      b. filtering and phagocytizing (processing and killing) antigens
      c. generating lymphocytes and monocytes.
   4. **Spleen** functions include:
      a. removing worn-out erythrocytes from blood
      b. storing blood and platelets
      c. filtering and purifying blood.
   5. The **tonsils, adenoids,** and other mucoid lymphatic tissues defend the body against microorganisms.
   6. In the **hematopoietic system,** bone marrow and lymphatic tissue produce blood cells, including those involved in immunologic defense (i.e., leukocytes). *Table 11-1* provides information on the types of leukocytes.

C. **Nonspecific immunologic defense** is a type of immunity effective against any harmful agent entering the body. The body's **natural immunity** can discriminate friend from foe or self from nonself but cannot distinguish between agents and pathogens. Natural mechanisms include the following:
   1. **Physical barriers.** Intact skin and mucous membranes prevent pathogens from gaining access to the body. Cilia of the respiratory tract filter and clear pathogens from the upper respiratory tract.
   2. **Chemical barriers.** Acidic gastric juices, enzymes in tears and saliva, and sebaceous and sweat secretions attempt to destroy invading bacteria and fungi.
   3. **Biologic response modifiers.** Interferon, a viricidal substance, counters viruses and activates other components of the immune system.
   4. **Actions of white blood cells** (See *Table 11-1.*)
      a. **Neutrophils** are first to arrive at the inflammatory injury.
      b. **Eosinophils** and **basophils** are activated in response to allergic reactions and stress.
      c. **Granulocytes** release cell mediators, such as histamine, bradykinin, and prostaglandins, and engulf the foreign toxins.
      d. **Monocytes** or **macrophages** function as phagocytic cells to engulf, ingest, and destroy foreign toxins.
   5. **Inflammatory response.** This mechanism is elicited in response to tissue injury or invading organisms. Mast cells release chemical mediators, which enhance the inflammatory response and produce the typical signs of infection (i.e., redness, edema, and

TABLE 11-1
Types of leukocytes

Cell type	Normal level	Characteristics	Function
Granulocytes	5,000 to 10,000/mm^3	■ Formed in bone marrow ■ Granular (under microscope)	■ Immediate response to cellular injury
Basophils	<1% of all leukocytes	■ Granules filled with heparin, histamine	■ Play role in inflammatory response
Eosinophils	2% to 4% of all leukocytes	■ Contain heparin, histamine	■ Play role in hypersensitivity reaction
Neutrophils	50% to 70% of all leukocytes	■ 12-hour lifespan; 2- to 4-hour lifespan with infection	■ Phagocytic ■ First cell to site of cellular injury ■ Contain lysosomes
Agranulocytes		■ Produced in lymphatic system ■ Nongranular (under microscope)	■ Fight infection
Lymphocytes	25% to 33% of all leukocytes	■ Classified as B cells or T cells	■ Phagocytosis ■ Release of lymphokines ■ Production of gamma-globulins ■ Cell-mediated reactions
Monocytes	4% to 6% of all leukocytes	■ Circulate in blood but also settle in tissue, where they are transformed into macrophages	■ Phagocytosis (can ingest larger particles than neutrophils; five times as many in one ingestion)

itching). Vasoconstriction and vasodilation also play a role in the inflammatory response.

6. **Natural killer cells.** These lymphocytes are responsible for immune surveillance and host resistance to infection.

7. **Complement.** This group of at least 20 circulating plasma proteins, made in the liver, are sequentially activated in the presence of an antigen.

   a. **Functions of complement**
   - Cell lysis
   - Opsonization, which involves making antigen more susceptible to phagocytosis
   - Chemotaxis, which involves inducing phagocytes to antigen
   - Agglutination, which involves clumping of antigens
   - Neutralization of viruses

   b. **Activation of complement** can occur in one of two basic ways:
   - **Classical.** Antigen-antibody complex activates C1 (first of circulating complement proteins).
   - **Alternate.** No antigen-antibody complex is required; complement can be initiated by the release of endotoxins and begins with C3.

D. Specific immunologic defense is a type of immunity effective against specific harmful agents entering the body. Immunity is a normal adaptive response designed to protect

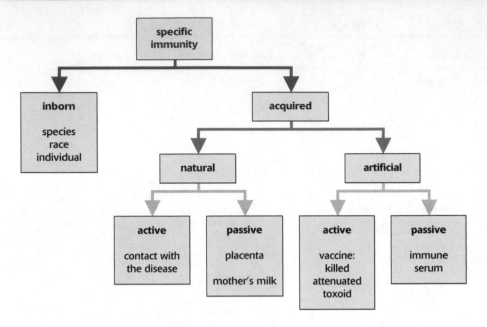

FIGURE 11-1
Types of specific immunity

the body against potentially harmful antigens (i.e., any substance recognized as foreign by the immune system).
1. **Types of immunity** (See *Figure 11-1*.)
    a. **Inborn immunity** is an inherited immunity of species (e.g., humans do not contract certain animal diseases), races, and individuals to certain diseases.
    b. **Acquired immunity** is immunity that develops as an individual encounters specific harmful agents. It may be natural (i.e., activated by the affected individual) or artificial (i.e., activated by vaccine) and active or passive.
    – Active immunity involves production of antibodies and sensitized lymphocytes in response to an antigen or immunization.
       - Memory cells do not secrete antibodies, but on re-exposure to the specific antigen, they develop into antibody-secreting plasma cells.
       - Important vaccines include an I.M. tetanus and diphtheria booster injection, which is required for adults at least every 10 years, and the hepatitis B vaccine, which is required for all health care workers. (See *Box 11-1*.)
    – Passive immunity is a temporary immunity acquired by introduction of antibodies or sensitized lymphocytes from another source (e.g., antibodies through placental circulation to a fetus, gamma globulin, antiserum from blood plasma of a person with acquired immunity). The body does not generate memory cells.
2. **The mechanisms of specific immunity** are of two types: humoral (B lymphocyte) and cell-mediated (T lymphocyte) immunity. These two types of specific immunologic responses discriminate self from nonself and distinguish among antigens.
    a. **Humoral immunity** involves the formation of antibodies by plasma cells in response to foreign proteins.

BOX 11-1
Vaccinations for adults

Hepatitis A
Recommended for travelers to locations where sanitation and hygiene are unsatisfactory and for people at high risk (i.e., homosexual men, I.V. drug users, health care personnel). Administered in two doses — first dose, then second dose 6 to 12 months after the first dose.

Hepatitis B
Recommended for people at high risk (i.e., health care personnel, hemodialysis clients.) Administered in three doses — first dose, second dose 1 month later, then third dose 5 months after the second dose.

Influenza "flu shot"
Recommended every fall for people age 65 or older; residents in long-term care facilities; individuals with heart or lung disease, diabetes, kidney disease or a compromised immune system; and for those who work with or live with any of these individuals.

Pneumococcal
Recommended one time for people age 65 or older and for people younger than age 65 who have certain chronic illnesses. For people with chronic respiratory disorders, a one-time revaccination dose after 5 years is recommended.

Tetanus diphtheria (Td) "tetanus shot"
Must have booster dose every 10 years after childhood immunizations. If none in childhood, must have three shots — first dose, then second dose 1 month later, then third dose 6 months after the second dose.

Varicella
Recommended for people who have never had chicken pox. Administered in two doses — first dose, then second dose 1 to 2 months after the first dose.

Encourage the client to consult his heath care provider to determine the need for recommended vaccines or vaccines required when traveling out of the United States.

- Humoral immunity functions primarily in type I, type II, and type III hypersensitivity reactions. (See section III.A.)
- B lymphocytes (so named because they were first identified in the avian bursa) are involved in antibody (i.e., immunoglobulin [Ig]) production.
- Unsensitized B cells proliferate and mature into plasma cells after exposure to antigen.
- Plasma cells differentiate into memory cells (which trigger a B-cell response on subsequent exposure to same antigen) and antibodies.
- Five types of antibodies are produced by the body:
  - IgG activates complement, enhances phagocytosis, crosses placenta (i.e., passive immunity), and is active in a second response (reinfection).
  - IgA is present in body fluids (i.e., blood, saliva, and tears; pulmonary, GI, prostatic, and vaginal secretions; and breast milk), prevents absorption of antigens from food, and protects against respiratory, GI, and genitourinary infections.
  - IgM is the first antibody produced in the immune response. It activates the complement system.
  - IgD may be required on B-cell surface for transformation into plasma cells, but its exact role is unclear.
  - IgE is associated with allergic and hypersensitivity reactions and possibly helps in defense against parasites.
- *b.* **Cell-mediated immunity** involves attack of microbes by special killer T cells formed from lymphocytes.
  - Cellular immunity functions primarily in delayed hypersensitivity reactions; rejection of transplants; and viral, fungal, and chronic infections.

– T lymphocytes (cells are thymus derived), on exposure to antigen, proliferate and differentiate into one of several types of T cells.
- Helper T cells (T4) assist B cells in humoral response to form antibodies.
- Suppressor T cells (T8) suppress B-cell synthesis of antibody production through a feedback mechanism.
- Memory T cells store future immune response to some antigen.
- Cytotoxic T cells directly attack antigen, altering cell membrane with resultant cell lysis.

3. **Stages of specific immune responses**
   a. **Recognition.** Circulating lymphocytes and macrophages recognize foreign material or antigens as nonself.
   b. **Proliferation.** Sensitized lymphocytes proliferate, differentiate, and mature into respective T and B cells.
   c. **Response.** Antibody is produced with specific T-cell action.
   d. **Effector.** Antigen is destroyed by antibody, which is produced by B-cell or cytotoxic T-cell action.

NURSING PROCESS OVERVIEW

II. THE IMMUNE SYSTEM

A. Assessment
   1. **Health history**
      a. **Elicit a description of the client's present illness and chief complaint,** including onset, course, duration, location, and precipitating and alleviating factors. Elicit a description of the client's overall health status, including immunizations status, usual childhood diseases, known allergies, and a history of past and present medications. Cardinal signs and symptoms indicating altered immunity are subsequently described.
      – **General**
        - Recurrent infections
        - Seasonal symptoms
        - Weight loss
        - Fever
      – **Head**
        - Itching, burning, watering eyes; vision problems; and eye infections
        - Recurrent ear infections
        - Rhinitis and sneezing
      – **Respiratory system**
        - Cough
        - Dyspnea
        - Recurrent infection
      – **Cardiovascular system**
        - Pain
        - Raynaud's phenomenon (i.e., extreme pallor and then cyanosis of extremities brought on by cold exposure)
      – **GI system**
        - Nausea and vomiting
        - Diarrhea

     Genitourinary system
- Recurrent infections
- Dysuria and hematuria

  – **Musculoskeletal system**
- Weakness and fatigue
- Inability to perform activities of daily living (ADLs)

  – **Neurologic system**
- Disorientation to name, date, and place
- Altered level of consciousness
- Paresthesias

  b. **Explore the client's health history for risk factors** associated with immune disorders, including not keeping up-to-date immunizations, exposure to infectious disease, and exposure to pollens, insects, and allergens.

2. **Physical examination**
   a. **Inspection**
   - Inspect skin and mucous membranes for rashes, lesions, dermatitis, purpura (subcutaneous bleeding), and any type of inflammation or drainage.
   - Assess the joints for tenderness, edema, and range of motion.
   - Inspect ears for drainage, inflammation, and scarring from ear infections.

   b. **Palpation**
   - Palpate the anterior and posterior cervical, axillary, and inguinal lymph nodes for enlargement.
   - Note the location, size, and consistency of lymph nodes. Document complaints of tenderness if the node is palpable.

   c. **Auscultation**
   - Auscultate lungs for abnormal lung sounds, such as wheezing, crackles, and rhonchi.
   - Auscultate heart sounds for abnormalities, such as palpitations and dysrhythmias.

3. **Laboratory and diagnostic studies**
   a. **Multi-allergen allergy testing** measures the increase and quantity of allergen-specific immunoglobulin (Ig) E antibodies and is done to identify allergens to which the client has immediate hypersensitivity.

   b. **T- and B-lymphocyte assays** evaluate the number of lymphocytes in the immune system.

   c. **Ig assays (IgG, IgA, IgM)** can detect and monitor immune deficiencies.

   d. **Serum complement assays** test for C3 and C4 complement when the total complement level is decreased.

   e. **Autoantibody tests**
   - Antinuclear antibody (ANA) test measures and differentiates ANAs associated with certain autoimmune diseases such as systemic lupus erythematosus.
   - Rheumatoid factor test measures for a macroglobulin type of antibody found in rheumatoid arthritis.

   f. **Radioallergosorbent test** is a radioimmunoassay that measures allergen-specific IgE.

   g. The **human immunodeficiency virus (HIV) test** determines the presence of HIV antibodies, which is the etiologic factor for acquired immunodeficiency syndrome (AIDS).

B. Nursing diagnoses
   1. Ineffective airway clearance
   2. Risk for infection

3. Acute or chronic pain
4. Impaired skin integrity
5. Deficient fluid volume
6. Deficient knowledge
7. Bathing or hygiene self-care deficit
8. Risk for injury
9. Ineffective coping

C. **Planning and outcome identification.** The goals for a client diagnosed with an immunologic disorder include improved airway clearance, prevention of infection, increased comfort, improvement and maintenance of skin integrity, increased knowledge regarding disease prevention and self-care, absence of complications and injury, and improved coping.

D. **Implementation**
   1. **Assess respiratory status,** including assessment of lungs, rate and depth of respirations, effort of breathing, use of accessory muscles, cyanosis, restlessness, anxiety, or any change in level of consciousness.
   2. **Minimize the risk of infection.**
      a. Instruct the client on ways to avoid infection, including the importance of personal hygiene and avoidance of people with infections and large crowds.
      b. Instruct the client to wash the affected area with warm water before applying topical creams; instruct him to wash his hands before and after administering topical creams.
   3. **Provide pain relief.** Assess the client's pain, rule out any complications, implement any nonpharmacologic interventions (e.g., ice, cold, massage) to relieve pain, administer pain medication, and evaluate the effectiveness of interventions.
   4. **Promote skin integrity.**
      a. Assess the skin and mucous membranes for any rashes, color changes, lesions, pallor, purpura, hydration and inflammation.
      b. Keep skin clean and dry. Do not use harsh soaps.
   5. **Maintain fluid balance.** Monitor the client's intake and output, and maintain 30 ml/hour urinary output; use a urometer to ensure accurate output. Assess for dehydration.
   6. **Provide client and family teaching.**
      a. Teach the client about the disease process and possible triggers.
      b. Teach the client measures to minimize or prevent exposure to the allergen. (See *Client and family teaching 11-1.*)
      c. Discuss emergency measures (e.g., use of epinephrine) and medication therapy, including the use of corticosteroids to reduce inflammation.
      d. Teach the client danger signs and symptoms to report, including respiratory distress and infection.
   7. **Promote self-care.** Assist the client with ADLs as needed, but promote independence. Use any energy-saving techniques available.
   8. **Prevent injury.** Instruct the client to wear identification tags or bracelets concerning allergies or disease.
   9. **Promote client and family coping.**
      a. Teach the client and his family ways to cope with chronic illness, including verbalization of feelings and ways to prevent exacerbations.
      b. Provide referrals to counselors and support groups.

CLIENT AND FAMILY TEACHING 11-1
Health education for allergy symptom control

Maintain a dust-free environment
- Reduce room contents to the barest minimum by removing drapes, curtains, blinds (use pull shades instead), and carpets.
- Wash woodwork and linoleum floors.
- Use wooden furniture, which allows for easier dusting.
- Use washable cotton materials.
- Wear a mask when cleaning.
- Cover the mattress with a hypoallergenic cover.
- Avoid wearing fabrics that cause itching.
- Decrease dust in the environment by using air conditioning, air cleaners, humidifiers, and dehumidifiers.

Reduce exposure to pollen
- Avoid barns, weeds, dry leaves, and grass.
- Avoid allergens and irritants, including dusts, fumes, odors, animals, and tobacco smoke.
- Avoid sprays, powders, and perfumes. Use hypoallergenic cosmetics.
- Wear a mask at times of increased exposures (e.g., windy days, mowing yard).
- Be aware of high pollen counts. Reduce exposure at these times and stay in air-conditioned areas.
- Ensure a smoke-free environment.
- Do not change detergents or soaps.

E. Outcome evaluation

1. The client displays no respiratory distress, as evidenced by an absence of chest tightness, wheezing, cyanosis, cough, and exaggerated expiratory effort.
2. The client shows no symptoms of opportunistic infection, such as fatigue, fever, night sweats, weight loss, and diarrhea.
3. The client verbalizes relief of joint pain and discomfort.
4. The client exhibits clean, dry skin that is free from rash, itching, burning, scaling, ulcerations and infection.
5. The client has intact skin and oral mucosa.
6. The client maintains adequate fluid and electrolyte balance and nutritional status.
7. The client can verbalize an understanding, preventive measures, and treatment of the disease process and the signs or symptoms that should be reported to the health care provider.
8. The client is able to care for himself and perform independent ADLs.
9. The client remains free from injury.
10. The client is able to verbalize appropriate coping mechanisms to control anxiety.

III. CATEGORIES OF IMMUNE DISORDERS

A. **Hypersensitivity reactions** are immune responses to allergens that result in tissue destruction.
1. **Type I (anaphylactic) reactions** are mediated by the immunoglobulin (Ig) E antibody, which promotes the release of histamine and other reactive mediators. These basophil or mast cells produce the characteristic symptoms of asthma or hay fever.
2. **Type II (cytotoxic) reactions** (e.g., hemolytic anemia) are mediated by IgG and IgM antibodies, which attach to cells (usually circulating blood elements) and cause cell lysis.
3. **Type III (immune complex) reactions** (e.g., rheumatoid arthritis, serum sickness) are mediated by antigen-antibody complexes that deposit in the lining of blood vessels or on tissue surfaces.
4. **Type IV (delayed hypersensitivity) reactions** (e.g., contact dermatitis, transplant rejection) are mediated by lymphokines released from sensitized T lymphocytes.

B. **Allergic disorders** are hypersensitive responses to an allergen to which an organism has previously been exposed and to which the organism has developed antibodies.
  1. Interaction between antigen and antibody typically results in one or more manifestations of tissue injury.
  2. IgE antibodies are formed by persons experiencing allergies who are genetically predisposed. Histamine and other mediators are released on reexposure to the allergen to which the person is sensitized.

C. **Autoimmune disorders** are conditions in which the body no longer differentiates self from nonself.
  1. Alterations in T cells or B cells produce autoantibodies and autosensitized T cells that cause tissue injury. These changes may involve one organ or many organ systems.
  2. The cause of autoimmune disorders remains unknown, but many theories exist.

D. **Immune deficiency** is defined as a congenital or acquired deficit in the immune system that makes the person susceptible to life-threatening opportunistic infection.
  1. In **congenital (primary) immunodeficiency,** the body produces inadequate amounts of one or more immune cells. Deficits can be humoral (B cell), cell-mediated (T cell), or combined.
  2. **Acquired (secondary) immunodeficiency** is attributed to various etiologies, including:
      a. immunosuppressive therapy, such as chemotherapeutic agents, corticosteroids, nonsteroidal anti-inflammatory agents, and irradiation
      b. age-related factors, such as deterioration in the thymus gland and T-cell functioning and a decreased number of suppressor T cells and helper T cells
      c. disruption of skin integrity, as occurs with burns and trauma
      d. nutritional deficits
      e. malignant processes, such as leukemia and lymphoma
      f. infectious processes, such as sepsis and acquired immunodeficiency syndrome.

IV. ALLERGIC RHINITIS

A. **Description.** Allergic rhinitis (i.e., hay fever) is an allergic reaction to inhaled airborne allergens characterized by seasonal occurrences. It is the most common form of respiratory allergy. Although children and adolescents have an especially high incidence, it occurs in all age groups.

B. **Etiology.** Allergic rhinitis is induced by airborne pollens. Common seasonal pollens include:
  1. tree pollens (e.g., oak, maple, and birch) in the spring
  2. grass pollens (e.g., sheep sorrel and plantain) in the summer
  3. weed pollens (e.g., ragweed) in the fall.

C. **Pathophysiology.** Allergic rhinitis occurs when immunoglobulin (Ig) E antibodies in the nasal mucosa combine with inhaled allergens on the mucosal surface. The nasal mucosa reacts by slowing of ciliary action, edema formation, and leukocyte infiltration. Tissue edema is a result of vasodilation and increased capillary permeability.

D. **Assessment findings**
  1. **Associated findings** may include a family history of allergies.

2. **Clinical manifestations**
   a. Itching, burning nasal mucosa
   b. Copious mucous secretions causing runny nose
   c. Red, burning, tearing eyes
   d. Sneezing
   e. Pale, boggy nasal mucosa
3. **Laboratory and diagnostic study findings**
   a. Nasal smears reveal eosinophils in nasal secretions.
   b. Peripheral blood counts reveal a lymphocyte count above total 1,200/ml.
   c. Total serum IgE determination shows an elevated serum level of IgE.
   d. Skin testing identifies the offending allergens.
   e. Radioallergosorbent test measures allergen-specific IgE. If antibodies are present, they combine with the radiolabeled allergens, which are compared with control values.

E. Nursing management

1. **Administer prescribed medications,** which may include antihistamines, decongestants, and topical corticosteroids. (See *Drug chart 11-1*, pages 288 to 290.)
2. **Encourage the client to use saline nasal sprays to soothe mucous membranes.** Advise the client to blow his nose before administering nasal medications.
3. **Prepare the client for immunotherapy,** which is prescribed only when IgE hypersensitivity to specific, unavoidable inhalant allergens (house dust and pollens) is demonstrated.
4. **Minimize the risk of infection.** (See section II.D.2.)
5. **Provide client and family teaching.** (See section II.D.6; also see *Client and family teaching 11-1*, page 285.)

V. ALLERGIC DERMATOSES

A. Description.
Allergic dermatoses is a group of inflammatory conditions caused by skin reaction to irritating or allergenic materials. They include allergic contact dermatitis and atopic dermatitis.

B. Etiology

1. **Allergic contact dermatitis** is produced by many substances. Common causes include exposure to poison ivy, topical medications, cosmetics, soaps, and industrial chemicals.
2. Although the cause of **atopic dermatitis** is unknown, the condition appears to be associated with a family history of allergic respiratory disorders (e.g., allergic rhinitis, asthma). Exacerbating factors may include irritants, infection, and certain allergens.

C. Pathophysiology

1. **Allergic contact dermatitis** involves delayed hypersensitivity and requires a latent period ranging from several days (for strong sensitizers such as poison ivy) to years.
2. **Atopic dermatitis** is a type I immediate hypersensitivity disorder resulting in large amounts of histamine in the skin, changes in lipid content of the skin, sebaceous gland activity, and diaphoresis. It most commonly begins in infancy or early childhood. It may subside spontaneously, to be followed by unpredictable exacerbations throughout life.

(Text continues on page 290.)

DRUG CHART 11-1
Medications for immune disorders

Classifications	Indications	Selected interventions
Adrenergics albuterol epinephrine isoetharine isoproterenol metaproterenol terbutaline	Relax smooth bronchial muscle and dilate airways	■ Instruct the client to inhale twice as follows: inhale once, wait 1 minute, and inhale once more.
Antibiotics aminoglycosides (gentamicin, tobramycin) amoxicillin erythromycin penicillin tetracycline	Prevent or treat infections caused by pathogenic microorganisms	■ Before administering the first dose, assess the client for allergies and determine whether culture has been obtained. ■ After multiple doses, assess the client for superinfection (thrush, yeast infection, diarrhea); notify the health care provider if these occur. ■ Assess the insertion site for phlebitis if antibiotics are being administered I.V. ■ To assess the effectiveness of antibiotic therapy, monitor the white blood cell count. ■ Monitor peaks and troughs for aminoglycosides.
Antidiarrheals attapulgite bismuth subsalicylate diphenoxylate and atropine loperamide	Absorb excess water from stool	■ To assess the effectiveness of the medication, record the number and consistency of stools. ■ Monitor intake and output, daily weight, and serum electrolyte levels.
Antiemetics benzquinamide dimenhydrinate trimethobenzamide hydrochloride promethazine scopolamine	Relieve nausea and vomiting by inhibiting medullary chemoreceptor triggers; drug choice depends on the cause of vomiting	■ Advise the client that this medication may cause drowsiness. ■ Because the medication may cause chemical irritation, administer by deep I.M. injection into a large muscle mass, if appropriate. ■ Measure emesis and maintain accurate intake and output; monitor for dehydration.
Antihistamines cetirizine chlorpheniramine maleate desloratadine diphenhydramine fexofenadine loratadine terfenadine	Inhibit histamine release by binding selectively to H_1 receptors	■ Teach the client to avoid alcohol, driving, or engaging in hazardous activities because the medication may cause drowsiness. (Some antihistamines are nonsedating. Make sure the client is knowledgeable of the medication's adverse effects.) ■ Encourage sucking on hard candy or ice chips for relief of dry mouth.

DRUG CHART 11-1

Medications for immune disorders *(continued)*

Classifications	Indications	Selected interventions
Antipruritic agents **Topical steroids** desoximetasone hydrocortisone triamcinolone **Topical anesthetics** benzocaine dibucaine	Relieve or prevent itching (may be topical steroids or anesthetics)	■ Advise the client to wash his hands before and after application. ■ Instruct the client to clean the affected area with warm water before application.
Antiretrovirals **Nucleoside reverse transcriptase inhibitors** didanosine zidovudine	Suppress synthesis of viral deoxyribonucleic acid by reverse transcriptase; first drugs used against human immunodeficiency virus (HIV) infection; remains a mainstay of treatment	■ The client must adhere closely to the prescribed dosing schedule. ■ All medications are oral, except I.V. zidovudine, which must be administered slowly.
Nonnucleoside reverse transcriptase inhibitors delavirdine nevirapine	Cause direct inhibition of HIV by binding to active center of reverse transcriptase	■ Instruct the client to take the medication 1 hour before or after food or antacids. ■ Inform the client to notify his health care provider if a rash occurs.
Protease inhibitors indinavir ritonavir	Bind to the active site of HIV protease, thereby preventing the enzyme from cleaving HIV polyproteins; the virus remains immature and noninfectious; when used in combination with reverse transcriptase inhibitors, viral load reduced to a level undetectable by current assays	■ Instruct the client to follow proper instructions when taking the medication; some must be taken on an empty stomach, and others must be taken with food. ■ Inform the client that all protease inhibitors may cause diabetes. (Inform the client of the signs and symptoms of diabetes and to notify his health care provider if these occur.)
Bronchodilators *(xanthine derivatives)* theophylline	Relax bronchial smooth muscle	■ Monitor serum level of theophylline (therapeutic level, 10 to 20 µg/ml). ■ Provide the medication at regular intervals, before meals, and with a full glass of water. ■ Instruct the client to notify his health care provider of irritability, restlessness, headache, insomnia, dizziness, tachycardia, palpitations, or seizures. ■ Do not crush sustained-release medication.
Corticosteroids inhaled — fluticasone; beclomethasone oral — hydrocortisone, methylprednisolone, prednisone) topical	Ensure a potent, local acting anti-inflammatory and immune modifier effect; also used to strengthen the biologic membrane, which inhibits capillary permeability and prevents leakage of fluid into the injured area and development of edema; exact mechanism unknown	■ Caution the client not to exceed the maximum daily dose of 4 sprays/nostril. ■ Instruct the client to rinse his mouth after each use to prevent nasal candidiasis. ■ Instruct the client to take the medication exactly as directed and to taper it rather than stop it abruptly, which could cause serious withdrawal symptoms leading to adrenal insufficiency, shock, and death.

(continued)

DRUG CHART 11-1
Medications for immune disorders (continued)

Classifications	Indications	Selected interventions
Corticosteroids (continued)		■ Forewarn the client that the medication may cause reportable cushingoid effects (weight gain, moon face, buffalo hump, and hirsutism) and may mask signs and symptoms of infection. ■ Instruct the client to wash his hands before and after topical application. ■ Instruct the client to wash the exposed area with warm water and to dry it thoroughly before applying the medication.
COX-2 inhibitors celecoxib rofecoxib	Inhibit the formation of substances that can cause joint and connective tissue problems	■ Instruct the client to report tinnitus, which is a sign of aspirin toxicity, to his health care provider.
Leukotriene receptor antagonist montelukast	Reduce inflammation in airways; used for prophylactic and maintenance drug therapy for chronic asthma	■ Instruct client to take medication in the evening without food. ■ Explain that the medication is not for acute asthma attacks.
Mast cell inhibitor cromolyn sodium	Inhibit mast cell, thereby releasing chemical mediators that result in bronchodilation and a decrease in airway inflammation	■ Teach the client to insert the capsule in a nebulizer device, exhale completely, place the mouthpiece between the lips, inhale deeply, hold his breath for 10 seconds, and then exhale. ■ Tell the client than an inhaler is used prophylactically before exercise, not in acute asthma attack.
Nonopioid analgesics Nonsteroidal anti-inflammatory drugs acetylsalicylic acid ibuprofen	Relieve pain, edema, and inflammation	■ Instruct the client to take with food to decrease GI upset. ■ Instruct the client to report signs and symptoms of GI distress (i.e., nausea, vomiting, bleeding) to his health care provider.
Vasopressors metaraminol norepinephrine	Rapidly restore blood pressure in anaphylaxis by producing vasoconstriction and stimulating the heart	■ Monitor the client's vital signs, intake and output, mental status, peripheral pulses, and skin color. ■ The client should be on telemetry and monitored continuously.

D. Assessment findings

1. **Associated findings.** Client history may reveal known or suspected exposure to an allergen.
2. **Clinical manifestations**
   a. **Allergic contact dermatitis**
      - Burning, itching, edema, and erythema of skin
      - Crusting, weeping lesions
      - Drying and peeling of the skin
      - Hemorrhagic bullae, possibly with severe responses
   b. **Atopic dermatitis**
      - Pruritus
      - Hyperirritability of the skin

– Excessive dryness of the skin
– Redness for 15 to 30 seconds after stroking, followed by pallor lasting for 1 to 3 minutes
3. **Laboratory and diagnostic study findings**
   a. **Allergic contact dermatitis.** Patch tests of the skin may clarify diagnosis with offending agents being identified.
   b. **Atopic dermatitis**
      – Serum immunoglobulin E levels are frequently elevated.
      – Skin biopsy shows nonspecific eczematous changes.

E. Nursing management
1. **Administer prescribed medications,** which may include antihistamines, antipruritics, or steroidal creams. (See *Drug chart 11-1*, pages 288 to 290.)
2. **Minimize the risk of infection.** (See section II.D.2.)
3. **Provide pain relief.** (See section II.D.3.)
4. **Promote skin integrity.** (See section II.D.4.)
5. **Promote client and family coping.** (See section II.D.9.)
6. **Provide client and family teaching.** (See section II.D.6; also see *Client and family teaching 11-1*, page 285.)
   a. Instruct the client to wear cotton fabrics and wash with a mild detergent.
   b. Advise the client to take daily baths to hydrate the skin.
   c. Encourage the client to use topical skin moisturizers.
   d. Advise the client to humidify dry heat during winter. Recommend that the client keep the room temperature at 68° to 70° F (20° to 21.1° C).

VI. ALLERGIC ASTHMA

A. Description. Allergic asthma is a chronic reactive respiratory disorder producing episodic, reversible airway obstruction. The estimated incidence is 3% to 8% of the population; more than one half of cases are found in children younger than age 10.

B. Etiology. Allergic asthma results from an immunologically mediated hypersensitivity to inhaled allergens, such as airborne pollens and molds, dust, and animal danders.

C. Pathophysiology. Although the pathologic mechanisms of allergic asthma remain somewhat unclear, the fundamental process presumably involves a reaction of sensitized immunoglobulin E antibodies to an inhaled allergen, with subsequent release of chemical mediators, such as histamine, slow-reacting substance of anaphylaxis, and eosinophil chemotactic factor of anaphylaxis. Obstruction results from constriction of bronchial smooth muscle, swelling of bronchial membranes, and hypersecretion of mucus.

D. Assessment findings
1. **Associated findings.** The client's health history may reveal a family history of allergic asthma and exposure to a known or suspected precipitating substance.
2. **Clinical manifestations**
   a. Chest tightness
   b. Prolonged, strenuous expirations
   c. Wheezing on expiration
   d. Buccal and peripheral cyanosis

  e. Cough, nonproductive at first, followed by violent coughing that produces thin, gelatinous mucus and is relieved by a bronchodilator

  f. Nausea and vomiting

  g. Anxiety

 3. Laboratory and diagnostic study findings

  a. Pulmonary function studies reveal airway obstruction and decreased peak expiratory flow rate.

  b. Radiologic or bronchoscopic examination may show hyperinflation and a flattened diaphragm.

  c. Arterial blood gas (ABG) analysis typically reveals the following:

   – Decreased partial pressure of arterial oxygen

   – Initially, decreased partial pressure of arterial carbon dioxide ($Paco_2$) and increased pH (respiratory alkalosis)

   – Later, increased $Paco_2$ and decreased pH (respiratory acidosis)

E. Nursing management (See section II.D.)

 1. Administer prescribed medications, which may include adrenergics, bronchodilators, leukotriene receptor antagonists, mast cell inhibitors, and oral corticosteroids. (See *Drug chart 11-1,* pages 288 to 290.)

 2. Provide nursing care during an acute attack.

  a. Administer adrenergics, which are the initial medications because they dilate bronchial smooth muscles, increase ciliary movements, and decrease the chemical mediators of anaphylaxis.

  b. Collaborate with respiratory therapy and administer oxygen, as prescribed.

  c. Elevate the head of the bed, and lean the client forward to provide maximum lung expansion and ease respiratory effort.

  d. Monitor respiratory rate and depth and auscultate lung sounds.

  e. Monitor ABGs for changes from baseline.

  f. Administer fluids because clients are usually dehydrated from diaphoresis.

  g. Provide reassurance to help relieve anxiety.

 3. Monitor for and take precautions to prevent complications, such as pneumothorax, pulmonary hypertension, right heart failure, and respiratory failure.

 4. Provide client and family teaching.

  a. Encourage the client to undergo testing to identify the cause of asthma attacks.

  b. Convey the importance of strict compliance with the therapeutic regimen.

  c. Discuss the need for increased fluid intake to thin bronchial secretions.

  d. Review stress-reduction methods.

  e. Provide additional teaching. (See *Client and family teaching 11-1,* page 285.)

 5. Provide referrals to the American Lung Association and the Asthma and Allergy Foundation of America. (See appendix A.)

VII. ANAPHYLAXIS

 A. Description. Anaphylaxis is an acute, life-threatening allergic reaction marked by rapidly progressive urticaria and respiratory distress that may result in anaphylactic shock.

 B. Etiology. Anaphylaxis results from ingesting (or other systemic exposure) to allergenic substances. Possible causative substances include:

  1. drugs (e.g., penicillin and other antibiotics, vaccines, hormones, salicylates, and local anesthetics)

2. foods (e.g., legumes, nuts, berries, seafood, and egg albumin)

3. sulfite-containing food additives

4. insect venom (e.g., wasp, hornet, honeybee, certain spiders).

C. Pathophysiology

1. Anaphylactic reaction requires previous sensitization to the triggering allergen, with production of specific immunoglobulin (Ig) E antibodies that bind to mast cells and basophils.

2. On reexposure, IgE reacts immediately with the allergen and triggers release of potent chemical mediators (e.g., histamine, eosinophil chemotactic factor of anaphylaxis) from basophils and mast cells. Concurrently, IgG or IgM activates release of complement fractions, and two other chemical mediators (i.e., bradykinin and leukotrienes) trigger profound vascular changes that can lead to vascular collapse (i.e., anaphylactic shock).

3. Anaphylaxis is a medical emergency because of the possibility of respiratory obstruction and vascular collapse. In severe cases, death may occur within 5 to 10 minutes of onset.

D. Assessment findings

1. Clinical manifestations depend on whether mediators remain local or are systemic.

　　a. **Local effects** include wheals with surrounding red flares and urticaria. Usually, local effects are not dangerous.

　　b. **Systemic manifestations**

　　　　– Intense urticaria and edema at the site of injection or injury, rapidly spreading to the face, hands, and other body areas

　　　　– Respiratory distress from bronchospasm, coughing, sneezing, or wheezing

　　　　– Arrhythmias, tachycardia or bradycardia, hypotension, and signs of circulatory collapse

　　　　– Nausea and vomiting, abdominal pain, and diarrhea

2. Laboratory and diagnostic study findings

　　a. Serum and urine histamine is elevated for a short time.

　　b. Serum tryptase, a mast cell enzyme marker for allergic and anaphylactic reactions, elevates 30 to 90 minutes after reaction onset.

E. Nursing management (See section II.D.)

1. Provide nursing care during an anaphylactic attack.

　　a. Establish a patent airway

　　b. Administer epinephrine, I.M. or subcutaneously, to constrict dilated blood vessels, raise the heart rate, improve myocardial contractility, and dilate the bronchioles. Use a tuberculin syringe to ensure exact dosage and monitor the client closely after administration.

　　c. Establish a patent I.V. line for drug and fluid administration.

　　d. Administer a high concentration of oxygen. Have a tracheostomy set at the bedside.

　　e. Monitor vital functions, evaluating blood pressure, pulse, respirations, arterial blood gas values, electrocardiogram, and urinary output.

　　f. Administer prescribed medications, which may include antihistamines, bronchodilators, vasopressors, and corticosteroids. (See *Drug chart 11-1*, pages 288 to 290.)

2. Teach preventive measures.

　　a. Encourage the client to avoid or eliminate any offending allergens.

　　b. Advise the client, who is sensitive to insect bites, to carry "anti-sting" kits.

　　c. Instruct the client to wear identification tags or bracelets.

3. Maintain safety precautions.

✋ *a.* Always keep the client in the office for 30 minutes after administering any new medication to determine if allergic reaction occurs.

b. Always check for known allergies before administering any prescribed or over-the-counter medication.

4. **Provide a referral** to MedicAlert. (See appendix A.)

VIII. RHEUMATOID ARTHRITIS

A. Description. Rheumatoid arthritis is a chronic, progressive disease involving inflammation of synovial joints. The incidence is three times greater in women than in men. Peak age of onset is between age 30 and 60, but the disease can develop at any age.

B. Etiology. Rheumatoid arthritis is apparently an autoimmune disorder; its cause is unknown. Exacerbations may be associated with increased physical or emotional stress.

C. Pathophysiology. Pathologic changes begin as inflammation and progress to destruction of joints, producing deformity and loss of motion. The disease may affect only joints or may extend to body organs and blood vessels.

D. Assessment findings

1. **Clinical manifestations**
   a. Edematous, warm, tender joints
   b. Limited range of motion in affected joints
   c. Generalized edema or nodules around affected joints
   d. Impaired mobility and ability to perform activities of daily living (ADLs)
   e. Fatigue, weakness, and anorexia
   f. In later stages, weight loss, fever, anemia, muscle atrophy, and Sjögren's syndrome

2. **Laboratory and diagnostic study findings**
   a. Radiographic studies reveal abnormalities such as progressive joint damage.
   b. Rheumatoid factor is present in more than 80% of clients.
   c. Erythrocyte sedimentation rate is significantly elevated.
   d. Red blood cell count and C4 complement component are decreased.

E. Nursing management. Care is directed at relieving pain and maintaining function.

1. **Administer prescribed medications,** which may include nonsteroidal anti-inflammatory drugs, aspirin, slow-acting antirheumatic medications, and corticosteroids. (See *Drug chart 11-1,* pages 288 to 290.)

2. **Provide pain relief.** Provide comfort measures, including massage and position changes. Apply hot or cold therapy to affected joints according to the client's needs. (See section II.D.3.)

3. **Promote self-care.** (See section II.D.7.)

4. **Promote client and family coping.** (See section II.D.9.)

5. **Promote adequate rest and sleep** to prevent fatigue; provide comfort measures, including a foam mattress and supportive pillows; and discuss energy conservation techniques.

6. **Encourage proper body alignment** to prevent contractures.

7. **Collaborate with the physical therapist** to design and provide the client with a physical therapy program, which begins after the acute phase resolves. Encourage a muscle activity program for self-care. Water exercises are excellent because water promotes buoyancy, which eases joint movements.

8. Recommend a weight reduction program, if appropriate.
9. **Collaborate with the occupational therapist and promote the use of braces, splints, and assistive mobility devices,** if appropriate.
10. **Discuss relaxation techniques,** such as imagery, self-hypnosis, biofeedback, diversionary activities, and distraction for pain management.
11. **Discuss maintaining optimal nutritional status.**
12. **Provide a referral** to the Arthritis Foundation. (See appendix A.)

IX. SYSTEMIC LUPUS ERYTHEMATOSUS

A. **Description.** Systemic lupus erythematosus (SLE) is a chronic systemic inflammatory disease affecting multiple body systems. Women are affected at least eight times more often than men, and women of childbearing age are particularly susceptible.

B. **Etiology.** SLE is thought to be an autoimmune disorder.

C. **Pathophysiology**

1. SLE involves markedly increased B-cell activity, hypergammaglobulinemia, autoantibody production, and decreased T-cell functions. Symptoms result from immune complex invasion of body systems. Disease progression, which is characterized by recurring remissions and exacerbations, is widely variable.
2. Prognosis is good with early detection and treatment; however, SLE can lead to potentially serious complications, including cardiovascular, renal, and neurologic problems and severe bacterial infections.

D. **Assessment findings**

1. **Clinical manifestations** may be insidious or acute; the client may remain undiagnosed for many years; clinical manifestations involve multiple body systems.
   a. **Musculoskeletal system**
      - Arthralgias and arthritis (synovitis)
      - Joint edema and tenderness
      - Pain on movement and morning stiffness
   b. **Integumentary system**
      - Subacute cutaneous lupus erythematosus results in a butterfly rash across the bridge of the nose and cheeks.
      - Discoid lupus erythematosus results in skin involvement that may be provoked by sunlight or artificial ultraviolet light.
      - Oral ulcers of the buccal mucosa and hard palate occur in crops and may accompany skin lesions.
   c. **Cardiovascular system**
      - Pericarditis
      - Papular, erythematous, and purpuric lesions on fingertips, elbows, toes, forearms, and hands
   d. **Respiratory system**
      - Pleural effusion
      - Pleuritis
   e. **Neurologic system**
      - Subtle changes in personality and cognitive ability
      - Commonly, depression and psychosis

     f. **Other systems**
- Lymphadenopathy
- With renal involvement, the glomeruli of kidneys are usually affected.

  2. **Laboratory and diagnostic study findings**
    a. Antinuclear antibody test result is positive.
    b. Red and white blood cell counts may be decreased, revealing thrombocytopenia, severe anemia, leukocytosis, and leukopenia.
    c. Anti-deoxyribonucleic acid cell test reveals a high titer.
    d. Urine testing reveals proteinuria and cellular casts in urine.

E. Nursing management (See section II.D.)
  1. **Administer prescribed medications**, which may include corticosteroids, nonsteroidal anti-inflammatory drugs, and salicylates to help control the joint pain and oral or topical corticosteroids to help with the rash. (See *Drug chart 11-1*, pages 288 to 290.) Antimalarial agents are used in some clients.
  2. **Maintain skin integrity,** which includes keeping the skin clean and dry, using mild soaps and lotions, and inspecting the skin for vasculitic lesions.
  3. **Perform a cardiovascular, respiratory, neurologic and musculoskeletal assessment** to identify and describe any systemic problems.
  4. **Provide meticulous mouth care.**
  5. **Arrange for a dietary consult** to ensure optimal nutrition while meeting the client's need for soft, easily tolerated foods.
  6. **Apply warm packs** as needed to relieve joint pain and stiffness.
  7. **Collaborate with the physical therapy department and encourage an appropriate exercise program** to help maintain mobility and strength.
  8. **Provide client and family teaching.**
    a. Encourage protection from the sun and ultraviolet light. Advise the client to avoid going out between 10:00 a.m. and 4:00 p.m., use sunscreen with a sun-protection factor of at least 30, wear a large hat and tight weave clothing, and refrain from using a tanning bed.
    b. Advise the client to consult a health care provider before receiving immunizations or taking birth control pills or over-the-counter drugs.
    c. Advise the client to avoid persons with contagious infections.
  9. **Provide a referral** to the Lupus Foundation of America. (See appendix A.)

X. ACQUIRED IMMUNODEFICIENCY SYNDROME

A. Description. Acquired immunodeficiency syndrome (AIDS) is a severe immunodeficiency caused by the human immunodeficiency virus (HIV), which allows normally benign organisms to flourish and cause disease. The virus causes cell death and a decline in immune function resulting in opportunistic infections, malignancies, and neurologic problems. These opportunistic conditions define the syndrome.

B. Etiology
  1. **HIV** is transmitted sexually, through direct contact with blood or blood products and some body secretions.
  2. **Persons at risk for contracting HIV**
    a. Anyone who engages in unprotected sexual activity with an infected partner.

   b. Recipients of transfused blood or blood components (uncommon since 1985, when blood screening was instituted).
   c. I.V. drug abusers
   d. Children (perinatally) of mothers with HIV
   e. Health care workers exposed to HIV by needle stick (The incidence for health care workers exposed to HIV by needle stick is estimated to be less than 1%.)

C. Pathophysiology. HIV is part of a group of viruses known as retroviruses, which carry genetic material in ribonucleic acid rather than deoxyribonucleic acid. HIV infects cells with CD4 lymphocytes (also called T4 or helper T cells). This infection causes cell death and a decrease in the immune function, resulting in opportunistic infections and neurologic problems. HIV can be isolated from blood, semen, saliva, tears, breast milk, and cerebrospinal fluid. After a variable course of about 10 years from the time of infection, 50% of infected persons develop AIDS. The incubation period of HIV varies, ranging from 6 months to 5 years, with an average of 2 years.

D. Assessment findings
   1. **Associated findings.** The client may report recurring viral and bacterial infections.
   2. **Clinical manifestations**
      a. Fatigue
      b. Fever and night sweats
      c. Weight loss
      d. Generalized lymphadenopathy
      e. Nonproductive cough and shortness of breath
      f. Skin lesions, dry skin, and pallor
      g. GI upset and chronic diarrhea
      h. Edema
      i. Visual impairment
      j. Painful oral lesions
      k. Bruising and bleeding tendencies
      l. Joint pain
      m. Opportunistic infections, such as *Pneumocystis carinii* pneumonia, mycobacterial infections, cryptococcal infection, toxoplasmosis, histoplasmosis, and cytomegalovirus infection
      n. Kaposi's sarcoma and AIDS-related lymphoma
      o. Neurologic deficits, such as AIDS dementia complex
      p. HIV wasting syndrome
   3. **Laboratory and diagnostic study findings**
      a. Enzyme-linked immunosorbent assay (ELISA) indicates exposure to or infection with HIV but does not diagnose AIDS.
      b. Western blot assay identifies HIV antibodies.
      c. SUDS screening test is only about 95% accurate but the results are available in 30 to 60 minutes. This test is useful when a health care worker sustains a needle stick injury; if the client's test comes back positive, the health care worker is started on prophylactic anti-retroviral medications.
      d. AIDS is diagnosed on clinical history, risk factors, physical examination, laboratory evidence of immune dysfunction, and positive ELISA or Western blot assay.

E. Nursing management. No cure or vaccine has been found, and treatment focuses on maintaining health and improving survival time.

1. **Administer prescribed medication,** which may include drug therapy for AIDS-related opportunistic infections, antiretroviral therapy, antidiarrheals, and antiemetics. (See *Drug chart 11-1,* pages 288 to 290.)

2. **Promote preventive measures related to the transmission of HIV.** This is a prime concern until a vaccine is found; researchers have reported that a vaccine is being investigated and tested for prevention of HIV transmission.
   a. Promote public education regarding HIV and AIDS. Teach clients and families to practice safe sex, avoid sharing needles, and avoid touching another's body fluids without protection.
   b. Inform HIV-infected clients that even though HIV is undetectable, the client may be infectious and should practice safe sex.
   c. Promote standard precautions to protect health care providers from exposure to the client's blood or body fluids and to protect the client from cross-contamination.

3. **Maintain skin integrity** by instructing the client to avoid scratching, strong perfumed soaps, and adhesive tapes; follow routine oral care; keep anal area as clean as possible; wear white socks to prevent foot problems; keep linens dry and clean; and apply protective barriers to the skin as necessary.

4. **Instruct the client about the promotion of normal bowel movements and prevention of diarrhea.** Instruct the client to monitor the quantity and volume of liquid stools and avoid bowel irritants, such as raw fruits, vegetables, spicy foods, and hot or cold foods.

5. **Promote infection prevention.** Discuss the importance of maintaining personal hygiene, keeping bathrooms and kitchens clean, avoiding exposure to individuals who are sick, avoiding smoking and alcohol, and getting adequate rest, activity, and a well-balanced diet.

6. **Teach energy conservation techniques,** such as sitting while doing morning care, using a shower chair, and arranging the home in a way to save time from walking or standing. In the hospital, put all necessary items within easy reach.

7. **Discuss ways the client and family can assist with mental status problems.** These include putting notes on the refrigerator or note boards, using calendars and clocks to orient the client to time and place, and assisting the client with paying bills, shopping, and other household activities.

8. **Teach methods for airway clearance.** These include turning, coughing, and deep breathing; increasing fluid intake to thin secretions; maintaining semi-Fowler's position; and using humidified oxygen if necessary.

9. **Help maintain nutritional status** by controlling nausea and vomiting; encouraging foods that are easy to swallow; encouraging oral hygiene before and after meals; promoting a high-protein, high-calorie diet; monitoring weight, intake, and output; monitoring fluid and electrolyte balance; and administering appetite stimulants.

10. **Monitor and manage complications of opportunistic infections.** Opportunistic infections — protozoan, fungal, bacterial and viral — occur because of immune suppression; they account for most of the clinical manifestations observed in AIDS. *Pneumocystis carinii* pneumonia is the most common.

11. **Teach ways to cope with chronic illness** to the client and his family. Always include the family in teaching and care, and provide family members with grief counseling. Discuss advanced directives and durable power of attorney for health care.

12. **Provide referrals** to the National Association of People with AIDS and Project Inform. (See appendix A.)

Study questions

1. Which nursing intervention should be included when teaching the client diagnosed with allergic rhinitis?
   1. Encouraging the client to use saline nasal sprays
   2. Discouraging nose blowing before administering nasal medication
   3. Advising use of a bronchodilator regularly, even if having no symptoms
   4. Instructing the client to carry epinephrine with him at all times

2. Which intervention should the nurse discuss with the client who has an allergic disorder and is requesting information for allergy symptom control? (Select all that apply.)
   1. Instructing the client to refrain from using air conditioning or humidifiers in the house
   2. Instructing the client to use curtains instead of pull shades over windows
   3. Instructing the client to cover the mattress with a hypoallergenic cover
   4. Instructing the client to wear a mask when cleaning
   5. Instructing the client to avoid using sprays, powders, and perfumes
   6. Instructing the client to change detergents frequently

3. Which intervention should the nurse implement when caring for a client diagnosed with *Pneumocystis carinii* pneumonia related to acquired immunodeficiency syndrome who is crying over the loss of friends and family members because they will not talk to him anymore?
   1. Advising the client not to worry, and telling him everything will be all right
   2. Asking the health care provider for a psychiatric consult to assess the client's mental functioning
   3. Sitting down and listening to the client's concerns and frustrations

   4. Telling the client that the friends probably were not true friends anyway

4. Which client statement indicates that the nurse's teaching about allergies has been successful?
   1. "I don't need to wear any type of mask when I'm cleaning my house."
   2. "I should stay in the house when there's a low pollen count outside."
   3. "I should avoid any types of sprays, powders, and perfumes."
   4. "I can wear any type of clothing that I want to as long as I wash it first."

5. A client diagnosed with rheumatoid arthritis (RA) complains about joints that always hurt, saying, "I just feel like staying in bed all day." Which discharge instruction would be aimed at maintaining as much function as possible?
   1. "Refrain from exercise because it only aggravates the disease process."
   2. "Apply elastic bandages to all joints to increase the pain threshold."
   3. "Maintain a supine position most of the day to prevent the stress of weight bearing."
   4. "Promote aquatic (water) exercises to enhance joint mobility."

6. A nurse sustained a dirty needle stick injury. Which diagnostic test would be ordered on the client?
   1. Enzyme-linked immunosorbent assay (ELISA)
   2. SUDS screening test
   3. Antibody titers
   4. Skin biopsy for Kaposi's sarcoma

7. After the first injection of an immunotherapy program, the nurse notices a large, red wheal on the client's arm, coughing, and expiratory wheezing. Which intervention should the nurse implement *first*?

1. Notifying the health care provider immediately
2. Administering I.M. epinephrine per protocol.
3. Beginning oxygen by way of nasal cannula
4. Starting an I.V. line for medication administration

8. Which intervention should the nurse implement for a client who is using a steroidal cream for allergic dermatoses?
   1. Applying an occlusive dressing over the inflamed area afterward
   2. Washing hands before and after applying the cream
   3. Avoiding washing the inflamed area before applying the cream
   4. Using alcohol to clean the inflamed area before applying the cream

9. Which clinical manifestation would cause the nurse to suspect that the client is diagnosed with systemic lupus erythematosus?
   1. Joint edema and tenderness
   2. Red, burning, tearing eyes
   3. Chest tightness with wheezing on expiration
   4. Fever and night sweats

10. Which instruction would be included in the teaching plan for a client diagnosed with systemic lupus erythematosus?
   1. "Wear large-brimmed hats when exposed to the sun."
   2. "Use tanning beds instead of sunbathing outside."
   3. "Remove all rugs, curtains, and dust-collecting items in home."
   4. "Carry injectable epinephrine at all times in case of exacerbation."

11. Which discharge instruction would be included in the care plan for a client diagnosed with atopic dermatitis?
   1. "Take weekly baths to avoid hydrating the skin."

2. "Add humidity to the dry air caused by dry heat during the winter."
3. "Keep the room temperature between 78° and 80° F."
4. "Apply hot or cold therapy to affected joints."

12. A client who was stung by a bee now exhibits redness and edema in the hand and forearm. The nurse's actions would be based on which *scientific* rationale?
   1. Baking soda is the best treatment for the edema from a bee sting.
   2. Hypersensitivity is possible; the client may need to buy an anti-sting kit.
   3. The client should not worry; people cannot develop an allergy to bee stings.
   4. The client needs regular checkups to obtain immunotherapy.

13. Which condition would the nurse suspect when a client complains of a runny nose, itching and burning eyes, and sneezing since visiting a friend who had a cat in the home?
   1. Allergic rhinitis
   2. Anaphylaxis
   3. Bronchitis
   4. Asthma

14. During the past 6 months, a client diagnosed with acquired immunodeficiency syndrome has had chronic diarrhea and has lost 18 pounds. Additional assessment findings include tented skin turgor, dry mucous membranes, and listlessness. Which nursing diagnosis focuses attention on the client's most immediate problem?
   1. Deficient fluid volume related to diarrhea and abnormal fluid loss
   2. Imbalanced nutrition: less than body requirements related to nausea and vomiting
   3. Disturbed thought processes related to central nervous system effects of disease
   4. Diarrhea related to the disease process and acute infection

15. Which dietary instruction would be included in the teaching plan for a client with acquired immunodeficiency syndrome who has chronic diarrhea, anorexia, a history of oral candidiasis, and weight loss?
1. "Follow a low-protein, high-carbohydrate diet."
2. "Eat three large meals per day."
3. "Include unpasteurized dairy products in the diet."
4. "Follow a high-protein, high-calorie diet."

16. Which instruction would be included in the discharge teaching plan for a client with rheumatoid arthritis who was prescribed nonsteroidal anti-inflammatory drugs (NSAIDS)?
1. "Expect to taper off the medication so that the adrenal gland will start functioning."
2. "Do not drive or engage in hazardous activities because you may get drowsy."
3. "Take the medication with food or meals to minimize stomach upset."
4. "Be sure to rinse your mouth with water before and after taking this medication."

Answer key

1. The answer is **1.**
For the client with allergic rhinitis, saline nasal sprays may be helpful in soothing mucous membranes, softening crusted secretions, and removing irritants. To achieve maximum relief, the client should blow the nose before administering any medication into the nasal cavity. The client diagnosed with asthma, not allergic rhinitis, may use bronchodilators. Carrying epinephrine would be appropriate for the client with an allergy to insect stings or certain foods such as shell fish.

2. The answers are **3, 4, 5.**
Using hypoallergenic covers and cosmetics will help reduce the chance of an allergic attack, wearing a mask while cleaning will help decrease the amount of dust entering the lungs, and avoiding sprays, powders, and perfumes will help decrease the chance of an allergic attack. The client should use air conditioning and humidfiers. Drapes, curtains, blinds, and carpets should be removed. The client should not change detergents or soaps.

3. The answer is **3.**
Crying is evidence that the client is beginning to express concerns to the nurse. In response, active, nonjudgmental listening would be most appropriate because it aids in the development of a trusting relationship. Advising the client not to worry or saying that everything will be all right provides false reassurance, which does not help the client cope. Further assessment is needed to determine whether a psychiatric consult should be considered. Telling the client that the friends were not true friends discounts the client's feelings and hinders the development of a therapeutic relationship.

4. The answer is **3.**
The goal of teaching a client with allergies focuses on avoidance of the offending agent and other triggers. The client with allergy problems should reduce any exposure to pollen (including avoiding barns, weeds, dry leaves, and grass), fumes, odors, sprays, powders, and perfumes. The client also should wear a mask when cleaning the house or working in the yard and stay inside when the pollen counts are high, not low. Any fabrics that cause itching should be avoided.

5. The answer is **4.**
Water exercises are excellent because water promotes buoyancy, which eases joint movement. Persons with RA should maintain an active exercise program to strengthen and

preserve muscle movement. Heat or cold applications, which promote circulation and reduce swelling, may help relieve pain, but elastic bandage wraps most likely would not be helpful.

6. The answer is **2.**
SUDS screening test results are available in 30 to 60 minutes. The test is performed on a client to determine if the health care worker with a dirty needle stick injury should begin antiretroviral treatment. ELISA test results indicate exposure to or infection with human immunodeficiency virus (HIV), but the test does not diagnose acquired immunodeficiency syndrome (AIDS). Antibody titers would not be appropriate to determine whether the health care worker has been exposed to HIV or hepatitis. Kaposi's sarcoma is usually associated with AIDS but not immediately after a needle stick.

7. The answer is **2.**
Immediately on noticing the client's signs and symptoms, the nurse would determine that the client is experiencing anaphylaxis to the injection. The first action is to give 0.2 to 0.5 ml of 1:1,000 epinephrine I.M. Notifying the health care provider, beginning oxygen administration, and starting an I.V. line follow after the initial injection of epinephrine is administered.

8. The answer is **2.**
The inflamed area is prone to infection. Before applying medication to it, the inflamed area and the hands should be washed. After application, the medication should be washed off the hands so that it will not be transferred to the eyes, skin, or other areas. The inflamed area usually is left open to air, or a light gauze dressing — not an occlusive dressing — is used. The inflamed area should be cleaned with water, not alcohol.

9. The answer is **1.**
Clinical features of systemic lupus erythematosus involve multiple body systems. When the musculoskeletal system is involved, the client exhibits joint tenderness, edema, and morning stiffness. Eyes that are red, burning, and tearing are commonly associated with allergic rhinitis (i.e., hay fever). Chest tightness and wheezing on expiration are associated with allergic asthma. Fever and nights sweats are manifestations of acquired immunodeficiency syndrome.

10. The answer is **1.**
The client diagnosed with systemic lupus erythematosus needs to modify his lifestyle. This includes avoiding sun and ultraviolet light exposure, especially between the hours of 10 a.m. and 4 p.m. The client also should wear tightly woven clothing. Regardless of the source, exposure to ultraviolet light, even by means of tanning beds, should be strictly avoided. Removing all dust-collecting items in the home is appropriate for a client diagnosed with asthma. Carrying injectable epinephrine is appropriate for a client who is allergic to insect stings or certain foods.

11. The answer is **2.**
Atopic dermatitis is an inflammatory condition involving a skin reaction to irritants or allergens. Adding humidity to the dry air caused by dry heat during the winter helps keep the skin hydrated and helps prevent itching and scratching. Daily bathing is necessary to hydrate the skin. The room temperature should be maintained between 68° and 70° F (20° and 21.1° C). Applying heat or cold therapy to affected joints is appropriate for a client diagnosed with rheumatoid arthritis.

12. The answer is **2.**
This client is demonstrating signs of a moderate reaction to the bee sting and may be hypersensitive and should have access to an anti-sting kit in the event he is stung again. The use of baking soda is ineffective in controlling the client's reaction. People can develop an allergy to bee stings. Immunotherapy is prescribed only when immunoglobulin E

hypersensitivity to specific inhalant allergens (e.g., house dust, pollens) that the client is unable to avoid is demonstrated.

13. The answer is **1.**
This client most likely is suffering from allergic rhinitis, an allergic reaction to inhaled airborne allergens. In this case, the friend's cat triggered the client's symptoms. Anaphylaxis is an acute, life-threatening allergic reaction marked by rapidly progressive urticaria and respiratory distress. Bronchitis and asthma produce symptoms in the lower respiratory tract, such as expiratory wheezing and chest tightness.

14. The answer is **1.**
Based on the client's assessment findings, the most immediate problem is dehydration because of the chronic diarrhea. The nursing diagnosis of deficient fluid volume is the priority, and interventions are geared to improving the client's fluid status. Although im-

balanced nutrition, disturbed thought processes, and diarrhea are involved, they assume a lower priority at this time.

15. The answer is **4.**
Dietary instructions should include the need for a high-protein, high-calorie diet. The patient should be taught to eat small, frequent meals and include low-microbial foods, such as pasteurized dairy products, washed and peeled fruits and vegetables, and well-cooked meats.

16. The answer is **3.**
Gastric upset is a common adverse effect of NSAIDS. The client should be instructed to take the medication with food or meals to minimize this effect. Corticosteroids, not NSAIDS, affect adrenal gland function and need to be tapered. Because NSAIDS do not cause drowsiness or stomatitis, the cautions about driving and rinsing the mouth are not appropriate.

12 Integumentary disorders

I. STRUCTURE AND FUNCTION OF THE INTEGUMENTARY SYSTEM

A. Structure

1. **The skin.** The body's largest organ, the skin has three layers: hypodermis (subcutaneous layer), dermis, and epidermis. (See *Figure 12-1*.)

   a. **Hypodermis**
   - The hypodermis, the innermost layer, provides a cushion between the skin layers and the muscles and the bones.
   - The hypodermis is composed of loose areolar connective tissue or adipose (fat) tissue, depending on its location in the body.

   b. **Dermis**
   - The dermis, the middle layer, primarily comprises collagen fibrils that provide mechanical strength to the skin.
   - The dermis also contains blood vessels, nerves, lymphatics, hair follicles, and sebaceous and sweat glands.
   - The dermis is composed of two layers:
     - The papillary layer, or upper layer, is composed primarily of loose connective tissue, small elastic fibers, and an extensive network of capillaries
     - The reticular layer, or lower layer, forms a dense bed of vascular connective tissue that includes nerves and lymphatic tissue.

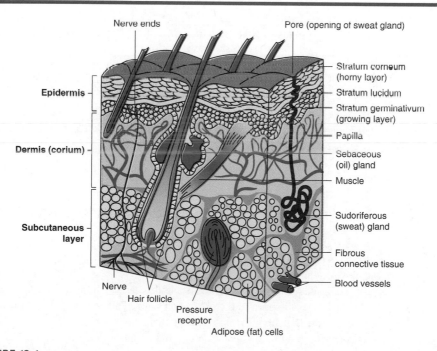

FIGURE 12-1
Anatomic structures of the skin

c. **Epidermis**
- The epidermis is a multilayered outer covering of the skin consisting of four layers throughout the body, except for the palms of the hands and soles of the feet, which have five layers.
- Each of the layers becomes more differentiated as it rises from the basal stratum germinativum layer to the outermost stratum corneum layer.
- The epidermis contains two main types of cells: melanocytes and keratinocytes.
  - **Melanocytes.** Scattered throughout the basal layer of the epidermis, melanocytes produce melanin, a pigment that shields deeper skin structures from sunlight. People of all races have basically the same number of melanocytes. Differences in skin color result from differences in the size and distribution of melanosomes produced by melanocytes.
  - **Keratinocytes** develop from cells in the basal layer and then mature and move to the skin surface (i.e., stratum corneum), where they flatten, dehydrate, and become keratinized. Alterations in this process account for many dermatologic problems.

2. **Epidermal appendages** are formed from epidermal cells located in the epidermis and dermis. Epidermal appendages include hair, nails, and sebaceous and sweat glands (i.e., apocrine and eccrine).

a. **Hair**
- Hair follicles are distributed on all skin surfaces, except the palms and soles.
- No new hair-producing structures are produced after birth.
- Most hair shafts are composed of three layers: the medulla (inner layer), the cortex (middle layer), and the cuticle (outer layer).
- Melanocytes produced at the base of each hair follicle determine hair color; an abundance of pigment produces dark color, and smaller amounts produce a lighter color.
- Hair growth
  - Hair growth occurs in phases: resting (telogen), growth (anagen), and atrophy (catagen). Scattered patterns of these phases keep the total number of hairs relatively constant.
  - Chemical, mechanical, or physiological factors can convert all hair to the atrophic phase, resulting in baldness.
  - Scalp hair grows about 1 cm per month.

b. **Nails**
- Nails are composed of keratinized (horny) layers of cells that arise from undifferentiated epithelial tissue called the matrix.
- The nail plate covers the distal portion of the digits; the nail root attaches to the matrix; the nail bed is the vascular bed under the nail plate; and the periungual tissues surround the nail plate and free edge of the nail.

c. **Sebaceous glands**
- The sebaceous glands are most prevalent and largest on the face, scalp, upper chest, and back (and absent from the palms and soles). They secrete sebum, a complex lipid mixture that empties into hair shafts.
- The male hormone androgen initiates and sustains sebum production.

d. Sweat glands
- Apocrine glands
  - Located in the axillae, areolae, groin, perineum, and circumanal and periumbilical regions, these large sweat glands are rudimentary structures with no known useful purpose.
  - They respond to autonomic, rather than thermal, stimulation. They produce odorless, viscous, milklike droplets that cause a distinctive body odor when acted on by the bacteria normally present on the skin surface.
- Eccrine glands
  - These small sweat glands, distributed in the skin all over the body, are true secretory glands that produce sweat, which functions in thermoregulation and other processes.
  - The sweat from the eccrine gland is a clear, aqueous solution containing 99% water and 1% solids. Hypotonic under normal conditions, a high rate of sweating may produce isotonic concentrations.
  - Sweat is released from the eccrine glands in response to elevated ambient temperature and elevated body temperature.
  - The rate of sweat secretion is under the control of the sympathetic nervous system.

B. Function
1. **Protective functions**
   a. The skin is responsible for the protection of underlying organs from the external environment.
   b. The normally acidic skin and perspiration protect against invasion by bacteria and foreign matter.
   - The skin surface normally is covered with microorganisms, especially such bacteria as *Staphylococcus epidermidis* and diphtheroids. Infection occurs when the balance between host and microorganisms is upset.
   - Healthy persons can develop bacterial skin infections, but predisposing factors, such as moisture, obesity, skin disease, systemic steroids and antibiotics, chronic disease, and diabetes mellitus, increase the risk.
   c. The thickened skin of the palms and soles provides a tough covering to protect from the constant trauma to these areas.
2. **Water balance**
   a. The epidermis (i.e., superficial stratum corneum) prevents the excessive loss of water and electrolytes from the internal body and retains moisture in the subcutaneous tissues.
   b. The skin allows evaporation of small amounts of water, called insensible perspiration, which is approximately 600 ml daily from a normal adult.
3. **Sensory functions**
   a. Receptor endings of nerves in the skin provide constant monitoring of the immediate environment. The primary functions of these receptors include sensing coldness, warmth, pain, and touch pressure.
   b. The density of receptors varies in different body areas; the fingertips and lips are high-density areas compared with the back.
   c. The skin contains various types of sensory endings. Each type of receptor nerve ending responds to only one kind of cutaneous sensation.
   - Naked nerve endings mediate all four sensory modalities.
   - Free nonmyelinated nerve endings mediate pain sensation.

    – Expanded tips on sensory nerve terminals mediate touch (i.e., Merkel's disks) and warmth (i.e., Ruffini endings).

    – Encapsulated nerve endings mediate pressure (i.e., Pacini's corpuscles), touch (i.e., Meissner's corpuscles), and cold (i.e., Krause's bulbs).

4. Vitamin D production

    a. Endogenous synthesis of vitamin D, which is critical for bone metabolism, occurs in the epidermis.

    b. Only a few minutes of sun exposure on a small body area are needed for vitamin D production.

5. Thermoregulatory functions

    a. The body continuously produces heat as a by-product of cellular metabolism. This heat is dissipated locally, primarily through the skin.

    b. The body's internal core temperature normally is maintained at a constant 99.7° F (37.6° C) through a balance between heat production and heat loss.

    c. Three primary processes are involved in heat loss from the body to the external environment:

      – *Radiation* is the body's ability to give off its heat to another object of lower temperature situated at a distance.

      – *Conduction* is the transfer of heat from the body to a cooler object in direct contact.

      – *Convection* is the bulk movement of warm air molecules away from the body.

    d. The rate of heat loss depends primarily on the skin's surface temperature, which depends on skin blood flow, regulated by neural mechanisms. Increased blood flow results in delivery of more heat to the skin and a greater rate of heat loss from the body; when body temperature falls, the skin's blood vessels constrict to reduce heat loss from the body.

    e. Perspiration facilitates heat loss from the body. Body temperature, environmental temperature and humidity, and neurologic factors such as response to emotional stress regulate it.

6. Immunologic functions

    a. Wheal and flare reaction

      – This immunologic function of the skin involves edema (i.e., wheal) and diffuse redness caused by increased temperature in the area from a stimulus.

      – The wheal is caused by increased capillary permeability. Trauma causes protein-containing fluid to leak out of capillaries locally to produce edema. Dilation of arterioles and venules (i.e., flares) constitutes normal reaction to injury.

    b. Reactions associated with release of histamine and bradykinin

      – Histamine causes contraction of bronchial smooth muscle, dilation of small venules and constriction of larger vessels, and increased secretion of gastric and mucosal cells.

      – Bradykinin contracts smooth muscles of the bronchi and blood vessels and causes increased permeability of the capillaries, resulting in edema.

    c. Immune complexes

      – Major deposition sites of immune complexes include the dermal-epidermal junction and dermal vessels of the skin.

      – Deposition of immune complexes leads to fixation and activation of complement at tissue sites.

– Vasodilation and increased permeability result from anaphylatoxin components of C3 and C5. Neutrophils and monocytes attracted by complement-generated chemotactic factors result in acute and perhaps chronic inflammation.

7. **Circulatory function**
   a. Changes in the cutaneous vascular system contribute significantly to systemic circulatory status.
   b. Skin color depends in part on the quantity of blood in the small vessels. Skin temperature depends chiefly on the rate of blood flow through the skin.
   c. Stimulation of sympathetic fibers supplying the skin causes vasoconstriction of cutaneous vessels. Interruption of these fibers results in vasodilatation of small arteries and arterioles.
   d. The cutaneous circulatory system also responds to such chemical agents as:
      – acetylcholine, which causes vasodilatation
      – norepinephrine, epinephrine, and vasopressin, which cause vasoconstriction.

8. **Aesthetic function.** The skin contributes to each person's unique appearance and identity. Skin defects or problems can have negative effects on a person's body image and self-esteem.

NURSING PROCESS OVERVIEW

 II. THE INTEGUMENTARY SYSTEM

A. Assessment
   1. **Health history**
      a. **Elicit a description of the client's present illness and chief complaint,** including onset, course, duration, location, and precipitating and alleviating factors. Elicit a description of the client's overall health status. Cardinal signs and symptoms indicating altered integumentary function are changes in size, formation, or texture of any type of skin lesion (e.g., mole, wart) or any type of disease or injury that causes the integrity of the skin to be penetrated.
      b. **Explore the client's health history** for risk factors associated with integumentary disease, including:
         – sun exposure (use of sunblocks)
         – exposure to irritants and radiation
         – allergic reactions to food, medications, and chemicals
         – inadequate intake of protein and vitamins A, B complex, C, and K.
   2. **Physical examination**
      a. **Inspection**
         – Assess skin color, texture, and turgor.
         – Assess the skin for abnormal growths, lesions, rashes, scars, or discoloration.
         – Observe for any areas of scaliness or dryness.
         – Assess for signs of skin infection.
         – Assess the skin for evidence of bleeding, ecchymosis, or increased vascularity.
         – Assess the scalp hair, eyebrows, eyelashes, and body hair for color and distribution.
         – Assess the fingernails and toenails, noting color of nails, shape, configuration, and consistency.
      b. **Palpation**
         – Palpate all nonmucous membrane surfaces for moisture and temperature.

      – Palpate the skin for peripheral or sacral edema.

      – Palpate the hair, noting the condition of hair from the scalp to the end of the hair.

      – Palpate the nail, noting the consistency.

  3. Laboratory and diagnostic studies

    a. **Skin cultures and microscopic examination** can identify infectious organisms. The lesion is cleaned, and a scalpel is used to remove scales from the margin of the lesion. Infected scales are viewed under a microscope, and the organism is isolated.

    b. **Skin biopsy** and **histologic examination** are done for cancer diagnosis.

    c. **Patch testing** is performed to identify substances to which the client has developed an allergy.

B. Nursing diagnoses

  1. Impaired skin integrity

  2. Acute pain

  3. Imbalanced nutrition: less than body requirements

  4. Risk for infection

  5. Impaired physical mobility

  6. Deficient knowledge

  7. Disturbed body image

  8. Ineffective coping

C. Planning and outcome identification. The major goals may include the maintenance of skin integrity; relief of discomfort; absence of complications, such as altered nutrition, infection, and impaired mobility; understanding the condition to enhance compliance with prescribed therapy; and improved body image and coping.

D. Implementation

  1. Enhance skin integrity.

    a. Assess the entire skin area, including the mucous membranes, scalp, and nails, for evidence of irritation or breakdown.

    b. Keep intact skin clean and dry; clean the skin with mild soap at least once daily.

    c. Protect skin folds and surfaces that rub together.

    d. Keep clothing and linen clean and dry.

    e. Protect hands by wearing gloves when using strong soaps, solvents, detergents, and other chemicals.

  2. Provide pain relief.

    a. To help relieve pruritus, humidify the room, maintain a cool temperature, remove excess bedding and clothing, and use soaps for sensitive skin.

    b. Encourage diversionary activities and relaxation techniques to ensure restful sleep and to alleviate discomfort.

  3. Promote nutritional balance.

    a. Encourage the client to consume foods rich in protein and vitamins A, B complex, C, and K.

    b. Encourage the client to increase fluid intake to 2 to 3 L per day, unless contraindicated.

  4. Prevent infection.

    a. Maintain careful handwashing, and wear gloves when handling or dressing any type of skin disorder.

    b. Implement standard precautions when applicable, and collaborate with the infection-control nurse.

CLIENT AND FAMILY TEACHING 12-1
Tips for a client with a skin disorder

- Maintain a cool environment to deter itching.
- Use mild soap or soap made for sensitive skin.
- Remove excess clothing or bedding to promote a cool environment.
- Wash all bed linens and clothing with mild soap.
- Protect skin from sun exposure, especially between 10 a.m. and 4 p.m., and use sunscreen with a sun protection factor of 30 or higher.
- Use vinyl gloves when being exposed to harsh detergents, soaps, or other chemicals.
- Take tepid, cooling baths or use a cool dressing for itching.
- Apply mild skin lotion to keep skin hydrated.
- Keep fingernails short and trimmed to prevent injury from scratching.

- Do not use commercial topical ointments unless prescribed by a health care provider.
- Bathe or shower only as absolutely necessary, using mild soap and rinsing thoroughly.
- Dry skin thoroughly after bathing by blotting gently and avoiding friction.
- Maintain a healthy, well-balanced diet.
- Apply topical steroidal and antibacterial ointment as prescribed; wash hands before and after application.
- Notify a health care provider if skin condition does not improve after 48 hours of treatment, if affected areas become more reddened with purulent drainage, or if the client has a temperature greater than 100° F (37.8° C).
- Express feelings about body image disturbance because of the skin disorder.

---

5. **Improve physical mobility.** Perform passive range-of-motion exercises, and encourage the client to perform active range-of-motion exercises at least three times daily.
6. **Provide client and family teaching.**
   a. Instruct the client on the principles of good nutrition and the importance of exercise, rest, and sleep in maintaining healthy intact skin.
   b. Instruct the client to report any change in skin lesions, including a change in size, texture, or contour.
   c. Instruct the client on the cause of the disorder and interventions aimed at preventing complications. Discuss medication administration.
   d. Provide additional teaching. (See *Client and family teaching 12-1.*)
7. **Improve coping and body image.**
   a. Encourage the client to verbalize feelings and identify effective coping strategies to deal with the illness.
   b. Encourage the client to ventilate feelings about the impact that the body change has had on self-concept and his relationships with others.

E. Outcome evaluation
1. The client exhibits intact or only minimally disrupted skin integrity.
2. The client's skin heals without inflammation or vesicular eruption and exhibits no sign of infestation.
3. The client reports no pain or discomfort.
4. The client maintains optimal nutritional balance to promote healing.
5. The client remains free from infection.
6. The client participates in physical therapy to maintain an optimal range of motion and function and to prevent contractures.
7. The client verbalizes important preventive measures to avoid complications associated with disorders of the integumentary system.
8. The client exhibits healthy adaptation to body image changes.
9. The client verbalizes feelings and is able to cope effectively with disorders of the integumentary system.

III. SEBORRHEIC DERMATITIS

A. Description. Seborrheic dermatitis is a chronic, inflammatory, scaling eruption characterized by periodic remissions and exacerbations. It most commonly develops in middle-aged or older people as multiple lesions occurring chiefly on the scalp, face, or trunk.

B. Etiology. Seborrheic dermatitis is associated with genetic predisposition and aggravated by physical or emotional stress.

C. Pathophysiology. Seborrhea refers to excessive production of sebum by sebaceous glands in areas where glands are normally found in large numbers (i.e., face, scalp, eyebrows, eyelids, ears, and groin). These areas have a predilection to seborrheic dermatitis because they have a high bacterial count. The area becomes inflamed, resulting in an oily form or dry form of seborrheic dermatitis. The inflamed area may develop a secondary *Candida* (yeast) infection in body creases and folds.

D. Assessment findings. Clinical manifestations may include:
1. scaling (i.e., dry, moist, or greasy), predominantly in areas where glands are normally found in large numbers (e.g., trunk, face, scalp) and in skin folds
2. patches of sallow, greasy-appearing skin with or without scaling and slight erythema
3. pruritus and pain.

E. Nursing management (See section II.D.)
1. **Administer prescribed medications,** which may include topical corticosteroids or antibiotics to allay the secondary inflammatory response. (See *Drug chart 12-1.*)
2. **Provide client and family teaching.**
   a. Instruct the client to treat dandruff by properly shampooing with medicated shampoo.
   b. Advise the client to remove any external irritants.
   c. Instruct the client to avoid excessive heat and perspiration.
   d. Caution the client that this is a chronic problem with remissions and exacerbations.
   e. Provide additional teaching. (See *Client and family teaching 12-1,* page 311.)

IV. NONINFECTIOUS INFLAMMATORY DERMATOSES

A. Description
1. **Psoriasis** is a chronic inflammatory disease marked by epidermal proliferation. The incidence is highest among whites.
2. **Exfoliative dermatitis** is a generalized scaling eruption of the skin characterized by progressive inflammation.
3. **Pemphigus vulgaris** is a serious autoimmune skin disease marked by blisters on the skin and mucous membranes.
4. **Toxic epidermal necrolysis (TEN)** is a rare, potentially fatal skin disorder marked by epidermal erythema, necrosis, and skin erosions.

B. Etiology
1. **Psoriasis** appears to be a hereditary defect.
2. **Exfoliative dermatitis** is caused by several factors, including:
   a. a secondary or reactive response to an underlying skin disease
   b. lymphoma disease (may accompany or precede lymphoma)

DRUG CHART 12-1
Medications for skin disorders

Classifications	Indications	Selected interventions
Antibiotics aminoglycosides (gentamicin, tobramycin) amoxicillin erythromycin penicillin tetracycline	Prevent or treat infections caused by pathogenic micro-organisms	▪ Before administering the first dose, assess the client for allergies and determine whether culture has been obtained. ▪ After multiple doses, assess the client for super-infection (thrush, yeast infection, diarrhea); notify the health care provider if these occur. ▪ Assess the insertion site for phlebitis if antibiotics are being administered I.V. ▪ To assess the effectiveness of antibiotic therapy, monitor the white blood cell count. ▪ Monitor peaks and troughs for aminoglycosides. ▪ Take tetracycline 1 hour before or 2 hours after consuming food or dairy products.
Topical antibiotics clindamycin erythromycin	Suppress the growth of *Propionibacterium acnes* and reduce surface free fatty acid levels	▪ Advise the client to wash his hands before and after application.
Antifungals griseofulvin	Treat superficial mycosis (fungal infection); administered orally	▪ Absorption is enhanced by taking the drug with a fatty meal.
Topical antifungals clotrimazole miconazole	Treat a variety of superficial mycosis (fungal infections)	▪ Advise the client to wash his hands before and after application. ▪ Instruct the client to clean the affected area with warm water before application.
Corticosteroids oral hydrocortisone, methylprednisolone, prednisone	Strengthen biologic membrane, inhibiting capillary permeability and preventing leakage of fluid into the injured area; also prevents development of edema; exact mechanism unknown	▪ Instruct the client to take the medication exactly as directed and to taper it rather than it stop abruptly, which could cause serious withdrawal symptoms leading to adrenal insufficiency, shock, and death. ▪ Forewarn the client that the medication may cause reportable cushingoid effects (weight gain, moon face, buffalo hump, and hirsutism) and may mask signs and symptoms of infection.
Topical corticosteroids desoximetasone hydrocortisone triamcinolone	Relieve or prevent inflammation and itching	▪ Advise the client to wash his hands before and after application. ▪ Instruct the client to clean the affected area with warm water before application.
Opioid analgesics codeine hydrocodone hydromorphone morphine propoxyphene	Relieve moderate to severe pain by reducing pain sensation, producing sedation, and decreasing the emotional upset often associated with pain; most often schedule II drugs	▪ Assess the pain for location, type, intensity, and what increases or decreases it; rate pain on scale of 1 (no pain) to 10 (worst pain). ▪ Rule out any complications. Is this pain routine or expected? Is this a complication that needs immediate intervention? ▪ Medicate according to pain scale findings. ▪ Institute safety measures — bed in low position, side rails up, and call light within reach. ▪ Evaluate the effectiveness of the medication in 30 minutes.

(continued)

DRUG CHART 12-1
Medications for skin disorders *(continued)*

Classifications	Indications	Selected interventions
Topical vitamin A tretinoin (Retin-A)	Seed cellular turnover, thereby clearing keratin plugs from the pilosebaceous ducts	▪ Caution the client to avoid sun exposure ▪ Explain to the client that noticeable improvement may take 8 to 12 weeks, during which time skin redness and peeling are common.
Other topical agents (e.g., coal tar products) anthralin preparations	Slow pathologic processes; retard overactive epidermis without affecting other tissues	▪ Apply with a tongue blade or gloved hand; do not apply to normal skin. ▪ Caution the client that anthralin, a coal tar derivative, temporarily stains the skin and clothing.

  c. severe reaction to various drugs (e.g., sulfonamides, penicillins, anticonvulsants, analgesics).
 3. Pemphigus vulgaris is an autoimmune disorder of unknown origin.
 4. TEN. The cause of this disorder is unknown. It may be a reaction to medications (i.e., antibiotics, anticonvulsants, butazones, and sulfonamides) or result from a viral infection.

C. Assessment findings
 1. Clinical manifestations depend on the specific disorder.
  a. **Psoriasis**
   – Profuse, erythematous scales or plaques, often covering large areas of the body
   – Pruritus and sometimes pain
   – Possibly arthritic symptoms (e.g., joint stiffness)
  b. **Exfoliative dermatitis**
   – Patchy or generalized erythematous eruption (initially), followed by characteristic scaling, possibly with hair loss and nail shedding
   – Possible severe fluid and electrolyte imbalance, anemia, and systemic infections
  c. **Pemphigus vulgaris**
   – Widespread bullae on the skin and mucous membranes that enlarge and rupture, leaving denuded areas that eventually form crusts
   – Possible fluid and electrolyte imbalance, systemic infection, or impaired nutrition, which may lead to critical illness requiring frequent hospitalization
  d. **TEN**
   – Formation of large, flaccid bullae in some areas, with shedding of large sheets of epidermis (along with toenails, fingernails, eyebrows, and eyelashes) in others
   – Possibly serious fluid and electrolyte imbalance and systemic infection that may lead to sepsis
 2. Laboratory and diagnostic study findings
  a. **Pemphigus vulgaris**
   – A skin biopsy and specimen from the blister demonstrates separation of the epidermal cells from each other (i.e., acantholysis).
   – Serum studies reveal circulating pemphigus antibodies.

h. TEN
- Skin biopsy from freshly denuded area reveals necrotic tissue.
- Serum studies detect atypical epidermal autoantibodies.

D. Nursing management

1. **Provide nursing care for the client with psoriasis.**
   a. **Administer prescribed medications,** which may include coal tar therapy and topical corticosteroids. (See *Drug chart 12-1.*)
   b. **Discuss and assist with the administration of additional medical treatments,** which may include coal tar shampoos, intralesional therapy (i.e., injection of medication directly into lesion), systemic cytotoxic medication, photochemotherapy, and occlusive dressing.
   c. **Enhance skin integrity.** (See section II.D.1.)
   d. **Prevent infection.** (See section II.D.4.)
   e. **Provide client and family teaching.** (See section II.D.6.)
      - Advise the client receiving systemic cytotoxic (e.g., methotrexate) therapy, which inhibits deoxyribonucleic acid synthesis in epidermal cells to speed the replacement of psoriatic cells, to continue taking the medication even if nausea and vomiting occur, to increase fluid intake to prevent nephrotoxicity, and to avoid alcoholic beverages.
      - Instruct the client to avoid sun exposure during photochemotherapy. This regimen of oral psoralens and phototherapy with ultraviolet A (PUVA) light decreases cellular proliferation. PUVA therapy results in photosensitivity, and the client should avoid exposure to sunlight during this time.
      - Be knowledgeable about treatment, and give the client written instructions.
2. **Provide nursing care for the client with exfoliative dermatitis.**
   a. **Administer prescribed medications,** which may include topical and systemic corticosteroids and systemic antibiotics. (See *Drug chart 12-1.*)
   b. **Monitor for fluid and electrolyte imbalance.** This is important because a considerable amount of water and protein are lost from the skin surface.
   c. **Observe the client for signs and symptoms of heart failure** because hyperemia and increased cutaneous blood flow can produce cardiac failure of high-output origin.
   d. **Enhance skin integrity.** (See section II.D.1.)
   e. **Prevent infection.** (See section II.D.4.)
   f. **Provide client and family teaching.** (See section II.D.6.)
3. **Provide nursing care for the client with pemphigus vulgaris.**
   a. **Administer prescribed medications,** which include high-dose corticosteroids. (See *Drug chart 12-1.*) Immunosuppressive agents, such as azathioprine or cyclophosphamide, may be prescribed to help control the disease and reduce the corticosteroid dose.
   b. **Enhance skin integrity.** Never use tape on the skin because it may cause more blisters. (See section II.D.1.)
   c. **Provide client and family teaching.** If plasmapheresis is recommended, explain that this treatment is a reinfusion of specially treated plasma cells that temporarily decreases serum antibody concentration. The success rate of the process varies. (See section II.D.6.)
   d. **Encourage meticulous oral hygiene** to keep the oral mucosa clean.
   e. **Institute measures to keep the client warm and comfortable** because hypothermia is common.

f. **Assess for and prevent infection.** (See section II.D.4.)

g. **Promote nutritional balance.** Encourage the client to increase oral intake and eat small, high-protein, high-calorie meals.

4. **Provide nursing care for the client with TEN.** (See section II.D.)

a. **Administer prescribed medications,** which may include systemic antibiotics and topical bacteriostatic agents, such as silver nitrate solution or nitrofurazone. These medications help prevent wound sepsis. (See *Drug chart 12-1,* pages 313 and 314.)

b. **Provide skin care,** which is priority because skin denudes easily. Be very gentle when turning and treating.

c. **Encourage careful oral hygiene** to keep the oral mucosa clean.

d. **Monitor the client for fluid and electrolyte imbalances.**

e. **Institute measures to prevent chilling** because the client is at risk for hypothermia. Use hypothermic blankets, ceiling-mounted heat lamps, and heat shields.

f. **Institute infection prevention measures.** Remember the major cause of death from TEN is infection.

5. **Provide additional teaching.** (See *Client and family teaching 12-1,* page 311.)

V. ACNE VULGARIS

A. **Description.** Acne vulgaris is an inflammatory disease of the sebaceous follicles. The incidence is highest at puberty, although it may occur as early as age 8 and can persist into adulthood.

B. **Etiology.** The cause appears to involve multiple factors, including genetics, hormonal factors, and bacterial infection. Diet does not affect incidence or severity.

C. **Pathophysiology.** Acne eruptions are initiated by increased sebum production activated by androgenic hormones. Sebum is secreted into dilated hair follicles containing normal skin bacteria, such as *Propionibacterium acnes.* The bacteria secrete the enzyme lipase, which reacts with sebum to produce free fatty acids to trigger inflammation. At the same time, keratin produced by the hair follicles combines with sebum to form plugs in dilated follicles.

D. **Assessment findings.** Clinical manifestations include closed comedones (i.e., whiteheads), open comedones (i.e., blackheads), papules, pustules, nodules, and cysts. Acne lesions appear primarily on the face, chest, shoulders, and upper back.

E. **Nursing management**

1. **Administer prescribed medications,** which may include acne products containing benzoyl peroxide (explain that these products initially cause skin redness and scaling but that the skin adjusts quickly); topical agents, such as vitamin A acid; and antibiotics such as tetracycline. (See *Drug chart 12-1,* pages 313 and 314.)

2. **Provide client and family teaching.** (See section II.D.6; also see *Client and family teaching 12-1,* page 311.)

a. Advise the client that heat, humidity, and perspiration exacerbate acne. Explain that uncleanliness, dietary indiscretions, menstrual cycle, and other myths are not responsible for acne.

b. Explain that it will take 4 to 6 weeks of compliance with the treatment regimen to obtain results.

c. Instruct the client to wash his face gently (do not scrub) with mild soap twice daily.

d. Instruct the client not to squeeze blackheads; not to prop hands on or rub the face; to wash hair daily and keep it off the face; and to use cosmetics cautiously, because some may exacerbate acne.

e. Instruct the female client to inform her health care provider if she is possibly pregnant. Some medication, such as systemic retinoic acid, have teratogenic effects, therefore a pregnancy test is required prior to treatment and strict birth-control measures are used throughout therapy.

VI. BACTERIAL INFECTIONS (PYODERMAS)

A. Description and etiology

1. **Impetigo** is a superficial skin infection caused by streptococci, staphylococci, or multiple bacteria. It is especially common among children living in poor hygienic conditions.
2. **Folliculitis** is a staphylococcal infection arising in hair follicles. It is commonly seen in the beard area of men who shave and on women's legs.
3. **Furuncle** (also known as a *boil*) is an acute inflammation arising deep in one or more hair follicles and spreading into the surrounding dermis.
4. **Carbuncle** is abscess of skin and subcutaneous tissue representing extension of a large, deep-seated furuncle that has invaded several follicles.

B. Pathophysiology

1. Bacterial infections of the skin may be primary or secondary.
2. Primary skin infections originate in previously normal-appearing skin and are usually caused by a single organism.
3. Secondary skin infections arise from a preexisting skin disorder or from disruption of the skin integrity resulting from injury or surgery.
4. The most common primary bacterial skin infections are impetigo and folliculitis. Folliculitis may lead to furuncles or carbuncles.

C. Assessment findings. Clinical manifestations vary depending on the specific infection.

1. **Impetigo** begins as small, red macules and rapidly progresses to discrete, thin-walled vesicles. These vesicles rupture and become covered with a loosely adherent, honey-yellow crust.
2. **Folliculitis** produces single or multiple, superficial or deep papules or pustules close to hair follicles.
3. A **furuncle** is marked by tenderness, pain, and surrounding cellulitis. After the furuncle localizes, a boggy center with a yellow or white head on the skin surface may be noted.
4. A **carbuncle** is marked by skin abscess along with systemic symptoms, such as fever, pain, prostration, and leukocytosis.

D. Nursing management

1. **Administer medications,** which may include systemic or topical antibiotics. (See *Drug chart 12-1,* pages 313 and 314.) Soak and wash lesions with mild soap solution to remove the central site of bacterial growth before applying topical antibiotics.
2. **Prevent infection and infection transmission.** (See section II.D.4.)
   a. Instruct the client not to squeeze a boil or pimple; the protective wall of induration that localizes the infection should not rupture or be destroyed.
   b. Instruct the client to bathe at least daily with bactericidal soap.

    c. Inform clients and families that impetigo is a contagious disease. Cleanliness is a priority. Encourage the use of separate towels for family members.

    d. Isolate drainage in severe cases of folliculitis, furuncles, or carbuncles. Cover the mattress and pillow with plastic material.

3. Promote comfort measures.

    a. I.V. fluids, fever sponges, and other supportive treatments are indicated for clients who are very ill or suffering with toxicity.

    b. Apply warm, moist compresses to increase vascularization and help with resolution of the furuncle or carbuncle.

4. Provide client and family teaching. (See section II.D.6; also see *Client and family teaching 12-1*, page 311.)

VII. FUNGAL SKIN DISEASES

A. Description and etiology. The most common fungal (mycotic) skin disorder is tinea.

  1. **Tinea pedis** is a fungal infection of feet known as athlete's foot, especially in those who use communal showers or swimming pools.

  2. **Tinea corporis** is a fungal infection that affects the face, neck, trunk, and extremities. Animal varieties (nonhuman varieties) cause an intense inflammatory reaction; these may be transmitted through contact with pets or pet objects.

  3. **Tinea capitis** is ringworm of the scalp and is a contagious fungal infection of the hair shafts and a common cause of hair loss.

  4. **Tinea cruris** is fungal infection of the groin, which may extend to the inner thighs and buttock area, also known as "jock itch." It most frequently occurs in young joggers, obese people, and those who wear tight underclothing.

  5. **Tinea unguium (i.e., onychomycosis)** is a chronic fungal infection of the toenails and less commonly of the fingernails. Usually caused by *Trichophyton* species or *Candida albicans*, it may represent lifetime fungal infection of the feet.

B. Pathophysiology. The fungal infections are caused by fungi, tiny representatives of the plant kingdom that feed on organic matter. They affect only the skin and its appendages in these skin disorders.

C. Assessment findings

  1. **Clinical manifestations** depend on the specific infection.

    a. **Tinea pedis** may appear as an acute (i.e., inflamed vesicles) or chronic (i.e., scaly, dusky, or red rash) infection on the soles of the feet or between the toes with client complaints of pruritus.

    b. **Tinea corporis** begins with erythematous macules advancing to rings of vesicles with central clearing; the lesions are found in clusters on the scalp, hair, or nails.

    c. **Tinea capitis** characteristically results in red, scaling patches in the scalp; small pustules or papules may be seen at the edges of the patches. Hair becomes brittle and breaks easily at the scalp.

    d. **Tinea cruris** manifests with small, red, scaly patches extending to circular plaques with elevated scaly or vesicular borders; clients complain of itching.

    e. In **tinea unguium,** the nails become thickened, friable (i.e., easily crumbled), and lusterless. Debris accumulates under the free edge of the nail and, ultimately, the nail plate separates. The entire nail may be destroyed.

2. **Laboratory and diagnostic study findings**
   a. Skin culture and sensitivity testing identify the causative organism.
   b. Under Wood's light, the infected hair appears fluorescent, which aids in diagnosing tinea capitis.

D. Nursing management (See section II.D.)
   1. **Provide general nursing care for fungal skin diseases,** which focuses on enhancing skin integrity, providing pain relief, preventing infection, and providing client and family teaching.
   2. **Provide nursing care for the client with tinea pedis.**
      a. Administer fungal foot sprays.
      b. Teach the client to keep his feet as dry as possible, including the area between the toes.
         – Small pieces of cotton can be placed between the toes at night to absorb moisture.
         – Socks should be made of absorbent white cotton, and hosiery should have cotton feet, because synthetic material does not absorb perspiration as well as cotton.
         – Instruct the client to apply talcum powder or antifungal powder twice daily.
         – Instruct the client to alternate shoes so they can dry completely before being worn again.
   3. **Provide nursing care for the client with tinea corporis.**
      a. Administer prescribed medications, which may include topical antifungal medication. (See *Drug chart 12-1,* pages 313 and 314.)
      b. Instruct the client to use a clean towel and washcloth daily.
      c. Instruct the client to thoroughly dry all skin areas and skin folds that retain moisture.
      d. Encourage the client to wear clean cotton clothing next to the skin.
      e. Instruct the client to be careful around pets and pet objects.
   4. **Provide nursing care for the client with tinea capitis.**
      a. Administer prescribed medications, including griseofulvin, an antifungal agent. (See *Drug chart 12-1,* pages 313 and 314.) Topical agents do not provide an effective cure because the infection occurs within the hair shaft and below the surface of the scalp.
      b. Instruct the client and his family to use separate combs and brushes and to avoid exchanging hats and other headgear.
      c. Encourage the client that all family members and household pets must be examined, because familial infections are relatively common.
   5. **Provide nursing care for the client with tinea cruris.**
      a. Administer prescribed medications, which may include topical antifungal medication. (See *Drug chart 12-1,* pages 313 and 314.)
      b. Instruct the client to avoid excessive heat and humidity as much as possible, including avoiding wearing nylon underwear, tight-fitting clothes, and wet bathing suits.
      c. Instruct the client to clean, dry, and dust the groin area with a topical antifungal agent.
   6. **Provide nursing care for the client with tinea unguium.**
      a. Administer prescribed medications, including griseofulvin, an antifungal, orally for up to 1 year. (See *Drug chart 12-1,* pages 313 and 314.)
      b. Advise the client that response to medication is poor at best; frequently when the treatment is stopped, the infection returns.

VIII. HERPES ZOSTER

A. **Description.** Herpes zoster (i.e., shingles) is an acute viral infection marked by painful vesicular skin eruptions. The incidence is greatest in adults older than age 50.

B. **Etiology.** Herpes zoster is caused by the varicella-zoster virus, which also causes varicella (chicken pox).

C. **Pathophysiology.** Herpes zoster results from reactivation of latent varicella-zoster virus that has lain dormant since a previous episode of varicella. The cause of reactivation is unknown.

D. **Assessment findings.** Herpes zoster is marked by painful vesicular eruptions along the route of inflamed nerves from one or more posterior ganglia. Eruption is preceded and accompanied by itching and pain, which may radiate over the entire region supplied by involved nerves.

E. **Nursing management**
   1. **Administer prescribed medications,** which include pain medications, topical lotions, and systemic corticosteroids. (See *Drug chart 12-1*, pages 313 and 314.) Acyclovir, an antiviral medication administered systemically, inhibits viral multiplication by affecting deoxyribonucleic acid. Forewarn the client that the drug helps manage disease but does not cure it or prevent it from spreading.
   2. **Prevent infection.** (See section II.D.4.)
   3. **Provide client and family teaching.** Teach the client to apply wet dressings or medication to the lesions. (See section II.D.6; also see *Client and family teaching 12-1*, page 311.)

IX. PARASITIC SKIN DISEASES

A. **Description and etiology**
   1. **Pediculosis,** infestation by lice, involves three different parasites:
      a. Pediculosis humanus capitis (head louse)
      b. Pediculosis humanus corporis (body louse)
      c. Phthirus pubis (pubic or crab louse).
   2. **Scabies** involves infestation by the itch mite, *Sarcoptes scabiei.*

B. **Pathophysiology**
   1. **Pediculosis.** Lice live on the host's skin surface and depend on the host for nourishment, feeding on human blood approximately five times daily. They inject their digestive juices and excrement into the host's skin and lay their eggs (i.e., nits) on hair shafts.
   2. **Scabies.** Adult itch mites burrow into the superficial layer of skin and lay two to three eggs daily for up to 2 months. Eggs hatch in 3 to 4 days; clinical symptoms are related to a sensitivity reaction as larvae emerge to the skin surface.

C. **Assessment findings**
   1. **Pediculosis** is marked by:
      a. itching
      b. excoriation from scratching
      c. possibly small, red papules in infested areas
      d. tiny, gray-white nits on hair shafts

2. **Scabies** is marked by:
   a. severe itching
   b. excoriated lesions possibly appearing as erythematous nodules
   c. possible secondary bacterial infection.

D. Nursing management (See section II.D.)

1. **Provide general nursing care for parasitic skin diseases,** which focuses on enhancing skin integrity, providing pain relief, preventing infection, and providing client and family teaching.
2. **Provide client and family teaching regarding measures to treat pediculosis.** Teach the client with lice (or a parent if the client is a child) to shampoo with lindane and remove nits with a fine-tooth comb.
3. **Provide client and family teaching regarding measures to treat scabies.** Teach the client how to use a scabicide, such as lindane or crotamiton. Explain that the scabicide is directly absorbed by the parasites. Instruct the client to wash scaling debris or crusts with warm, soapy water and dry the area thoroughly before applying medication. Leave the medication on for 12 to 24 hours and then wash thoroughly.
4. **Teach precautions to prevent future infestations.**
   a. Wash all bedding and clothing in hot water and dry it using the hot cycle of the clothes dryer.
   b. Never share hair brushes, combs, or hats.

X. PRESSURE ULCERS

A. Description. Pressure ulcers (i.e., decubitus ulcers, pressure sores) are localized areas of cellular necrosis on the skin and subcutaneous tissue.

B. Etiology

1. Pressure ulcers result from excessive pressure on body areas, particularly over bony prominences.
2. Older adults are especially susceptible because of:
   a. decreased skin thickness
   b. decreased vascularity of dermal layer, which slows tissue repair and healing capacity.
3. Major risk factors include decreased or limited activity, immobility, malnutrition, incontinence, and impaired circulation and sensation.
4. Other risk factors from related conditions may include fever with diaphoresis, radiation therapy, anemia, and dehydration.

C. Pathophysiology

1. Excessive pressure on the skin interrupts normal circulatory function by constricting cutaneous and subcutaneous blood vessels. Impaired circulation leads to tissue anoxia, necrosis, and ulceration.
2. Ulcer severity depends on the intensity and duration of pressure ulcers.

D. Assessment findings

1. **Clinical manifestations** vary according to the stage in which the ulcer is classified. The appearance of purulent drainage or foul odor suggests an infection.
   a. **In stage I,** the reddened area is an area of nonblanchable erythema, tissue edema, and congestion, and the client complains of discomfort.

       b. **In stage II,** the reddened area exhibits a break in the skin through the epidermis or dermis; an abrasion, blister, or shallow crater may be seen.

       c. **In stage III,** the ulcer extends into the subcutaneous tissue; a deep crater with or without undermining of adjacent tissues is noted along with necrotic tissue, eschar, and exudate.

       d. **In stage IV,** the ulcer extends into the underlying structures, including the muscle and possibly the bone.

   2. Laboratory and diagnostic study findings. Wound culture or biopsy may identify infective organisms and guide choice of antimicrobial therapy.

E. **Nursing management.** The focus is *prevention* of pressure ulcers. Nursing neglect is a primary reason for the development of pressure ulcers. (See section II.D.)

   1. Assess the client's risk for pressure ulcers by using assessment tools such as the Braden Scale. The Braden Scale has demonstrated reliability, validity, sensitivity, and specificity in predicting pressure ulcer risk.

   2. Administer prescribed medications, which may include pain medication and antibiotics. (See *Drug chart 12-1,* pages 313 and 314.)

   3. Administer prescribed treatment, which may include hydrophilic powders, beads, or gels. Collaborate with a wound-care specialist.

   4. Relieve pressure.

       a. Turn the client every 2 hours, using the prone position if possible.

       b. Avoid positioning the client on the ulcerated side.

       c. Teach wheelchair push-ups if appropriate.

       d. Use pressure-relieving devices (e.g., convoluted foam mattress, air-fluidized therapy) as necessary.

   5. Prevent skin friction.

       a. Use anatomic pads when necessary.

       b. Use a lift sheet to prevent dragging the client across the bed.

   6. Prevent shearing force on the skin.

       a. Elevate the head of the bed 30 degrees when not contraindicated.

       b. Provide a foot board to prevent sliding down in bed.

       c. Help the client maintain appropriate body position and alignment.

   7. Keep skin clean and dry. If necessary, apply a fecal incontinence bag or external urine collection device.

   8. Do not massage reddened areas because increased tissue damage may result.

   9. Promote wound healing.

       a. Provide pressure relief.

       b. Provide nutritional support.

       c. Perform mechanical debridement with wet-to-dry dressing, if indicated.

       d. Discuss and assist with preparations for surgical debridement, if indicated.

 10. Provide client and family teaching.

       a. Teach measures to help prevent recurrence.

       b. Instruct the client in wound care and infection control measures.

       c. Teach the client about sources of supplies.

 11. Provide referrals to wound-care clinics and home health care agencies.

XI. BURNS

A. **Description and etiology.** Burns are skin injuries resulting from heat, electric current, chemicals, friction, or excessive sunlight exposure. Based on the standard depth of injury classification, burns are first, second, or third degree. The following must be considered when determining depth of burn:
   1. History of how the injury occurred
   2. Causative agent, such as flame or a scalding liquid
   3. Temperature of burning agent
   4. Duration of contact with the agent
   5. Thickness of the skin.

B. **Pathophysiology**
   1. Burns are caused by transfer of energy from a heat source to the body.
   2. Tissue destruction (i.e., skin and mucosa of upper airways) results from coagulation, protein denaturation, or ionization of cellular contents from a thermal, radiation, or chemical source.
   3. Pathophysiologic changes result from major burns during the initial burn-shock period. Changes include tissue hypoperfusion and organ hypofunction secondary to decreased cardiac output, followed by a hyperdynamic and hypermetabolic phase.

C. **Assessment findings.** Clinical manifestations depend on the depth of the burn.
   1. **First-degree (superficial) burns (e.g., sunburn)**
      a. Superficial tissue destruction involving the epidermis only
      b. Local pain and erythema; blisters are absent for about 24 hours
      c. Mild to absent systemic response
      d. Rapid healing (normally 3 to 5 days) without scarring
      e. First-degree burns generally do not require treatment, except in the case of large burns of infants or elderly persons.
   2. **Second-degree (partial-thickness) burns**
      a. Tissue destruction involving the epidermis and part of the dermis
      b. Skin appearing red to pale ivory and moist
      c. Formation of wet, thin-walled blisters immediately after injury
      d. Intact tactile and pain sensors
      e. Healing in 21 to 28 days with variable amount of scarring
   3. **Third-degree (full-thickness) burns**
      a. Tissue destruction involving the epidermis, dermis, and underlying subcutaneous tissue
      b. Injury appearing white, cherry red, or black; the injury may or may not contain deep blisters or visible thrombosed veins
      c. Dry, hard, leathery appearance due to loss of epidermal elasticity
      d. Marked edema and decreased elasticity, which may necessitate escharotomies of circumferential burns within the first few hours after the injury
      e. Painless to touch because of destruction of all superficial nerve endings in skin

D. **Nursing management (See section II.D.)**
   1. **Teach about or provide emergency care at the scene of the burn,** when appropriate.
      a. Eliminate the source of the burn, depending on cause.
         – **Flame.** If clothes are smoldering, wet them using any available water, or smother flames using a blanket, rug, or coat.

- **Scald.** Pour cool liquid over the area, and remove clothing.
- **Chemicals.** Remove clothing from involved areas, and dilute the chemical by flushing the area with copious amounts of water; if eyes are involved, flush each eye with at least 1 L of lactated Ringer's or other solution.
- **Tar, asphalt, or melted plastic.** Cool area by flushing with water. Do not attempt to remove material unless the airway is compromised. (Solvents may be used after initial assessment to soften product and facilitate removal.)
- **Electric current.** Do not touch a person still in contact with an electrical source. If safe, move the person away from the electrical source without touching the source.

b. Cool the burn for several minutes. Do not use ice.

c. Remove restrictive objects.

d. Cover the wound with sterile dressing or a clean, dry cloth.

e. Apply the ABCs of trauma: airway, breathing, circulation.

f. Prevent shock by initiating I.V. fluid therapy immediately.

g. Ensure that the client avoids oral intake and is placed in an upright position to prevent aspiration of vomitus, because nausea and vomiting typically occur as a result of paralytic ileus, which results from the stress of the injury.

h. Transport the client to the nearest emergency medical center. Note the time of the burn (needed for resuscitation).

2. **Assess for and treat smoke-inhalation injury.** Support pulmonary function through early intubation and volume ventilator-assisted respiration with optimal positive end-expiratory pressure, large tidal volume, and the lowest possible inspired oxygen concentration.

3. **Assess for and treat carbon monoxide inhalation.** Administer 100% oxygen, as prescribed, until the arterial blood gas determination demonstrates adequate oxygenation, and perform frequent neurologic assessment until hypoxia resolves.

4. **Provide pain relief.** Assess the client's pain, rule out complications, medicate or intervene as appropriate, institute safety measures (e.g., side rails up, call light within reach), and evaluate the effectiveness of pain medication. Premedicate the client prior to any whirlpool or debriding.

5. **Monitor acid-base balance and electrolyte levels.** Intervene as necessary to correct imbalances.

6. **Take special actions for electrical burns**.
   a. Apply a cervical collar, and place the client on a spinal board as soon as possible. (Severe contractions produced by electrical current passing through the body may injure the spinal cord.)
   b. Monitor for cardiac arrest or arrhythmias for at least 24 hours after the injury.
   c. Assess for and treat myoglobinuria resulting from massive soft-tissue destruction accompanying a major electrical injury. Administer I.V. infusion of lactated Ringer's solution at a rate to maintain urine output (100 ml/hour for adults or 2 ml/kg/hour for children) until urine clears.
   d. Prepare the client for early surgical exploration and wound debridement after cardiovascular stabilization. Debridement is performed every 48 to 72 hours until wound closure is complete.
   e. Prepare the client for amputation, if indicated. Amputation is necessary in more than 90% of electrical injuries because of the extensive damage caused by the electrical current.

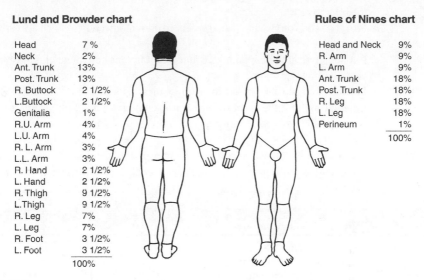

Lund and Browder chart

Head	7 %
Neck	2%
Ant. Trunk	13%
Post. Trunk	13%
R. Buttock	2 1/2%
L.Buttock	2 1/2%
Genitalia	1%
R.U. Arm	4%
L.U. Arm	4%
R. L. Arm	3%
L.L. Arm	3%
R. Hand	2 1/2%
L. Hand	2 1/2%
R. Thigh	9 1/2%
L.Thigh	9 1/2%
R. Leg	7%
L. Leg	7%
R. Foot	3 1/2%
L. Foot	3 1/2%
	100%

Rules of Nines chart

Head and Neck	9%
R. Arm	9%
L. Arm	9%
Ant. Trunk	18%
Post. Trunk	18%
R. Leg	18%
L. Leg	18%
Perineum	1%
	100%

FIGURE 12-2

Two methods of charting burn injuries are known as the Lund and Browder chart and the Rules of Nines chart. These methods assign numerical values to body surface areas. The Rule of Nines assigns values in the amount of nine and multiples of nine. By both methods, the total body surface area totals 100%.

 f. Discuss potential late complications of electrical injury (e.g., corneal cataracts, ataxic gait abnormalities, associated neurologic problems).

7. **Monitor and treat potential complications,** which include acute respiratory failure, distributive shock, acute renal failure, compartment syndrome, paralytic ileus, and a Curling ulcer.

8. **Monitor for and treat burn shock,** which occurs in all clients with a major burn injury. The sequence begins within minutes of injury and leads to death from hypovolemic shock unless treated appropriately.

9. **Estimate the burn size** using the Rule of Nines chart or the Lund and Browder chart. (See *Figure 12-2*.)

10. **Provide appropriate fluid resuscitation, based on the Parkland formula** (4 ml of lactated Ringer's solution × % of total body surface area burned × kg body weight = total fluid requirement for 24 hours postburn). Provide one half of the total administered in the first 8 hours after the burn, one fourth of the total administered in the second 8 hours after the burn, and the last one fourth administered in the third 8 hours after the burn.

11. **Estimate the adequacy of fluid resuscitation** based on urine output of 30 ml/hour. Increase or decrease fluid to maintain hourly urine output.

12. **Provide infection prevention measures.** Clean and debride the wound, and apply topical antimicrobial agents and dressings. Medicate the client 20 to 30 minutes before a dressing change or medication application.

13. **Teach the client about planned skin grafting procedures, as indicated.** Third-degree burns require skin grafting with the client's own skin (i.e., autograft) because all dermal elements have been destroyed and cannot regenerate.

14. **Promote optimum recovery.**

326 INTEGUMENTARY DISORDERS

a. Ensure optimum nutrition. Total parenteral nutrition (TPN) is often administered. (See chapter 21.)

b. Provide meticulous wound management to prevent infection and achieve early wound coverage.

c. Initiate physical therapy to regain and maintain optimal range of motion and prevent contractures.

d. Provide psychosocial support to promote mental health.

e. Carefully monitor the client to detect problems early. Provide appropriate interventions to minimize complications.

f. Provide family-centered care to promote integrity of the family unit as it meets the demands of the rehabilitating burn client over several years.

g. Encourage postdischarge follow-up for several years of reconstructive therapy as needed.

Study questions

1. Which clinical manifestation would lead the nurse to suspect that the client has psoriasis?
1. Profuse, erythematous scales often covering large areas of the body
2. Patchy eruptions with possible hair loss and nail shedding
3. Widespread bullae on the skin and mucous membranes
4. Shedding of large sheets of epidermis along with toenails and eyebrows

2. Which instruction should be included in the teaching plan for the client receiving oral prednisone as treatment for an inflammatory skin disorder?
1. "Take the medication at night to prevent nocturia."
2. "Do not discontinue the medication abruptly."
3. "Notify your health care provider if you lose weight."
4. "Stop taking the medication when the inflammation is gone."

3. Which outcome is expected when evaluating adequate fluid replacement in a burn client based on the Parkland formula for fluid resuscitation?
1. The client received 2 ml/kg body weight × total body surface area (TBSA) burned over the first 24 hours after the burn.

2. The client received 4 ml lactated Ringer's solution × % TBSA burned × kg body weight over the first 24 hours after the burn.

3. The client received 4 ml/kg body weight × % TBSA burned over the first 36 hours after the burn.

4. The client received 1 ml/kg body weight × % TBSA burned over the first 24 hours after the burn.

4. Before debriding a second-degree burn wound on the left lower leg, which intervention should the nurse implement?
1. Applying lindane to the affected area
2. Medicating the client with an opioid analgesic
3. Administering acyclovir I.V.
4. Applying a topical antimicrobial ointment

5. Which nursing intervention should the nurse include to prevent pressure ulcers?
1. Turning the client every 8 hours
2. Avoiding the use of a lift sheet
3. Using pressure-relieving devices
4. Keeping the head of the bed flat

6. Which pressure ulcer stage would the nurse use to document a client's pressure ulcer that extends into the subcutaneous tissue with a deep crater involving some of the adjacent tissue?

1. Stage I
2. Stage II
3. Stage III
4. Stage IV

7. Which instruction should be included when completing discharge teaching for a client with a skin disorder?
1. "Maintain a warm environment."
2. "Use sunscreen with a sun-protection factor (SPF) of less than 10."
3. "Wash with mild soap."
4. "Follow a high-carbohydrate diet."

8. A client asks the nurse, "What is toxic epidermal necrolysis?" Which is the nurse's *best* response?
4. "A rare, potentially fatal skin disorder causing reddened, dead, eroded skin."
2. "An autoimmune disease that causes blisters on the skin and mucous membranes."
3. "An inflammatory condition affecting the sebaceous follicles."
4. "An acute viral infection that causes markedly painful skin eruptions."

9. A client with acne vulgaris says, "I try to keep my skin clean. I scrub my face every night, but the blackheads will not go away." Which would be the nurse's best response?
1. "Why do you scrub you face?"
2. "You need a stronger soap when you scrub."
3. "You want the blackheads to go away."
4. "Uncleanliness is not the problem with acne."

10. Which would the health care provider suspect after noticing a loosely adherent, honey-yellow colored lesion around the client's nose?
1. Impetigo
2. Folliculitis
3. Furuncle
4. Carbuncle

11. When evaluating the effectiveness of client teaching about health promotion and maintenance behaviors regarding skin care, which action demonstrates that the client understood the teaching?
1. The client stays unprotected in the sun between 12 p.m. and 4 p.m.
2. The client avoids repeated exposure to irritants and allergens.
3. The client is exposed to repeated low-dose radiation.
4. The client avoids excessive sun exposure if he is middle-aged.

12. Which instruction would be appropriate for a client diagnosed with tinea pedis?
1. "Wear white cotton socks."
2. "Use your own comb or brush."
3. "Use a clean towel and washcloth daily."
4. "Avoid wearing tight-fitting clothing."

13. At the scene of a burn injury, which intervention is the *first* priority in treating a client who has sustained a partial-thickness burn to the left hand?
1. Applying ice packs to the burned area
2. Applying petroleum jelly to the burned area
3. Immersing the client's left hand in cool water
4. Immediately taking the client to the emergency department

14. Which would be the nurse's best response when the client asks, "What does it mean if I have a first-degree burn?"
1. "You have destroyed your dermis and epidermis."
2. "You have destroyed your skin and the underlying subcutaneous tissue."
3. "You have superficial tissue destruction involving the epidermis only."
4. "You will probably have some scarring after healing occurs."

15. An 84-year old client who had a motor vehicle accident is on strict bedrest. Which interventions should the nurse implement? (Select all that apply.)

1. Keeping the client in the prone position as much as possible
2. Turning, coughing, and having the client deep-breathe every two hours
3. Decreasing the client's fluid intake to 1000 ml/day
4. Assessing the client's skin, especially boney prominences, every shift
5. Massaging any reddened areas found on the client.
6. Performing active and passive range-of-motion (ROM) exercises to extremities

16. Which nursing intervention would be appropriate for a client who has had an electrical burn?
    1. Monitoring the client for arrhythmias for at least 24 hours
    2. Flushing the burned area with copious amounts of cool water
    3. Supporting pulmonary function through early intubation
    4. Administering 100% oxygen based on arterial blood gas (ABG) results

Answer key

1. The answer is **1.**
Psoriasis is marked by profuse, erythematous scales or plaques, often covering large areas of the body. The client also may complain of pruritus, pain, and possibly of arthritic symptoms such as joint stiffness. Patchy eruptions with possible hair loss and nail shedding are associated with exfoliative dermatitis. Widespread bullae on the skin and mucous membranes generally indicate pemphigus vulgaris. Shedding of large sheets of epidermis along with toenails and eyebrows suggest toxic epidermal necrolysis.

2. The answer is **2.**
Prednisone is a systemic corticosteroid. If stopped abruptly, adrenal insufficiency may result and lead to shock and death. Dosage must be tapered gradually. Prednisone does not cause increased urination or weight loss. Adverse effects include moon face, weight gain, and other cushingoid effects. The dosage must be decreased gradually, not stopped when inflammation is resolved.

3. The answer is **2.**
An appropriate outcome when using the Parkland formula for fluid resuscitation is based on this formula: 4 ml of lactated Ringer's solution $\times$ % TBSA burned $\times$ kg body weight = total fluid requirement for 24

hours after the burn. One half of total is given in the first 8 hours after the burn, one fourth of total given in second 8 hours after the burn, and the last one fourth given in the third 8 hours after the burn. One or 2 ml/kg of body weight would be inadequate. All three parameters must be addressed — kilograms of body weight, percent of TBSA burned, and the first 24 hours — to evaluate the adequacy of fluid resuscitation.

4. The answer is **2.**
Debridement and dressing changes are very painful for the client with a burn wound. The nurse should medicate the client before the procedure. Lindane is the treatment of choice for lice. Acyclovir is the treatment of choice for herpes zoster (i.e., shingles). A topical antimicrobial is appropriate after debridement, not before treatment.

5. The answer is **3.**
Pressure on the skin can be minimized by using pressure-relieving devices, such as convoluted foam mattresses and air-fluidized therapeutic devices. The client should be turned at least every 2 hours. A lift sheet should be used when moving a client to prevent dragging the client across the bed and causing skin breakdown or raw areas. The head of the bed should be elevated 30 degrees

to prevent a shearing force on the skin (unless contraindicated by the pathologic condition).

6. The answer is **3.**
An ulcer that extends into the subcutaneous tissue with a deep crater involving some of the adjacent tissue describes a stage III ulcer. Stage I describes a reddened area of nonblanchable erythema, stage II describes a reddened area exhibiting a break in the skin through the epidermis or dermis, and a stage IV ulcer extends into the underlying structures, including the muscle and possible the bone.

7. The answer is **3.**
Mild soaps or soaps made for sensitive skin should be used because these contain no detergents, dyes, or hardening agents that can further irritate the skin. A cool environment, not warm, should be maintained to deter itching. A sunscreen with an SPF of 30 or above should be used. A healthy, well-balanced diet should be encouraged.

8. The answer is **1.**
Toxic epidermal necrolysis is a rare, potentially fatal skin disorder marked by epidermal erythema, necrosis, and skin erosions. Pemphigus vulgaris is an autoimmune disease that causes blisters on the skin and mucous membranes. Acne vulgaris is an inflammatory condition that affects the sebaceous follicles. Herpes zoster is an acute viral infection that causes painful skin eruptions.

9. The answer is **4.**
The client's statement reflects a lack of knowledge about acne. The nurse's best response provides information. The client needs to be informed that acne is not caused by dirt or uncleanliness and that he should avoid scrubbing the face constantly. The nurse should not ask "Why?" of the client. "Why?" questions may be interpreted as accusatory and block further communication and instruction. The client with acne should use a mild soap. Asking the client whether he wants the blackheads to go away may be more appropriate after the information is provided. This question may help elicit additional information about the client's feelings of self-esteem and body image.

10. The answer is **1.**
The appearance of a loosely adherent, honey-yellow colored lesion indicates impetigo, a superficial skin infection caused by streptococci, staphylococci, or multiple bacteria. Folliculitis produces papules or pustules close to hair follicles. A furuncle is a boil. A carbuncle is an abscess of the skin and subcutaneous tissue representing an extension of a furuncle.

11. The answer is **2.**
Avoidance of exposure to irritants and allergens is recommended to prevent skin cancer and other skin disorders. It is recommended that individuals of all ages, not just those who are middle-aged, have protection against the sun and that they avoid exposure to the sun during the time when the sun is strong, if possible. Any radiation (high or low) should be avoided.

12. The answer is **1.**
Tinea pedis is athlete's foot. White cotton socks help with this condition because synthetic material does not absorb perspiration as well as cotton. Using his or her own comb or brush is appropriate for tinea capitis (i.e., ringworm of the scalp); using a clean towel and washcloth daily is appropriate if the client has tinea corporis (i.e., ringworm of the body). Tight fitting clothing should be avoided if the client has tinea cruris (i.e., jock itch).

13. The answer is **3.**
Immersing the left hand in cool water gives immediate and striking relief from pain, retards the burning process, and restricts local tissue edema and damage. Ice may worsen the tissue damage and lead to hypothermia in clients with large burns. Petroleum

jelly, ointments, and salves should not be used; they may cause further damage. The burn must be treated immediately to stop the burning process; then the client may be taken to the emergency department.

14. The answer is **3.**
The nurse's best response is to explain that a first-degree burn is a superficial burn. Characteristics of a first-degree burn (i.e., sunburn) include superficial tissue destruction involving the epidermis only; local pain and erythema; blisters absent for about 24 hours; mild to absent systemic response; and rapid healing, usually over 3 to 5 days. Destruction of the dermis and epidermis occurs with a second-degree (partial-thickness) burn. Destruction of the skin and underlying subcutaneous tissue and scarring after healing characterize a third-degree (full-thickness) burn.

15. The answers are **2, 4, 6.**
The client on strict bedrest is at risk for developing pressure sores and other complications of immobility, therefore the nurse should turn, cough, and have the patient deep-breathe to prevent pneumonia and pressures sores, should assess the skin for signs of skin breakdown, and perform ROM exercises. Keeping the client prone will not prevent complications of immobility. The client should increase fluid intake to prevent pneumonia and constipation. Reddened areas should not be massaged because massage can cause skin breakdown.

16. The answer is **1.**
With an electrical burn, the electrical current passes through the client's body, possibly altering the electrical conduction system of the heart. The client is at risk for arrhythmias and requires close monitoring for the first 24 hours. Flushing the area would be appropriate for a burn resulting from tar, asphalt, or melted plastic. Supporting pulmonary function with early intubation is appropriate for a client who has experienced smoke inhalation. Administering 100% oxygen based on ABG results is appropriate for a client with carbon monoxide inhalation.

13 *Neurologic disorders*

I. STRUCTURE AND FUNCTION OF THE NERVOUS SYSTEM

The nervous system may be categorized according to structure or function. Structurally, the nervous system is divided into the central nervous system (i.e., brain and spinal cord) and the peripheral nervous system (i.e., cranial and spinal nerves). Functional divisions include the somatic (voluntary) and visceral (involuntary) nervous systems. This chapter is organized according to structural classifications.

A. **Central nervous system, cranial**

  1. **Structures**

     a. **Protective structures**

        - **Cranium and meninges.** The brain is enclosed within the bones of the cranium and covered by three meningeal layers: dura mater (outer), arachnoid mater, and pia mater (inner).
        - **Cerebrospinal fluid (CSF)**
          - CSF is a clear liquid that circulates in the subarachnoid space.
          - CSF is manufactured in the choroid plexus of the ventricular system. Ventricular structures include the lateral, third, and fourth ventricles; the aqueduct of Sylvius; and the foramina of Luschka and Magendie.
          - Between 500 and 700 ml of CSF is manufactured daily, but only 150 ml is circulating at any one time. Excess CSF is absorbed through the arachnoid villi into the venous system.

     b. **The brain.** Categorized into four distinct areas, the brain includes the cerebrum, cerebellum, brain stem, and diencephalon.

        - The **cerebrum** is divided into left and right hemispheres by the falx, an indentation of the dura.
          - The **lobes,** contained within each cerebral hemisphere, are described as frontal, temporal, parietal, and occipital. (See *Figure 13-1.*)
          - The **cortex** contains the outer nervous tissue (i.e., gray matter) of the cerebrum. The basal ganglia, four masses of gray matter located deep in the cerebral hemisphere, encompass the caudate nucleus, putamen, globus pallidus, and substantia nigra.
        - The **cerebellum** is divided into left and right hemispheres, which are connected by the vermis. It is located in the posterior fossa and is separated from the cerebral hemispheres by a fold of dura mater, the tentorium cerebelli.
        - The **brain stem** is divided into the medulla oblongata, pons, and midbrain. It is located in the posterior fossa. Extending for the entire length of the brain stem is a diffuse mass of gray matter called the reticular formation.
        - The **diencephalon** includes the thalamus, located on either side of the third ventricle; hypothalamus, located anterior and inferior to the thalamus; and pituitary gland, located beneath the brain in the pituitary fossa of the sphenoid bone.
        - **Supratentorial structures** (i.e., cerebral hemispheres and the diencephalon) are above the tentorium and infratentorial structures (i.e., pons, cerebellum, and medulla) and lie below the tentorium. The tentorium acts as a hammock, supporting the occipital lobes above the cerebellum. It forms a tough septum that divides the cranial cavity.
        - **Vascular supply** to the brain is provided from the basilar artery, formed from the union of two vertebral arteries, and the internal carotids. These two systems join to form the circle of Willis.

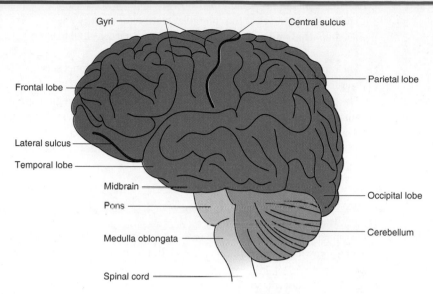

FIGURE 13-1
View of the external surface of the brain showing the lobes and key parts

2. **Function**
   a. **Protective structures**
   - **The cranium and meninges** protect the brain from injury and infection.
   - **The tentorium** helps stabilize cranial structures within the skull.
   - **CSF** forms a watery cushion, which protects the fragile nervous tissue from blows and other trauma, carries nutrients to cells, and transports waste from cells.
   b. **Brain**
   - **Cerebrum**
     - **Frontal lobe.** The prerolandic area of the frontal lobe is the brain's center of foresight, abstract thinking, and judgment. The postrolandic area controls voluntary motor movements.
     - The **temporal lobe** is the center of memory and contains visual and auditory association areas.
     - The **parietal lobe** controls sensory functions, such as recognition of pain, temperature, and pressure and perception of body and limb position.
     - The **occipital lobe** is the center of visual function.
     - The **limbic lobe** is the center of emotions, drives, and basic survival functions.
   - The **cerebellum** is involved in coordination of muscle movements and maintenance of equilibrium and muscle tone.
   - **Brain stem**
     - The **medulla oblongata** contains several vital centers, including those for respiration, heart rate, vomiting, and hiccuping.
     - In the **pons,** the pneumotaxic system controls respiratory patterns.
     - The **mid-brain** contains nuclei that are reflex centers involved in vision and hearing.
     - The **reticular activating system** (RAS) maintains alertness and sleep-wake cycles.

- **The diencephalon**
  - The **thalamus** serves as the chief relay station for sensory fibers.
  - The **hypothalamus** helps regulate body temperature, fluid balance, and some endocrine functions.
  - The **pituitary gland** is the chief regulator of endocrine functions.
- **Vascular supply**
  - The brain uses about 20% of total cardiac output. An **autoregulation mechanism** maintains blood flow to the brain despite changes in systemic pressure. Trauma can disrupt this mechanism.
  - The **blood-brain barrier** prevents many toxic substances in the blood stream from entering the brain.

B. Central nervous system, spinal
  1. Structure
     a. **Protective coverings**
       - The spinal cord is encased within the vertebral column, which consists of 31 vertebrae in cervical, thoracic, lumbar, sacral, and coccygeal segments. (See *Figure 13-2.*)
       - The cervical, thoracic, and lumbar vertebrae are separated by disks. The disk's outer covering is called the annulus; the inner part is the nucleus pulposus.
       - Like the brain, the spinal cord is covered by meninges and surrounded by CSF.
     b. The **spinal cord and brain stem** form a continuous structure extending from the cerebral hemispheres and serve as a connection between the brain and the periphery.
       - **Major descending tracts** in the spinal cord include the lateral corticospinal (pyramidal) tract, the posterior tract, and the spinothalamic tract.
       - **Major ascending tracts** include the lateral spinothalamic and ventral spinothalamic tracts and the posterior columns. Fibers of the lateral spinothalamic tract cross in the brain stem.
       - The **gray matter** (looks like the letter "H") consists of two dorsal (posterior) horns and two ventral (anterior) horns; it surrounds the central canal of the cord.
       - The **white matter,** composed of myelinated fiber tracts, is located on each side of the cord and is divided into three regions: the posterior, lateral, and anterior columns.
       - **Vascular supply** is provided from the radicular arteries and posterior and anterior spinal arteries.
  2. Function
     a. **Protective covering**
       - The vertebral column protects the cord and helps maintain an upright body position.
       - The three connective tissue membranes covering and protecting the central nervous system structures are meninges.
         - The dura mater is the outermost layer.
         - The arachnoid mater is the middle meningeal layer.
         - The pia mater clings tightly to the surface of the brain and spinal cord.
     b. **Spinal cord**
       - **Spinal tracts**
         - The **lateral corticospinal tract** transmits impulses controlling voluntary motor movement (i.e., conducts motor impulses to the anterior horn cells from the opposite side of the brain).

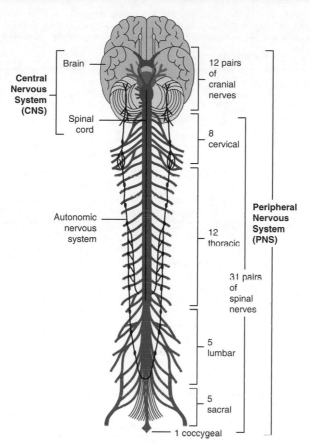

FIGURE 13-2
Parts of the nervous system, including the spinal cord and spinal nerves

- The **posterior tract** conducts sensation, principally the perception of touch, pressure, vibration, position, and passive motion from the same side of the body; these fibers cross to the opposite side in the medulla oblongata.
- The **spinothalamic tract** transmits pain and temperature impulses to the thalamus and cortex; these fibers cross to the opposite side immediately after entering the spinal cord.

C. Peripheral nervous system: Structure and function

1. **Cranial nerves.** The peripheral nervous system contains 12 pairs of cranial nerves, which control various functions. (See *Table 13-1,* page 336.) The nuclei of many cranial nerves are located in the brain stem. (See *Figure 13-2.*)
2. **Spinal nerves.** The peripheral nervous system contains 33 pairs of spinal nerves exiting through vertebral foramina, which control various functions. There are 8 cervical, 12 thoracic, 5 lumbar, 5 sacral, and 4 or 5 coccygeal segments. (See *Figure 13-2.*)

TABLE 13-1
Cranial nerves

Cranial nerve	Function
Olfactory (I)	Sense of smell
Optic (II)	Visual acuity
Occulomotor (III)	Regulation of eye movements
Trochlear (IV)	Regulation of eye movements
Trigeminal (V)	Facial sensation, corneal reflex, mastication
Abducens (VI)	Regulation of eye movements
Facial (VII)	Facial muscle movement, facial expression, tear and saliva secretion
Vestibulocochlear (VIII)	Hearing and equilibrium
Glossopharyngeal (IX)	Taste: posterior third of tongue
Vagus (X)	Pharyngeal contraction; movement of vocal cords, soft palate; movement and secretion of thoracic and abdominal viscera
Spinal accessory (XI)	Movement of sternocleidomastoid and trapezius muscles
Hypoglossal (XII)	Movement of tongue

    a. **Roots.** Each spinal nerve is attached to the spinal cord by dorsal or ventral roots.
       – **Dorsal roots** are formed by sensory (afferent) fibers. These nerve fibers transmit impulses from the periphery toward the central nervous system.
       – **Ventral roots** are formed by the two types of motor (efferent) fibers.
         - **Somatic fibers** terminate in skeletal muscle.
         - **Autonomic fibers** innervate cardiac smooth muscle and glands.
3. **Neurons** are highly specialized nerve cells that transmit messages (i.e., nerve pulses) from one part of the body to another. Each muscle fiber is under voluntary control through a combination of two nerve cells: the upper and lower motor neurons.
    a. The **upper motor neuron,** located in the motor cortex, is formed by the motor pathways from the brain to the spinal cord as well as from the cerebrum to the brain stem.
    b. The **lower motor neuron,** located in the anterior horn of the spinal cord, receives the impulse in the posterior part of the cord and runs to the myoneural junction that terminates in the muscle.
    c. **Dendrites** are neuron processes that conduct impulses toward the cell body.
    d. **Axons** are neuron processes that transmit nerve impulses away from the cell body and synapse in an axonal terminal where neurotransmitters are released into the extracellular space. A myelin sheath protects and insulates the fibers and increases the transmission rate of the nerve impulses.
    e. **Reflex arcs** are rapid, predictable, and involuntary responses to stimuli. Autonomic reflexes regulate activity of smooth muscle, such as heart rate, pupillary reflex, digestion, elimination, and sweating. Somatic reflexes include all reflexes that stimulate the skeletal muscles, such as pulling your foot off a tack.

II. THE NERVOUS SYSTEM

A. Assessment

1. **Health history**

   a. **Explore the client's health history for risk factors** associated with neurologic disease, including unsafe behavior (e.g., driving too fast, driving while drinking, diving into unknown waters), atherosclerosis, and family history.

   b. **Elicit a description of the client's present illness and chief complaint,** including onset, course, duration, location, and precipitating and alleviating factors. Cardinal signs and symptoms indicating altered neurologic function include altered level of consciousness (LOC), lethargy, restlessness, and confusion.

2. **Physical examination**

   a. **Overview**

      – Neurologic assessment involves assessing neurologic system intactness, with particular emphasis on sensation, motor ability (including coordination), alertness, and cognition. Neurologic assessment also should include assessment of pupils, reflexes, vital signs, and respiratory pattern.

      – Various assessment tools (e.g., Glasgow Coma Scale) may be used to assess the client's LOC. (See *Figure 13-3*, page 338.)

      – In the presence of specific disorders or nursing diagnoses, additional assessments or more in-depth assessment of specific areas may be done. The acuity of the client's condition determines the necessary frequency of neurologic checks.

   b. **Sensory function**

      – With the client blindfolded, touch all levels of each extremity, and ask him to identify the different pressure points.

      – Ask the client if he feels numbness, tingling, or other abnormal sensations.

      – Assess whether the client with decreased arousal moves the extremities in response to pressure or more intense stimuli.

      – Evaluate each extremity, and note any deficits.

   c. **Motor function**

      – Ask the client to grasp your hands and to push against his palms with his feet.

      – Evaluate muscle strength.

      – Have the client lift each arm and foot.

      – Evaluate the client's ability to walk. Assess posture, gait, and coordination.

      – To assess fine motor coordination, have the client touch your fingertip and then his own nose.

      – In a client with decreased arousal, assess movement in response to pressure or more intense stimuli.

   d. **Alertness** (level of arousal and orientation)

      – Speak the client's name. If he does not respond, speak louder, shake him, and finally apply a slightly painful stimulus. Notice whether he opens his eyes or responds verbally.

      – Ask a responsive client to state his name, the place, and the date, along with other questions that can provide data on the level of orientation.

   e. **Cognition** (including judgment)

      – Determine whether the client can follow commands.

      – Ask questions to evaluate memory (recent and past).

FIGURE 13-3
The Glasgow Coma Scale

The Glasgow Coma Scale is the standard for evaluating level of consciousness. In clients unable to respond verbally because of tracheal intubation, the score would contain a T rather than a numeral. In clients with eyes closed by edema, the score would be noted by a C.

Action	Response	SCORE
Eyes open	Spontaneously	4
	To speech	3
	To pain	2
	No response	1
Best verbal response	Oriented	5
	Confused	4
	Inappropriate words	3
	Incomprehensible words	2
	No response	1
Best motor response	Obeys commands	6
	Localized pain	5
	Flexion withdrawal	4
	Abnormal flexion	3
	Abnormal extension	2
	Flaccid	1
	Total	

   – Determine the client's ability to calculate simple numeric problems.
   f. **Pupils.** Evaluate pupil size and response to light, along with equality of response.
   g. **Reflexes**
   – Determine the presence or absence of the corneal and gag reflexes.
   – Assess such common reflexes as biceps, brachioradialis, triceps, patellar, and ankle reflexes. Reflexes are graded as 4+ (hyperactive with sustained clonus), 3+ (hyperactive), 2+ (normal), 1+ (hypoactive), and 0 (absent).
3. **Laboratory and diagnostic studies**
   a. **Magnetic resonance imaging** uses a powerful magnetic field to obtain images of different areas of the body that are used to identify cerebral abnormalities.
   b. **Computed tomography** provides cross-sectional views of the brain and helps to identify pathologies, such as tumors, hematomas, and edema.

     c. **Angiography** is an X-ray study of the cerebral circulation after a contrast agent has been injected into a selected artery that allows visualization of vascular problems, tumors, and hematomas.

     d. **Electroencephalography** evaluates the brain's electrical activity (i.e., alpha, beta, theta, and delta waves). It is used primarily in the diagnosis of epilepsy and brain death.

     e. **Ventriculography** demonstrates the ventricular system by injection of contrast media (usually air) directly into a ventricle. It is used when infratentorial lesions are suspected.

     f. **Lumbar puncture** involves inserting a needle into the subarachnoid space to obtain data on cerebrospinal fluid (CSF), CSF pressure, and possible infection.

     g. **CSF analysis** should reveal clear CSF, which contains 15 to 45 mg of protein per 100 ml, 50 to 80 mg glucose per 100 ml, and no red blood cells and has a specific gravity of 1.007.

     h. **Myelography** involves radiography after injection of a possibly irritating contrast medium into the spinal column to detect tumors, disk abnormalities, or other spinal cord problems.

     i. **Intracranial pressure (ICP) monitoring** involves inserting a catheter into the cranium to measure pressure within the lateral ventricle, the subarachnoid space, and the epidural space.

B. Nursing diagnoses

1. Ineffective cerebral tissue perfusion
2. Acute or chronic pain
3. Ineffective airway clearance
4. Disturbed thought process
5. Risk for injury
6. Risk for infection
7. Impaired physical mobility
8. Feeding, dressing or grooming, bathing or hygiene self-care deficit
9. Impaired verbal communication
10. Deficient knowledge
11. Disturbed body image
12. Ineffective coping

C. Planning and outcome identification. The major goals for the client diagnosed with a neurologic disorder include achievement of neurologic homeostasis to improve cerebral tissue perfusion; pain relief; maintenance of normal ventilation and gas exchange; improvement of thought processes; prevention of injury, infection, and complications of immobility; ability to perform self-care activities; achievement of some sort of communication; understanding of disease process and treatment; and improved body image and coping.

D. Implementation

1. **Promote measures to ensure adequate tissue perfusion.**

     a. Complete a neurologic assessment on the client every 2 hours, including the Glasgow Coma Scale. (See *Figure 13-3.*)

     b. Monitor vital signs closely and frequently.

     c. Keep the head of the bed elevated at least 30 degrees.

2. **Provide pain relief.** Assess the client's pain, rule out complications, medicate or intervene as appropriate, institute safety measures (e.g., side rails up, call light within reach), and evaluate the effectiveness of pain medication.

3. **Promote measures to maintain adequate airway.** Encourage the client to turn, cough, and deep-breath frequently; use incentive spirometry. Assess the adequacy of alveolar ventilation by taking frequent measurements of the respiratory rate, vital capacity, and inspiratory force.

4. **Enhance the client's thought process.** Encourage activities directed at redeveloping the client's ability to solve problems and meet basic needs.

5. **Promote measures to prevent injury.**
   a. Assess neurologic status for signs of ICP.
   b. Institute measures for seizure activity per facility protocol.
   c. Promote measures that keep the client calm and quiet, and avoid using restraints at all costs.
   d. Assess the client's ability to swallow, and take precautions to prevent aspiration.

6. **Protect the client from infection.** Monitor the client's vital signs, assess for signs and symptoms of infection, and monitor the white blood cell count.

7. **Prevent complications of immobility.**
   a. Maintain skin integrity by turning the client on a regular schedule; protect pressure points as needed, changing moist or wet linens immediately and lifting (not pulling) the client when changing his position in bed.
   b. Provide passive range-of-motion exercises to prevent contractures from prolonged immobility. (See *Client and family teaching 13-1.*)

8. **Promote self-care.**
   a. Assist the client with activities of daily living (ADLs).
   b. Collaborate with other health care members to maintain the client's independence and ability to perform ADLs.

9. **Maximize effective communication.**
   a. Assess the client and his family to identify ways for the client to communicate effectively.
   b. Listen closely to the client.
   c. Allow the client time to communicate needs.
   d. Have the client blink or wiggle his fingers for yes and no questions or allow other gestures.
   e. Use a communication board or pictures.
   f. Encourage lip reading.
   g. Give simple commands with gestures, such as pointing to objects.
   h. Eliminate extraneous stimuli when communicating (e.g., turn off the television).
   i. Anticipate the client's needs during an acute exacerbation.

10. **Provide client and family teaching.** Provide explanations for the cause, treatment, and expected course of the neurologic disorder.

11. **Promote measures to enhance body image.** Encourage the client to verbalize feelings about body image and self-concept changes.

12. **Promote client and family coping.** Encourage the client and family to verbalize feelings and refer to appropriate resources as needed.

E. **Outcome evaluation**
1. The client has adequate cerebral tissue perfusion as evidenced by being alert and oriented, follows verbal commands, and answers questions correctly.
2. The client reports reduced pain; facial expression and body movements reflect increased comfort.
3. The client demonstrates absence of lung infections or infiltrates.
4. The client demonstrates improvement in cognitive functioning and problem solving.

CLIENT AND FAMILY TEACHING 13-1
Range-of-motion exercises

- Instruct the client to perform range-of-motion (ROM) exercises at least four times each day, moving the joint through its range of motion at least three times.
- The client and his family should be taught how to perform ROM exercises so that exercises can be continued at home or be performed more often in the facility. It will also make the family feel useful and helpful in the care of their loved one.
- Encourage the client to perform active (client completes independently) ROM exercises, but discuss assisted (the client receives help from another person) and passive (another person does the exercise for the client) ROM exercises.
- Instruct the client or his family that the joint to be exercised is supported, the bones above the joint are stabilized, and the body part distal to the joint is moved through the joint's ROM.
- Instruct the client or his family that the joint should not be moved beyond its free ROM and should be stopped at the point of pain.

- Have a return demonstration to ensure that exercises are done correctly:
  – Move each arm from the side of the body to above the head and back down to the side of the body.
  – Move each arm forward and upward until it is alongside the head.
  – Bend both wrists so that the palms are toward the forearms.
  – Extend and flex each finger.
  – Move the leg outward from the body as far as possible and then return it to the normal position.
  – Bend the hip by moving the leg as far forward as possible; the knee should be toward the head.
  – Straighten the leg and then raise the leg off the bed.
- Instruct the client to be in a comfortable position on a firm mattress in the supine position.
- Explain the importance of these exercises in preventing contractures in clients with neurologic deficits or prolonged bed rest.

5. The client exhibits no signs or symptoms of increased ICP.
6. The client does not have accidents and remains injury free.
7. The client is afebrile and has no signs or symptoms of local or systemic infection.
8. The client does not develop complications from immobility; skin remains intact, and no deep vein thrombosis, respiratory problems, or contractures occur.
9. The client demonstrates the ability to perform ADLs to the maximum of his functional capacity.
10. The client is able to effectively communicate physical and emotional needs to family members, significant others, and health care providers.
11. The client's family verbalizes understanding of the client's condition and demonstrate the willingness and ability to assist him in functioning at his optimal level.
12. The client acknowledges his entire body and shows no evidence of unilateral neglect.
13. The client and his family demonstrate a positive attitude and coping mechanisms.

III. INCREASED INTRACRANIAL PRESSURE

A. **Description.** Increased intracranial pressure (ICP) is the result of the amount of brain tissue, intracranial blood volume, and cerebrospinal fluid (CSF) within the skull at any time. Normal ICP depends on the position of the client and is 15 mm Hg or less. Increased intracranial pressure is more than 15 mm Hg.

B. **Etiology.** ICP may increase in cases of head injury, stroke, inflammatory lesions, brain tumor, or intracranial surgery. Any type of injury to the head may lead to increased ICP.

C. **Pathophysiology**

1. The only three things in the skull are brain tissue, blood, and CSF. If any abnormality (e.g., edema from trauma, brain tumor) occurs in the adult skull (i.e., closed cavity), there is no room for expansion, which results in neurologic deficits because of the increased

pressure in the closed cavity. The body compensates for this increased pressure or decompensates.

2. Compensatory mechanisms for maintaining ICP within normal limits include:
   a. increased CSF absorption
   b. shunting of blood to the spinal subarachnoid space
   c. decreased CSF production.

3. Failure of these compensatory mechanisms results in decompensation with the following sequence of events:
   a. Decreased cerebral blood flow with inadequate perfusion
   b. Increased partial pressure of carbon dioxide and decreased partial pressure of oxygen, leading to hypoxia
   c. Vasodilation and cerebral edema
   d. Further increases in ICP.

D. Assessment findings

1. **Clinical manifestations**
   a. Lethargy is the earliest sign; altered level of consciousness, restlessness, slowing of speech, and delay in response to verbal suggestions are other early indicators.
   b. Pupil changes (e.g., fixed, dilated, slowed response, inequality)
   c. Increasing systolic blood pressure with stable or falling diastolic pressure and bradycardia, called the Cushing reflex
   d. Bradypnea, irregular breathing pattern
   e. Hyperthermia, a late sign of increasing ICP
   f. Focal neurologic signs, such as visual changes (e.g., blurred or double vision, photophobia), muscle weakness or paralysis, decreased response to pain stimulus, a positive Babinski's sign, decerebrate or decorticate posturing, and flaccidity
   g. Headache

2. **Laboratory and diagnostic study findings**
   a. ICP monitoring reveals an ICP greater than 15 mm Hg.
   b. Magnetic resonance imaging, radiographs, and computed tomography may identify the cause of the increased pressure (e.g., tumor, ischemic area).

E. Nursing management (See section II.D.)

1. **Administer prescribed medications,** which may include osmotic diuretics, corticosteroids, analgesics, and sedatives. (See *Drug chart 13-1.*)
2. **Monitor neurologic status,** including vital signs, level of consciousness (LOC), oculomotor nerve function, and motor and sensory status.
3. **Provide safety measures** when administering sedatives and analgesics that may depress respiration and decrease LOC.
   a. Reduce or eliminate noxious stimuli.
   b. Elevate the head of the bed 30 degrees.
   c. Hyperoxygenate the client before suctioning.
4. **Maintain a patent airway.** Suction as needed, and position the client to prevent airway obstruction.
5. **Manage hyperthermia.**
   a. Provide only minimal bed coverings and clothing.
   b. Use a hypothermia blanket; avoid rapid cooling.
   c. Administer antipyretics as prescribed.
   d. Force fluids unless contraindicated.

DRUG CHART 13-1
Medications for neurologic problems

Classifications	Indications	Selected interventions
Anticholinergic agents benztropine mesylate procyclidine trihexyphenidyl	Block cholinergic receptor sites to inhibit the action of acetylcholine	▪ Instruct the client to take the medication after meals to minimize GI upset. ▪ Advise the client to increase his fluid intake to prevent constipation (an adverse effect). ▪ Explain to the client that this medication may cause drowsiness.
Anticholinesterase agents neostigmine pyridostigmine	Inhibit the breakdown of acetylcholine (a substance associated with muscle tone)	▪ Administer the medication at the same time daily to ensure maximum strength available for activity. ▪ Administer the medication with food to minimize GI distress. ▪ In the case of an overdose, have the antidote atropine on hand.
Anticoagulants oral warfarin sodium	Prevent recurrence of emboli (no effect on emboli that are already present)	▪ Monitor the International Normalized Ratio, for which the therapeutic level is 2 to 3. Antidote is AquaMEPHYTON (vitamin K). ▪ Instruct the client to report bruising, unexplained bleeding, or dark, tarry stools; use a soft bristle toothbrush; be cautious when using sharp objects or machinery; wear a medi-alert bracelet; and notify any health care provider (e.g., dentist, pharmacist) that he is on an anticoagulant. ▪ If bleeding occurs, instruct the client to apply direct pressure to the wound; if bleeding does not stop after 5 minutes of direct pressure, tell him to get medical help.
Anticonvulsants carbamazepine phenobarbital phenytoin	Control seizure activity by an unknown mechanism	▪ Inform the client that the medication may cause drowsiness, and advise avoiding activities that require mental alertness and coordination. ▪ Caution the client not to stop the medication abruptly, because doing so may trigger seizure activity. ▪ Teach the client to perform regular oral hygiene and seek regular dental care to control gingival problems and other oral adverse effects. ▪ Urge the client to carry medical identification. ▪ Instruct the client to report signs of serious adverse effects, such as rash or flulike symptoms. ▪ Monitor therapeutic serum drug levels.
Antihistamines diphenhydramine	Inhibit acetylcholine and allay tremors with a mild sedative effect	▪ Direct the client to take the medication with food to minimize GI distress. ▪ Suggest that the client drink plenty of water, chew sugarless gum, or suck sour, hard candy to relieve dry mouth.
Antiparkinson agents levodopa	Improve transmission of voluntary nerve impulses to the motor cortex by stimulating dopamine receptors	▪ Instruct the client to report overdose signs, such as muscle or eye twitching, at once. ▪ Tell the client not to take the medication with food but to eat food 30 minutes after the dose to minimize GI distress. ▪ Discuss precautions to prevent or minimize orthostatic hypotension. *(continued)*

DRUG CHART 13-1
Medications for neurologic problems *(continued)*

Classifications	Indications	Selected interventions
Antiplatelets aspirin dipyridamole ticlopidine	Suppress platelet aggregation; principal indication is prevention of thrombosis in arteries	▪ Instruct the client to take the medication daily with food. ▪ Instruct the client to report any tinnitus, GI bleeding, or gastric upset; encourage enteric-coated aspirin.
Corticosteroids hydrocortisone methylprednisolone prednisone solu-medrol	Strengthen biologic membrane, which inhibits capillary permeability and prevents leakage of fluid into the injured area and development of edema (exact mechanism unknown)	▪ Instruct the client to take the medication exactly as directed and to taper discontinuation rather than stop it abruptly, which could cause serious withdrawal symptoms leading to adrenal insufficiency, shock, and death. ▪ Forewarn the client that the medication may cause reportable cushingoid effects (weight gain, moon face, buffalo hump, and hirsutism) and may mask signs and symptoms of infection. ▪ Administer I.V. delivery during times of acutely increased intracranial pressure.
Muscle relaxants baclofen carisoprodol diazepam methocarbamol	Act in the central nervous system to relieve spasticity; within the spinal cord, it suppresses active reflexes involved in regulation of muscle movement	▪ Warn the client that these medications cause drowsiness initially but diminish with continued use. ▪ Instruct the client to avoid hazardous activities; and to not mix these medications with alcohol or other depressants.
Nonopioid analgesics acetaminophen	Treat mild to moderate pain; blocks the generation impulse through peripheral medanism	▪ Inform the client that the medication may be purchased over the counter. ▪ Caution the client that overdose may be toxic to the liver.
Nonsteroidal anti-inflammatory drugs ibuprofen idomethacin ketorolac naproxen salicylates	Reduce the inflammatory process, thereby reducing pain	▪ Instruct the client to administer the medication with food to minimize upset. ▪ Inform the client that the medication may have an anticoagulant effect. ▪ Instruct the client to report tinnitus (ringing in ears), which is a sign of ASA toxicity.
Opioid analgesics codeine hydrocodone hydromorphone morphine propoxyphene	Relieve moderate to severe pain by reducing pain sensation, producing sedation, and decreasing the emotional upset often associated with pain; most often schedule II drugs	▪ Assess the pain for location, type, intensity, and what increases or decreases it; rate pain on a scale of 1 (no pain) to 10 (worst pain). ▪ Rule out complications. Is this pain routine or expected? Is this a complication that needs immediate intervention? ▪ Medicate according to the pain scale findings. ▪ Institute safety measures—bed in low position, side rails up, and call light within reach. ▪ Evaluate the effectiveness of pain medication in 30 minutes.
Osmotic diuretic mannitol	Decrease cerebral edema in head trauma by drawing water across intact membranes, thereby reducing the volume of brain and extracellular fluid	▪ Monitor fluid and electrolyte balance. ▪ Maintain accurate intake and output records. ▪ Observe I.V. preparation for crystals before use; always use a filter needle.

DRUG CHART 13-1
Medications for neurologic problems *(continued)*

Classifications	Indications	Selected interventions
Sedatives phenobarbital	Depress central nervous system (CNS) activity, thereby reducing restlessness and agitation, as in clients with cerebral aneurysm	■ Administer I.V. medication by a large vein to avoid extravasation. ■ Monitor vital signs closely, because sedative drugs depress CNS and respiratory activity and may mask decreasing level of consciousness. ■ Institute safety precautions—side rails up and call light within reach.

---

6. **Prevent infection** by using sterile technique for wound care, insertion of the ICP monitoring device, and by keeping the monitoring system intact.
7. **Maintain fluid and electrolyte balance.**
   a. Monitor the client's skin turgor, mucous membranes, serum, and urine osmolarity for signs of dehydration.
   b. Monitor strict intake and output through an indwelling Foley catheter. Use a urometer if necessary.
8. **Promote measures to prevent complications.**
   a. Institute measures to prevent Valsalva's maneuver (e.g., straining, coughing, constipation) because of increased ICP.
   b. Institute seizure precautions. (See section VI.)
   c. Monitor for complications of ICP, which include brain-stem herniation, diabetes insipidus, and syndrome of inappropriate antidiuretic hormone.
9. **Help orient the client and reduce confusion.**
   a. Reduce external stimuli.
   b. Provide for adequate rest.
   c. Give simple directions.
   d. Provide familiar objects in the client's environment.

IV. HEAD TRAUMA

A. **Description**
   1. Head trauma refers to direct or indirect impact to the head that produces some degree of brain injury. Common types of head trauma include:
      a. closed head injuries (i.e., concussion, contusion, or laceration)
      b. intracranial hemorrhage (i.e., epidural, subdural, or intracerebral hematoma)
      c. skull fractures (open or closed).
   2. Head trauma causes 80,000 to 100,000 deaths each year in the United States. Another 700,000 cases require hospitalization.

B. **Etiology.** Common causes of head trauma include falls, automobile accidents, beatings, and blunt object and missile injury (e.g., gunshot or stab wounds).

C. **Pathophysiology.** Injury to the head may result in bleeding or edema in response to the injury and may result in increased intracranial pressure (ICP). (See section III.)

D. **Assessment findings**
   1. **Clinical manifestations** of head trauma depend on the type, site, and extent of injury.

a. A common manifestation is loss of consciousness, ranging from a few minutes to 1 hour or longer.

b. Cerebrospinal otorrhea (i.e., cerebrospinal fluid [CSF] draining from the ear) and cerebrospinal rhinorrhea (i.e., CSF draining from nose) may be present. This is determined by a positive glucose reading on a dextrose stick or halo sign (i.e., blood surrounded by a yellowish stain).

c. An area of ecchymosis may exist over the affected area.

2. **Laboratory and diagnostic study findings**

a. Computed tomography may reveal the area that is contused or injured.

b. Radiographs may reveal skull fractures.

E. Nursing management (See section II.D.)

1. **Provide nursing management for ICP.** Assess all drainage from the nose and ears for CSF; watch for the halo sign or test drainage with a dextrose stick for glucose. (See section III.E.) In cases where ICP cannot be controlled medically, a burr hole may be used to remove subdural or epidural hemotomas. In extreme cases, a craniotomy may be performed to remove the hemotomas.

2. **Establish and maintain a patent airway** by keeping the head of the bed elevated 30 degrees, instituting effective suctioning procedures, and monitoring arterial blood gases.

3. **Provide ongoing assessment.** Assess blood and urine electrolytes and osmolarity.

4. **Provide adequate nutrition** and possible nasogastric tube feedings if cerebrospinal fluid rhinorrhea is not present.

5. **Promote coping.** Collaborate with rehabilitation members to identify activities directed at redeveloping the client's ability to devise new problem-solving strategies.

6. **Provide referrals** to the National Rehabilitation Information Center for Independence. (See appendix A.)

V. CEREBROVASCULAR DISORDERS

A. Description. This group of disorders involves disruption of blood supply to the brain.

1. **Stroke,** also known as *cerebrovascular accident,* is a sudden loss of brain function resulting from disruption of the blood supply to a part of the brain. The most common site of stroke is the middle cerebral artery. About one half of the survivors sustain permanent neurologic deficits.

2. **Transient ischemic attack (TIA)** is a transient or temporary episode of neurologic dysfunction caused by decreased blood supply to the brain. This disorder is considered a warning sign of stroke. The most common site of TIA is at the bifurcation of the common carotid artery.

3. **Cerebral aneurysm** is a dilation of the walls of a cerebral artery resulting from a weakness in the arterial wall. The most common type is berry aneurysm. The most common site is in the anterior portion of the circle of Willis, usually at a vessel junction.

B. Etiology

1. **Stroke** results from thrombosis (most common), embolism, and vessel rupture or spasm.

2. **TIA** results from occlusion of an intracranial or extracranial artery, commonly associated with atherosclerosis.

3. **Cerebral aneurysm** results from a weakness in a vessel wall because of a congenital defect or a degenerative process, such as hypertension or atherosclerosis.

C. Pathophysiology

1. In a **stroke,** the sudden interruption of blood supply to areas of the brain results in cerebral anoxia and impaired cerebral metabolism, which permanently damages brain tissue and produces focal neurologic deficits of varying severity.
2. In a **TIA**, there is a temporary decrease in blood flow to a specific region of the brain, but there is no necrosis of brain tissue. The symptoms (lasting seconds to hours) produce transient neurologic deficits that completely clear within 12 to 24 hours.
3. A **cerebral aneurysm** is prone to rupture, which causes blood to leak into the subarachnoid space (and sometimes into brain tissue, where it forms a clot), resulting in increased intracranial pressure (ICP) and brain tissue damage.

D. Assessment findings

1. **Clinical manifestations** depend on the disorder.
   a. **Stroke.** Clinical manifestations depend on the artery affected, the severity of damage, and the extent of collateral circulation that develops. Common signs and symptoms include:
   – hemiplegia and sensory deficits
   – aphasia (Impairment may be in speaking, listening, writing, or comprehending; most cases are mixed expressive and receptive.)
   – homonymous hemianopia
   – unilateral neglect of paralyzed side
   – bladder impairment
   – possible respiratory impairment
   – impaired mental activity and psychological effects.
   b. **TIA.** Manifestations may include:
   – temporary loss of consciousness or dizziness
   – paresthesias
   – garbled speech.
   c. **Cerebral aneurysm.** A client with a nonruptured cerebral aneurysm often is asymptomatic or reports nonspecific symptoms, such as headache or blurred vision. Aneurysm rupture produces various manifestations, which may include:
   – signs and symptoms of increased ICP (see section III.D)
   – severe headache
   – nuchal rigidity and pain on neck movement
   – photophobia and possible blurred vision
   – irritability and restlessness
   – slight temperature elevation.
2. **Laboratory and diagnostic study findings**
   a. Carotid angiography reveals a narrowing of the carotid artery.
   b. Computed tomography and magnetic resonance imaging reveal the location and extent of the necrotic brain tissue.

E. Nursing management (See section II.D.)

1. Provide nursing care during the acute phase (48 to 72 hours) of stroke.
   a. Administer medications, which may include osmotic diuretics, corticosteroids, and anticonvulsants. To prevent further development, oral anticoagulant and antiplatelet agents may be prescribed. (See *Drug Chart 13-1,* pages 343 to 345.)
   b. Monitor for increased ICP. (See section III.)
2. Provide nursing care during the rehabilitation phase of stroke.

a. Collaborate with the entire health care team to assist the client in returning to preillness functioning. Always include the client's family.

b. Enhance communication as described in section II.D.9.

c. Plan the client's care to allow for adequate periods of uninterrupted rest. Schedule therapy sessions after rest periods.

d. Provide a balanced diet, and assist the client with eating if necessary. Allow sufficient time for meals, place food so that the client can see it, and provide foods that are easy to handle.

e. Maximize the client's opportunities for social interaction.

f. Consider the client's interests when planning daily activities.

g. Teach the client how to use a walker, cane, or wheelchair as appropriate.

h. Collaborate with the occupational therapist to develop and assist the client in using assistive devices to achieve activities of daily living as independently as possible.

i. Encourage the client to wear simplified clothing (e.g., slacks with front-opening snaps, apparel with Velcro closures).

j. Discuss necessary home adaptations (e.g., wheelchair ramps, shower seat, bathroom modifications).

k. Assist the client with personal hygiene as necessary (e.g., hair washing and brushing, makeup application, shaving).

l. Teach and assist with or perform range-of-motion (ROM) exercises to help maintain muscle tone and prevent contractures. (See *Client and family teaching 13-1*, page 341.)

m. Encourage the client to touch the paralyzed side and to participate in passive ROM exercises as appropriate.

n. Ensure correct positioning to prevent contractures. Prevent hip reduction by positioning the client on his side with his hips slightly flexed and in as natural a position as possible; use a prone position if possible; and prevent shoulder adduction by placing pillow in the axilla.

o. **Turn the client every 2 hours to prevent impaired skin integrity and contractures, and include the prone position at least 15 to 30 minutes several times each day.**

p. Assist the client with attaining bladder control; analyze the client's usual voiding patterns and offer a urinal or bedpan on schedule.

q. Help reduce pain and promote comfort.
   - Administer analgesics as prescribed.
   - Position the client to decrease discomfort.
   - For a client with subarachnoid hemorrhage, reduce external stimuli, move him slowly, and turn his neck gently.

r. Prepare the client for surgical intervention as appropriate, which may include:
   - carotid endarterectomy for a client experiencing TIA
   - craniotomy for surgical clipping of aneurysm.

s. Teach the client's family:
   - effective communication techniques
   - new ways of interacting with the client after discharge
   - ways to encourage the client in self-feeding
   - safety precautions (e.g., keeping the client's environment clear of obstacles).

t. Provide referrals to the National Institute of Neurological Disorders and Stroke, National Stroke Association, and National Rehabilitation Information Center for Independence. (See appendix A.)

VI. SEIZURE DISORDERS

A. Description

1. **Seizure** refers to paroxysmal, uncontrolled, excessive firing of hyperexcitable neurons in the brain. A seizure is not a disease entity in itself but rather an indicator of underlying pathology. Epilepsy is a chronic disorder characterized by unprovoked seizure activity.

2. **Types of seizures**
   a. Tonic-clonic (grand mal)
   b. Absence (petit mal)
   c. Complex (temporal lobe; psychomotor)
   d. Jacksonian

B. Etiology. About 50% of cases of epilepsy are idiopathic, for which no underlying pathology can be identified. Possible causes include:

1. birth trauma
2. head trauma
3. brain tumor
4. meningitis, encephalitis, or brain abscess
5. metabolic disorders (e.g., hypoglycemia, phenylketonuria)
6. cerebrovascular disorders.

C. Pathophysiology

1. After a task is completed, nerve-cell impulses should cease. Sometimes these nerve-cell impulses continue firing even after the task is finished. During the continued firing of nerve-cell impulses, the parts of the body controlled by the errant cells may perform erratically. These erratic physical movements are called seizures.

2. Seizures are classified as partial (e.g., complex, Jacksonian), arising from a localized area of the brain, or generalized (e.g., tonic-clonic, absence), marked by widespread electrical abnormality in the brain.

3. Status epilepticus refers to continued seizure activity, a medical emergency treated with medications.

D. Assessment findings. Clinical manifestations depend on the type of seizure.

1. **Tonic-clonic seizures** are marked by:
   a. generalized seizure activity, with no focal onset and lasting about 2 minutes
   b. possible prodrome of a vaguely uneasy feeling, aura
   c. loss of consciousness, with falling if upright at onset
   d. muscle contraction (including jaw clenching) and possibly periods of apnea (in the tonic phase)
   e. rhythmic, forceful movement of extremities, excessive salivation, and rapid pulse (in the clonic phase)
   f. possible incontinence
   g. stupor for 5 to 10 minutes after the clonic phase.

2. **Absence seizures** are characterized by:
   a. generalized seizure activity, with no focal onset and occurring primarily in children
   b. momentary (10- to 30-second) loss of consciousness, marked by a glassy stare but usually no falling
   c. possibly occurring repeatedly over the course of a day.

3. In **complex seizures,** the client exhibits altered behavior (e.g., automatisms, unusual sensations, delusions) but is not aware of what is happening.

4. **Jacksonian seizures** begin in one part of the body (e.g., twitching of one side of the face or abnormal movements of one hand) and may progress to a generalized tonic-clonic seizure.

E. Nursing management (See section II.D.)

1. **Administer prescribed medications,** which include anticonvulsants. (See *Drug chart 13-1,* pages 343 to 345.)

2. **Provide nursing care during a seizure.**

   a. Institute seizure precautions as per facility protocol.
   - Pad all side rails (controversial).
   - Place an oral airway at the head of the bed (controversial).
   - Make sure all staff know the client is at risk for seizures.
   - Keep the bed in low position with side rails elevated.
   - Do not allow the client to take a tub bath and stay with him during a shower.

   b. Provide ongoing assessment.
   - Observe and record the client's movements and behavior before, during, and after the seizure. Document incontinence, frothing, and guttural sounds.
   - Note the parts of the body affected by seizure activity.
   - Note the duration of seizure activity.

   c. Provide privacy for the client. Protect the client from injury by placing him in a side-lying position, moving furniture, and protecting the head. Do not restrain him.

   d. If teeth are not clinched, insert an oral airway; do not insert anything if teeth are clinched; do not put fingers in the client's mouth.

3. **Provide nursing care after a seizure (postictal).**

   a. Keep the client in a side-lying position to prevent aspiration.
   b. Maintain a patent airway.
   c. If the client is confused, help reorient him. If the client is tired, provide a quiet, restful environment.
   d. Provide client and family teaching covering:
   - aura or indications of seizure
   - necessary lifestyle modifications, such as getting adequate sleep, abstaining from alcohol, and using relaxation techniques
   - the need for social interaction opportunities
   - the need to carry an identification card or jewelry listing the diagnosis and medication
   - importance of taking medications as prescribed.

   e. Encourage the client's family to avoid being overprotective.
   f. Provide a referral to the Epilepsy Foundation. (See appendix A.)

VII. SPINAL CORD INJURIES

A. Description. Spinal cord injures include fractures, contusions, or compression of the vertebral column with damage to the spinal cord. Common sites of injury include the cervical spine and the junction of the thoracic and lumbar areas (T12 and L1).

B. Etiology. Causes of spinal cord injury include motor vehicle accidents, diving accidents, falls, sports injuries, and gunshot wounds.

C. Pathophysiology

1. Spinal cord injuries can result from flexion, extension, rotation, compression, or a combination of these mechanisms.
2. Injury may directly damage the cord, or vertebral fracture or dislocation can be a potential source of cord injury, in which case inappropriate movement can cause permanent damage.
3. Cord injury may be complete, involving total cord transection, or incomplete, with partial transection or other damage.
4. Damage ranges from mild, transient cord concussion to immediate and permanent quadriplegia.
5. With cord damage, spinal shock (i.e., areflexia) may occur. Subsequently, loss of motor, sensory, and autonomic activity below the level of injury may result in a decrease of blood pressure. The parts of the body below the level of the cord lesion are paralyzed, without sensation or diaphoresis. This condition may persist for several days to months after injury.

D. Assessment findings

1. **Clinical manifestations**
   a. Common immediate symptoms of spinal cord injury include pain and paresthesias or, conversely, loss of sensation; altered motor function ranging from paresis to paralysis; and possibly loss of consciousness.
   b. Neurologic damage depends on the level of cord injury. Edema may temporarily increase deficits.
   – Below C4: loss of motor and sensory function from the neck down, including independent respiratory function and bowel and bladder control
   – Below C6: loss of motor and sensory function below the shoulders; loss of bowel and bladder control; impaired intercostal muscle function
   – Below C8: loss of motor control and sensation to parts of the arms and hands; loss of bowel and bladder control
   – Below T6: loss of motor control and sensation below the mid-chest but with motor control and sensation preserved in the arms and hands; loss of bowel and bladder control
   – Below T12: loss of motor control and sensation below the waist; loss of bowel and bladder control
   – Below L2: loss of motor control and sensation in the legs and pelvis; loss of bowel and bladder control
   – Below L4: loss of motor control and sensation in parts of the thighs and legs; loss of bowel and bladder control.
2. **Laboratory and diagnostic study findings**
   a. Spinal radiography can locate the area of cord damage.
   b. Computed tomography can locate the area of cord damage and search for other injuries that often accompany spinal trauma.

E. Nursing management (See section II.D.)

1. **Provide emergency treatment.**
   a. Do not move the client until adequate personnel and equipment are available.
   b. Keep the neck aligned.
   c. Immobilize the head and neck.
   d. Maintain a patent airway (i.e., oxygen therapy, arterial blood gases, and pulse oximeter); with cervical injury, ascending edema may cause respiratory difficulty.

2. **Administer prescribed medications,** which may include high-dose corticosteroids (i.e., reduces disability if given within 8 hours of injury), osmotic diuretics, muscle relaxants (e.g., baclofen), and dextran (i.e., prevents the blood pressure from dropping and improves capillary blood flow). (See *Drug chart 13-1,* pages 343 to 345.)

3. **Assist with immobilization and reduction of dislocations and stabilization of the cervical vertebral column** by applying skeletal traction (i.e., skeletal tongs such as Gardner-Wells tongs or Crutchfield tongs) or halo traction. Nursing care includes:
   a. caring for the client on a Stryker frame or CircOlectric bed
   b. ensuring that weights hang freely and do not interfere with traction; never remove weights
   c. cleaning tong insertion sites and assessing for infection
   d. instituting measures to prevent skin breakdown.

4. **Prepare the client for surgery** if appropriate — usually for repair of fractures or dislocations to stabilize the spinal column. (See chapter 21.)

5. **Prevent complications of immobility.**
   a. Perform passive range-of-motion (ROM) exercises on paralyzed limbs to maintain joint mobility. (See *Client and family teaching 13-1,* page 341.)
      - Position feet against a padded footboard, or use high-top tennis shoes to prevent footdrop.
      - Apply trochanter rolls from the crest of the ilium to the mid-thigh of both legs to prevent external rotation of the hip joints.
      - When turning the client every 2 hours, always maintain body alignment and log roll the client.
   b. Teach the client active ROM exercises to maintain or increase strength and mobility in the upper extremities. (See *Client and family teaching 13-1,* page 341.)
   c. Provide nursing care to prevent such complications as deep vein thrombosis, pressure ulcers, contractures, constipation, and pneumonia.

6. **Prepare the client and his family for ambulation and home maintenance management.**
   a. Work with other disciplines in securing needed assistive devices. Teach the client transfer skills if appropriate.
   b. Collaborate with the client's family to identify ways to adapt the home environment to the client's needs.

7. **Teach the client and his family signs and symptoms of impending autonomic hyperreflexia (dysreflexia) episodes, which occur with cord lesions above T6.**
   a. They are characterized by severe, pounding headaches with paroxysmal hypertension; profuse diaphoresis; nasal congestion; and bradycardia.
   b. They are triggered by distended bladder (most common), distended bowel, and pain stimulation.
   c. The nurse must intervene immediately in this emergency situation, place the client in the sitting position, empty the bladder immediately, assess for fecal impaction, assess for any other trigger and, if there is no decrease in blood pressure, seek emergency help (to administer antihypertensive medication).

8. **Promote normal bowel and bladder elimination.**
   a. Promote measures to prevent constipation, and encourage the client to establish a regular bowel routine.
      - Advise the client to set a schedule for defecation, preferably 15 to 20 minutes after a meal.
      - Provide a warm liquid before defecation time.

- Encourage the client to ingest sufficient dietary roughage and adequate fluids and to avoid foods that can cause constipation.
- Encourage the client to attempt defecation in the sitting position, if possible.
  b. Provide bladder care to prevent urine stasis.
- Schedule frequent times for voiding.
- Maintain an adequate fluid intake but avoid fluids before bedtime.
- Identify and use triggering mechanisms that can stimulate voiding.
- Perform intermittent bladder catheterization as appropriate.
9. **Promote client and family coping.** Evaluate the client's and family members' coping strategies, and teach new strategies if needed. Encourage the client and his family to verbalize concerns.
10. **Provide information on alternative means for achieving sexual satisfaction** as appropriate.
11. **Provide a referral** to the National Spinal Cord Injury Association. (See appendix A.)

VIII. INTERVERTEBRAL DISK HERNIATION

A. Description. Intervertebral disk herniation is a disorder involving impingement of a vertebral disk's nucleus pulposus on spinal nerve roots, causing pain and possible neuromuscular deficit.

B. Etiology. A herniated disk can result from:
1. degenerative disorders
2. trauma
3. congenital predisposition.

C. Pathophysiology. Rupture of the annulus pulposus (i.e., disk's outer ring) allows part of the nucleus pulposus (i.e., soft, gelatinous inner portion) to protrude and press against spinal nerve roots, producing symptoms. Herniation can occur anywhere along the vertebral column but is most common in the lumbar area.

D. Assessment findings
1. **Clinical manifestations** vary with the location and degree of herniation and the course of its progression. Common signs and symptoms of herniated disk include:
   a. back pain (in lumbar herniation, often with radiation down the posterior thigh and leg), exacerbated by coughing, sneezing, or straining
   b. various degrees of motor and sensory impairment (e.g., muscle weakness, and diminished deep tendon reflexes in the lower extremities)
   c. pressure on the sciatic nerve can produce severe, sometimes debilitating pain and, if chronic, possible motor and sensory changes (in lumbar disk herniation).
2. **Laboratory and diagnostic study findings**
   a. Straight-leg raising test or the LeSegue test result is positive.
   b. Computed tomography, magnetic resonance imaging, or myelography may reveal the location of herniation.

E. Nursing management (See section II.D.)
1. **Administer prescribed medications,** which may include muscle relaxants and opioid or nonopioid analgesics. (See *Drug chart 13-1,* pages 343 to 345.)
2. **Provide pain relief.**
3. **Provide ongoing assessment.**
   a. Assess the site, nature, course, and progress of back pain.

   b. Monitor motor and sensory status.
4. **Provide conservative management if indicated.**
   a. Encourage bed rest.
   b. Position the client with the head of the bed elevated 30 degrees and knees slightly flexed.
   c. Apply heat.
   d. Instruct the client in appropriate exercises to increase muscle strength around the spinal cord (e.g., pelvic tilts, straight-leg raises).
5. **Maximize functional abilities.**
   a. Prevent complications of immobility.
   b. Promote self-care.
6. **Provide perioperative and postoperative care** if laminectomy is ordered to remove protruding disk fragments. (See chapter 21). Provide the following postoperative care:
   a. Assess strength, sensation, and movement of extremities.
   b. Promote measures to maintain adequate airway.
   c. Protect the client from infection.
   d. Keep the client in proper body alignment when in bed (provide a firm mattress) and when turning (use log-rolling).
   e. Encourage the client to wear well-fitted, safe walking shoes when ambulating.
   f. Teach proper body mechanics to prevent injury.
   g. Caution the client to avoid slippery surfaces and activities that can involve sudden back movements.
7. **Provide client and family teaching.**
8. **Promote client and family coping.**

IX. MULTIPLE SCLEROSIS

A. **Description.** Multiple sclerosis (MS) a progressively disabling demyelinating disease affecting nerve fibers of the brain and spinal cord and marked by periodic exacerbations and remissions. Incidence is greater for women than men and is highest in temperate climates. Onset is typically between ages 20 and 40.

B. **Etiology.** The cause of MS is unknown. Theories suggest that myelin damage is the primary event and that it results from a viral infection early in life that becomes apparent as an autoimmune process later in life. It is believed that a defective immune response has a major role in the pathogenesis of MS.

C. **Pathophysiology**
   1. MS produces patches of demyelination throughout the central nervous system, resulting in myelin being lost from the axis cylinders and degeneration of the axons themselves.
   2. The plaques in the involved area become sclerosed, interrupting the flow of nerve impulses and resulting in a variety of manifestations, depending on which nerves are affected.
   3. Periodic and unpredictable exacerbations and remissions mark the course of MS.
   4. Prognosis varies. MS can cause rapid, sometimes fatal, disability, but about 70% of clients lead active, productive lives with long periods of remission.

D. **Assessment findings**
   1. **Clinical manifestations** of MS vary widely but may include:

      a. visual problems, such as diplopia, blurred vision, and nystagmus

      b. motor dysfunction, such as muscle weakness that typically worsens throughout the day, paralysis, spasticity, hyperreflexia, tremors, and gait ataxia

      c. fatigue

      d. bladder or bowel incontinence

      e. mental changes, such as mood swings, irritability, and depression.

  2. Laboratory and diagnostic findings

      a. Lumbar puncture and cerebrospinal fluid (CSF) analysis may reveal elevated CSF gamma globulins.

      b. Magnetic resonance imaging may confirm the presence of demyelinating plaques.

E. Nursing management (See section II.D.)

  1. Administer prescribed medications, which may include corticosteroids and muscle relaxants (i.e., baclofen). (See *Drug chart 13-1,* pages 343 to 345.) Hormones such as corticotropin may be prescribed to stimulate the release of adrenal cortex hormones, which help to improve nerve conduction. Instruct the client to notify the health care provider if serious adverse effects, such as fluid retention, muscle weakness, abdominal pain, or headache, occur.

  2. Promote measures to avoid fatigue.

      a. Assess the client's sleep and rest patterns.

      b. Encourage adequate rest.

      c. Assist the client in planning lifestyle modifications to decrease stress and fatigue and maximize functional abilities.

      d. Encourage relaxation and coordination exercises to improve muscle efficiency.

  3. Maximize functional abilities.

      a. Assess the nature and degree of neuromuscular deficits and their effect on the client's routine activities.

      b. Prevent complications of immobility.

      c. Promote self-care.

      d. Maximize effective communication.

  4. Encourage the use of an eye patch if diplopia occurs.

  5. Provide appropriate care during exacerbations (e.g., help the client establish bladder and bowel control, prevent and treat muscle spasticity).

  6. Promote measures to maintain adequate air way.

  7. Provide client and family teaching.

  8. Promote measures to enhance body image.

  9. Promote client and family coping, which may be compromised because of the chronic, progressive disease process.

  10. Provide referrals to the National Multiple Sclerosis Society, Multiple Sclerosis Foundation, and Multiple Sclerosis Association of America. (See appendix A.)

X. PARKINSON'S DISEASE

A. Description. Parkinson's disease is a progressive neurologic disorder resulting from the degeneration of basal ganglia in the cerebrum. The second most common neurologic disorder in the elderly, Parkinson's disease affects about 1 of 100 persons older than age 60. The incidence is higher among men than women.

B. Etiology. The cause of Parkinson's disease is unknown. Suspected causes include:

  1. viral infection

      2. chemical toxicity

      3. cerebrovascular disease

      4. effects of drugs, such as major tranquilizers and reserpine.

C. Pathophysiology

      1. Dopamine, a neurotransmitter secreted by the basal ganglia, is essential to extrapyramidal function. Depletion of dopamine diminishes normal neuromuscular-inhibiting mechanisms, leading to the characteristic neurologic deficits associated with parkinsonism, such as bradykinesia, muscle rigidity, and resting tremor.

      2. Progressive deterioration continues for about 10 years; death commonly results from pneumonia or another infection.

D. Assessment findings. Clinical manifestations include:

      1. tremor (An early sign, tremors commonly affect the hands and are more prominent at rest [i.e., resting or "pill rolling" tremor.])

      2. impaired movement to include bradykinesia, akinesia, and dyskinesia

      3. rigidity marked by decreased muscle tone and stiffness, with jerky movements (i.e., "cogwheel rigidity")

      4. fatigue and muscle weakness

      5. stooped posture and shuffling gait marked by arm swinging

      6. impaired ability to turn in bed and rise from chair

      7. masklike facial expression and decreased blinking reflex

      8. autonomic manifestations, such as oily skin (i.e., seborrhea) and excessive perspiration

      9. dysphagia (i.e., difficulty with swallowing) and drooling

      10. monotone speech, and impaired articulation (i.e., dysarthria)

      11. constipation resulting from decreased fluid intake and autonomic dysfunction

      12. depression and withdrawal.

▨ E. Nursing management (See section II.D.)

      1. **Administer prescribed medications,** which may include antiparkinson medications, anticholinergics, and antihistamines. (See *Drug chart 13-1,* pages 343 to 345.) Amantadine hydrochloride, an antiviral agent, is prescribed early in treatment to reduce rigidity, tremors, and bradykinesia. A monoamine oxidase inhibitor, selegiline shows promise in slowing progression of the disease.

      2. **Prepare the client for stereotaxic surgery** to reduce tremors and rigidity if indicated.

      3. **Promote measures to maintain a adequate airway.**

      4. **Promote methods to ease difficulty with swallowing if indicated.** Encourage semisolid diet.

      5. **Maximize functional abilities.**

         a. Improve mobility and prevent complications of immobility.

            – Encourage daily exercise, stretching exercises, and special walking techniques to offset the shuffling gait.

            – Instruct the client in ways to prevent constipation (e.g., increase fluids, maintain high-fiber diet, follow regular bowel routine).

         b. Promote self-care.

         c. Maximize effective communication.

      6. **Provide client and family teaching.**

      7. **Promote measures to enhance body image.**

      8. **Promote client and family coping.**

✋ *a.* Include the family in teaching, and counsel family members to learn techniques to reduce stress, to obtain periodic relief from responsibilities, and to express feelings of frustration, anger, or guilt.

b. Address issues of depression with the client; encourage counseling and possible administration of antidepressants.

9. **Provide referrals** to the American Parkinson Disease Association and National Parkinson Foundation. (See appendix A.)

XI. AMYOTROPHIC LATERAL SCLEROSIS

A. Description. Amyotrophic lateral sclerosis (ALS) is a progressively debilitating and eventually fatal disease involving degeneration of motor neurons. ALS affects 2 to 7 of every 100,000 persons, affecting men more than women. Onset typically occurs between ages 40 and 70.

B. Etiology. The cause of ALS is unknown.

C. Pathophysiology

1. ALS is marked by progressive destruction of motor cells in the anterior gray horns and pyramidal tract; upper and lower motor neurons are affected. As motor neurons die, the muscle cells they supply undergo atrophic changes. Progressive paralysis results.

2. Prognosis varies. Most ALS clients die within 3 to 10 years of onset, usually from secondary causes such as pneumonia.

D. Assessment findings

1. **Clinical manifestations** vary with the location of affected motor neurons and disease stage and may include:

a. progressive weakness, atrophy, spasticity, and tremors of upper extremities, followed by involvement of lower extremities and then respiratory muscles

b. fatigue

c. impaired speech, chewing, and swallowing

d. breathing difficulty

e. depression.

2. **Laboratory and diagnostic study findings.** Electromyographic studies of the affected muscles indicate reduction in the number of functioning motor units.

▦ **E. Nursing management (See section II.D.)**

1. **Maximize functional abilities.**

a. Prevent complications of immobility.

b. Promote self-care.

c. Maximize effective communication.

2. **Ensure adequate nutrition.**

3. **Prevent respiratory complications.**

a. Promote measures to maintain adequate airway.

b. Promote measures to enhance gas exchange, such as oxygen therapy and ventilatory assistance.

c. Promote measures to prevent respiratory infection.

4. **Provide intellectually stimulating activities,** because the client typically experiences no cognitive deficits and retains mental abilities.

5. **Provide client and family teaching.**

6. **Promote measures to enhance body image.**
7. **Promote client and family coping** as the client and his family deal with the poor prognosis and the grieving process.
8. **Provide referrals** to the Amyotrophic Lateral Sclerosis Association and the Les Turner Amyotrophic Lateral Sclerosis Foundation. (See appendix A.)

XII. MYASTHENIA GRAVIS

A. **Description.** Myasthenia gravis is a progressive disorder affecting neuromuscular transmission of impulses in voluntary muscles. The incidence is 1 case per 25,000 persons and is higher among women than men. Initial symptoms typically occur between ages 20 and 40.

B. **Etiology.** Myasthenia gravis is thought to result from an autoimmune response.

C. **Pathophysiology**
1. In myasthenia gravis, acetylcholine receptor (ACHR) antibodies interfere with impulse transmission across myoneural junctions. This causes abnormal weakness and fatigability of skeletal muscle, particularly of the eyes, face, jaw, and neck, and may involve muscles of upper extremities and respiratory muscles.
2. The disorder follows an unpredictable course of periodic exacerbations and remissions. Drug therapy allows many clients to lead normal lives; however, progressive weakness of respiratory muscles may cause life-threatening respiratory distress or myasthenic crisis.

D. **Assessment findings**
1. **Clinical manifestations**
   a. Abnormal weakness of any striated muscle (particularly of the face, neck, arms, and hands), typically worsening after activity and improving with rest
   b. Severe fatigue
   c. Drooping facial muscles and ptosis
   d. Diplopia
   e. Impaired chewing and swallowing
   f. Breathing difficulty because of weak respiratory muscles
2. **Laboratory and diagnostic study findings**
   a. Positive Tensilon test result confirms the diagnosis.
   b. Serum anti-ACHR antibodies are present.

E. **Nursing management**
1. **Administer prescribed medications,** which may include anticholinesterase agents. (See *Drug chart 13-1*, pages 343 to 345.)
2. **Assist the client undergoing medical procedures,** such as plasmapheresis (i.e., plasma exchange produces a temporary reduction in the titer of circulating antibodies) or thymectomy (i.e., decreases formation of anti-ACHR antibodies), if indicated.
3. **Prevent problems associated with swallowing difficulty.** Provide small, frequent meals, and keep suctioning equipment readily available.
4. **Prevent problems associated with respiratory function.**
   a. Promote measures to maintain adequate airway. Encourage effective coughing, chest physiotherapy, and suctioning to remove secretions. (See section II.D.3.)
   b. Monitor pulmonary function tests.
5. **Encourage adjustments in lifestyle to prevent fatigue.**
   a. Plan adequate rest periods throughout the day, and set realistic daily schedules.

b. Administer medications 30 minutes before activities.
6. **Maximize functional abilities.**
   a. Prevent complications of immobility. (See section II.D.7.)
   b. Promote self-care. (See section II.D.8.).
   c. Maximize effective communication. (See section II.D. 9.)
7. **Prevent problems associated with impaired vision resulting from ptosis of eyelids.** Encourage the client to tape eyes open for short intervals, instill artificial tears, and wear sunglasses when outside.
8. **Be prepared for emergency treatment of myasthenic or cholinergic crisis.** Determine the type of crisis by administering I.V. edrophonium. If the crisis is myasthenic, improvement is noticed temporarily, and if cholinergic, there is no improvement. Treat myasthenic crisis with I.V. anticholinesterase. Treat cholinergic crisis with atropine.
9. **Provide client and family teaching.** (See section II.D.10.)
10. **Promote measures to enhance body image.** (See section II.D.11.)
11. **Promote client and family coping.** (See section II.D.12.)
12. **Provide a referral** to the Myasthenia Gravis Foundation of America. (See appendix A.)

XIII. GUILLAIN-BARRÉ SYNDROME

A. Description. Guillain-Barré syndrome is an acute, rapidly progressive form of polyneuritis producing muscle weakness and mild sensory disturbances. It can develop at any age but is most common between ages 30 and 50. The incidence is about equal among men and women.

B. Etiology. Guillain-Barré syndrome is a postinfectious polyneuritis of unknown origin that commonly follows febrile illness.

C. Pathophysiology
1. Segmental demyelination of peripheral nerves causes inflammation and degeneration in sensory and motor nerve roots.
2. Most clients experience spontaneous and complete recovery, although mild deficits may persist.

D. Assessment findings
1. **Clinical manifestations**
   a. Respiratory or GI infection (usually occurs 1 to 4 weeks before the onset of symptoms)
   b. Ascending paralysis starting in the legs (Paresis in the legs is usually the initial manifestation.)
   c. Motor weakness progressing to involve the entire peripheral nervous system, including respiratory muscles
   d. Paresthesias
   e. Progression may involve total or partial paralysis.
2. **Laboratory and diagnostic study findings.** Lumbar puncture and cerebrospinal fluid (CSF) analysis may reveal elevated levels of CSF proteins.

E. Nursing management (See section II.D.)
1. **Explain all procedures and care measures to help reduce the client's anxiety.**
2. **Monitor respiratory status if respiratory muscles are involved.** Mechanical ventilation may be necessary.

3. **Maximize functional abilities.**
   a. Prevent complications of immobility, such as deep vein thrombosis, constipation, contractures, and pressure ulcers. (See *Client and family teaching 13-1,* page 341.)
   b. Maximize effective communication. The client may need to use blinking of eyes when unable to move upper extremities.
4. **Promote adequate nutrition to prevent muscle wasting.**
   a. Encourage soft foods that are easy to swallow.
   b. If the client is unable to swallow, the client may need nasogastric tube feedings.
5. **Assist with plasmapheresis,** if prescribed.
6. **Provide a referral** for the Guillain-Barré Syndrome Foundation International. (See appendix A.)

XIV. MENINGITIS

A. **Description.** Meningitis is an infection or inflammation of the meninges covering the brain and spinal cord. Children are more prone than adults because of their greater propensity for respiratory infection.

B. **Etiology**
   1. Bacterial meningitis most often results from previous infection with *Neisseria meningitis, Streptococcus pneumoniae,* or *Haemophilus influenzae.*
   2. Aseptic meningitis may be caused by viral infection or other causes.

C. **Pathophysiology**
   1. Infective organisms that enter the brain quickly disseminate through the meninges and into the ventricles. Dissemination may result in:
      a. meningeal congestion
      b. cerebral edema
      c. increased intracranial pressure (ICP)
      d. generalized inflammation with exudate formation
      e. hydrocephalus if exudate blocks ventricular passages.
   2. Prognosis is good with early detection and prompt treatment; however, untreated meningitis or delayed treatment commonly proves fatal, particularly for children and elderly persons.

D. **Assessment findings**
   1. **Clinical manifestations**
      a. Headache and fever
      b. Altered level of consciousness
      c. Signs of meningeal irritation, such as nuchal rigidity, positive Brudzinski's and Kernig's signs, exaggerated deep tendon reflexes, and opisthotonos
      d. Signs and symptoms of increased ICP. (See section III.C.)
   2. **Laboratory and diagnostic study findings.** Cultures of cerebrospinal fluid identify infecting organisms.

E. **Nursing management (See section II.D.)**
   1. **Administer prescribed medications,** which include I.V. antibiotics. If seizures occur, anticonvulsants are prescribed. If cerebral edema occurs, osmotic diuretics are prescribed. (See *Drug chart 13-1,* page 343 to 345.)

2. **Prevent respiratory complications resulting from altered consciousness.** Implement such measures as oxygen therapy, arterial blood gases, pulmonary toileting, and pulse oximetry.

3. **Apply a hypothermia blanket** to relieve hyperthermia, as prescribed.

4. **Promote measures to help prevent recurrence of meningitis.**
    a. Persons in close contact with the client should be considered for prophylactic antibiotic therapy if appropriate.
    b. Administer vaccinations as indicated. A vaccination can be administered to prevent meningitis in pediatric clients; one type is currently prescribed for military recruits.

5. **Intervene as appropriate to reduce increased ICP.** (See section III.E.)

XV. BELL'S PALSY

A. **Description.** Bell's palsy is a disorder of the facial nerve (cranial nerve VII) producing unilateral facial paresis or paralysis. It affects all age groups but is most prevalent in persons younger than age 60.

B. **Etiology.** Bell's palsy results from facial nerve inflammation, most commonly because of infection, vascular disorders, or local trauma. In some cases, an autoimmune reaction may be involved.

C. **Pathophysiology**
   1. The inflamed, edematous facial nerve becomes compressed, causing paresis or paralysis of facial muscles.
   2. In most clients, spontaneous recovery occurs within 3 to 5 weeks. Partial recovery may leave the client with facial contractures.

D. **Assessment findings.** Clinical manifestations include:
   1. drooping mouth on one side, possibly with drooling
   2. possible pain
   3. inability to close the eyelid on the affected side.

E. **Nursing management**
   1. **Administer prescribed medications,** which may include corticosteroids. (See *Drug chart 13-1, pages 343 to 345.*)
   2. **Provide small, frequent feedings of soft foods.**
   3. **Provide eye care.** Teach the client to close his lids periodically and to use artificial tears.
   4. **Provide care for facial muscles.**
      a. Apply a facial sling to support facial muscles.
      b. Massage facial muscles gently and apply heat.

XVI. HYPERTHERMIA

A. **Description.** Hyperthermia (i.e., heat stroke) is an abnormally high body temperature caused by heat stress. Exertional heat stroke, caused by exercise in extreme heat and humidity, can cause death.

B. **Etiology**
   1. Exposure to high-humidity heat waves
   2. Age extremes

3. Debilitating disease
4. Impaired self-care ability
5. Certain drugs (e.g., major tranquilizers, anticholinergics, diuretics, propranolol)
6. Exertional heat stroke in healthy individuals during sports or work activities

C. **Pathophysiology.** Hyperthermia occurs when the body's heat-regulating mechanisms fail. Most heat-related deaths occur in elderly persons because their circulatory systems are unable to compensate for stress imposed by heat. Exertional heat stroke results because of inadequate heat loss.

D. **Assessment findings**
   1. **Clinical manifestations**
      a. Hyperpyrexia
      b. Altered level of consciousness (LOC): confusion, delirium, or coma
      c. Hot, dry skin with absence of sweating
      d. Tachycardia and tachypnea
      e. Hypotension
      f. Possibly, vomiting and diarrhea
   2. **Laboratory and diagnostic study findings.** Serum aspartate transaminase, lactate dehydrogenase, and creatinine kinase levels may be grossly elevated.

E. **Nursing management (See section II.D.)**
   1. **Reduce the client's body temperature rapidly.**
      a. Immerse the client in cool water.
      b. Sponge the client with cool water.
      c. Use a hypothermia blanket.
      d. Administer iced saline lavage.
   2. **Provide ongoing assessment.** Monitor vital signs, electrocardiographic findings, LOC, central venous pressure, and intake and output.
   3. **Promote circulation** by massaging the client.
   4. **Initiate I.V. fluids and oxygen therapy** as indicated.
   5. **Admit the client to the intensive care unit.**

XVII. COGNITIVE IMPAIRMENT DISORDERS

A. **Description**
   1. Cognitive impairment disorders are a group of chronic, progressive, organic mental disorders resulting in deterioration of the cognitive processes; most common are Alzheimer's disease and multi-infarct dementia.
   2. Alzheimer's disease accounts for more than 50% of dementias and affects 2% to 4% of persons older than age 65. Incidence increases with age, particularly after age 75. Multi-infarct dementia accounts for about 15% of cases of dementia; incidence is greater among men than women, and the onset generally is earlier than in Alzheimer's disease.

B. **Etiology**
   1. The cause of Alzheimer's disease is unknown, but many theories exist:
      a. Toxic chemical excess
      b. Autoimmune mechanism
      c. Slow virus mechanism
      d. One or more faulty genes.

2. Multi-infarct dementia results from cerebrovascular disease producing multiple small cerebral infarctions.

C. Pathophysiology

1. **Alzheimer's disease** is a chronic and irreversible disease characterized by specific neurologic and biochemical changes including:

   a. neurofibrillary tangles, granulovacuolar degeneration of neurons, and senile or neuritic plaques, primarily in the cerebral cortex

   b. brain atrophy, with widened cortical sulci and enlarged cerebral ventricles

   c. decreased acetylcholine production.

2. **Multi-infarct dementia.** Pathologic changes include multiple areas of extensive localized softening along with various changes in cerebral vessels.

D. Assessment findings

1. **Clinical manifestations**

   a. **Alzheimer's disease.** Signs and symptoms are highly variable and may include:

   - early, subtle changes such as forgetfulness, recent memory loss, and poor concentration, which the client may be able to hide

   - later, more overt signs of impaired cognition (e.g., severe memory loss and forgetfulness; inability to hold a conversation, think abstractly, or formulate concepts; poor hygiene and grooming and inappropriate dress; inability to perform instrumental activities of daily living [ADLs])

   - behavioral changes, such as depression, anxiety, wandering, impulsive behavior, catastrophic reactions, imitation, emotional lability, and withdrawal.

   b. **Multi-infarct dementia.** Clinical manifestations include:

   - dizziness, headaches

   - confusion

   - patchy memory loss

   - hallucinations and delusions

   - focal neurologic signs (e.g., muscle weakness, dysreflexia, dysarthria).

2. **Laboratory and diagnostic study findings**

   a. Computed tomography, electroencephalography, and positron emission tomography are useful in excluding hematomas, brain tumors, stroke, normal-pressure hydrocephalus, and atrophy but are not reliable in making a definitive diagnosis of Alzheimer's disease.

   b. Autopsy is the definitive diagnosis of Alzheimer's disease.

E. Nursing management (See section II.D.)

1. **Administer prescribed medications,** such as tacrine HCl, which slows progression of Alzheimer's disease by maintaining the availability of dopamine but with very toxic hepatic effects. These medications are more effective when administered early in the disease. There are no medications effective in preventing the progression of disease.

2. **Provide initial and ongoing assessments.**

   a. Record the client's usual daily routine as well as words and behaviors used to communicate ADL needs; validate this information with a reliable second source in a separate interview, and chart words and techniques that "get through" to the client.

   b. Request that a family member stay with the client if the client wanders or cannot be sent to diagnostic tests alone; avoid sedation and restraints whenever possible.

   c. Assign the client to a room that maximizes the potential for observation and is not next to an exit or stairwell (if the client is prone to wandering).

    d. Orient the client to the room and the unit; mark the room and bedside area with familiar belongings.

    e. Attach an ID bracelet; alert others to wandering (e.g., special clothing, care plan, posted notice).

    f. Determine if the client has an advance directive or a durable power of attorney for health care. (If so, obtain a copy.)

3. Maximize effective communication.

    a. Use short sentences, simple words, gestures, and written or pictorial cues, if needed; explain and repeat instructions unless this increases distress.

    b. Maintain a calm demeanor and a consistent approach.

    c. Avoid excessive questioning and confrontation.

    d. Break down instructions into simple components.

    e. Support the anxious or depressed client.

    f. Attempt to analyze behavior for meaning.

4. Maximize environmental safety.

    a. Install alarms on stairwells.

    b. Institute injury, fire, and poisoning precautions.

    c. Provide adequate lighting in all rooms.

    d. Keep the bed in a low position or place the mattress on the floor (side rails may pose a hazard).

    e. Place a wanderer's bracelet on the client.

    f. Intervene as necessary to manage evening agitation (i.e., "sun-downing"); provide a night light, soft music, and supervision.

    g. Create a limited-access, safe unit to obviate activity restriction and decrease the need for supervision, if indicated.

5. Promote optimal functioning.

    a. Fit daily diagnostic and therapeutic procedures into the client's usual schedule as possible.

    b. Assign consistent caregivers.

    c. Establish a daily routine for care, maintaining the client's preadmission sleep-wake cycle if possible and desirable.

    d. Provide a clock, calendar, and daily schedule in the room (but avoid pressuring the client for accuracy).

    e. Prompt for ADLs with memory aids and verbal cues, and encourage performance within the limits of ability (avoiding pressure for performance, which could trigger catastrophic reaction).

    f. Focus the client on simple, repetitive, and purposeful activities with sequencing of skills.

    g. Monitor the client for adverse effects of drug therapy.

    h. Encourage ambulation and other exercise.

    i. Ensure good grooming and personal hygiene.

    j. Use distraction to alter undesirable behavior, break episodes of preservation, or remove from harm.

    k. Intervene as necessary to calm an agitated client.

    l. Limit stimuli (e.g., noise, people, caffeine).

    m. Regularly assess the skin, gums, teeth, and feet for breakdown and infection, and provide good skin and mouth care.

    n. Maximize opportunities for social interaction.

    o. Provide touch, respect, affection, praise, and the opportunity for choice.

6. **Optimize nutrition and fluid balance.**
    a. Monitor food and fluid intake, noting increased or decreased hunger and thirst.
    b. Remind the client to eat regularly.
    c. Provide small, frequent meals with high-calorie supplements if appropriate.
    d. Match food consistency to the client's chewing and swallowing ability.

7. **Optimize elimination.**
    a. Make sure the client knows where the bathroom is to encourage its use.
    b. Monitor bowel-elimination patterns.
    c. Prevent constipation.
    d. Give periodic reminders to urinate.
    e. Schedule toileting based on voiding pattern.
    f. Provide protective pants as indicated.

8. **Provide discharge planning.**
    a. Begin discharge planning on the client's admission to the hospital.
    b. Determine whether the client will be discharged to home alone, to live with family, or to a long term care facility; evaluate whether independent living could be hazardous to the client.
    c. As indicated, assist the client's family in arranging for a long-term care center, day care, or respite care.
    d. Encourage regular health care after discharge.
    e. Document all client information on transfer forms to promote continuity of care.
    f. Teach home caregivers to assist the client with ADLs as needed and to provide any special care required.
    g. Refer the client and family to community agencies, legal and financial counseling, and the Alzheimer's Association and Alzheimer's Disease Education and Referral Center. (See appendix A.)

XVIII. SUBSTANCE ABUSE

A. Description. Substance abuse refers to misuse of specific substances intended to alter mood or behavior.

B. Etiology. Commonly abused substances, which are often used in combination, include:
1. alcohol
2. opioids
3. hallucinogens
4. amphetamines
5. barbiturates.

C. Assessment findings
1. **Clinical manifestations** of substance abuse vary widely, depending on the substance and the amount ingested. Common signs and symptoms include:
    a. signs of central nervous system depression or stimulation
    b. altered temperature (hypothermia or hyperthermia)
    c. respiratory depression or tachypnea
    d. hallucinations
    e. seizure activity
    f. abnormal pupil size and response
    g. nausea and vomiting.

2. **Laboratory and diagnostic study findings**
   a. Blood urea nitrogen and serum creatinine levels may be elevated.
   b. Arterial blood gas values may reveal acidosis or alkalosis.
   c. Serum or urine analysis may identify the substance.

D. Nursing management (See section II.D.)

1. **Treat the client suffering from drug overdose.**
   a. Monitor cardiovascular status.
   b. Control airway, ventilation, and oxygenation. (Insertion of a cuffed endotracheal tube may be necessary.)
   c. Aid in elimination of drugs from the body.
      – Remove the ingested drug from the stomach with syrup of ipecac or gastric lavage as ordered; prevent aspiration in a client with absent gag or cough reflexes by first intubating him.
      – Administer the specific drug antidote (e.g., naloxone for opioid overdose; activated charcoal only after emesis or lavage).
      – Assist with hemodialysis or peritoneal dialysis as indicated.
   d. Start I.V. fluid infusion as indicated.

2. **Promote client and family coping.**
   a. Develop a supportive, empathic rapport, and attend the client at all times.
   b. Arrange consultation with psychiatrist or drug or alcohol treatment program before discharge.

3. **Refer the client and family** to support groups such as Alcoholics Anonymous. (See appendix A.)

Study questions

1. When monitoring a client for early signs of increasing intracranial pressure, the nurse should be particularly alert for which assessment data?
1. Pupillary changes
2. Difficulty arousing the client
3. Decreasing blood pressure
4. Elevated temperature

2. Which nursing intervention should the nurse implement for a client experiencing a tonic-clonic seizure?
1. Placing a tongue blade between the client's clenched teeth
2. Elevating the client's head at least 30 to 60 degrees
3. Protecting the extremities from contact with other objects
4. Firmly restraining the arms and legs alongside the body

3. Which clinical manifestation would alert the nurse to the possibility of meningitis?
1. Unilateral mouth drooping
2. Postactivity muscle weakness
3. Impaired speech and swallowing
4. Nuchal rigidity

4. Which clinical manifestations would the nurse expect to assess in a client diagnosed with Guillain-Barré syndrome?
1. Headache and nuchal rigidity
2. Unilateral mouth drooping and pain
3. Severe fatigue and diplopia
4. Leg paresis and paresthesia

5. A client has sustained a severe head injury and damaged the prefrontal lobe. Which complication should the nurse expect to assess in the client?

1. Visual impairment
2. Swallowing difficulty
3. Impaired judgment
4. Hearing impairment

6. A client who was in a motor vehicle accident was admitted to the intensive care unit (ICU) with severe head trauma. What nursing interventions should the ICU nurse implement when caring for the client? (Select all that apply.)
   1. Administering osmotic diuretics as prescribed
   2. Hypooxygenating the client before suctioning
   3. Encouraging the client to perform Valsalva's maneuver every 4 hours
   4. Keeping the bed flat at all times
   5. Reducing or eliminating noxious stimuli
   6. Instituting seizure precautions

7. Which statement would be included in the teaching plan for the client scheduled for a carotid angiography?
   1. "You will receive general anesthesia before the needle is inserted."
   2. "The test will take several hours to complete."
   3. "You may feel a burning sensation when the contrast dye is injected."
   4. "There are relatively few serious complications with this procedure."

8. After a stroke, which statement by the client indicates that teaching about passive range-of-motion (ROM) exercises has been sucessful?
   1. "I do these exercises by myself with the supervision of the nurse."
   2. "The nurse can help me do them if I have trouble doing them on my own."
   3. "I should sit at the side of the bed to perform the exercises."
   4. "The nurse performs the exercises without any help from me."

9. Which intervention would have priority when providing emergency care to a client with a possible cervical spinal injury?
   1. Monitoring vital signs every 5 minutes
   2. Placing the neck in position of flexion
   3. Checking to see if the client can move his toes
   4. Immobilizing the head and spine in proper alignment

10. Which response by the nurse would be most appropriate for a client with aphasia who states, "I want a ..." and then stops?
   1. Waiting for the client to complete the sentence
   2. Immediately showing the client various objects in the environment
   3. Leaving the room and coming back later
   4. Beginning naming objects the client could be referring to

11. Which statement by the nurse would be appropriate when assisting a client with a neurologic disorder who has the nursing diagnosis of altered thought processes with self-care deficits?
   1. "What would you like to do first: brush your teeth?"
   2. "Where is your toothbrush?"
   3. "When would you like to have your bath?"
   4. "Do you want to brush your teeth or have me do it for you?"

12. Which position would be most appropriate for a client with right-sided paralysis after a stroke?
   1. Side lying with hips slightly flexed and pillows in the axilla
   2. Semi-Fowler's position, with hands tightly holding a washcloth
   3. Supine with two large pillows under the head and a footboard
   4. Prone for at least 2 hours with trochanter rolls and a footboard

13. In assisting a client diagnosed with multiple sclerosis (MS), which topic would be important to include in client teaching?
1. Effect of stress and fatigue on symptoms
2. Need for small, frequent meals
3. Need for strenuous exercise
4. Positive effect of a high-protein diet

14. When teaching the client diagnosed with myasthenia gravis about anticholinesterase medications, which intervention should the nursing include in the discussion?
1. Giving instructions to take medication 30 minutes before eating meals
2. Explaining that atropine is used to determine a myasthenic or cholinergic crisis
3. Discussing the importance of tapering the dose when discontinuing this medication
4. Discussing the need to avoid exposure to ultraviolet rays of the sun with this medication

15. Which statement describes the halo sign exhibited by a client with a head injury?
1. Presence of glucose in ear drainage
2. Cerebral artery dilation because of a weakness in the arterial wall
3 Cerebrospinal fluid (CSF) leakage of blood surrounded by a yellow stain
4. Temporary neurologic dysfunction from decreased cerebral blood supply

16. In which area would the nurse expect loss of motor control and sensation if the client experienced a spinal cord injury below the level of L4?
1. Below the mid-chest
2. Parts of the arms and hands
3. Legs and pelvis
4. Parts of the thighs and legs

Answer key

1. The answer is **2.**
The first sign of pressure on the reticular activating system in the brain stem is a decrease in responsiveness, evidenced by difficulty in arousing the client. Pupillary changes occur later. Systolic blood pressure increases, not decreases, with increased intracranial pressure. Temperature changes vary and may not be present even with severe decreases in responsiveness.

2. The answer is **3.**
Because of the tonic-clonic motions, protecting the client by moving objects so that the arms and legs do not hit them and placing a soft object under the head are the most important immediate interventions. Trying to force a tongue blade or other object into the mouth may damage the teeth. Nothing is gained by elevating the client's head, because breathing will return to normal after the activity stops. Restraining movement may result in injury or stiffness after the seizure.

3. The answer is **4.**
Meningitis results in meningeal irritation. Signs of meningeal irritation include nuchal rigidity, positive Brudzinski's and Kernig's signs, exaggerated deep tendon reflexes, and opisthotonos. Unilateral mouth drooping suggests Bell's palsy. Muscle weakness, especially after activity, suggests myasthenia gravis. Impaired speech and swallowing may suggest amyotrophic lateral sclerosis or be the result of a stroke.

4. The answer is **4.**
Common signs and symptoms of Guillain-Barré syndrome include leg paresis (usually the initial manifestation); motor weakness progressing to involve the entire peripheral nervous system, including respiratory mus-

cles; and paresthesias. A client diagnosed with meningitis exhibits nuchal rigidity and complains of a headache. Unilateral mouth drooping and pain occur with Bell's palsy. Diplopia along with severe fatigue is seen in a client diagnosed with myasthenia gravis.

5. The answer is **3.**

A number of areas of the brain are involved in cognition and thinking, but damage to the prefrontal area usually results in impaired judgment and insight. Vision problems may occur with pathology in the occipital lobe or in the pituitary area (i.e., optic chiasm). Swallowing problems result from damage to cranial nerve IX in the brain stem. Hearing impairment commonly occurs with damage to cranial nerve VIII.

6. The answers are **1, 5, 6.**

Because the client with severe head trauma is at risk for increased intracranial pressure (ICP), osmotic diuretics are administered to help reduce cerebral edema, seizure precautions are instituted, and safety measures — such as reducing noxious stimuli — should be instituted until normal neurologic status is restored. The client should be hyperoxygenated prior to suctioning, Valsalva's maneuver would increase ICP, and the head of the bed should be elevated to 30 degrees.

7. The answer is **3.**

Providing a client with information about expected sensations often helps decrease anxiety. The contrast medium commonly causes a burning sensation as it passes through the cerebral arteries. Clients rarely receive general anesthesia for angiography. The test usually takes less than an hour. Various serious complications, such as airway obstruction and vasospasm with sensory and motor deficits, may occur after an angiogram.

8. The answer is **4.**

Passive ROM exercises are defined as those performed by one person to the joints of a client, without any help from the client. The client's performance of the exercises is called active ROM. Performing the exercises by himself with some assistance if trouble is encountered is referred to assisted ROM. ROM exercises are usually done *in* bed but can be done anywhere.

9. The answer is **4.**

The most important consideration when dealing with a client who has a possible cervical spinal injury is to immobilize the head and spine in alignment to prevent possible fractures or dislocated bone from damaging the spinal cord. Monitoring the client's vital signs is important but secondary to immobilization. Flexing the neck can cause spinal cord damage. Clients with suspected spinal injuries should avoid movement until spinal cord damage is ruled out.

10. The answer is **1.**

The client with aphasia may need additional time to select the proper words when speaking. It is essential for the nurse to allow the client time to complete the sentence. Showing or naming various objectives and leaving the room are inappropriate responses. Actions such as these often lead to additional client frustration, anxiety, and feelings of low self-esteem.

11. The answer is **2.**

Because the client has problems with altered thought and has self-care deficits, the nurse needs to make the decisions. Simple questions and directions are most appropriate. This client probably is not capable of making decisions at this time. Asking what the client wants to do first, when he would like to have his bath, or whether he wants to brush his own teeth or have the nurse do it for him require the client to make a decision. These types of questions are inappropriate in this situation.

12. The answer is **1.**

For a client with right-sided paralysis after a stroke, the client should be placed on his side with the hips slightly flexed in as natural a position as possible and with pillows placed in the axillary area to prevent adduction. A semi-Fowler's position may cause too great a degree of hip flexion. Having the client's hands tightly holding a washcloth could lead to contractures. The supine position is avoided to minimize the risk of aspiration, and placing too many pillows under the head may interfere with breathing and pull the rest of the body out of alignment. Although the prone position should be used if possible, it should be used only for 15 to 30 minutes several times each day.

13. The answer is **1**.
Studies have shown that stress and fatigue adversely affect the course of MS. The teaching plan needs to address these topics. Teaching stress-management techniques and helping the client adjust her schedule to ensure adequate rest are beneficial. Small, frequent feedings are not a priority for a client with MS. Vigorous exercise can lead to fatigue, possibly exacerbating the disease. Increased protein intake is not associated with MS treatment.

14. The answer is **1**.
Anticholinesterase agents inhibit the breakdown of acetylcholine, providing the client with more strength for activities such as eating. The medication should be taken daily at the same time to ensure maximum strength available for activity. Tensilon is used to determine the type of crisis. Atropine is the antidote for cholinergic crisis. Anticholinesterase medications are prescribed for life, and tapering is not suggested. Anticholinesterase medications do not cause photosensitivity.

15. The answer is **3**.
A halo sign refers to the leakage of CSF that appears bloody and is surrounded by a yellow stain. The presence of glucose in ear drainage denotes otorrhea. Cerebral artery dilation because of a weakness in the arterial wall describes a cerebral aneurysm. Temporary neurologic dysfunction because of a decrease in cerebral blood supply refers to a transient ischemic attack.

16. The answer is **4**.
With a spinal cord injury below the level of L4, the client typically experiences loss of motor control and sensation in parts of the thighs and legs. Loss of motor control and sensation from below the mid-chest occurs in clients with a spinal cord injury below T6, but motor control and sensation are preserved in the arms and hands. Loss of motor control and sensation to parts of the arms and hands is seen in a client with injury below C8. With all these injuries, bowel and bladder control is lost.

14

Eye, ear, nose, sinus, and throat disorders

I. EYES

A. **Structures.** Anatomically, the eye can be divided into three layers, or coats (i.e., outer, middle, and inner), and the refractive media. (See *Figure 14-1.*)

1. **The outer, protective layer**
   a. The **sclera** is the white, opaque, fibrous connective tissue.
   b. The **cornea** is the anterior continuation of the sclera, which is transparent and avascular.

2. **The middle, vascular layer** (i.e., uveal tract)
   a. The **choroid** is a thin, pigmented membrane containing blood vessels that supply eye tissues.
   b. The **ciliary body** is the anterior continuation of the choroid containing muscles that change the shape of the lens to focus vision.
   c. The **iris** is the central extension of the ciliary body, consisting of two muscles and a central opening, the pupil, which constricts and dilates to regulate the amount of light entering the eye's interior (i.e., constricts with strong light and near vision, dilates with dim light and far vision).

3. The **inner, neural layer** (i.e., retina) contains layers of nerve cells, including rods and cones, that translate light waves into neural impulses for transmission to the brain.

4. **Refractive media**
   a. The **cornea** is the transparent layer that forms the external coat of the anterior portion of the eye.
   b. The **aqueous humor** is watery fluid filling the eye's anterior chamber that serves as a refracting medium and maintains the hydrostatic intraocular pressure.
   c. The **lens** is a biconvex crystalline body located behind the pupil that changes shape for accommodation (i.e., focusing).

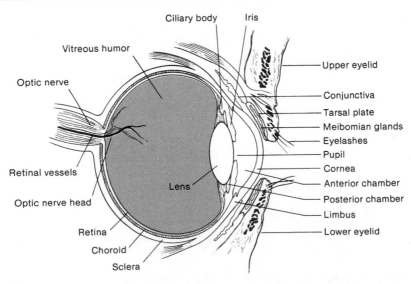

FIGURE 14-1
Transverse section of the eye

Source: Fuller J., and Schaller-Ayers, J. *Health Assessment: A Nursing Approach,* 3rd ed. Philadelphia: Lippincott Williams & Wilkins, 2000.

      d. The **vitreous humor** is a jelly-like substance filling the posterior cavity behind the lens, acting as a refractive medium and maintaining the shape of the eye.

B. Function

1. Vision depends on a complex coordination of ocular structures that mediate passage of light rays reflected from an external object to the retina and transmit visual images to the brain for interpretation.
2. Normally, light passes through the refractive media to the retina, where an inverted and reversed image forms.
3. In the retina, rods and cones convert the projected image into nerve impulses and transmit them to the optic nerve.
4. Impulses travel along the optic nerve to the brain's optic chiasm and then to the cerebral cortex, where they are interpreted as sight.

NURSING PROCESS OVERVIEW

 II. THE EYES

A. Assessment

1. **Health history**

   a. **Elicit a description of the client's present illness and chief complaint,** including onset, course, duration, location, and precipitating and alleviating factors. Cardinal signs and symptoms include:
   - decreased visual acuity
   - blurred vision
   - decreased color perception
   - pain in the eye.

   b. **Explore the client's health history for risk factors** associated with eye disorders, including:
   - family history of eye disease
   - systemic medical conditions
   - sports injuries
   - laser surgery
   - blows to the head
   - vitamin A deficiency
   - certain medications.

2. **Physical examination**

   a. **Inspection**
   - Assess for head tilting, squinting, or other noticeable postural characteristics.
   - Assess for symmetry in the appearance of the eyes.
   - Inspect the eyebrows and eyelashes for distribution of hair growth.
   - Inspect the eyelid for ptosis, redness, lesions, and edema.
   - Assess the sclera for whiteness.
   - Inspect the cornea for transparency, smoothness, shininess, and brightness.
   - Assess for the blink reflex.

   b. **Measurement of vision**
   - The visual fields confrontation test evaluates the peripheral extent of visual fields (other than central reading vision). Normal findings include 60 degrees nasally, 50 degrees upward, 90 degrees temporally, and 70 degrees downward.

- In vision testing, Snellen's chart is used to evaluate visual acuity, and newsprint is used to assess near vision. Normal visual acuity is considered to be 20/20, in which the numerator represents the distance from the person to chart and the denominator the distance at which a normal eye can read the line; the larger the denominator, the poorer the vision.
- Used to prescribe corrective lenses, the refraction test requires the person to read a Snellen's chart through various corrective lenses to measure errors of focus: myopia (i.e., nearsightedness), hyperopia (i.e., farsightedness), and astigmatism (i.e., inability to focus horizontal and vertical rays on retina).

3. **Laboratory and diagnostic studies**
    a. **Culture and smears of eye exudate** are performed to identify presence and type of bacteria.
    b. **Computed tomography** visualizes the globes, extraocular muscles, and optic nerves.
    c. **Radioisotopic scanning** is used to locate tumors, lesions, and hemorrhaging in the optic body.
    d. A **tonometer** measures intraocular pressure (IOP), which normally ranges from 12 to 21 mm Hg.
    e. **Ophthalmoscopic examination** evaluates blood vessels and structures of the posterior eye (i.e., fundus), detecting retinal changes caused by neurologic or vascular conditions.
    f. **Ultrasonography** aids in the diagnosis of trauma and intraorbital tumors and helps to determine gross outline changes in the eye.
    g. **Slit-lamp examination** permits microscopic magnification of anterior ocular structures.

B. **Nursing diagnoses**
    1. Disturbed visual and sensory perception
    2. Acute pain
    3. Risk for injury
    4. Dressing or grooming self-care deficit
    5. Deficient knowledge
    6. Anxiety

C. **Planning and outcome identification.** The major goals for the client diagnosed with an eye disorder may include prevention of further visual deterioration; pain relief; injury prevention; independence in self-care activities; knowledge of the disease process, treatment, and eye care; and control of anxiety.

D. **Implementation**
    1. **Promote measures that addresses the client's visual disorder.**
        a. Use large, bold letters for printed client-education materials and signs. Avoid muted colors, especially in the blue and green spectrum; a sharp color contrast from background promotes readability.
        b. Protect the client from injury: Keep paths clear of obstacles, provide adequate lighting, and avoid glare.
        c. The nurse should identify herself when approaching the client.
        d. Insert a notation regarding the client's visual deficit in the care plan.
        e. Keep the client's belongings and essential equipment in consistent locations within the client's visual field.

CLIENT AND FAMILY TEACHING 14-1
Guidelines for eye care

- Recommend that the client have his eyes checked yearly by an ophthalmologist.
- Advise the client to always wash his hands thoroughly before touching or rubbing his eyes.
- Instruct the client to read instructions carefully before using cleaning fluids, detergents, or harsh chemicals.
- Instruct the client to wear glasses, goggles, or safety glasses to protect eyes when around dust particles, flying fragments, fumes, and harsh chemicals.
- Instruct the client to wear safety glasses for sports, especially raquetball, tennis, baseball, and basketball.
- Instruct the client to wear protective caps or helmets when playing sports, such as ice hockey, skating, and football.

- Advise the client to be extremely careful when using explosive fireworks or to avoid their use entirely.
- Suggest that the client, when mowing the lawn or doing garden work, pick up all rocks, stones, and branches. Tell him to also avoid low-hanging branches and refrain from letting anyone stand on the mower.
- Instruct the client to irrigate his eyes immediately with warm water or saline if they come into contact with chemicals.
- Advise the client to wear a hat or sunglasses when out in the sun and not to look directly into the sun.

---

   f. Help the client obtain assistive devices (e.g., magnifying lenses, large-print books) as necessary.

   g. Teach the client the importance of annual eye examinations.

2. Promote measures to prevent or decrease pain and discomfort.

   a. Apply bilateral patching, which helps limit eye movement (i.e., eyes move in synchrony), relieving pain.

   b. Reduce lighting, because light causes pain in many eye conditions.

   c. Instruct the client to avoid reading or watching TV when having eye pain.

   d. Assess the client's eye pain, rule out any complications that require immediate intervention, administer prescribed analgesics or antibiotics, and evaluate the effectiveness of the nursing interventions.

3. Promote measures that help prevent and care for injuries to the eye.

   a. Teach the client measures to prevent eye injuries as detailed in *Client and family teaching 14-1.*

   b. If the client has ophthalmic trauma, apply a light dressing over both eyes (do not apply pressure) because movement of the eyes should be kept at a minimum.

   c. If the client has a nonpenetrating foreign body in the eye, lift the upper lid over the lower lid, allowing the lashes of the lower lid to brush the object off the inside of the upper lid. If this does not work, irrigate the eye.

   d. If the client has a foreign body penetrating the eye, notify the ophthalmologist. *Do not remove the foreign body.* The eye is anesthetized, and the foreign object is then removed. In some circumstances, surgery may be required.

   e. If the client has a corneal abrasion, apply a pressure eye patch to immobilize the lid and promote comfort and healing. For extensive abrasions, bilateral patching and bed rest may be prescribed.

   f. If the client has a chemical burn, irrigate the eye with copious amounts of physiologic solution or water immediately for at least 20 minutes.

   g. If the client has blunt trauma to the eye, apply cold compresses and rule out further trauma.

   h. If the client has a ruptured globe (i.e., eyeball), cover the eye with an eye shield, and notify the ophthalmologist immediately. *Do not touch the eye or administer eye drops.*

4. **Encourage the client to carry out as much self-care as possible to promote a feeling of self-sufficiency.**
   a. Assist the client with activities of daily living (ADLs) as needed.
   b. Ensure that any medication bottles or instructions are labeled in large letters and used where there is plenty of light.
   c. Assist the client's family with preparing the home for the client's condition, removing all obstacles, obtaining any assistive devices available, and discussing how to handle emergency situations and a wide variety of other potential problems.
   d. When blindness is permanent, reeducation in ADLs may be performed by specially trained personnel or persons with similar conditions and concerns.

5. **Instruct the client about the correct way to prepare for instillation of eye drops.**
   a. Explain the importance of keeping all eye medications sterile.
   b. Instruct the client to not use unlabeled, cloudy, or discolored solutions.
   c. Instruct the client to avoid contact with the eye to prevent contaminating the medication bottle or tube tip.
   d. Instruct the client to treat each eye separately (i.e., separate medication and equipment); treat the uninfected eye first to avoid cross contamination.

6. **Instruct the client about the correct way to instill eye drops.**
   a. Teach the client to follow the health care provider's instructions for administration of eye drops in the proper eye; OS indicates the left eye, OD indicates the right eye, and OU indicates both eyes.
   b. Tilt the client's head back slightly, and expose the lower conjunctival sac by pulling down gently on the cheekbone.
   c. Have the client look up.
   d. Resting a hand on the client's forehead for support to prevent eye injury during administration, instill the prescribed amount of medication onto the lower conjunctiva.
   e. Close the lid gently and press on the nasal-lacrimal canal (i.e., inner canthus) to prevent systemic drug absorption and resulting adverse effects.
   f. Wipe excess secretions with a sterile cotton ball, wiping from the inner to the outer canthus.

7. **Instruct the client about the correct way to instill eye ointment.**
   a. Follow the same basic procedure as for instilling eye drops.
   b. Have the client close the lid and roll the eye after instillation.

8. **Instruct the client about the correct way to apply an eye patch.**
   a. Have the client close both eyes during patch application.
   b. Apply the patch and secure it with two strips of tape extending from the mid-forehead to the lateral cheekbone.
   c. Never apply pressure unless prescribed; if pressure is indicated, use two or three pads and more tape.
   d. Never change an eye patch without a health care provider's order.

9. **Instruct the client about the correct way to apply an eye shield.**
   a. Apply an eye shield, alone or over an eye patch, to protect the eye from pressure or irritation.
   b. Rest the shield on the bony prominences of the brow, cheek, and nose, and secure it in place with strips of transparent tape in the same manner as for an eye patch (i.e., medial top to lateral bottom).

10. **Promote measures that help decrease anxiety when loss of sight occurs.**
    a. Encourage the client to ventilate feelings of anxiety, fear, and depression, which are common reactions to loss of sight, whether temporary or permanent.
    b. Assess and encourage the client to participate in diversionary activities (e.g., radio, tape player, books on tape).
    c. If blindness is permanent, encourage to the client to get a seeing-eye dog to increase independence, which helps decrease anxiety.
    d. Allow the client time to grieve when blindness is permanent.
11. **Provide preoperative nursing interventions for the client undergoing eye surgery.**
    a. Explain expected preoperative procedures (e.g., sedation, local or general anesthetic) to reduce anxiety associated with the unfamiliar and unexpected.
    b. For the same reason, explain what to expect postoperatively (e.g., eye-patch application, prescribed positioning, activity restrictions, ophthalmic medication use, measures to prevent increased IOP, a small amount of serous drainage and subjunctival hemorrhage postoperatively, eyelid edema for several days).
12. **Provide postoperative nursing interventions for the client undergoing eye surgery.**
    a. Take precautions to prevent increased IOP.
       – Instruct the client to lie on the unoperated side.
       – Advise the client to avoid constipation (e.g., by administering stool softeners).
       – Encourage the client to avoid sneezing or coughing (or to cough with the mouth open, if necessary).
       – Administer an antiemetic to a client who is nauseous to prevent vomiting.
       – Wash the client's hair, when allowed, with the neck hyperextended rather than flexed.
       – Instruct the client to avoid excessive exertion, such as lifting and pushing objects.
    b. Take precautions to prevent injury.
       – Orient the client to the hospital environment.
       – Keep a call bell and other needed items within the client's reach and in a consistent place.
       – Keep the bed in a low position with the side rails up.
       – Provide adequate room light or dim lights if the client experiences photophobia.
       – Assist the client with ambulation, if indicated.
       – Advise the client not to rub the eyes or touch an eye patch.
    c. Relieve postoperative discomfort with proper positioning and analgesics as prescribed; avoid opiates, which may cause vomiting or constipation.
    d. Instruct the client to report any sharp pain or feelings of pressure in the eye, which may indicate hemorrhage, increased IOP, or infection. Instruct the client to report signs and symptoms of additional complications, such as coughing, marked restlessness, or any eye pain unrelieved by analgesics.
    e. Promote mobility within postoperative restrictions; post any prescribed activity restrictions on the client's bed.
    f. Prevent sensory deprivation.
       – Provide sensory stimulation (e.g., talk to the client often, provide a radio or TV, encourage frequent visitation by family and friends).
       – Frequently reorient the client to the environment and the date and time of day.
    g. Promote adequate nutrition; assist the client with eating and drinking, as necessary, to ensure adequate intake and to prevent choking and aspiration.
    h. Teach appropriate self-care measures, which may include:
       – not removing an eye patch unless specifically ordered

- wearing an eye shield at night or when lying down
- taking sponge baths or showers without getting water on the face
- wearing dark glasses and dimming room lights if experiencing photophobia or using dilating drops
- taking medications as prescribed.

13. **Provide referrals** to the American Foundation for the Blind and Lighthouse International. (See appendix A.)

E. Outcome evaluation

1. The client exhibits positive adjustment to altered vision and rehabilitative requirements and adheres to activity and positioning requirements.
2. The client reports an adequate comfort level after surgery.
3. The client remains free of eye and other injuries.
4. The client is able to maintain independence in ADLs.
5. The client verbalizes an understanding of prescribed medications, demonstrates appropriate administration technique of eye medications, and verbalizes the importance of carrying medical identification and of avoiding activities that can increase IOP.
6. The client displays low anxiety during the period of visual impairment.

III. RETINAL DETACHMENT

A. Description. Retinal detachment is a separation of the retina from the choroid in the posterior eye. It most commonly affects persons older than age 40.

B. Etiology. Retinal detachment may result from trauma, age-related degenerative changes, or cataract removal.

C. Pathophysiology

1. Retinal layers separate from the choroid, creating a subretinal space. Vitreous fluid seeps between these layers, disrupting choroidal blood supply.
2. Detachment may be partial, causing various degrees of visual deficits, or total, causing blindness in the affected eye.

D. Assessment findings

1. **Clinical manifestations**
   a. Recurrent flashes of light and floating spots initially
   b. Progressive blurring of vision in the affected eye, followed by visual field deficits, with the area of visual loss depending on the area of detachment
   c. Anxiety, confusion, and fear of becoming blind
2. **Laboratory and diagnostic study findings.** Ophthalmoscopic examination may reveal an area of gray, opaque retina, possibly with folds, holes, or tears.

E. Nursing management (See section II.D.)

1. **Discuss and provide written information regarding surgical options,** which may include:
   a. creating localized chorioretinal adhesions to reapproximate the retina and choroid through cryotherapy, photocoagulation, or laser surgery
   b. sealing the retina to the choroid with scleral buckling surgery
   c. injecting an intraocular gas bubble to promote adhesion.
2. **Promote measures that limit mobility to prevent further injury.**

a. Position the client in bed preoperatively as prescribed (usually with the detached area dependent), and instruct the client to avoid lying face down, stooping, or bending.

b. Enforce bed rest for 1 day postoperatively, with the client positioned supine or on the unoperated side unless otherwise directed.

3. Promote measures that assist with the client's adaptation to the perceptual impairment.

a. Preoperatively, patch both eyes if detachment threatens the macula.

b. Administer sedation as prescribed, promote comfort and relaxation, and minimize eye strain.

c. Administer prescribed medications, which may include adrenergic agonist agents (mydriatic) and anticholinergic (cycloplegic) agents. (See *Drug chart 14-1, pages* 380 and 381.)

4. Provide postoperative care.

a. Patch the affected eye for 1 to 4 hours.

b. Encourage visitors, socialization, sensory stimulation, and diversionary activities.

c. Administer mild analgesics for discomfort, and apply cool or warm compresses to edematous eyelids.

5. Instruct the client on discharge instructions.

a. Discuss allowed and restricted activities.

b. Discuss prescribed positions.

c. Instruct the client on the resumption of activity, including resuming activities of daily living gradually and as tolerated, commonly resuming light work in 3 weeks and normal activity in 6 weeks; avoiding heavy lifting, deep bending, or stooping (possibly for life); and avoiding bumping or otherwise injuring the head.

IV. GLAUCOMA

A. Description

1. Glaucoma refers to a group of disorders characterized by abnormally elevated intraocular pressure (IOP), which can damage the optic nerve.

2. Types include:

   a. chronic open-angle glaucoma

   b. acute closed-angle (or narrow-angle) glaucoma.

3. The second most common cause of blindness in the United States, glaucoma affects about 2% of the population older than age 40.

B. Etiology. Glaucoma may be congenital, inherited, or related to previous trauma.

C. Pathophysiology

1. In **chronic open-angle glaucoma,** obstruction to outflow of aqueous humor through the trabecular meshwork into Schlemm's canal leads to increased IOP. It usually is bilateral. Increased IOP eventually destroys optic nerve function, causing blindness.

2. **Acute closed-angle glaucoma** results in increased IOP because of obstructed outflow of aqueous humor. However, acute closed-angle glaucoma typically involves sudden, complete, unilateral closure, with pupil dilation stimulated by a dark environment, emotional stress, or mydriatic drugs. It is considered a medical emergency; delay in treatment leads to blindness within several days of onset.

DRUG CHART 14-1
Medications for eye, ears, nose, sinus, and throat disorders

Classifications	Indications	Selected interventions
Adrenergic agonists (mydriatic agents) epinephrine (dipivefrin converts to epinephrine in the eye) phenylephrine	Diagnose and treat ophthalmic disorders; cause pupillary dilatation but does not cause paralysis of the ciliary body	▪ Instruct the client to wear sunglasses until the medication wears off. ▪ Instruct the client to avoid driving or operating hazardous machinery until the medication wears off. ▪ Instruct the client about the correct administration of eye drops.
Antibiotics amoxicillin erythromycin penicillin	Prevent or treat infections caused by pathogenic microorganisms	▪ Before administering the first dose, assess the client for allergies and determine whether culture has been obtained. ▪ After multiple doses, assess the client for superinfection (thrush, yeast infection, diarrhea); notify the health care provider if these occur. ▪ Instruct the client to take all of his prescribed medication, even if he is feeling better.
Topical gentamicin	Treat infection of the eyes	▪ Be sure to obtain a specimen for culture before use.
Antibiotic-steroid combinations tobramycin with dexamethasone	Decrease nonpyrogenic inflammation and help prevent infection in eyes	▪ Instruct the client to clean exudate from the eyes before administering the medication.
Anticholinergics atropine cyclopentolate scopolamine	Diagnose and treat of ophthalmic disorders; produce cycloplegia, which causes paralysis of the ciliary body; produce mydriasis, which dilates pupils	▪ Instruct the client to wear sunglasses until the the medication wears off. ▪ Instruct the client to avoid driving or using hazardous machinery until the drug wears off. ▪ Instruct the client about the correct administration of eye drops.
Antiemetics chlorpromazine HCl droperidol trimethobenzamide HCl	Relieve nausea and vomiting by inhibiting medullary chemoreceptor triggers	▪ Advise the client that this medication may cause drowsiness. ▪ Instruct the client on safety issues.
Antihistamines dimenhydrinate meclizine	Treat Ménière's disease by suppressing vestibular activity, thereby decreasing vertigo, nausea, and vomiting	▪ Instruct the client to avoid hazardous activities. ▪ Instruct the client to take the medication with food to decrease GI distress. ▪ Instruct the client to chew sugarless gum to relieve dry mouth.
Antitussives dextromethorphan hydrobromide hydrocodone	Suppress cough	▪ Instruct the client to read over-the-counter product labels to ensure the medication is appropriate for symptoms. ▪ Instruct the client to stay well hydrated and to avoid smoking.
Beta-blockers betaxolol HCl metipranolol	Treat glaucoma by decreasing production of aqueous humor	▪ Monitor the client's heart rate and blood pressure. ▪ Instruct the client about the correct administration of eye drops.

DRUG CHART 14-1

Medications for eye, ears, nose, sinus, and throat disorders *(continued)*

Classifications	Indications	Selected interventions
Carbonic anhydrase inhibitors acetazolamide	Treat glaucoma by lowering intraocular pressure by decreasing production of aqueous humor	■ Inform the client that this medication may cause malaise, anorexia, and fatigue and to continue the medication if these adverse effects occur. ■ Instruct the client to administer the medication orally as prescribed.
Cholinergics pilocarpine	Treat glaucoma by constricting pupils and promoting outflow of aqueous humor	■ Warn the client that visual acuity is decreased in environments with low lighting. ■ Use with caution in clients who have urinary tract obstruction. ■ Instruct the client about the correct administration of eye drops.
Decongestants oxymetazoline pseudoephedrine HCl	Treat nasal decongestion by causing blood vessels to constrict, thereby relieving congestion	■ Instruct the client to read product labels to ensure appropriate over-the-counter medications for symptom control. ■ Instruct the client to inform health care providers about the use of over-the-counter medications.
Hyperosmotics glycerin mannitol	Treat angle-closure glaucoma by elevating plasma osmolality and enhancing flow of water into the extracellular fluid, thereby reducing intraocular pressure	■ Because this is a medical emergency, try to calm and reassure the client. ■ Instruct the client to administer orally as prescribed.
Opioid and nonopioid analgesics acetaminophen codeine propoxyphene	Relieve moderate pain by reducing pain sensation, producing sedation, and decreasing emotional upset often associated with pain; often schedule II drugs	■ Instruct the client to take the medication before the pain is severe. ■ Instruct the client to avoid hazardous activities.
Steroids prednisolone acetate	Decrease eye inflammation	■ Monitor the client for signs of corneal ulceration. ■ Advise the client not to share eye drops with others.
Vasodilators methantheline niacin tolazoline	Treat Ménière's disease by relaxing vascular smooth muscle, thereby reducing tinnitus	■ Instruct the client on ways to prevent orthostatic hypotension. ■ Instruct the client to remain on bed rest during an acute attack when taking this medication.

D. Assessment findings
 1. **Clinical manifestations**
  a. **Chronic open-angle glaucoma**
   – No early symptoms
   – Insidious visual impairment, blurring
   – Diminished accommodation
   – Gradual loss of peripheral vision (tunnel vision)

- Mildly aching eyes
- Halos around lights later with elevated IOP

b. **Acute closed-angle glaucoma**
- Transitory attacks of diminished visual acuity
- Colored halos around lights
- Reddened eye with excruciating pain
- Headache
- Nausea and vomiting

2. Laboratory and diagnostic study findings
a. Tonometry detects elevated IOP.
b. Slit-lamp examination reveals abnormalities in the anterior vitreous humor.

E. Nursing management (See section II.D.)
1. **Administer prescribed medications,** which may include cholinergics (miotics), beta blockers, and carbonic anhydrase inhibitors. (See *Drug chart 14-1,* pages 380 and 381.)
2. **Provide information about laser trabeculoplasty,** if medication therapy proves ineffective.
3. **Provide information regarding management of acute closed-angle glaucoma.**
   a. Discuss preoperative and postoperative teaching for immediate surgical opening of the eye chamber.
   b. Prepare to administer carbonic anhydrase inhibitors I.V. or I.M. to restrict production of aqueous humor.
   c. Prepare to administer osmotic agents.
   d. Discuss and prepare the client for surgical or laser peripheral iridectomy after the acute episode is relieved.
   e. Discuss and prepare the client for prophylactic peripheral iridectomy of the unaffected eye before discharge.
4. **Teach the client about specific safety precautions.**
   a. Instruct the client to avoid mydriatics such as atropine, which may precipitate acute glaucoma in a client with closed-angle glaucoma.
   b. Instruct the client to carry prescribed medications at all times.
   c. Instruct the client to carry a medical identification card or wear a bracelet stating his type of glaucoma and need for medication.
   d. Instruct the client to take extra precautions at night (e.g., use handrails, providing extra lighting to compensate for impaired pupil dilation from miotic use).

V. CATARACTS

A. Description. Cataract formation is a gradual, progressive opacity of the lens or lens capsule that leads to visual loss.

B. Etiology
1. The most common cause of cataracts is aging; about 85% of persons older than age 80 experience this problem to some degree.
2. Other possible causes include trauma, drug or chemical toxicity, genetic defects, and secondary effects of other diseases.

C. Pathophysiology. Altered nutrient metabolism within the lens triggers cataract formation. The lens becomes cloudy and has reduced accommodative power. Light rays cannot pass through the opaque lens to the retina, causing vision loss.

D. Assessment findings

1. **Clinical manifestations**
   a. Progressively worsening blurred vision
   b. Cloudy-appearing lens
   c. No pain or eye redness
2. **Laboratory and diagnostic study findings.** Ophthalmoscopic and slit-lamp examination confirm diagnosis.

E. Nursing management (See section II.D.)

1. **Provide preoperative nursing care for extraction of the cataract,** which may be extracapsular or intracapsular.
   a. Explain to the client that this surgery is usually done on an outpatient basis.
   b. Discuss and administer preoperative medications, which may include I.V. sedation, adrenergic agonists, and hyperosmotic agents. (See *Drug chart 14-1*, pages 380 and 381.)
2. **Provide postoperative nursing care.**
   a. Instruct the client to remain in a semi-Fowler's position or on the nonoperative side.
   b. Explain the importance of keeping a patch or protective shield on the affected eye.
   c. Promote measures to relieve postoperative discomfort with analgesics and atropine eye drops as prescribed. Instruct the client to report severe eye pain immediately; this may indicate increasing intraocular pressure or hemorrhage.
3. **Provide postoperative discharge teaching,** which usually occurs a few hours after surgery.
   a. Inform the client that the surgeon will change the patch on the second postoperative day.
   b. Discuss the need for eye protection by instructing the client to wear glasses during daytime hours (sunglasses at first) and to use an eye shield at night to prevent eye rubbing. Also tell the client to avoid straining, to lie on the back or unaffected side when in bed, to read only in moderation, and to maintain a sedentary lifestyle for 2 weeks.
   c. Instruct the client to turn his head to the side to scan the entire visual field to compensate for impaired peripheral vision.
   d. Instruct the client on how to administer steroid-antibiotic eye drops. Caution the client that the medication may initially cause sensitivity to bright light. (See *Drug chart 14-1*, pages 380 and 381.)
   e. Instruct the client to notify the health care provider if eye pain occurs after administration (i.e., possible indication of underlying glaucoma).

VI. EARS

A. Structures

1. **External ear**
   a. Structures of the external ear include the auricle, external auditory canal, and tympanic membrane, also called *the eardrum.* (See *Figure 14-2*, page 384.)
   b. The auricle and external auditory canal receive and direct sound waves to the tympanic membrane.
2. **Middle ear** communicates with mastoid air cells of the temporal bone.
   a. **Ossicles** (i.e., malleus, incus, and stapes) move and conduct sound waves from the external ear to inner ear.

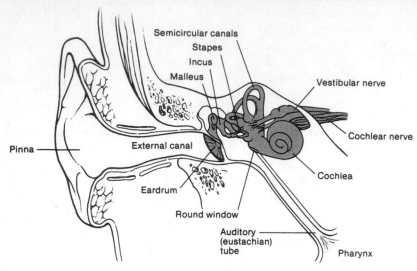

FIGURE 14-2
Structures of the ear

Source: Fuller J., and Schaller-Ayers, J. *Health Assessment: A Nursing Approach,* 3rd ed. Philadelphia: Lippincott Williams & Wilkins, 2000.

  b. The **eustachian tube** connects the middle ear to the nasopharynx and equalizes pressure on both sides of the tympanic membrane.
 3. Inner ear (i.e., labyrinth)
  a. The **vestibule** contains receptors that respond to the position of the head as it relates to gravity.
  b. The **cochlea** contains the organ of Corti (i.e., receptor end organ of hearing).
  c. **Semicircular canals** contain sensory organs of equilibrium.
 4. The **acoustic nerve** (cranial nerve VIII) connects the cochlea, semicircular canals, and vestibular receptors with the brain.

B. **Function.** The ears are involved in hearing and position sense (i.e., balance and equilibrium).
 1. Hearing
  a. Sound waves are directed by the external ear through the external auditory meatus, where they strike the tympanic membrane, causing it to vibrate.
  b. These vibrations trigger movement of the ossicles in the middle ear, whose stapes transmit the vibrations through the fluid in the inner ear to the cochlea and the organ of Corti.
  c. Movement in the organ of Corti stimulates the sensory ends of the cochlear branch of the acoustic nerve (cranial nerve VIII), which sends impulses to the temporal lobe for interpretation as sound.
 2. Position sense. Fluid in the semicircular canals of the inner ear responds to body movement by stimulating nerve cells that line the canals. These cells transmit impulses through the vestibular branch of the acoustic nerve to the brain for maintenance of balance and equilibrium.

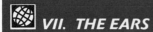

VII. THE EARS

A. Assessment

1. **Health history**

   a. **Elicit a description of the client's present illness and chief complaint,** including onset, course, duration, location, and precipitating and alleviating factors. Cardinal signs and symptoms include:
   - the client's reporting "trouble with hearing"
   - ear pain or discharge from ear
   - tinnitus or "ringing in the ears"
   - complaints of dizziness or incoordination.

   b. **Explore the client's health history** for risk factors associated with ear disorders, including:
   - age
   - heredity
   - allergies
   - upper respiratory infection
   - head trauma
   - excessive environmental noise or music
   - certain ototoxic medications.

2. **Physical examination**

   a. **Inspection**
   - Inspect the auricle and surrounding tissues for size, symmetry, and angle of attachment to head.
   - Inspect external canal for lesions, dryness, cleanliness, and redness.
   - Inspect ear canal for any bloody drainage, cerebrospinal fluid, pus, or serous fluid.
   - Tympanic membrane (eardrum) inspection involves straightening the external auditory canal of an adult by pulling the auricle up and back while tilting the client's head slightly; normal findings include an intact, shiny, pearly gray, and concave membrane that moves with swallowing.
   - Nose and throat assessment should accompany ear assessment because infection in these areas may lead to ear problems.

   b. **Palpation.** Palpate the area around the ear and palpate the auricle for pain or discomfort.

3. **Laboratory and diagnostic studies**

   a. An **otoscopic examination** is used to examine the external auditory canal and tympanic membrane.

   b. **Hearing acuity screening** is done by having the client identify the point near the ear at which he can hear a whispered voice or ticking watch; normally, the client should hear the sound at a distance of about 2 feet.

   c. **Weber's test** evaluates bone conduction with a tuning fork placed on the midline of the head; normally, the tone is heard equally in both ears by bone conduction.

   d. The **Rinne test** uses a tuning fork to evaluate air conduction and bone conduction; normally, air conduction is greater than bone conduction (i.e., positive Rinne result).

   e. **Audiometry,** the measurement of hearing acuity, should be performed by an audiologist certified by the American Speech and Hearing Association.

B. Nursing diagnoses
1. Disturbed auditory and sensory perception
2. Risk for injury
3. Impaired verbal communication
4. Acute pain
5. Deficient knowledge
6. Social isolation
7. Anxiety

C. Planning and outcome identification. The major goals for the client diagnosed with an ear disorder include adjustment to altered sensory perception, absence of injury or vertigo, ability to communicate effectively, freedom from pain or discomfort, knowledge of the disease process and treatment, and absence of social isolation and anxiety.

D. Implementation
1. **Promote measures that aid in maximizing the client's auditory sensory or perceptual functioning.**
   a. When hearing loss is permanent, encourage the client to participate in aural rehabilitation, which includes auditory training, speech reading, speech training, and use of hearing aids.
   b. Discuss the possibility of using a hearing aid; include advantages, types, care of the hearing aid, and cost of the hearing aid.
   c. Discuss the possibility of obtaining a hearing guide dog to increase the client's independence.
   d. Discuss assistive devices for the hearing impaired, including phone and television devices provided at no cost to the client.
2. **Protect the client from injury.**
   a. Instruct the client in hearing-protection measures.
      – Protect the ears from loud noises with such items as plugs or muffs.
      – Chew gum or suck hard candy when flying to open the eustachian tube and allow air into the middle ear.
      – **Never insert any object into the auditory canal beyond the extent of vision.**
      – Do not insert an object smaller than the finger into the ear.
      – Blow the nose with the mouth open and both nostrils open to prevent forcing contaminated material into the middle ear.
   b. Discuss with the client and his family hazards in the home environment that must be modified to provide a safe environment (e.g., installing a flashing light on the doorbell, telephone and smoke alarms).
   c. Assist the client with vertigo by assisting with ambulation, keeping side rails up on the bed, and providing the client with a safe environment.
3. **Promote measures that enhance effective communication.**
   a. A hearing-impaired client may be inaccurately labeled as demented because of impaired communication. Be sure to record the client's hearing deficit on the chart and care plan.
   b. Work with the client to develop a means of communication that is effective and mutually satisfying (e.g., lip reading, writing).
   c. Avoid startling the client; get the attention of the client before speaking.
   d. When talking to the hearing-impaired client:
      – devote full attention to what he is saying
      – speak slowly and distinctly in a low-pitched, clear voice, but do not yell

- minimize background noise
- do not try to appear to understand if unable
- try to determine the essential meaning of what is being said; use nonverbal cues.

    e. Instruct the client in the use and care of a hearing aid, if indicated.

    f. Assist the client in obtaining assistive devices (e.g., amplifying mechanisms as necessary).

4. Promote measures that help prevent or decrease pain and discomfort.

    a. Instruct the client on the correct way to administer prescription analgesics, which may be prescribed for the first 48 to 72 hours.

    b. Explain to the client that it may be necessary to insert a wick into the ear canal to keep the canal open so that liquid medication can be administered.

    c. Instruct the client to avoid putting anything in his ear and to avoid putting his head under water until ear pain or infection is resolved.

    d. Instruct the client not to put heat or cold applications to the ear.

5. Provide the client with self-care instructions.

    a. Instruct the client to avoid getting the ear wet to prevent infection.

    b. Instruct the client to avoid persons with upper respiratory infections.

    c. Instruct the client to avoid bending, straining, and flying until allowed in the postoperative period.

    d. Instruct the client to take the full course of prescribed medications, even after symptoms are relieved.

    e. Instruct the client to pull the top of the ear up and back when instilling ear drops (this straightens the ear canal).

    f. Instruct the client to take care to prevent burns with a hair dryer if the auricle is numb.

6. Promote measures that prevent social isolation for a client with impaired hearing.

    a. Do not rely on the hospital's intercom system.

    b. Do not exclude the client from conversations in the room.

7. Minimize anxiety. Assess the client's level of anxiety by allowing him to ventilate feelings and assisting him to identify coping skills and stress-management techniques.

8. Prepare a client undergoing ear surgery for postoperative expectations and requirements.

    a. Inform the client that hearing may not improve noticeably until edema decreases and packs are removed.

    b. Explain expected postoperative restrictions on positioning and movement.

    c. Instruct the client not to sneeze, cough, blow the nose, or touch the ear or dressing until allowed.

9. Take steps to prevent injury from postoperative complications.

    a. Monitor for signs and symptoms of infection (e.g., temperature elevation, headache, drainage).

    b. Do not disturb the inner dressing.

    c. Avoid applying pressure to the ear or ear dressing, which could dislodge a graft or prosthesis.

    d. If the client experiences vertigo, note nystagmus and record the direction of eye movement and effects of position changes.

    e. Observe for signs of facial nerve injury (e.g., inability to frown, wrinkle forehead, close eyes, bare teeth, pucker lips). (*Note:* Injury may be temporary because of edema, or it may be permanent.)

    f. Protect the eye if facial nerve injury occurs.

g. Instruct the client to report tinnitus, fluctuating hearing, or vertigo.

10. **Promote mobility within postoperative restrictions.**

   a. Maintain bed rest for up to 48 hours.

   b. Position the client in the side-lying position with the operative ear up to prevent displacement of the graft; with operative ear down to enhance drainage; or on the unoperated side to minimize nausea and vomiting.

11. **Relieve postoperative discomfort and guard against injury.**

   a. Maintain the prescribed position.

   b. Keep the bed rails up, and assist the client with ambulation.

   c. Teach the client to use hand rails (vertigo may threaten safety) and avoid contraindicated or sudden movements.

   d. Avoid jarring the client or the bed.

   e. Instruct the client to breathe deeply through an open mouth.

   f. Medicate for pain or nausea as indicated.

   g. Provide a light or liquid diet to control nausea as necessary.

12. **Provide referrals** to the National Institute on Deafness and Other Communication Disorders and Self-Help for Hard of Hearing People. (See appendix A.)

E. Outcome evaluation

1. The client modifies lifestyle to decrease disability and exert maximum control and independence within limits posed by impaired hearing.

2. The client demonstrates understanding of effective ear care, hearing-protection measures, and remains free from injury.

3. The client is able to effectively communicate with others.

4. The client reports relief of pain and discomfort.

5. The client verbalizes an understanding of the disorder, self-care, and ways to modify home and work environments to maintain safety.

6. The client socializes with family, friends, and maintains an active social life within limits imposed by the hearing impairment.

7. The client verbalizes a decrease in anxiety.

VIII. CONDUCTIVE HEARING LOSS

A. Description. Conductive hearing loss refers to various problems involving impaired passage of sound from the external ear and the inner ear. Specific conditions include:

1. cerumen impaction

2. external otitis media

3. serous otitis media

4. suppurative otitis media

5. otosclerosis.

B. Etiology

1. **Cerumen impaction** usually occurs in persons who naturally produce large amounts of cerumen.

2. **External otitis media** may be caused by infection (bacterial or fungal), excessive moisture in the auditory canal (swimmer's ear), and trauma.

3. **Serous otitis media** may result from eustachian-tube obstruction, sudden changes in atmospheric pressure, allergy, and viral disease.

4. **Suppurative otitis media** may follow viral disease, tympanic-membrane perforation, or prolonged forceful nose blowing. It is most common in infants and young children because of their immature and relatively poorly draining eustachian tubes.

5. **Otosclerosis** appears to be a hereditary condition; it affects women twice as often as men and typically develops between ages 15 and 30.

C. Pathophysiology

1. **Cerumen impaction** in the external ear can block sound from reaching the tympanic membrane.

2. **External otitis media** involves inflammation of the external ear, with crust formation and edema in the auditory canal.

3. **Serous otitis media** involves sterile fluid accumulation in the middle ear. It may be acute or chronic; frequent recurrences can threaten hearing.

4. **Suppurative otitis media** involves pus accumulation in the middle ear and possibly extending into adjacent structures. Chronic recurrence may lead to tympanic-membrane perforation.

5. **Otosclerosis** involves spongy bone growth over the normal bony labyrinth, causing the footplate of the stapes to become fixed in the oval window of the otic capsule.

D. Assessment findings

1. **Clinical manifestations**

   a. **Cerumen impaction** is often visible; the client demonstrates some degree of hearing loss.

   b. **External otitis media** results in itching, pain, and watery or purulent discharge.

   c. **Serous otitis media** is manifested by a plugged feeling in the ear, reverberation of the client's own voice, and hearing loss.

   d. **Suppurative otitis media** typically produces:
   - throbbing ear pain
   - fever, hearing loss, nausea, and vomiting
   - feeling of increased pressure in the ear
   - bright red, bulging or retracted tympanic membrane
   - possible tympanic-membrane rupture with discharge (i.e., otorrhea).

   e. **Otosclerosis** may be marked by mixed hearing loss or sensorineural hearing loss, and tinnitus.

2. **Laboratory and diagnostic findings**

   a. In **otitis media**, the otoscope findings depend on the stage of disease.
   - In the first stage, the tympanic membrane is retracted.
   - In the second stage, the tympanic membrane's blood vessels dilate and appear red.
   - During the third stage, the tympanic membrane becomes red, thickened, and bulging, with a loss of landmarks.
   - If the tympanic membrane spontaneously perforates, pus and blood drain from the ear.

   b. In **otosclerosis**, reduced air conduction compared with bone conduction is noted on the Rinne test.

E. Nursing management (See section VII.D.)

1. **Instruct the client about the correct way to remove impacted cerumen.**

   a. Soften cerumen with instilled peroxide or glycerol preparations.

   b. Instruct the client to irrigate the ear in 2 or 3 days to remove the wax.

   c. Instruct the client keep otic solution in the ear for 15 minutes by tilting the head sideways or by putting cotton in the ear.

      d. Instruct the client to notify the health care provider if inflammation or irritation occurs.

      e. Instruct the client not to use the solution for more than 4 consecutive days.

  2. Provide care to a client with tympanic-membrane perforation.

      a. Maintain strict asepsis.

      b. Do not irrigate the ear.

      c. Protect from water contamination by having the client wear ear plugs and a bathing cap.

      d. Recognize that the client is at risk for labyrinthitis or meningitis.

      e. Use a message board if necessary.

      f. Insert a hearing aid if indicated.

  3. Treat external otitis media with topical antibiotics and steroids, gentle debridement, and acid–alcohol solutions to sterilize the auditory canal as prescribed.

  4. Discuss, prepare, and assist a client with serous otitis media for a myringotomy, which is an incision into the tympanic membrane to relieve pressure and remove pus.

  5. Provide nursing interventions for the client with suppurative otitis media.

      a. Provide prescribed treatments for a client with suppurative otitis media, which may include systemic antibiotics (for at least 7 days), nasal decongestants, and analgesics. (See *Drug chart 14-1*, pages 380 and 381.)

      b. Discuss, prepare, and assist the client with suppurative otitis media for surgery.

        – Mastoidectomy is the removal of the mastoid bone.

        – Myringoplasty is the repair of perforated tympanic membrane.

        – Tympanoplasty is a procedure involving the replacement or rebuilding of middle-ear structures.

  6. Discuss, prepare, and assist the client with otosclerosis for surgery, as indicated.

      a. Stapedectomy is the replacement of diseased ossicles with prostheses.

      b. Fenestration is the creation of a new window into the labyrinth to provide a new pathway for sound.

IX. MÉNIÈRE'S DISEASE

  A. **Description.** Ménière's disease is a chronic disorder of the inner ear involving sensorineural hearing loss, severe vertigo, and tinnitus.

  B. **Etiology.** The cause of Ménière's disease is unknown; it is associated with aging and may follow middle-ear infection or head trauma.

  C. **Pathophysiology**

    1. Ménière's disease appears to involve overproduction or decreased absorption of endolymph, with resultant degeneration of vestibular and cochlear hair cells.

    2. Recurrent attacks result in progressive sensorineural hearing loss (especially low tones), usually unilateral in nature.

  D. **Assessment findings**

    1. Clinical manifestations

      a. Sudden episodes of severe whirling vertigo, with an inability to stand or walk; an episode may last up to several hours.

      b. Buzzing tinnitus (worsens before and during an episode)

      c. Nausea, vomiting, and diaphoresis

      d. Possibly, brief loss of consciousness with nystagmus

    2. **Laboratory and diagnostic findings.** Audiometric testing reveals sensorineural hearing loss.

E. Nursing management (See section VII.D.)

1. **Provide nursing care during an acute attack.**
   - *a.* Provide a safe, quiet, dimly lit environment, and enforce bed rest.
   - *b.* Provide emotional support and reassurance to alleviate anxiety.
   - *c.* Administer prescribed medications, which may include antihistamines, antiemetics and, possibly, mild diuretics. (See *Drug chart 14-1,* pages 380 and 381.)
2. **Instruct the client on self-care instructions to control the number of acute attacks.**
   - *a.* Discuss the nature of the disorder.
   - *b.* Discuss the need for a low-salt diet.
   - *c.* Explain the importance of avoiding stimulants and vasoconstrictors (e.g., caffeine, decongestants, alcohol).
   - *d.* Discuss medications that may be prescribed to prevent attacks or self-administration of appropriate medications during an attack, which may include anticholinergics, vasodilators, antihistamines and, possibly, diuretics or nicotinic acid. (See *Drug chart 14-1,* pages 380 and 381.)
3. **Discuss, prepare, and assist the client with surgical options.**
   - *a.* A labyrinthectomy is the most radical procedure and involves resection of the vestibular nerve or total removal of the labyrinth performed by the transcanal route, which results in deafness in that ear.
   - *b.* An endolymphatic decompression consists of draining the endolymphatic sac and inserting a shunt to enhance the fluid drainage.

X. STRUCTURE AND FUNCTION OF THE NOSE, SINUS, AND THROAT

A. Structures (See *Figure 14-3,* page 392.)

1. The **nasal passages,** or turbinates, are three bony structures (i.e., superior, middle, and inferior) located between the roof of the mouth and the frontal, ethmoid, and sphenoid bones of the skull.
2. The **four paranasal sinuses** (i.e., frontal, maxillary, ethmoidal, and sphenoidal) are air cavities located around and draining into the nasal turbinates.
3. The **pharynx,** or throat, is a tubelike structure that connects the nasal and oral cavities to the larynx, which is the transition between the upper and lower airways.
4. The **larynx,** or voice organ, is a cartilaginous epithelium-lined structure that connects the pharynx and the trachea.
   - *a.* The **epiglottis** is a valve flap of cartilage that covers the opening to the larynx during swallowing.
   - *b.* The **glottis** is the opening between the vocal cords in the larynx.
   - *c.* The **thyroid cartilage** is the largest cartilage in the trachea, and part of it forms the Adam's apple.
   - *d.* The **cricoid cartilage** is the only complete cartilaginous ring in the larynx and is located below the thyroid cartilage.
   - *e.* The **vocal cords** are ligaments controlled by muscular movements that produce vocal sounds.
5. The **palatine tonsils** are connected to the palatine arches, which are located on either side of the uvula.

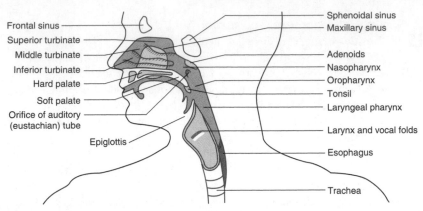

FIGURE 14-3
Cross-section of the nasal cavity, pharynx, larynx, and tonsils

      6. The **adenoids,** or pharyngeal tonsils, are located in the roof of the nasopharynx.

B. Function

      1. The **nasal passages** contain cilia, which are tiny hairs that filter, warm, and humidify inspired air. Enervated by the olfactory nerve (cranial nerve I), the nose provides the function of olfaction (smell); the senses of taste and smell are closely related.

      2. The **sinuses** produce mucus for the nasal cavity and give timbre and resonance to the voice.

      3. The **pharynx** is a common passageway for food, fluids, and air.

      4. The **larynx** permits vocalization and protects the lower airway from foreign substances and facilitates coughing.

      5. The **palatine tonsils** and **adenoids,** or pharyngeal tonsils, are important links in the chain of lymph nodes, guarding the body from invasion by organisms entering the nose and throat.

NURSING PROCESS OVERVIEW

 XI. THE NOSE, SINUS, AND THROAT

A. Assessment

      1. **Health history**

         a. **Elicit a description of the client's present illness and chief complaint,** including onset, course, duration, location, and precipitating and alleviating factors. Cardinal signs and symptoms indicating altered nose, sinus, and throat function include:

            – difficulty swallowing

            – cough

            – sore throat

            – fever and difficulty breathing.

         b. **Explore the client's health history for risk factors** associated with nose, sinus, and throat disorders, including:

            – allergies

- alcohol and tobacco use
- activities that cause a forceful blow to face
- upper respiratory infections.

2. **Physical examination**

   a. **Inspection**
   - Assess olfaction by having the client identify various odors.
   - Insert speculum blades 0.5″ (1.3 cm) into the nares while resting the index finger on the side of the client's nose.
   - Inspect for pallor, edema, masses, polyps, and redness.
   - Inspect the nasal mucosa for redness and discharge.
   - Examine the posterior pharynx with a warmed mirror (to prevent fogging) and tongue depressor, instructing the client to open the mouth wide and take a deep breath to flatten the posterior tongue.
   - Observe color and symmetry; note any exudate, ulcerations, or edema.

   b. **Palpation**
   - Palpate the frontal and maxillary sinuses for tenderness.
   - Palpate the neck for enlarged lymph nodes.
   - Palpate the neck to assess position and mobility of the trachea; lateral deviation may indicate a mass in the neck or mediastinum.

3. **Laboratory and diagnostic study findings.** Sinus radiographs are obtained to rule out other local or systemic disorders.

B. Nursing diagnoses

1. Ineffective breathing pattern
2. Risk for injury
3. Acute pain
4. Deficient knowledge
5. Anxiety

C. Planning and outcome identification.
The major goals for the client diagnosed with a nose, sinus, or throat disorder may include maintenance of a patent airway; absence of injury; pain relief; knowledge of the disorder, treatment, and preventive measures; and a decrease in anxiety level.

D. Implementation

1. **Promote measures that maintain a patent airway.**

   a. Humidify the environment with room vaporizers or inhaling steam.

   b. Keep the client in semi-Fowler's position.

   c. Increase fluid to help thin secretions.

2. **Promote measures that help prevent injury.**

   a. Instruct the client to eat thickened fluids to help prevent choking.

   b. Encourage the client to wear protective face gear when engaging in physical activities that may traumatize the nose.

   c. Instruct the client not to put any foreign objects in his mouth.

   d. Instruct the client to chew food completely before swallowing.

3. **Promote pain relief measures.**

   a. Administer and encourage the client to take analgesics to help relief discomfort.

   b. Encourage the client to avoid hot, cold, or spicy foods.

4. **Provide verbal and written instructions** on the course of disease, its treatment, and preventive measures to help prevent recurrence.

    5. Minimize anxiety. Encourage the client to ventilate feelings and identify ways to effectively deal with anxiety.

E. Outcome evaluation

1. The client maintains a patent airway.
2. The client reports no further upper respiratory system injury.
3. The client reports adequate relief of pain and discomfort.
4. The client verbalizes an understanding of the course of illness, its treatment, medication used to treat the illness, and signs and symptoms to report to the health care provider.
5. The client remains calm and exhibits decreased anxiety.

XII. SINUSITIS

A. Description. Sinusitis is an inflammation of the nasal sinuses that can be acute or chronic.

B. Etiology

1. **Acute sinusitis** develops as a result of an upper respiratory tract infection, particularly a viral infection or an exacerbation of allergic rhinitis.
2. The cause of **chronic sinusitis** is not clear.

C. Pathophysiology

1. In **acute sinusitis,** nasal congestion (caused by inflammation, edema, and transudation of fluid) leads to obstruction of sinus cavities, which is an excellent medium for bacterial growth.
2. **Chronic sinusitis** usually is caused by chronic nasal obstruction from discharge and edema of the nasal mucous membrane.

D. Assessment findings

1. **Clinical manifestations**
   a. **Acute sinusitis**
       – Pressure and pain over the sinus area
       – Purulent nasal secretions
   b. **Chronic sinusitis**
       – Cough due to the constant dripping of thick discharge backward into the nasopharynx
       – Chronic headaches in the periorbital area and facial pain most pronounced on awakening
       – Nasal stuffiness
       – Fatigue
2. **Laboratory and diagnostic findings.** Sinus radiographic studies reveal inflammation of the sinuses.

E. Nursing management (See section XI.D.)

1. **Promote measures that relieve pain and discomfort.**
   a. Administer prescribed antibiotics and nasal decongestants. (See *Drug chart 14-1,* pages 380 and 381.)
   b. Provide the client with heated mist and saline irrigations to help open blocked passages.
2. **Provide oral and written information to promote drainage.**
   a. Instruct the client to inhale steam (e.g., steam bath, hot shower, facial sauna).

b. Instruct the client to increase fluid intake.

c. Instruct the client to apply hot wet packs to facial area.

3. Provide the client with education to prevent sinus infections.

a. Instruct the client to avoid allergens when suspected.

b. Instruct the client to avoid people with respiratory-tract infections.

c. Instruct the client to seek medical attention if upper respiratory symptoms persist longer than 7 to 10 days.

d. Instruct the client to notify the health care provider if nasal discharge is discolored or foul smelling and when fever, severe headache, or stiff neck occurs.

XIII. PHARYNGITIS

A. Description. Pharyngitis is an inflammation of the throat that can be acute or chronic.

B. Etiology

1. **Acute pharyngitis** is caused by a viral organism; the most common is group A *Streptococcus* (i.e., "strep throat").

2. **Chronic pharyngitis** is common in adults who work or live in dusty surroundings, use their voice to excess, suffer from chronic cough, and habitually use alcohol and tobacco.

C. Pathophysiology

1. In **acute** and **chronic pharyngitis,** the pharynx becomes infected by a virus or bacteria and becomes inflamed.

2. **Chronic pharyngitis** is one of the following three types:

a. **Hypertrophic pharyngitis** is characterized by general thickening and congestion of pharyngeal mucous membrane.

b. **Atopic pharyngitis,** a late stage of hypertrophic pharyngitis, is characterized by a thin, whitish, glistening, and sometimes wrinkled membrane.

c. **Chronic granular pharyngitis,** or "clergyman's sore throat," is marked by numerous edematous lymph follicles on the pharyngeal wall.

D. Assessment findings

1. **Clinical manifestations**

a. **Acute pharyngitis**

– Fiery red pharyngeal membrane and tonsils

– Lymphoid follicles are edematous and flecked with exudate

– Enlarged and tender cervical lymph nodes

– Fever, malaise, and sore throat

b. **Chronic pharyngitis**

– Constant sense of irritation or fullness in the throat

– Mucus collects in the throat and can be expelled by coughing

– Difficulty in swallowing

2. **Laboratory and diagnostic findings.** Culture and sensitivity of the throat identify bacterial infection.

E. Nursing management (See section XI.D.)

1. **Promote measures that decrease pain and discomfort.**

a. Prepare to administer prescribed antibiotics, analgesics, antitussives, and decongestants (See *Drug chart 14-1*, pages 380 and 381.)

b. Encourage the client to gargle with warm saline gargles and use throat lozenges.

c. Instruct the client that the temperature of saline should be sufficiently high to be effective and should be as hot as the client can tolerate.

d. Instruct the client to apply an ice collar to severe sore throats.

e. Instruct the client on proper mouth care.

2. **Promote measures that ensure adequate nutritional and fluid balance.**

   a. Instruct the client to have a liquid or soft diet.

   b. Encourage the client to increase fluid intake to 2,000/ml per day.

   c. Discourage the client from eating spicy foods and drinking juices that are acidic.

   d. If the client is unable to drink, fluids may be administered I.V.

3. **Provide oral and written instructions for treatment and prevention.**

   a. Instruct the client to take all antibiotics, even if he is feeling better.

   b. Encourage the client to avoid exposure to irritants, smoking, secondhand smoke, and exposure to cold and alcohol.

   c. Encourage the client to avoid contact with individuals with upper respiratory infections.

   d. Encourage the client to use a disposable mask when exposed to environmental and occupational pollutants.

XIV. TONSILLITIS AND ADENOIDITIS

A. Description
1. **Tonsillitis** is an inflammation of the tonsils.
2. **Adenoiditis** is an inflammation of the adenoids.

B. Etiology
1. **Tonsillitis** is caused most commonly by group A *Streptococcus*.
2. **Adenoiditis** frequently accompanies acute tonsillitis.

C. Pathophysiology
1. **Tonsillitis.** The inflammation of the tonsils occurs when bacteria attack the lymphoid tissue on the tonsils.
2. **Adenoiditis.** The inflammation of the adenoids results from bacteria attacking the abnormally large lymphoid tissue mass near the center of the posterior wall of the nasopharynx.

D. Assessment findings
1. **Clinical manifestations**
   a. **Tonsillitis**
      – Sore throat
      – Fever
      – Snoring
      – Difficulty swallowing
   b. **Adenoiditis**
      – Mouth breathing
      – Earache and draining ears
      – Frequent head colds
      – Foul-smelling breath
      – Noisy respirations
2. **Laboratory and diagnostic findings.** Culture and sensitivity results for the throat can identify the bacterial infection.

E. Nursing management (See section XI.D.)

1. **Provide nursing interventions for pharyngitis** as detailed in section XIII.E.
2. **Prepare the client for a tonsillectomy or adenoidectomy** if repeated attacks of tonsillitis and adenoiditis occur or if hypertrophy of the tonsils and adenoids could cause obstruction.
3. **Provide postoperative nursing care.**
   a. Provide continuous nursing observation because of the chance of hemorrhage.
   b. Position the client in the prone position with the head turned to the side to allow for drainage from the mouth and pharynx.
   c. Apply an ice collar to the neck.
   d. Notify the surgeon if any of the following occur:
      – The client vomits large amounts of bright red blood at frequent intervals.
      – The pulse increases, the blood pressure decreases, the temperature increases, or the client becomes restless.
4. **Provide oral and written instructions for treatment and prevention.**
   a. Instruct the client on the signs and symptoms of hemorrhage that require immediate intervention.
   b. Encourage the client to use alkaline mouthwashes and warm saline solutions to cope with the thick mucus that may be present.
   c. Encourage the client to use a liquid or semi-liquid diet for several days after surgery.
   d. Encourage the client to eat sherbets and gelatins and avoid spicy, hot, cold, acidic, or rough foods.
   e. Instruct the client to avoid milk and milk products (e.g., ice cream), because they tend to increase the amount of mucus produced.

XV. EPISTAXIS

A. Description. Epistaxis is a severe nosebleed.

B. Etiology

1. Epistaxis may be spontaneous or may result from trauma (usually nose picking).
2. It also may be associated with chemical irritation, acute or chronic infection (e.g., rhinitis, sinusitis), purpura, leukemia and other blood dyscrasias, hypertension, anticoagulant therapy, or deviated septum.

C. Pathophysiology

1. In children, epistaxis usually originates in the anterior nose and tends to be mild; in adults, it tends to originate in the posterior nose and be more severe.
2. Slight to moderate epistaxis usually causes no complications; severe bleeding (i.e., persisting longer than 10 minutes after pressure is applied) may cause blood loss up to 1 L/hour.

D. Assessment findings

1. **Clinical manifestations**
   a. Bleeding through the nares and blood trickling into the oropharynx
   b. Blood in the corners of eyes (through the lacrimal ducts)
   c. Blood in the auditory canal if the tympanic membrane is perforated
2. **Laboratory and diagnostic findings.** Nasal inspection with a bright light and speculum may locate the source of bleeding.

E. Nursing management (See section XI.D.)

1. **Provide nursing interventions to control bleeding.**
   a. Have the client sit upright, breathe through the mouth, and refrain from talking.
   b. Compress the soft outer portion of the nares against the septum for 5 to 10 minutes.
   c. Instruct the client to avoid nose blowing during or after the episode.
   d. If pressure does not control bleeding, prepare to assist the health care provider in inserting an anterior packing or posterior packing as appropriate. Keep scissors and a hemostat on hand to cut the strings and remove the packing in the event of airway obstruction.

2. **Provide ongoing assessment to monitor for bleeding.**
   a. Inspect for blood trickling into the posterior pharynx.
   b. Observe for hemoptysis, hematemesis, and frequent swallowing or belching.
   c. Instruct the client not to swallow but to spit out any blood into emesis basins.
   d. Monitor the client's vital signs.

3. **Provide oral and written instructions for treatment and prevention.**
   a. Discuss ways to prevent epistaxis, including avoiding forceful nose blowing, straining, high altitudes, and nasal trauma.
   b. Instruct the client to have adequate humidification to prevent drying of nasal passages.
   c. Instruct the client on the proper way to stop bleeding.
   d. Instruct the client to not put anything up the nasal passages.
   e. Instruct the client to contact a health care provider if the bleeding does not stop.

XVI. FOREIGN-BODY ASPIRATION

A. Description. Foreign-body aspiration occurs when there is a partial or total occlusion of the larynx or lower airway by an aspirated object.

B. Etiology
1. Children may aspirate a variety of objects.
2. Food is the most common cause of airway obstruction in adults.

C. Pathophysiology
1. Objects may be aspirated into the upper airway or lower airway (i.e., below the larynx). Aspirated objects can enter the right main bronchus.
2. Complete airway obstruction may rapidly lead to cardiopulmonary arrest.

D. Assessment findings
1. Signs of respiratory distress
2. Weak, ineffective cough
3. High-pitched noises on inspiration
4. Clutching of neck with hands
5. Inability to speak with complete obstruction
6. Cyanosis and loss of consciousness (may occur with complete obstruction)

E. Nursing management (See section XI.D.)
1. **Provide immediate nursing interventions if the client can speak** (indicating partial airway obstruction).
   a. Position for optimal ventilation.
   b. Encourage coughing.

     c. Do not hit the client on the back; leave him alone, and let him expel the foreign object.
2. **Provide immediate nursing interventions if the client cannot speak** (indicating complete obstruction).
     a. Call for help immediately.
     b. Perform abdominal thrust (Heimlich) maneuver; use lower sternal thrust for a client who is obese or pregnant.
     c. Remove an object in the larynx with a finger or forceps by laryngoscopy.
     d. Prepare the client and assist with removal of object in the lower airway through bronchoscopy.
     e. Prepare the client, and assist with emergency cricothyroidotomy if necessary.
3. **Promote measures to help relieve anxiety.**
     a. Do not leave the client unattended.
     b. Encourage the client to resume a normal breathing pattern and to talk about the episode after obstruction is relieved.

Study questions

1. Which intervention would the nurse perform to prevent systemic adverse effects from drug absorption during eyedrop instillation?
1. Applying pressure on the eyelid rim
2. Applying pressure on the inner canthus
3. Having the client close his eyes tightly
4. Placing the client in the supine position for a few minutes

2. Into which position would the nurse place a client diagnosed with a retinal detachment at the inner aspect of the right eye?
1. Fowler's position
2. Supine with a small pillow
3. Right-side lying
4. Left-side lying

3. Which medication would be the most appropriate analgesic for a client complaining of periocular aching after a surgical repair of a detached retina?
1. Acetaminophen
2. Codeine
3. Meperidine
4. Morphine

4. Which clinical manifestation would the nurse expect the client diagnosed with "strep throat" to exhibit?

1. A fiery red pharyngeal membrane and fever
2. Pain over the sinus area and purulent nasal secretions
3. Foul-smelling breath and noisy respirations
4. Weak cough and high-pitched noise on respirations

5. During the nursing history, which assessment data would the nurse expect the client scheduled for surgical correction of chronic open-angle glaucoma to report?
1. Seeing flashes of light and floaters
2. Recent motor vehicle crash while changing lanes
3. Complaints of headaches, nausea, and redness of the eyes
4. Increasingly frequent episodes of double vision

6. Which intervention would be included in the care plan for a client diagnosed with epistaxis?
1. Performing several abdominal thrust (Heimlich) maneuvers
2. Compressing the nares to the septum for 5 to 10 minutes
3. Applying an ice collar to the neck area
4. Encouraging warm saline throat gargles

7. Which assessment data would the nurse expect when collecting the nursing history from a client with cataracts?
1. Eye pain
2. Floaters
3. Eye redness
4. Blurred vision

8. Which nursing intervention would be included in the care plan for the client with an acute exacerbation of Ménière's disease?
1. Instructing the client on the correct way to remove impacted cerumen
2. Speaking slowly and distinctly in a low-pitched, clear voice without yelling
3. Providing a safe, quiet, dimly lit environment with enforced bed rest
4. Instructing the client to pull the top of the ear up and back to instill eardrops

9. Which assessment data would the nurse expect as the chief complaint from a client who is experiencing an acute exacerbation of Ménière's disease?
1. Vertigo
2. Dizziness
3. Severe ear pain
4. Sudden deafness

10. The nurse is administering 2 drops of medication in OS prior to ophthalmic surgery. Which interventions should the nurse implement? (Select all that apply.)
1. Instructing the client to look up prior to administering the medication
2. Administering the medication into the right eye
3. Administering the medication into the upper conjunctiva
4. Pulling the left ear up and back prior to administering the medication
5. Wiping the excess medication from the inner to the outer canthus
6. Pressing on the nasal-lacrimal canal

11. Which diet would be most appropriate to discuss with the client diagnosed with Ménière's disease?

1. Low-protein
2. Low-sodium
3. High-fiber
4. High-potassium

12. After nasal surgery with posterior packing in place, which assessment data would alert the nurse to the possibility of active bleeding?
1. Appearance of anxiety
2. Discoloration around the eyes
3. Frequent swallowing
4. Black, tarry stool

13. Which assessment data would cause the nurse to suspect serous otitis media?
1. Bright red, bulging or retracted tympanic membrane and fever
2. Inflammation of the external ear and crust formation on the auditory canal
3. Sensorineural hearing loss and complaints of tinnitus
4. Plugged feeling in the ear and reverberation of the client's own voice

14. Which intervention should the nurse implement first for a client who is choking and cannot speak?
1. Calling for help immediately
2. Leaving the client alone to clear his throat.
3. Telling the client to adequately humidify the house
4. Trying to determine what the client is choking on

15. Which statement by a client diagnosed with Ménière's disease who has had a labyrinthectomy of the left ear indicates that he understands the discharge teaching concerning the surgery?
1. "I should be able to hear fairly well after the edema in my ear subsides."
2. "I will be totally deaf in my left ear, but the dizziness will be gone."
3. "I should remove the inner ear packing in exactly 3 days."
4. "I should lubricate the skin around my stoma with petroleum jelly."

16. Which medication would be contraindicated in a client with chronic open-angle glaucoma?
1. Atropine
2. Pilocarpine
3. Timolol
4. Betaxolol

Answer key

1. The answer is **2.**
Systemic absorption and subsequent adverse effects may occur if the medication enters the nasolacrimal canal. The nurse therefore applies pressure to the inner canthus, causing occlusion of this canal and minimizing the risk for systemic adverse effects. Applying pressure on the eyelid rim would not occlude this canal. Having the client close his eyes tightly may cause some of the medication to be expelled. Positioning has no effect on the flow of medication into the nasolacrimal canal and subsequent absorption.

2. The answer is **4.**
When retinal detachment occurs, the client is positioned so that the area of detachment is dependent. For this client, the left-side lying position is used. Positioning the client in the Fowler, supine, or right-side lying positions would not place the detached area in a dependent position.

3. The answer is **1.**
Because the discomfort is typically mild after surgery to repair a detached retina, a mild analgesic such as acetaminophen would be used. Codeine is constipating and may lead to straining and increased intraocular pressure (IOP). Meperidine often causes nausea and vomiting, further adding to the client's level of discomfort, and vomiting may lead to increased IOP. Morphine causes nausea, vomiting, and constipation, which should be avoided after eye surgery.

4. The answer is **1.**
Strep throat, or acute pharyngitis, results in a red throat, edematous lymphoid tissues,

enlarged lymph nodes, fever, and sore throat. Pain over the sinus area and purulent nasal secretions would be evident with sinusitis. Foul-smelling breath and noisy respirations indicate adenoiditis. A weak cough and high-pitched noisy respirations are associated with foreign-body aspiration.

5. The answer is **2.**
Typically, the client with chronic open-angle glaucoma experiences a gradual loss in peripheral vision leading to tunnel vision. Being involved in a motor vehicle crash while changing lanes suggests the disorder. The client may experience insidious blurring, decreased accommodation, mild aching eyes and, eventually, halos around the lights as intraocular pressure increases. Flashes of light and floaters are characteristic of retinal detachment. Nausea, headache, and eye redness are seen with an episode of acute (sudden) closed-angle closure. Double vision occurs when one eye has a lens and the other is aphakic.

6. The answer is **2.**
When a client experiences epistaxis, the nurse should compress the soft outer portion of the nares against the septum for approximately 5 to 10 minutes. The client should sit upright, breathe through the mouth, and refrain from talking. Performing abdominal thrusts is appropriate for the client with a foreign-body aspiration. Applying an ice collar to the neck is commonly done for a client after a tonsillectomy. Warm saline throat gargles are appropriate for the client with pharyngitis.

7. The answer is **4.**
Cataracts lead to progressive worsening and

blurring of vision. Eye pain and redness, common with glaucoma, are not present with cataracts. Floaters are characteristic of retinal detachment.

8. The answer is **3.**
Ménière's disease is a chronic disorder of the inner ear involving sensorineural hearing loss, severe vertigo, and tinnitus. Typically, the client experiences sudden episodes of severe whirling vertigo with an inability to stand or walk, buzzing tinnitus that worsens before and during an episode, nausea, vomiting, and diaphoresis. The client's safety must be ensured along with decreasing exposure to extraneous stimuli. This is accomplished by providing the client with a quiet, dimly lit environment and bed rest. Instructions about removing cerumen are appropriate for the client with a cerumen impaction. Speaking slowly and distinctly in a low-pitched, clear voice without yelling is appropriate for clients experiencing a hearing loss. Clients with Ménière's disease are not deaf during acute exacerbations. However, hearing loss may occur after repeated episodes. Ear drops are not the treatment of choice for an acute attack of Ménière's disease.

9. The answer is **1.**
Ménière's disease is characterized by sudden, severe episodes of vertigo during which the client has a sensation of spinning. Dizziness is not vertigo and must be distinguished from true rotational vertigo. A feeling of pressure but not pain is also characteristic, and hearing loss is progressive, not sudden.

10. The answers are **1, 5, 6.**
The nurse is administering medication into the left eye (OS) for ophthalmic surgery, which includes instructing the client to look up, administering the medication into the lower conjunctiva, pressing on the nasal-lacrimal canal to prevent systemic drug absorption, and wiping excess secretions with a sterile cotton ball from the inner to outer canthus. The abbreviation for right eye is OD and both

eyes is OU.

11. The answer is **2.**
It is thought that Ménière's disease is caused by edema of the semicircular canals. A low-sodium diet is often prescribed in conjunction with diuretic therapy. Protein intake should have no relation to Ménière's disease, but hypoproteinemia may aggravate edema. Fiber and potassium have not been identified as instrumental in the development of Ménière's disease.

12. The answer is **3.**
After nasal surgery, drainage trickling down the posterior pharynx (seen with a flashlight) accompanied by frequent swallowing, belching, or hematemesis indicate continued bleeding. Anxiety is common because of the necessity to breathe through the mouth. Discoloration around the eyes occurs with surgical trauma and is to be expected. Tarry stools indicate previous, but not current, bleeding.

13. The answer is **4.**
Serous otitis media is manifested by a plugged feeling in the ear, reverberation of the client's own voice, and hearing loss. A bright red, bulging or retracted tympanic membrane and fever suggest suppurative otitis media. Inflammation of the external ear and crust formation on the auditory canal suggest external otitis media. Sensorineural hearing loss and tinnitus indicate otosclerosis.

14. The answer is **1.**
Because the client cannot speak, a total airway obstruction has occurred. The client is in acute distress and requires emergency treatment. Leaving the client alone to clear the throat would be appropriate for a client with a partial airway obstruction, as evidenced by choking but with an ability to speak. Adequate home humidification is appropriate for the client with recurrent epistaxis or nasal congestion. It does not matter what the client is choking on.

15. The answer is 2.

A labyrinthectomy is the most radical procedure for Ménière's disease. It involves resection of the vestibular nerve or total removal of the labyrinth by the transcanal route. Although this procedure controls the disorder, it results in deafness in the affected ear. With this procedure, inner ear packing is not used, and a stoma is not created.

16. The answer is 1.

Mydriatics such as atropine may precipitate acute glaucoma in a client with closed-angle glaucoma and should be avoided. Pilocarpine, a cholinergic agent, and timolol and betaxolol, beta blockers, are used to treat glaucoma.

15 *Musculoskeletal disorders*

I. STRUCTURE AND FUNCTION OF THE MUSCULOSKELETAL SYSTEM

A. Structure

1. **Bones.** The body contains 206 different bones.
   - *a.* **Types of osseous tissue**
     - **Compact bone** is dense and looks smooth and homogeneous.
     - **Spongy bone** is composed of small, needlelike pieces of bone and lots of open space.
   - *b.* **Bone classification** according to shape
     - **Long bones** (e.g., femur, humerus, radius)
     - **Short bones** (e.g., tarsals, carpals)
     - **Flat bones** (e.g., skull, sternum, ribs, ilium)
     - **Irregular bones** (e.g., mandible, vertebrae, ear ossicles)
   - *c.* **A long bone has several components.** (See *Figure 15-1.*)
     - The **diaphysis** (i.e., shaft) makes up most of the bone's length and is composed of compact bone.
     - The **periosteum** is a fibrous connective membrane that covers and protects the diaphysis.
     - The **epiphyses** are the ends of the long bone that consist of thin layers of compact bone enclosing an area filled with spongy bone.
     - The **epiphyseal line,** a thin line that spans the epiphysis, looks different from the rest of the bone. It is the remnant of the epiphysial plate that closes when the growing bone has reached its full length.

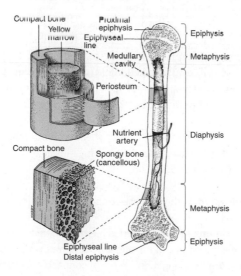

FIGURE 15-1
A long bone shown in longitudinal position

Source: Bullock B.L., and Henze, R. L. *Focus on Pathophysiology.* Philadelphia: Lippincott Williams & Wilkins, 2000.

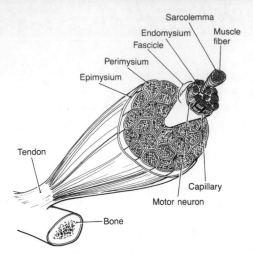

FIGURE 15-2
Structures of the skeletal muscle from muscle to bundle of fibers to single muscle fiber or cell

Source: Bullock B.L., and Henze, R.L. *Focus on Pathophysiology.* Philadelphia: Lippincott Williams & Wilkins, 2000.

   d. **Bone marrow** is vascular tissue located in the medullary (shaft) cavity of long bones and flat bones. Yellow marrow is primarily a storage area for adipose tissue, and red marrow (located in sternum, ilium, vertebrae, and ribs) produces red and white blood cells. (See chapter 18.)
   e. The **skeleton** is divided into two parts.
      – The **axial skeleton** forms the longitudinal axis of the body in the skull, the vertebral column, and the bony thorax.
      – The **appendicular skeleton** is composed of 126 bones of the limbs and the pectoral and pelvic girdles, which attach to the limbs of the axial skeleton.
2. **Articulations** (i.e., joints)
   a. **Synarthroses** (fibrous) are fixed joints (e.g., skull sutures).
   b. **Amphiarthroses** (cartilaginous) are slightly movable joints (e.g., vertebral joints).
   c. **Diarthroses** (synovial) are freely movable joints (e.g., mandible, vertebrate, ear ossicles).
   d. The **joint capsule** is a tough, fibrous sheath surrounding the articulating bone.
3. **Skeletal muscle** (striated muscle) is the only muscle type subject to conscious (voluntary) control. (See *Figure 15-2*.)
   a. The **sarcolemma** is the oval nuclei just beneath the plasma membrane.
   b. The **endomysium** is the delicate connective tissue sheath that encloses each muscle fiber.
   c. The **perimysium** is a coarse fibrous membrane that wraps around muscle fibers.
   d. The **fascicle** is a bundle of muscle fibers covered with connective tissue.
   e. The **epimysium** is a tougher overcoat of connective tissue that binds many fascicles together.
4. **Ligaments** are strong, fibrous connective tissues that bind bones.
5. **Tendons** are strong, fibrous, nonelastic connective tissue extending from muscle sheaths. (See *Figure 15-2*.)

6. **Cartilage** is a nonvascular, supporting connective tissue composed of various cells and fibers.
   a. **Hyaline cartilage** is a pearly, blue cartilage that covers articular bone surfaces.
   b. **Fibrocartilage** consists of a white, tough, fibrous tissue found in the knee.
   c. **Yellow cartilage** is an elastic, fibrous cartilage found in the larynx and external ear.

B. Function
1. **Bone functions**
   a. Protection of vital organs
   b. Support for body tissue
   c. Assistance in movement through leverage and attachment for muscles
   d. Hematopoiesis (i.e., red blood cell production)
   e. Storage of mineral salts
2. **Articulations** (joints) hold bones together securely but give the rigid skeleton mobility.
   a. **Ball and socket joints** permit full freedom of movement (e.g., hip, shoulder).
   b. **Hinge joints** permit bending in one direction only (e.g., elbows, knees).
   c. **Saddle joints** allow movement in two planes at right angles to each other (e.g., base of the thumb).
   d. **Pivot joints** are characterized by the articulation between the radius and the ulna, allowing turning motion.
   e. **Gliding joints** allow for limited movement in all directions.
   f. The **joint capsule,** which is lined with a synovial membrane, secretes a lubricating and shock-absorbing fluid (i.e., synovial fluid) into the joint capsule.
3. **Skeletal muscle functions**
   a. Facilitation of voluntary body movement through contraction.
   b. Maintenance of body posture.
   c. Production of body heat.
4. **Ligaments** provide joint stability and allow restricted joint movement
5. **Tendons** bind muscles to bones.
6. **Cartilage functions**
   a. Absorption of weight, shock, stress, and strain
   b. Protection of bones, joints, and joint tissue

NURSING PROCESS OVERVIEW

 ## II. THE MUSCULOSKELETAL SYSTEM

A. Assessment
1. **Health history**
   a. **Elicit a description of the client's present illness and chief complaint,** including onset, course, duration, location, and precipitating and alleviating factors. Cardinal signs and symptoms indicating altered musculoskeletal function include:
      – moderate to severe pain
      – inability to move body part
      – localized edema
      – altered sensation to affected area
      – contour deformity and asymmetry
      – contusions.

  b. **Explore the client's health history** for risk factors associated with musculoskeletal disorders, such as:
  – medical conditions or medications that would cause dizziness, falls, or injuries
  – environmental or physical conditions or unsafe behavior that would cause injuries
  – decreased dietary intake of essential nutrients for bone formation
  – history of infrequent exercise and sedentary lifestyle
  – family history of musculoskeletal problems.

2. **Physical examination**
  a. **Inspection**
  – Note upright body alignment, including posture.
  – Assess bone discrepancies, including contour, length, alignment, and symmetry.
  – Assess the client's ability to move each joint through its range of motion, noting smoothness, pain, crepitus, and clicks.
  – Note the client's gait, including coordination, rhythm, stride, and balance.
  – Assess the joint alignment, including symmetry, size, shape, contour, stability, tenderness, heat, and edema.
  – Note muscle discrepancies, including hypertrophy, atrophy, fasciculation, and spasms.

  b. **Palpation**
  – Palpate muscle mass, including shape, size, contour, symmetry, and firmness.
  – Palpate muscle strength, including symmetry, resistance, and contractility.

3. **Laboratory and diagnostic studies**
  a. **Roentgenography** (e.g., radiography, radiographs, photographic images) detects musculoskeletal structure, integrity, texture, or density problems. It also allows evaluation of disease progression and treatment efficacy.
  b. A **bone scan** detects skeletal trauma and disease by determining the degree to which the matrix of the bone "takes up" a bone-seeking radioactive isotope.
  c. **Arthrography** is the injection of a radiopaque substance or air into the joint cavity to identify acute or chronic tears of the joint capsule or supporting ligaments for the knee, shoulder, ankle, hip, or wrist.
  d. **Arthrocentesis** allows analysis of synovial fluid, blood, or pus aspirated from a joint cavity.
  e. **Myelography** is injection of a contrast agent into the subarachnoid space of the spine to detect herniation, tumor, and congenital or degenerative conditions of the spinal canal.
  f. **Electromyography** measures muscle electrical impulses for diagnosis of muscle or nerve disease.
  g. **Biopsy** (i.e., aspiration, punch, needle, or incision) studies bone, synovium, or muscle tissue.
  h. **Computed tomography scans** show soft tissue, bone, and the spinal cord in three-dimensional, cross-sectional images.
  i. **Magnetic resonance imaging** allows study of soft tissue in multiple planes of the body.
  j. **Complete blood count** analysis identifies anemias, hemorrhage, infections, neoplastic conditions, lupus erythematosus, blood dyscrasias, allergies, stress, and other conditions.
  k. **Alkaline phosphatase studies** identify increases in osteoblastic activity and inflammatory conditions.

    l. **Creatinine phosphokinase elevation** may identify skeletal muscle necrosis, atrophy, or trauma.

    m. **Lactate dehydrogenase evaluation** may identify skeletal muscle damage.

    n. **Serum calcium studies** may help to identify bone loss density.

    o. **C-reactive protein test** is used for evaluating the severity and course of an inflammatory process, such as a bacterial infection or rheumatic disease.

    p. **Rheumatoid factor** measures the presence of a macroglobulin type of antibody found in rheumatoid arthritis and other connective tissue diseases.

B. Nursing diagnoses

1. Acute or chronic pain
2. Ineffective peripheral tissue perfusion
3. Impaired physical mobility
4. Risk for infection
5. Risk for injury
6. Bathing or hygiene, dressing or grooming, feeding, or toileting self-care deficit
7. Deficient knowledge
8. Anxiety

C. Planning and outcome identification.
The goals of the client diagnosed with a musculoskeletal disorder include pain relief, maintenance of adequate tissue perfusion, improved physical mobility, prevention of infection and injury, achievement of maximum level of self-care, understanding the treatment regimen, and decreased anxiety.

D. Implementation

1. **Perform a neurovascular assessment.** (Remember the six Ps: pain, pulse, pallor, paresthesia, paralysis, polar.)

    a. **Assess pain,** which signals the beginning of muscle ischemia.
- Assess pain on a scale of 1 (no pain) to 10 (worst pain).
- Rule out complications that require medical intervention.
- Take an action: Medicate; use nonpharmacologic interventions, such as relaxation, massage, and guided imagery; or call the health care provider.
- Institute appropriate safety measures.
- Evaluate the effectiveness of the medication or nursing intervention.

    b. **Assess pulses,** pulselessness indicates disruption of arterial blood flow
- Assess various locations, including radial, brachial, pedal, posterior tibial, popliteal, and femoral pulses. Always mark pulses with an X.
- Document pulse strength using a scale of 0 to 4+: 0, no pulse; 1+, weak; 2+, normal; 3+, strong; 4+, bounding.
- Use a Doppler device to verify pulselessness.

    c. **Assess for pallor,** which indicates disruption of arterial blood flow. Check capillary refill time, which should be less than 3 seconds.

    d. **Assess for paresthesia;** nerve function may be disrupted by nerve compression.
- Determine whether the client experiences numbness, tingling, or the sensation that the foot is asleep.
- Ascertain whether the client feels pinching or touching of an extremity.
- Determine whether the client can feel dull or sharp touch sensation.

    e. **Assess for paralysis;** increasing edema causes nerve compression.
- Determine whether the client can move and lift the affected extremity.
- Ascertain whether the client can push the affected extremity against pressure.

CLIENT AND FAMILY TEACHING 15-1
Guidelines for the client with a musculoskeletal disorder

- Instruct the client to keep the affected extremity elevated above the level of the heart as much as possible to help decrease edema.
- Instruct the client to apply ice to the affected extremity to help decrease edema and decrease pain.
- Instruct the client to perform range-of-motion exercises for all unaffected extremities.
- Ensure safe use of treatment modalities, such as slings, walkers, and crutches.
- Encourage the client to perform activities of daily living within therapeutic limits of the musculoskeletal disorder.
- Encourage the client to take pain medications when pain is at a 3 or 4 on a pain scale of 1 (no pain) to 10 (worst pain); instruct on other comfort measures, such as guided imagery, relaxation techniques, and biofeedback.

- Instruct the client to notify the health care provider if any of the following occur:
  – Increased pain not relieved with prescribed medications
  – Skin cold to touch
  – Increased edema of affected extremity
  – Inability to move fingers, toes on affected extremity
  – Any tingling, numbness or abnormal sensation in affected extremity
  – Any diminished capillary refill.
- After removal of an immobilizer device, instruct the client to exercise the affected extremity as prescribed to return it to normal function.

    f. **Assess for polar** (i.e., coldness), which indicates disrupted arterial blood flow.
- Determine whether the client's extremity feels cool or has a bluish color.
- Note whether the client complains of a cold extremity.

2. **Provide pain relief.**
    a. Elevate the injured extremity above the level of the client's heart for the first 24 hours or as directed.
    b. Apply cold packs, as ordered, for the first 24 hours.

3. **Promote mobility.** Assist the client with active and passive range-of-motion exercises for unaffected body parts to help maintain function.

4. **Prevent infection.** Monitor the client's vital signs, assess for signs and symptoms of infection, and monitor the white blood cell count.

5. **Protect the client from injury.** Instruct the client in and request a return demonstration of safe transferring, ambulating, and sitting techniques to prevent further injury from immobilization or assistive devices.

6. **Promote the client's participation in self-care activities within limitations of the injury and treatment regimen.**

7. **Provide client and family teaching.**
    a. Provide explanations for the cause, treatment, and expected course for the client with a musculoskeletal disorder.
    b. Provide additional teaching as detailed in *Client and family teaching 15-1*.

8. **Minimize anxiety.** Assist the client with identifying and addressing feelings of anxiety to include therapeutic conversation, distraction therapy, or medication if needed.

E. Outcome evaluation

1. The client reports reduced pain and states appropriate measures to enhance comfort and promote healing.

2. The client exhibits adequate tissue perfusion and sensory function in the affected area.

3. The client has improved physical mobility as evidenced by the ability to transfer himself safely and the ability to use assistive devices properly.

4. The client has no signs or symptoms of systemic or local infection.

5. The client resumes normal activity without further injury after healing.

6. The client demonstrates proper performance of prescribed rehabilitative exercises and safety precautions to prevent reinjury.
7. The client maintains independence in self-care within limits of the injury and treatment plan.
8. The client participates in self-care activities and activities of daily living as much as possible.
9. The client verbalizes knowledge about the prescribed medications, cast care, dietary modifications, and other prescribed treatments.
10. The client states signs and symptoms of further complications to watch for and report to the health care provider.
11. The client reports a decrease in anxiety.

III. FRACTURES

A. **Description.** A fracture is a traumatic injury interrupting bone continuity. Fractures are classified according to type and extent. (See *Figure 15-3*, page 412.)
   1. **Closed simple, uncomplicated fractures** do not cause a break in the skin.
   2. **Open compound, complicated fractures** involve trauma to surrounding tissue and a break in the skin.
   3. **Incomplete fractures** are partial cross-sectional breaks with incomplete bone disruption.
   4. **Complete fractures** are complete cross-sectional breaks severing the periosteum.
   5. **Comminuted fractures** produce several breaks of the bone, producing splinters and fragments.
   6. **Greenstick fractures** break one side of a bone and bend the other.
   7. **Spiral (torsion) fractures** involve a fracture twisting around the shaft of the bone.
   8. **Transverse fractures** occur straight across the bone.
   9. **Oblique fractures** occur at an angle across the bone (less than a transverse).

B. **Etiology**
   1. Fractures can result from crushing force or direct blow.
   2. Torsion fractures can occur from a sudden twisting motion; persons with osteoporosis are at particular risk.
   3. Extremely forceful muscle contraction can cause fractures.
   4. Pathological fractures result from a weakness in bone tissue, which may be caused by neoplasm or a malignant growth.

C. **Pathophysiology**
   1. **Fracture occurs** when stress placed on a bone exceeds the bone's ability to absorb it.
   2. **Stages of normal fracture healing** include:
      a. inflammation
      b. cellular proliferation
      c. callus formation
      d. callus ossification
      e. mature bone remodeling.
   3. **Potential complications of fracture include:**
      a. life-threatening systemic fat embolus, which most commonly develops within 24 to 72 hours after fracture

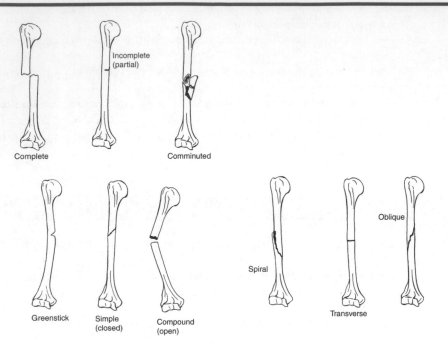

FIGURE 15-3
Fractures associated with long bones

Source: Bullock B.L., and Henze, R.L. *Focus on Pathophysiology.* Philadelphia: Lippincott Williams & Wilkins, 2000.

       b. compartment syndrome, which is a condition involving increased pressure and constriction of nerves and vessels within an atomic compartment

       c. nonunion of the fracture side

       d. arterial damage during treatment

       e. infection and possibly sepsis

       f. hemorrhage, possibly leading to shock.

D. Assessment findings

    1. Clinical manifestations

       a. Pain

       b. Edema

       c. Tenderness

       d. Abnormal movement and crepitus

       e. Loss of function

       f. Ecchymoses

       g. Visible deformity

       h. Paresthesias and other sensory abnormalities

    2. Laboratory and diagnostic study findings. Radiographs and other imaging studies may identify the site and type of fracture.

E. Nursing management (See section II.D.)

    1. Administer prescribed medications, which may include opioid or nonopioid analgesics and prophylactic antibiotics for an open fracture. (See *Drug chart 15-1.*)

> **DRUG CHART 15-1**
> # Medications for musculoskeletal problems

Classifications	Indications	Selected interventions
Antibiotics aminoglycosides (gentamicin, tobramycin) amoxicillin erythromycin penicillin tetracycline	Prevent or treat infections caused by pathogenic microorganisms	■ Before administering the first dose, assess the client for allergies and determine whether culture has been obtained. ■ After multiple doses, assess the client for super-infection (thrush, yeast infection, diarrhea); notify the health care provider if these occur. ■ Assess the insertion site for phlebitis if antibiotics are being administered. ■ To assess the effectiveness of antibiotic therapy, monitor the white blood cell count. ■ Monitor peaks and troughs for aminoglycosides.
Anticoagulants, subcutaneous Low-dose heparin (5,000 units)	Prophylactically prevent deep vein thrombosis; heparin activates antithrombin III, which inactivates newly formed factor Xa and thrombin	■ Administer subcutaneously in abdomen 1″ (2.5 cm) away from umbilicus. ■ Do not aspirate; do not massage. ■ Not necessary to monitor activated partial thromboplastin time because of short half-life.
Antiresorptive therapy	Decrease bone absorption of calcium	■ Instruct the client to continue with other therapies to help prevent and control complications of osteoporosis.
alendronate	Inhibit bone resorption by osteoclasts	■ Instruct the client to take the medication before breakfast with a full glass of water. ■ Instruct the client to remain upright for at least 30 minutes after breakfast.
calcitonin	Inhibit osteoclastic bone resorption	■ Instruct the client on the correct administration of nasal spray or subcutaneous route.
estrogen	Decrease bone reabsorption but not bone mass in women who have had ovaries removed or premature menopause	■ Instruct the client to perform breast self-examinations and have pelvic examinations routinely because increased rates of breast and endometrial cancers are adverse effects.
Low-molecular-weight (LMW) heparin enoxaparin	Prophylactically inactivate factor Xa (works same as heparin, but LMW molecules are short)	■ Administer in the anterolateral abdominal wall. ■ Do not aspirate; do not massage. ■ Insert an air bubble into the syringe. Not necessary to monitor partial thromboplastin time.
Nonopioid analgesics acetaminophen	Treat mild to moderate pain; blocks the generation blocks impulse through peripheral medanism	■ Inform the client that the medication may be purchased over the counter. ■ Caution the client that overdose may be toxic to the liver.
Nonsteroidal anti-inflammatory drugs ibuprofen idomethacin ketorolac naproxen salicylates	Reduce the inflammatory process, thereby reducing pain	■ Instruct the client to administer the medication with food to minimize upset. ■ Inform the client that the medication may have an anticoagulant effect. ■ Instruct the client to report tinnitus (ringing in ears), which is a sign of aspirin toxicity.

(continued)

DRUG CHART 15-1
Medications for musculoskeletal problems *(continued)*

Classifications	Indications	Selected interventions
Nonopioid analgesics (continued) **COX-2 inhibitors** nabumetone rofecoxib	Decrease inflammation in clients with severe arthritic conditions	▪ Inform the client to notify the health care provider of all prescription and over-the-counter medications
Opioid analgesics codeine hydrocodone hydromorphone morphine propoxyphene	Relieve moderate to severe pain by reducing pain sensation, producing sedation, and decreasing the emotional upset often associated with pain; most often schedule II drugs	▪ Assess the pain for location, type, intensity, what increases or decreases it; rate pain on scale of 1 (no pain) to 10 (worst pain). ▪ Rule out complications. Is this pain routine or expected? Is this a complication that needs immediate intervention? ▪ Medicate according to pain scale findings. ▪ Institute safety measures — bed in low position, side rails up, and call light within reach. ▪ Evaluate effectiveness of pain medication in 30 minutes.
Uric acid synthesis inhibitor allopurinol	Reduce the amount of uric acid delivered to the kidneys by inhibiting uric acid production	▪ Instruct the client to increase his fluid intake to at least 2,000 ml per day. ▪ Inform the client to notify the health care provider if a rash or fever develops.
Uricosuric drugs probenecid sulfinpyrazone	Act on renal tubules to inhibit reabsorption of uric acid; excretion of uric acid is increased, and hyperuricemia is reduced	▪ Instruct the client to take the medication with food. ▪ Instruct the client to increase his fluid intake to at least 2,000 ml per day.
Vitamins and minerals calcium supplements vitamin D	Increase bone density	▪ Instruct the client to swallow oral preparations intact, without crushing or chewing.

2. **Prevent infection.** Cover any breaks in the skin with clean or sterile dressings.
3. **Provide care during client transfer.**
   a. Immobilize a fractured extremity with splints in the position of the deformity before moving the client; avoid straightening the injured body part if a joint is involved.
   b. Support the affected body part above and below the fracture site when moving the client.
4. **Provide client and family teaching.**
   a. Explain prescribed activity restrictions and necessary lifestyle modifications because of impaired mobility.
   b. Teach the proper use of assistive devices, as indicated.
   c. Provide additional teaching as detailed in *Client and family teaching 15-1,* page 410.
5. **Provide appropriate nursing interventions associated with prescribed treatment modalities.** (See sections X, XI, and XII.)
6. **Prevent and manage potential complications.**

🖐 *a.* Observe for symptoms of life-threatening fat embolus, which include personality changes, restlessness, dyspnea, crackles, white sputum, and petechiae over the chest and buccal membranes. Assist with respiratory support, which must be instituted early.

🖐 *b.* Observe for symptoms of compartment syndrome, which include deep, unrelenting pain; hard edematous muscle; and decreased tissue perfusion with impaired neurovascular assessment findings. If necessary, discuss and assist with prescribed treatments, including fasciotomy, bivalve cast, or release of constrictive dressings.

c. Monitor closely for signs and symptoms of other complications.

IV. OSTEOPOROSIS

A. Description. Osteoporosis is a disorder of bone metabolism in which there is a reduction of total bone mass, making bones abnormally prone to fracture. It affects 25% of older adults, and the greatest incidence occurs among white females between ages 50 and 70.

B. Etiology. Osteoporosis may be iatrogenic or secondary to other disorders. Predisposing factors include postmenopausal status, long-term corticosteroid use, prolonged immobilization, and nutritional deficiency.

C. Pathophysiology. In osteoporosis, the rate of bone loss (i.e., resorption) exceeds bone formation, resulting in a decrease in total bone mass. Bones affected by osteoporosis lose calcium and phosphate salts, resulting in porous, brittle bones that are susceptible to fractures.

D. Assessment findings
1. **Clinical manifestations**
   a. Fractures, particularly vertebral compression fractures, hip fractures, and long bone fractures
   b. Pain
   c. Visible deformity (e.g., kyphosis)
   d. Loss of height
   e. Constipation
2. **Laboratory and diagnostic study findings**
   a. Radiographic and bone-density studies reveal loss of bone density in clients with 25% to 40% bone demineralization.
   b. Serum calcium, phosphorus, and alkaline phosphatase levels are within normal ranges.

E. Nursing management (See section II.D.)
1. **Administer prescribed medications,** which may include antiresorptive therapy, non-opioid analgesics, and calcium supplements. (See *Drug chart 15-1,* pages 413 and 414.)
2. **Prevent fractures.** Use caution when turning, lifting, and transferring the client to prevent fracture.
3. **Promote spinal stability** by applying a lumbosacral corset, if indicated; avoid appliances that can decrease mobility.
4. **Provide client teaching.**
   a. Encourage increased intake of foods high in calcium (e.g., milk, cheese, salmon, spinach, broccoli, rhubarb), vitamin D, fiber, and protein.

b. Teach knee flexion and muscle-relaxing exercises.

c. Teach the client to move the trunk as a unit and maintain good posture and body mechanics.

d. Instruct the client to perform range-of-motion exercises at least twice daily.

e. Suggest that the client sleep on a firm, nonsagging mattress.

f. Encourage a regular, moderate exercise regimen (e.g., walking, swimming, low-impact aerobics).

g. Teach the client about the disease process and prevention of progression.

h. Teach safety measures to prevent injury from falls.

V. OSTEOMYELITIS

A. Description. Osteomyelitis is a severe pyogenic bone infection.

B. Etiology

1. Osteomyelitis can result from trauma or secondary infection (most commonly with *Staphylococcus aureus*). It tends to affect persons with low resistance or with decreased blood flow to a trauma site.

2. Blood-borne (hematogenic) osteomyelitis is more common in children after a throat infection. Osteomyelitis resulting from trauma or orthopedic surgical procedures is more common in older persons.

C. Pathophysiology

1. Circulation of infectious microbes through the bloodstream to susceptible bone leads to inflammation, increased vascularity, and edema.

2. The organisms grow, pus forms within the bone, and abscess may form. This deprives the bone of its blood supply, eventually leading to necrosis.

D. Assessment findings

1. **Clinical manifestations**
   a. Localized bone pain
   b. Tenderness, heat, and edema in the affected area
   c. Guarding of the affected area
   d. Restricted movement in affected area
   e. Systemic symptoms
      – High fever and chills in acute osteomyelitis
      – Low-grade fever and generalized weakness in chronic osteomyelitis
   f. Purulent drainage from a skin abscess

2. **Laboratory and diagnostic study findings**
   a. White blood cell count reveals leukocytosis.
   b. Erythrocyte sedimentation rate is elevated.
   c. Blood culture identifies the causative organism.
   d. Radiograph and bone scan demonstrate bone involvement in advanced disease.

E. Nursing management (See section II.D.)

1. **Administer prescribed medications,** which may include opioid or nonopioid analgesics and antibiotics. (See *Drug chart 15-1*, pages 413 and 414.)

2. **Protect the affected extremity from further injury and pain** by supporting the limb above and below the affected area.
3. **Promote healing and tissue growth.**
   a. Provide local treatments as prescribed (e.g., warm saline soaks, wet to dry dressings).
   b. Provide a diet high in protein and vitamins C and D.
   c. Referral to a wound care clinic may be necessary.
4. **Prepare the client for surgical treatment,** such as debridement, bone grafting, or amputation, as appropriate.
5. **Provide additional teaching** as detailed in *Client and family teaching 15-1,* page 410.

VI. DISLOCATIONS

A. Description. Dislocation is displacement of a bone from its normal articulation with a joint. Common sites of dislocation include the shoulder, elbow, wrist, digits, hip, knee, ankle, and vertebrae.

B. Etiology. A dislocation may be congenital (e.g., congenital hip displacement) or may result from trauma (e.g., abnormal twisting) or disease of surrounding joint tissue (e.g., Paget's disease).

C. Pathophysiology. Traumatic dislocation may cause severe stress to associated joint structures, interrupting blood supply and causing nerve damage. If untreated, this may lead to avascular necrosis or nerve palsy in the affected area.

D. Assessment findings
1. **Clinical manifestations**
   a. Pain
   b. Visible disruption of joint contour
   c. Edema
   d. Ecchymoses
   e. Impaired joint mobility
   f. Change in extremity length
   g. Change in axis of dislocated bones (i.e., rotation)
   h. In severe dislocation, circulatory or sensory changes of the affected joint and limb
2. **Laboratory and diagnostic study findings.** Radiographic findings may confirm the dislocation.

E. Nursing management (See section II.D.)
1. **Administer prescribed medications,** which may include opioid or nonopioid analgesics. (See *Drug chart 15-1,* pages 413 and 414.)
2. **Prevent further injury.**
   a. Immobilize the affected joint during transport to medical care.
   b. Keep the joint immobilized as prescribed, using bandages, splints, a cast, or traction.
3. **Assist the health care provider in reducing displaced parts as necessary.**
4. **Provide client teaching** as described in *Client and family teaching 15-1,* page 410.

VII. OSTEOARTHRITIS

A. **Description.** Osteoarthritis is a slowly progressive, degenerative joint disease characterized by variable changes in weight-bearing joints. The most common form of arthritis, osteoarthritis affects both sexes about equally, with onset usually after age 40.

B. **Etiology.** Osteoarthritis is associated with obesity, aging, trauma, genetic predisposition, and congenital abnormalities.

C. **Pathophysiology**

1. Osteoarthritis starts with asymmetric cartilage loss, which leads to abnormal forces on the joint. It causes deterioration of the joint cartilage and formation of reactive new bone at joint margins and in subchondral areas. Soft tissue imbalance, joint malalignment, and bony hypertrophy can result.
2. Disability varies from the limitation of finger movement to severe hip and knee degeneration.
3. Progression is also variable; joints with minor deterioration may remain stable for years.

D. **Assessment findings**

1. **Clinical manifestations**
   a. Pain and muscle spasms, which are more pronounced after exercise, at night, and in the early morning
   b. Limited motion in affected joints
   c. Joint "grating" with movement
   d. Flexion contractures, primarily in the hip and knee
   e. Joint tenderness and Heberden's nodes in interphalangeal joints
2. **Laboratory and diagnostic study findings.** Radiographs may reveal a narrowing of joint space (because cartilage is not radiographic).

E. **Nursing management (See section II.D.)**

1. **Administer prescribed medications,** which may include analgesics and nonsteroidal anti-inflammatory drugs such as COX-2 inhibitors. (See *Drug chart 15-1,* pages 413 and 414.)
2. **Provide nonpharmacologic comfort measures.**
   a. Apply warm compresses or diathermy to sore joints.
   b. Massage surrounding muscles, not over inflamed joints.
   c. Promote adequate rest and reduction of stress.
   d. Maintain nonjudgmental attitude and respect the client's right to choose any alternative treatment for pain relief.
3. **Position the client to prevent flexion deformity** using a foot board, splints, sandbags, wedges, or pillows as needed. Remove splints routinely, if used, to exercise joints.
4. **Plan activities that promote optimal function and independence.**
5. **Refer the client to physical and occupational therapy,** as indicated. A physical therapist may prescribe and implement modified weight-bearing exercises within the client's tolerance level. An occupational therapist may help with self-management strategies.
6. **Prepare the client for surgical treatment,** as indicated. (See section XII.)
7. **Provide referrals** to the Arthritis Foundation. (See appendix A.)

VIII. GOUTY ARTHRITIS

A. Description. Gouty arthritis is a metabolic disease marked by urate crystal deposits in joints throughout the body, causing local irritation and inflammatory responses. For the most part, it affects men older than age 30.

B. Etiology. Gouty arthritis is linked to a genetic deficit in purine metabolism.

C. Pathophysiology

1. Gout is characterized by formation of tophus deposits in soft tissues and urate crystals in joint synovia. It primarily affects joints in the feet (especially the great toe) and legs, but it may strike in any joint.

2. The disorder follows a variable course of periodic attacks, often with long symptom-free periods between attacks. Eventually, it can lead to chronic disability and, in some cases, severe hypertension and progressive renal failure.

D. Assessment findings

1. **Clinical manifestations**

    a. Sudden attacks, usually at night, with periodic remissions and exacerbations

    b. Pain, usually monarticular, acute, crushing, and pulsating

    c. Joint edema and inflammation

    d. Intolerance to the weight of bed linens over the affected joint

    e. Pruritus or skin ulceration over the affected joint

    f. Signs of renal involvement (e.g., oliguria, low back pain, hypertension) in severe disease

2. **Laboratory and diagnostic study findings**

    a. Arthrocentesis reveals urate crystals in synovial fluid.

    b. Serum uric acid level is increased.

    c. Radiograph may show joint damage in advanced disease.

E. Nursing management (See section II.D.)

1. **Administer prescribed medications,** which may include nonsteroidal antiinflammatory drugs, uric acid synthesis inhibitors, and uricosuric agents. Colchicine may be prescribed for acute attack and used in small doses for prevention. Nausea, vomiting, and diarrhea are toxic effects of colchicine and should be reported to the health care provider. (See *Drug chart 15-1,* pages 413 and 414.)

2. **Promote measures to prevent exacerbations.**

    a. Urge the client to drink 2 to 3 L of fluid daily and to report any decrease in urine output.

    b. Teach the client about dietary modifications to limit foods high in purine (e.g., organ meats, anchovies, sardines, shellfish, chocolate, meat extracts).

3. **Provide measures to promote comfort and reduce pain.**

    a. Maintain strict bed rest for 24 hours after an attack.

    b. Provide a bed cradle to keep bed linen off affected joints to help reduce pain.

4. **Provide client teaching** as detailed in *Client and family teaching 15-1,* page 410.

IX. SPRAINS AND STRAINS

A. Description

1. A **sprain** is a complete or incomplete tear in the supporting ligaments surrounding a joint. Common locations include the ankle, knee, wrist, thumb, shoulder, neck, and lower back.

2. A **strain** is an overstretching injury to a muscle or tendon. Commonly affected areas are the groin, hamstring, calf, shoulder and back muscles, and the Achilles tendon.

B. Etiology

1. **Sprains** commonly result from a wrenching or twisting motion that disrupts the stabilizing action of ligaments.

2. **Strains** typically result from excessively vigorous movement in understretched or overstretched muscles and tendons.

C. Pathophysiology.
The affected ligament is unable to stabilize the joint when the client is applying weight and attempting to mobilize the affected joint. Blood vessels may be ruptured and edema produced.

D. Assessment findings

1. **Clinical manifestations**

   a. **Sprains**
   - Pain and discomfort, especially on joint movement
   - Edema, possibly ecchymoses
   - Decreased joint motion and function
   - Feeling of joint looseness with severe sprain

   b. **Strains**
   - Pain (In acute strain, pain may be sudden, severe, and incapacitating. With chronic strain, pain may be manifested as a gradual onset of soreness and tenderness.)
   - Edema
   - Ecchymoses developing several days after injury

2. **Laboratory and diagnostic study findings.** Radiographs are commonly done to rule out fracture or dislocation.

E. Nursing management (See section II.D.)

1. **Administer prescribed medications,** which may include nonopioid analgesics. (See *Drug chart 15-1,* pages 413 and 414.)

2. **Provide nursing care for a client who sustains a sprain.**

   a. Elevate or immobilize the affected joint, and apply ice packs immediately.

   b. Assist with tape, splint, or cast application, as necessary.

   c. Prepare the client with a severe sprain for surgical repair or reattachment, if indicated.

3. **Provide nursing care for a client suffering muscle or tendon strain.**

   a. Instruct the client to allow the muscle or tendon to rest and repair itself by avoiding use for approximately 1 week and then by progressing activity gradually until healing is complete.

   b. Teach appropriate stretching exercises to be performed after healing to help prevent reinjury.

   c. Prepare the client for surgical repair in severe injury.

4. **Provide additional teaching** as detailed in *Client and family teaching 15-1,* page 410.

X. CAST APPLICATION

A. Description

1. **Casts** are solid dressings applied to a limb or other body part.
   a. **Short arm casts** extend from below the elbow to the proximal palmer crease.
   b. **Long arm casts** extend from the axillary fold to the proximal palmer crease.
   c. **Short leg casts** extend from below the knee to the base of the toes.
   d. **Long leg casts** extend from the upper third of the thigh to the base of the toes.
   e. **Spica casts** extend from the midtrunk to cover one or both extremities.
   f. **Body casts** encase the trunk of the body.
   g. **Splints** are bivalved casts that provide immobilization and allow for edema.
2. **Casts are applied to:**
   a. immobilize a body part in a specific position
   b. exert uniform compression to soft tissue
   c. provide for early mobilization of unaffected body parts
   d. correct or prevent deformities
   e. stabilize and support unstable joints.
3. **Several types of materials are used to make casts.**
   a. **Plaster casts** mold very smoothly to the body's contours. The cast initially emits heat and takes about 15 minutes to cool and 24 to 72 hours to dry. It must be handled carefully until dry.
   b. **Fiberglass casts** are dry in 10 to 15 minutes and can bear weight 30 minutes after application.
   c. **Polyester-cotton knit casts** take about 7 to 10 minutes to dry and can withstand weight bearing almost immediately.

B. Assessment. Assess the following before and after cast application:

1. **Evaluate the client's pain,** noting severity, nature, exact location, source, and alleviating and exacerbating factors.
2. **Access neurovascular status.**
3. **Inspect for and document any skin lesions, discoloration, or no removable foreign material.**
4. **Evaluate the client's ability to learn essential procedures,** such as applying slings correctly, crutch walking, or using a walker.

C. Nursing management (See section II.D.)

1. **Prepare the client for cast application.**
   a. Explain the procedure and what to expect.
   b. Obtain informed consent if surgery is required.
   c. Clean the skin of the affected part thoroughly.
2. **Assist the health care provider during application of the cast as needed.**
3. **After cast application, provide cast care.**
   a. Support an exposed cast with the palms of your hands to prevent indentations.
   b. Ensure that the stockinet is pulled over rough edges of the cast.
   c. Elevate the casted extremity above the level of the heart.
   d. Provide covering and warmth to uncasted areas.
   e. Expose the fresh plaster cast to circulating air, uncovered, until dry (24 to 72 hours). Expose the fresh synthetic cast until it is completely set (about 20 minutes).
   f. Instruct the client to avoid wetting the cast. Instruct him to dry a synthetic cast with a hair dryer on cool setting if it gets wet.

4. **Initiate pain relief measures if indicated.**
   a. Encourage position changes.
   b. Elevate the affected body part.
   c. Provide analgesics as appropriate. (See *Drug chart 15-1,* pages 413 and 414.)
   d. Promote nonpharmacologic pain relief measures, such as guided imagery, relaxation, and distraction.
5. **Observe for signs and symptoms of cast syndrome with clients who are immobilized in large casts,** such as a body or hip spica cast. Report abdominal pain and distention, nausea and vomiting, elevated blood pressure, tachycardia, and tachypnea, which are physiologic effects of cast syndrome. Any client who is claustrophobic is at risk for psychological cast syndrome, which includes acute anxiety and possible irrational behavior.
6. **Provide nursing care for compartment syndrome,** if indicated. Observe for signs and symptoms and discuss and assist with treatments.
7. **Notify the health care provider immediately if signs or symptoms of other neurovascular complications occur.**
8. **Notify the health care provider if "hot spots" occur along the cast; they may indicate infection under the cast.**
9. **Provide client and family teaching.**
   a. Encourage isometric exercises to strengthen muscles covered by the cast. Promote muscle-strengthening exercises for the upper body if crutches are to be used.
   b. Advise the client to promptly report cast breaks and signs and symptoms of complications (i.e., circulatory compromise, cast syndrome, and hot spots).
   c. Warn the client against inserting sharp objects (e.g., coat hanger to scratch itchy skin) under the cast. Instruct him to use a soft bristle tooth brush or cool air from a hair dryer to help alleviate the itch.
   d. Teach the client appropriate cast care, depending on the type of cast.
   e. Encourage safety precautions (e.g., avoid walking on wet floors, watch throw rugs, be careful with stairs).
   f. Teach the client skin care and muscle-strengthening exercises for the affected body part after cast removal.
   g. Encourage mobility and active participation in self-care.
   h. Provide additional teaching as shown in *Client and family teaching 15-1,* page 410.
   i. Reinforce health care provider instructions on the amount of weight bearing allowed.
10. **Ensure proper technique and procedure in cast removal.**

XI. TRACTION APPLICATION

A. Description

1. **Traction** is an orthopedic treatment that involves placing tension on a limb, bone, or muscle group using various weight and pulley systems.
   a. **Straight or running traction** (e.g., Buck's traction, pelvic traction) involves a straight pulling force in one plane.
   b. **Balanced suspension traction** (e.g., pelvic sling, Thomas leg splint) involves exertion of a pull while the limb is supported by a hammock or splint held by balanced weights, which allows for some mobility without disruption of the line of pull. (See *Figure 15-4.*)
   c. **Skin traction** (e.g., Buck's traction, pelvic traction) involves weight applied and held to the skin with a Velcro splint.

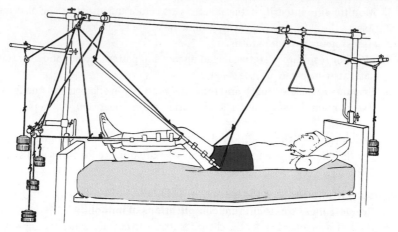

FIGURE 15-4
Balanced suspension traction with a Thomas leg splint is commonly used to stabilize a fractured femur.

Source: Smeltzer, S.C., and Bare, B.G. *Brunner and Suddarth's Textbook of Medical-surgical Nursing*, 10th ed. Philadelphia: Lippincott Williams & Wilkins, 2003.

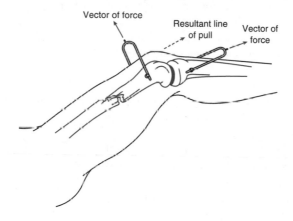

FIGURE 15-5
Skeletal traction may be applied in different directions to achieve the desired therapeutic line of pull. Adjustments in applied forces may be prescribed over the treatment period.

       d. Skeletal traction involves weight applied and attached to metal inserted into bone (e.g., pins, wires, tongs). (See *Figure 15-5.*)

  2. Traction is applied to:
      a. decrease muscle spasms
      b. reduce, align, and immobilize fractures (e.g., femur fractures that cannot be immobilized in a cast)
      c. correct or prevent deformity
      d. increase space between joint surfaces.

B. Assessment. Assess the client for the following while in traction:

1. **Monitor skin integrity** of the affected part before and after traction placement.
2. **Assess the skin,** especially bony prominences, for breakdown.
3. **Assess neurovascular status.**
4. **Monitor respiratory status,** including rate and pattern, breath and lung sounds, and ability to cough and breathe deeply.
5. **Evaluate muscle strength and tone and mobility** in affected and unaffected areas.
6. **Assess mental status,** noting level of orientation, effectiveness of coping, and behavior.
7. **Regularly check the condition of the traction equipment:** ropes, pulleys, and weights.
8. **For the client in skeleton traction, assess the pin site for signs and symptoms of infection.**

C. Nursing management (See section II.D.)

1. **Promote measures to prevent complications of immobility.**
   a. Place a bedboard under the client's mattress to ensure extra firm support.
   b. Turn and reposition the client regularly within the limitations of traction.
   c. Prevent constipation by increasing the client's fluid intake to 2,000 to 2,500 ml/day, and provide a balanced diet high in fiber.
2. **Promote skin integrity.**
   a. Use a special mattress to preserve skin integrity.
   b. Keep bed linen free of wrinkles to prevent skin breakdown.
   c. Provide frequent skin care to areas of potential pressure.
   d. Inspect skin traction for signs of skin breakdown. Assess areas over traction tape for tenderness or skin irritation. Always apply weights after the client is in the traction apparatus, and remove the weights before removing the traction apparatus.
   e. Inspect skeletal traction sites for signs of irritation or infection. Assess pin entrance and exit sites and areas surrounding pin sites at least twice each day. Clean pin sites as prescribed; never remove weights.
3. **Provide client teaching.**
   a. Encourage active exercises for unaffected body parts.
   b. Encourage the use of a trapeze, if indicated.
   c. Promote deep-breathing exercises hourly.
4. **Promote self-care within traction limitations.**

XII. ORTHOPEDIC SURGERY

A. Description. Orthopedic surgery refers to various surgical procedures involving the skeletal system and its joints, muscles, and associated structures.

1. **Specific procedures**
   a. **Open reduction** involves reduction and alignment of a fracture through a surgical opening.
   b. **Internal fixation** involves stabilization of a reduced fracture with screws, plates, nails, or pins.
   c. **Bone graft** involves placement of bone tissue for healing, stabilization, or replacement.
   d. **Arthroplasty** involves joint repair through a small arthroscope to avoid a large incision.

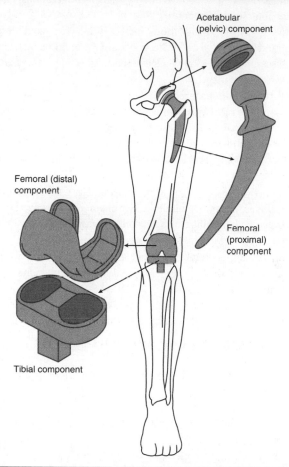

Acetabular
(pelvic) component

Femoral (distal)
component

Femoral
(proximal)
component

Tibial component

FIGURE 15-6
Hip and knee replacement

e. **Arthrodesis** involves immobilization of the joint through fusion.

f. **Joint replacement** involves replacement of joint surface with metal or plastic materials.

 – Total hip replacement involves replacement of the ball and socket of a severely damaged hip joint. (See *Figure 15-6.*)

 – Total knee replacement involves replacement of tibial, femoral, and patellar joint surfaces of a severely damaged knee joint. (See *Figure 15-6.*)

g. **Tendon transfer** involves movement of a tendon insertion to improve function.

h. **Tenotomy** involves cutting tendon.

i. **Fasciotomy** involves removal of muscle fascia, relieving constriction.

j. **Osteotomy** involves alignment of bone by removal of a wedge.

2. **Purpose of orthopedic surgery**

 a. Reconstruct diseased or injured musculoskeletal structures

 b. Replace a diseased or damaged bone or joint

 c. Remove a diseased or damaged bone or joint

 d. Repair an injured bone or joint

B. Assessment

 1. **Preoperative assessment**

    a. Elicit the client's medical history (e.g., past operations, responses to surgery medications and treatments).

    b. Identify current medications and conditions (e.g., colds, infections, steroids).

    c. Assess nutritional and hydration status: protein, calorie, and fluid intake.

    d. Assess the client's knowledge of the surgical procedure and treatment regimen.

    e. Assess skin integrity.

2. Postoperative assessment

    a. Assess the client's cardiovascular, respiratory, integumentary, fluid and electrolyte, and nutritional and hydration status.

    b. Assess the client's neurovascular status.

    c. Assess for joint dislocation (e.g., shortened extremity, increasing discomfort, impaired movement).

    d. Assess for infection (i.e., pain, fever, redness, edema, and dislocation).

    e. Assess for thromboembolism. (See chapter 7, section IV.)

    f. Assess and maintain the safety and effectiveness of the orthopedic apparatus.

3. Laboratory and diagnostic studies. Before surgery, the client should be in the most optimal condition, but because of trauma, this may not always be possible.

    a. Blood studies should reveal normal hemoglobin, hematocrit, and white blood cell count levels.

    b. Blood clotting studies should reveal normal clotting times.

    c. Radiographs should be normal and show no signs of infiltrate.

C. Nursing management (See section II.D.)

1. Provide preoperative care.

    a. Reinforce the health care provider's explanations of the surgery and related procedures.

    b. Provide meticulous skin preparation using aseptic technique as prescribed.

    c. Acquaint the client with postoperative treatment devices, procedures, exercises, and other measures.

    d. Provide routine preoperative nursing care. (See chapter 21.)

2. Provide postoperative care.

    a. Administer opioid or nonopioid analgesics, prophylactic antibiotics, and subcutaneous anticoagulants. (See *Drug chart 15-1,* pages 413 and 414.)

    b. Monitor blood loss at the operative site. Suction drainage as necessary. Monitor the incision site for infection.

    c. Perform regular neurovascular assessment.

    d. Turn and reposition the client, and exercise the unaffected body parts every 2 hours or as prescribed.

    e. Elevate the operative extremity to minimize edema.

    f. Encourage early ambulation and progressive weight bearing as prescribed.

    g. Develop an individualized exercise program within the client's limitations.

    h. Instruct the client in the proper use of assistive devices, if indicated.

    i. Encourage a well-balanced diet with increased protein and vitamin intake.

    j. Apply a sequential compression device and antiembolism stockings to help prevent deep vein thrombosis.

    k. Provide other routine postoperative nursing measures. (See chapter 21.)

    l. Position the client with a total hip replacement supine and on the unoperated side, supporting the entire operative leg in abducted position with an abductor pillow to prevent external rotation of the leg.

m. For the client with a total knee replacement, monitor the response to the continuous passive motion machine on the operative leg.
n. Provide client and family teaching.
– Instruct the client to pivot on the affected leg when turning.
– Teach the proper use of a walker or crutches; consult with a physical therapist as needed.
– Instruct the client to avoid activities causing hip flexion beyond 90 degrees (e.g., sitting in low chairs, riding in small cars) for 6 to 12 weeks after hip surgery. Encourage the client to obtain a raised toilet seat for use after discharge to prevent inappropriate hip flexion.
– Instruct the client who has had hip surgery to sit with the knees apart and to avoid crossing the legs.
– Assist in client teaching for stretching, exercise, and rest.
– Teach the client the signs and symptoms of joint and surgical complications (e.g., displacement, infection, bleeding) and to promptly notify his health care provider if any occur.
– Teach the client the importance of avoiding hyperflexion of the knee, jogging, jumping, heavy lifting, and obesity.
– Provide additional teaching as detailed in *Client and family teaching 15-1*, page 410.

Study questions

1. A client is admitted to the emergency department after a roller-blading accident and has a cast applied to the left lower leg for a fractured ankle. What instruction should the nurse include in her discharge teaching? (Select all that apply.)
1. "Keep the left leg in the dependent position as much as possible."
2. "Notify the health care provider if experiencing tingling or numbness of the left foot."
3. "Do not put anything down the cast if there is itching."
4. "Demonstrate the proper way to walk with crutches."
5. "Elevate your left foot to decrease swelling."
6. "It is normal to feel hot spots over the cast."

2. Which intervention should have priority for a client whose left arm is grossly deformed with ends of the humerus protruding through the skin?
1. Applying gentle traction to the area to align the fractured bone ends
2. Covering the broken skin and bone ends with a clean material
3. Securing a tight, clean covering around the broken skin and bone ends
4. Immediately splinting the deformed arm above the elbow at the fracture site

3. Which complication would the nurse suspect when assessing a client with a fractured femur and pelvis who becomes restless, exhibits dyspnea, and has petechiae over the chest area and crackles on auscultation?
1. Compartment syndrome
2. Deep vein thrombosis (DVT)
3. Fat embolism
4. Osteomyelitis

4. Which assessment data would indicate the effectiveness of analgesic medications for osteoarthritis?
1. The client has increased motion in joints with contractures.
2. The client's Heberden's nodes have disappeared.

3. The client reports decreased pain after exercise and at night.

4. The client demonstrates the ability to perform activities of daily living (ADLs).

5. For the client in a hip spica cast, which statement would alert the nurse to the potential complication of cast syndrome?
   1. "My skin is sensitive in warm, dry environments."
   2. "I become very upset when I feel confined in small spaces."
   3. "I had developed an infection after I had my appendix removed."
   4. "I felt more pain in my hip yesterday than I do today."

6. Which food would the nurse instruct the client with gouty arthritis to avoid when starting a low-purine diet?
   1. Citrus fruits
   2. Green vegetables
   3. Organ meats
   4. Fresh fish

7. Which assessment data would the nurse include when performing a neurovascular assessment on a client with a short left leg cast?
   1. Blood pressure (BP) and respiratory rate
   2. Pulse oximeter reading and arterial blood gases (ABGs)
   3. Level of consciousness (LOC) and pupillary size
   4. Pulse and polar

8. The health care provider orders Buck's traction for the client with a fractured hip. The nurse should plan for which traction applications?
   1. Balanced suspension skeletal traction
   2. Running skeletal traction
   3. Running skin traction
   4. Balanced suspension skin traction

9. Which intervention should the nurse implement when caring for a client with a fractured hip following application of Buck's traction?

1. Turning and repositioning the client with pillows every hour to prevent deformity
2. Cleaning the traction application site every 8 hours to improve circulation
3. Assessing pin sites every hour for signs and symptoms of infection
4. Assessing the neurovascular function in the affected leg every 2 hours

10. A client diagnosed with degenerative joint disease caused by osteoarthritis is scheduled for a total hip replacement of the right leg. What would be the nurse's *primary* concern?
   1. Local and systemic infections
   2. Self-care and ability to perform activities of daily living (ADLs)
   3. Response to pain medications
   4. Range of motion (ROM) in the affected joint

11. Which intervention would the nurse use to maintain the correct position of the client's right leg after a right total hip replacement?
   1. Placing an abductor wedge or pillows between the legs
   2. Using sandbags or pillows to keep the leg adducted
   3. Elevating the affected leg on two pillows or supports
   4. Positioning the client supine and on the operative side

12. When discussing physical activities with the client who has just undergone a right total hip replacement, which instruction should the nurse provide?
   1. "Avoid weight bearing until the hip is completely healed."
   2. "Intermittently cross and uncross your legs several times daily."
   3. "Pivot on the affected leg when transferring to the chair."
   4. "Limit hip flexion to only 45 to 60 degrees."

13. Which signs and symptoms indicate the need to decrease or stop the dosage of colchicine for the client experiencing an acute gout attack?

1. Bleeding gums and bruising
2. Vomiting and diarrhea
3. Gastric irritation and heartburn
4. Blurred vision and tinnitus

14. Which assessment finding would cause the nurse to suspect compartment syndrome in a client who received a long leg cast on the left leg 8 hours earlier and who complained of unrelenting pain that remained severe even after receiving pain medication?

1. Diminished capillary refill and cyanotic nail beds on the left leg
2. Warm, tender left calf and increased size of the left calf muscle
3. Ability to insert two fingers into the distal and proximal portion of the cast
4. Low-grade temperature and bilateral wheezing on lung auscultation

15. Which assessment finding would the nurse expect in a client diagnosed with osteomyelitis?

1. Leukocytosis and localized bone pain
2. Negative blood culture results and normal temperature
3. Hyperuricemia and pruritus
4. Petechiae over the chest and abnormal arterial blood gas (ABG) results

16. Which instruction would the nurse include in the discharge teaching for the client diagnosed with a left ankle sprain?

1. "Elevate the left leg, and apply ice packs periodically."
2. "Notify the health care provider if bruising occurs around the left ankle."
3. "Take colchicine every 8 hours to help with the pain."
4. "Keep the left leg in the continuous passive motion device."

Answer key

1. The answers are **2, 3, 4, 5.**
Tingling or numbness indicates neurovascular compromise that requires immediate intervention. Putting anything down the cast could cause a break in the skin integrity. The client will be using crutches. Elevating the foot will decrease edema. The foot should not be placed in the dependent position because that will increase edema. Hot spots are not normal; they may indicate infection under the cast and should be reported to the health care provider.

2. The answer is **2.**
The fracture described is an open, compound fracture, involving protrusion of the bone ends and a break in the skin. The immediate priority when caring for this fracture is to prevent movement until the limb is immobilized. First, the wound should be covered with a clean (or sterile if available) dressing to prevent further contamination. Next, the limb is splinted, moving the injured area as little as possible. No attempts to align or re-

duce the fracture, such as with gentle traction, should be made. The bone fragments should not be touched or pushed back into place. Using a tight, clean covering is inappropriate because it may act as a tourniquet, cutting off necessary blood flow. Splinting is done only after the area is protected from further contamination.

3. The answer is **3.**
The assessment findings of restlessness, dyspnea, chest petechiae, and crackles strongly suggest a fat embolism. The presenting features of fat embolism typically include cerebral disturbances manifested by mental status changes, tachypnea, dyspnea, crackles, wheezes, and large amounts of thick, white sputum. Compartment syndrome is associated with cyanotic nail beds; paresthesias; throbbing, unrelenting pain; and hard, swollen muscle. DVT usually manifests with swelling, warmth, and tenderness in the affected area. Osteomyelitis would be suspected if the client exhibited localized bone pain, tenderness,

heat, swelling, restricted movement, and fever and chills.

4. The answer is **3.**
Clients with osteoarthritis experience increased joint pain after exercise, at night, and in the early morning. Pain medication should relieve the pain during these times. Effectiveness of analgesia would be indicated by the client's reports of decreased pain in these areas. Increased motion in joints with contractures, disappearance of Heberden's nodes, and ability to perform ADLs are not specifically related to or reflective of analgesic effectiveness.

5. The answer is **2.**
Cast syndrome, which may involve physiologic or psychological manifestations, may occur in clients who are immobilized in large casts, such as a body or hip spica cast. Clients who report problems with claustrophobia are at risk for this complication. Cast syndrome associated with psychological manifestations is exhibited as a claustrophobic reaction involving acute anxiety and possible irrational behavior. Physiologic effects may include tachypnea, diaphoresis, dilated pupils, tachycardia, and elevated blood pressure related to the acute anxiety. Skin sensitivity in warm environments and a history of infection after surgery would alert the nurse to the client's potential risk for infection. Feeling more pain in the hip on the previous day is indicative of healing, not cast syndrome.

6. The answer is **3.**
Clients with gouty arthritis have a disorder of purine metabolism with abnormal amounts of urates in the body. Foods high in purine that should be avoided are organ meats, anchovies, sardines, shellfish, chocolate, and meat extracts. Citrus fruits, green vegetables, and fresh fish, which are not high in purine, are important to a well-balanced diet.

7. The answer is **4.**
A neurovascular assessment involves assessment of six areas (i.e., the six Ps): pallor, pulses, polar (i.e., coldness), pain, paresthesia, and paralysis. BP, respiratory rate, pulse oximeter reading, and ABG values are a part of a cardiopulmonary assessment. LOC and pupillary size are assessment data included in a neurologic assessment.

8. The answer is **3.**
The client has a fractured femur and needs the continuous traction pull to immobilize the fracture until surgery is performed. Buck's traction is an extension traction that exerts a straight pull on the leg. The traction is applied to the skin of the lower leg using a Velcro splint boot. Balanced suspension traction involves exertion of a pull while the limb is supported by balanced weights, which allows for some mobility without disruption of the line of pull. In balanced suspension skeletal traction, the weight is applied and attached to metal inserted into bone (e.g., pins, wires, tongs), whereas balanced suspension skin traction involves the use of a sling or similar device. Straight or running skeletal traction involves a straight pulling force in one plane through metal, such as pins, wires, or tongs inserted into the bone.

9. The answer is **4.**
Buck's traction is a type of skin traction. The priority here is neurovascular checks, which should be done every 2 hours for a client in traction to allow for early detection and prompt intervention if complications arise. A client in traction should be turned and positioned correctly about every 2 hours unless he is placed on a special mattress or device to prevent pressure ulcers. The traction tape should remain in place, but the area should be palpated to determine tenderness caused from pressure, decreased circulation, or nerve pressure. The nurse should check the ropes, pulleys, and weights for proper alignment and traction pull every 8 hours. Because Buck's traction is skin traction, there are no pin sites to inspect.

10. The answer is **1.**

Infection is a major concern for any client undergoing orthopedic surgery. It can be especially harmful for clients with joint replacements, because infection may prevent the client from achieving a functional joint postoperatively, possibly necessitating another surgical procedure. Although self-care, ability to perform ADLs, response to pain medications, and ROM may be important factors to assess, infection is the primary concern.

11. The answer is **1.**

After total hip replacement, the client should be kept flat while in a recumbent position with the affected extremity in an abducted position. This is accomplished by placing an abduction wedge or pillows between the client's legs. Adduction of the affected leg could cause dislocation of the hip replacement. Hip flexion should never extend beyond 45 to 60 degrees when elevating the leg or while sitting. The client should be turned only 45 degrees on the unoperated side, with full support to the operative leg to keep it in the abducted position.

12. The answer is **4.**

After a total hip replacement, the client should be taught to limit hip flexion to 45 to 60 degrees and to avoid activities that cause hip adduction (i.e., crossing legs), flexion beyond 90 degrees (i.e., sitting in low chairs or on low toilet seats), and rotation (i.e., pivoting on the affected leg). Progressive weight-bearing exercises are encouraged early, depending on health care provider's orders. Crossing the legs causes hip adduction, which is contraindicated after hip-replacement surgery. Pivoting on the affected leg causes rotational movement, also contraindicated after hip-replacement surgery.

13. The answer is **2.**

Anti-inflammatory medications such as colchicine are commonly prescribed to control acute attacks of gout. Because larger doses and high blood levels are needed, doses are usually prescribed to the maximum level tolerated, determined by the appearance of signs such as nausea, vomiting, and diarrhea. Bleeding gums, bruising, gastric irritation, heartburn, blurred vision, and tinnitus are signs and symptoms representing adverse effects of aspirin and must be addressed separately (e.g., giving enteric-coated tablets to reduce gastric irritation).

14. The answer is **1.**

Clinical manifestations of compartment syndrome may include diminished capillary refill; cyanotic nail beds; pulselessness distal to the involved area; deep, throbbing, unrelenting pain in affected area; and paresthesias and paralysis distal to the involved area. A warm, tender left calf and increased size of the left calf muscle indicate deep vein thrombosis. The nurse should be able to insert two fingers under the proximal and distal ends of the cast. Low-grade temperature and bilateral wheezing are signs unrelated to compartment syndrome.

15. The answer is **1.**

Osteomyelitis causes localized bone pain, tenderness, heat, and swelling at the affected area; high fever; increased white blood cell count and erythrocyte sedimentation rate; and positive blood culture results. Hyperuricemia and pruritus are associated with gouty arthritis. Petechiae over the chest and abnormal ABG results would suggest a fat embolism.

16. The answer is **1.**

Elevating the affected extremity and applying ice help decrease edema. Ecchymoses (i.e., bruising) is a common sign of sprains. The health care provider does not need to be notified. Colchicine is prescribed for an acute attack of gouty arthritis, not for a sprain. Using a continuous passive motion device is appropriate for a client with a total knee replacement.

16 Liver, biliary, and pancreatic disorders

I. STRUCTURE AND FUNCTION OF THE HEPATIC SYSTEM

A. Structure

1. **Liver** (See *Figure 16-1.*)

   a. The liver is the largest glandular organ of the body. It is located in the right upper abdominal quadrant, under the right diaphragm.

   b. The liver is divided into four lobes: left, right, caudate, and quadrate. The lobes are further subdivided into smaller units known as lobules.

   c. The liver contains several cell types, including hepatocytes (e.g., liver cells) and Kupffer's cells (e.g., phagocytic cells that engulf bacteria).

   d. Bile is continuously formed by hepatocytes (about 1 L/day). Bile comprises water, electrolytes, lecithin, fatty acids, cholesterol, bilirubin, and bile salts.

   – Bilirubin is pigment derived from the breakdown of hemoglobin. Hepatocytes remove bilirubin from the blood and conjugate it with glucuronic acid, which results in conjugated bilirubin being secreted into bile.

   – Bile salts, which are synthesized by hepatocytes from cholesterol, are required for emulsification of fats in the intestines. Bile salts are then reabsorbed in the distal ileum and returned to the liver through the portal vein to be used again.

   e. Blood supply to the liver is from the portal vein (75%), which drains the GI tract, and from the hepatic artery (25%).

2. **Biliary system** (See *Figure 16-1.*)

   a. **Canaliculi,** the smallest bile ducts located between liver lobules, receive bile from hepatocytes. The canaliculi form larger bile ducts, which lead to the hepatic duct.

   b. The **hepatic duct** from the liver joins the cystic duct from the gallbladder to form the common bile duct, which empties into the duodenum.

   c. **Oddi's sphincter** controls the flow of bile into the intestine.

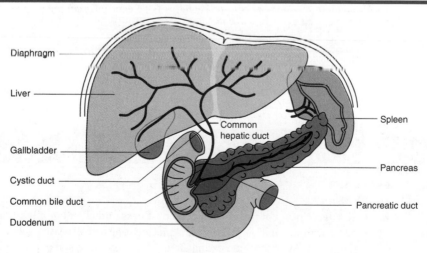

FIGURE 16-1
Liver and biliary system

    d. The **gallbladder** is a hollow, pear-shaped organ attached to the liver under the right lobe. The gallbladder normally holds 30 to 50 ml of bile and can hold up to 70 ml when fully distended.

  3. **Pancreas** (See *Figure 16-1,* page 433.)

    a. A slender, fish-shaped organ, the pancreas lies horizontally in the abdomen behind the stomach and extends roughly from the duodenum to the spleen.

    b. The functional pancreatic exocrine units are the secreting acini, which are arranged in lobules with channels that extend to the main lobular duct. The acini normally produce between 1,200 and 3,000 ml of pancreatic juice daily.

B. Function:

  1. **Liver** functions include:

    a. regulating blood glucose level by making glycogen, which is stored in hepatocytes

    b. synthesizing glucose from amino acids of lactate through gluconeogenesis

    c. converting ammonia produced from gluconeogenetic by-products and bacteria to urea

    d. synthesizing plasma proteins, such as albumin, globulins, clotting factors, and lipoproteins

    e. breaking down fatty acids into ketone bodies

    f. storing vitamins and trace metals

    g. affecting drug metabolism and detoxification

    h. secreting bile.

  2. **Biliary system** functions include:

    a. draining bile from hepatocytes to the gallbladder by way of the biliary tree

    b. storing bile in the gallbladder and releasing it to the duodenum, which is mediated by the hormone cholecystokinin.

  3. **The pancreas** has endocrine and exocrine functions. Endocrine functions are discussed in chapter 9, and exocrine functions are described subsequently in this chapter.

    a. The pancreas produces pancreatic juice, which is controlled by the vagus and two hormones (e.g., pancreozymin and secretin). Pancreatic juice contains three types of digestive enzymes.

      – Amylase hydrolyzes carbohydrate to disaccharides.

      – Lipase hydrolyzes fat to fatty acids and glycerol.

      – Trypsin, a proteolytic enzyme, splits proteins.

    b. The pancreas also secretes water and bicarbonate to neutralize gastric juice.

NURSING PROCESS OVERVIEW

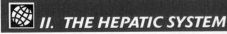

II. THE HEPATIC SYSTEM

A. Assessment

  1. **Health history**

    a. **Elicit a description of the client's present illness and chief complaint,** including onset, course, duration, location, and precipitating and alleviating factors. Cardinal signs and symptoms indicating altered hepatic, biliary, and pancreatic function include:

      – jaundice

      – changes in urine and stool color

      – vague to severe abdominal pain, especially after eating high fatty foods

      – abdominal tenderness and distention.

   b. **Explore the client's health history for risk factors** associated with hepatic, biliary, and pancreatic disorders, including:
- alcohol consumption
- high-fat diet
- infectious agents
- malnutrition.

2. **Physical examination**

  a. **Inspection**
- Inspect the abdomen for contour, pigmentation and color, scars, and striae.
- Assess for any visible masses, peristalsis, and pulsations.

  b. **Palpation**
- Palpate the liver to assess for consistency and firmness, pain, shape and nodules.
- Lightly palpate all four quadrants for masses, pain, and any abnormalities and then follow with deep palpation.

  c. **Percussion**
- Percuss all four quadrants in a systematic manner, beginning with the right lower quadrant, then right upper quadrant, crossing over to the left upper quadrant, and moving down to the left lower quadrant.
- Assess liver size by percussing the upper and lower liver borders.
- Record the level at which the lower border descends below the right costal margin.

  d. **Auscultation**
- Auscultate bowel sounds in all four quadrants.
- Auscultate for any abdominal bruits.

3. **Laboratory and diagnostic studies**

  a. **Liver**
- **Liver function tests** identify the degree of liver failure and include:
  - alkaline phosphatase level
  - alanine aminotransferase, also known as *serum glutamic-pyruvic transaminase;* and aspartate aminotransferase, also known as *serum glutamic-oxaloacetic transaminase*
  - serum proteins
  - direct and indirect bilirubin
  - serum ammonia
  - clotting factors
  - serum lipids
  - partial thromboplastin time
  - prothrombin time.
- **Liver biopsy,** sampling of liver tissue by needle aspiration for histologic analysis, can establish a diagnosis of specific liver disease.
- **Computed tomography (CT)** can detect neoplasms, cysts, abscesses, and hematomas.
- **Angiography** can visualize hepatic circulation or masses.
- **Splenoportography** can determine adequacy of portal blood flow.
- **Liver scan** can demonstrate liver size and shape.

  b. **Biliary system**
- **Ultrasonography** can detect calculi (e.g., gallstones) or a dilated common bile duct.
- **Radionuclide imaging** of the biliary tree and gallbladder can aid diagnosis of acute cholecystitis.

- **Cholecystography** can detect gallstones and assess the gallbladder's ability to fill, concentrate, and contract.
- **Endoscopic retrograde cholangiopancreatography (ERCP)** permits direct visualization of structures by inserting a flexible fiberoptic endoscope into the esophagus to the descending duodenum and then injecting a contrast material through a cannula into the biliary tree. Monitor for return of the gag reflex and for esophageal bleeding.
- **Percutaneous transhepatic cholangiography** is useful in distinguishing jaundice caused by liver disease.

c. **Pancreas**
- **Blood studies** include serum amylase level, lipase level, and white blood cell count (all of which are important aids in diagnosing pancreatitis) and serum bilirubin levels (which may be elevated in pancreatic dysfunction).
- **Radiographic studies** of the abdomen and chest may differentiate pancreatitis from other disorders.
- **Ultrasonography** and **CT scanning** can identify increased pancreas size and detect pancreatic cysts, pseudocysts, or tumors.
- **Stool analysis** evaluates fat content. Normally around 20%, fat content of stool may range from 50% to 90% in pancreatic disease.
- **ERCP** is the most helpful study in the diagnosis of pancreatitis; it also enables tissue biopsy for analysis and differentiates pancreatitis from carcinoma.

B. Nursing diagnoses
1. Acute pain
2. Imbalanced nutrition: less than body requirements
3. Excess or deficient fluid volume
4. Risk for infection
5. Risk for impaired skin integrity
6. Activity intolerance
7. Deficient knowledge
8. Disturbed thought processes
9. Disturbed body image

C. Planning and outcome identification. The major goals for a client diagnosed with a hepatic, biliary, or pancreatic disorder include relief of pain and discomfort, improved nutritional and fluid status, decreased potential for injury and infection, maintenance of skin integrity, increased activity tolerance, understanding of disease process and treatment, and improved mental status and body image.

D. Implementation
1. **Provide pain relief.** Assess the client's pain, rule out complications, medicate or intervene as appropriate, institute safety measures (side rails up, call light with reach), and evaluate the effectiveness of pain medication.
2. **Promote nutritional balance.**
   a. Assess nutritional status through diet history, provide appropriate diet for condition, and collaborate with a dietitian.
   b. Provide oral hygiene before meals.
   c. Ensure a pleasant environment for meal times.
3. **Provide ongoing assessment.**
   a. Assess all emesis and stool (e.g., bright red blood, occult blood, steatorrhea).
   b. Measure and record daily weight, intake and output, and abdominal girth.

CLIENT AND FAMILY TEACHING 16-1
Guidelines for a client diagnosed with liver dysfunction

- Instruct the client to keep his fingernails short, not to scratch himself, and to wear socks over his hands to protect skin integrity.
- Instruct the client to avoid harsh soaps and use emollient lotions.
- Encourage the client to take an Aveeno bath or small doses of Benadryl for itching.
- Instruct the client to use a soft toothbrush, avoid sharp objects, and blow his nose gently.
- Instruct the client to apply direct pressure for 5 minutes if bleeding occurs; if bleeding does not stop, tell him to notify his health care provider immediately.

- Instruct the client to notify his health care provider if untoward bleeding occurs (e.g., when brushing teeth, in urine).
- Instruct the client about a low-sodium diet. Advise him to avoid salt, salty foods, and canned or frozen foods. Encourage him to discuss salt substitutes with a health care provider; some products contain ammonia, which could precipitate hepatic encephalopathy.
- Warn the client to avoid the use of alcohol.
- Instruct the client to discuss prescription and over-the-counter medications with a health care provider before taking them.
- Instruct the client in proper handwashing techniques.

---

    c. Monitor and assess vital signs every 4 hours; watch for changes from baseline values.

    d. Assess for signs and symptoms of infection.

4. **Promote measures to increase activity tolerance.** Assist with selecting and pacing of activities, encourage rest, and assist with performing activities and hygiene when fatigued.

5. **Protect skin integrity.** Institute measures that help prevent skin breakdown, such as turning the client every 2 hours and using pressure-relieving devices.

6. **Enhance mental status.** Assess the client's level of consciousness, keep the client oriented to environment, and instruct the client to report mental confusion or lethargy at once.

7. **Provide client and family teaching.**

    a. Instruct the client on the cause of the disorder, signs and symptoms to report to a health care provider, interventions aimed at preventing complications, and appropriate administration of medications.

    b. Provide health education as detailed in *Client and family teaching 16-1.*

8. **Promote a positive body image.** Encourage the client to verbalize feelings about body image and self-concept changes.

E. Outcome evaluation

1. The client reports decreased pain with minimal discomfort.

2. The client maintains nutritional status, maintains adequate fluid and nutrient intake, and verbalizes understanding of dietary recommendations to help control symptoms.

3. The client maintains adequate electrolyte imbalance, has no change in weight or abdominal girth, and maintains adequate intake and output.

4. The client displays no evidence of infection or injury.

5. The client exhibits intact, uncompromised skin integrity with no evidence of jaundice.

6. The client reports decreased fatigue with activity.

7. The client verbalizes understanding of preventive measures, self-care to maintain health status, and understanding of the disorder and procedures used.

8. The client demonstrates improved mental status and increased level of consciousness.

9. The client verbalizes feelings about body image and self-concept.

III. CIRRHOSIS

A. **Description.** Cirrhosis is a chronic, degenerative liver disease marked by diffuse destruction and fibrotic regeneration of hepatic cells. It is classified as Laennec, posthepatic, or biliary cirrhosis. The incidence of cirrhosis is twice as high among men as women. Peak incidence occurs between ages 40 and 60.

B. **Etiology**
1. **Laennec's cirrhosis** is commonly caused by alcoholism and chronic nutritional deficiencies.
2. **Biliary cirrhosis** is caused by bile duct disorders that suppress bile flow.
3. **Posthepatic cirrhosis** is caused by various types of hepatitis.

C. **Pathophysiology**
1. In cirrhosis, liver cells are injured or destroyed and replaced with scar tissue. Regeneration of liver tissue is patchy, resulting in a characteristic "hobnail" appearance.
2. Fibrosis and other changes in hepatocytes and reticular cells, as well as vascular and bile duct changes, lead to decreased blood and bile flow. Obstructed blood flow results in portal hypertension and esophageal varices.
3. Impaired hepatic functions include gluconeogenesis, detoxification of drugs and alcohol, bilirubin metabolism, vitamin absorption, and hormonal metabolism.

D. **Assessment findings**
1. **Clinical manifestations**
   a. Enlarged, firm liver
   b. Chronic dyspepsia
   c. Constipation or diarrhea
   d. Gradual weight loss
   e. Ascites
   f. Splenomegaly
   g. Spider telangiectases
   h. Dilated abdominal blood vessels
   i. Signs and symptoms of portal hypertension (late)
2. **Laboratory and diagnostic study findings**
   a. Liver biopsy detects destruction and fibrosis of liver tissue.
   b. Liver scan reveals abnormal thickening and masses.
   c. Liver function test results for alanine aminotransferase, aspartate aminotransferase, and lactate dehydrogenase levels are elevated.
   d. Serum protein levels reveal hypoalbuminemia.
   e. Prothrombin time is elevated.

E. **Nursing management (See section II.D.)**
1. **Promote adequate nutrition.** Ensure a nutritious, high-protein diet supplemented with vitamins as prescribed.
2. **Protect the client from injury.**
   a. Prevent threats to skin integrity. Turn the client every 2 hours. Use mild, soft soaps.
   b. Minimize the risk of bleeding. Do not use sharp objects. Apply pressure if the client is bleeding.
   c. Minimize metabolic derangements that can cause further deterioration of mental status. Restrict dietary protein, limit visitors, and orient the client to date, time, and place.

    d. Institute safety measures, such as raising side rails and assisting with ambulation.

  3. **Develop a nursing care plan** to address the complications of liver failure (e.g., jaundice, portal hypertension, hepatic encephalopathy, bleeding esophageal varices).

  4. **Provide health education** as described in *Client and family teaching 16-1,* page 437.

  5. **Provide referrals** to the American Liver Foundation and Alcoholics Anonymous. (See appendix A.)

IV. JAUNDICE

A. Description. Jaundice is a symptom or syndrome characterized by increased bilirubin concentration in blood. It is classified as hemolytic, hepatocellular, or obstructive. Jaundice may also be hereditary.

B. Etiology

  1. **Hemolytic jaundice**
    a. Transfusion reaction
    b. Hemolytic anemia
    c. Severe burns
    d. Autoimmune hemolytic anemia

  2. **Hepatocellular jaundice**
    a. Hepatitis
    b. Yellow fever
    c. Alcoholism

  3. **Obstructive jaundice**
    a. **Extrahepatic** obstruction may be caused by bile-duct plugging from gallstones, an inflammatory process, tumor, or pressure from an enlarged gland.
    b. **Intrahepatic** obstruction may result from pressure on channels from inflamed liver tissue or exudate.

C. Pathophysiology

  1. **Hemolytic jaundice,** caused by increased destruction of red blood cells, results in the inability to excrete bilirubin as quickly as it forms.

  2. **Hepatocellular jaundice** results from the inability of diseased liver cells to clear normal amounts of bilirubin because of defective uptake, consumption, or transport mechanisms.

  3. **Obstructive jaundice** causes bile deposition in the skin, mucous membranes, and sclera, which results in characteristic yellow tinging of these structures.

D. Assessment findings

  1. **Clinical manifestations**
    a. Dark, foamy urine due to increased bile in the urine
    b. Light or clay-colored stools due to lack of bile in the small bowel
    c. Pruritus due to increased bile acids in the skin
    d. Inability to tolerate fatty foods due to absence of bile in the small intestine
    e. Mild to severe illness with other symptoms, such as anorexia, fatigue, nausea, weakness and, possibly, weight loss

  2. **Laboratory and diagnostic study findings**
    a. Conjugated bilirubin (direct) is normal or elevated.
    b. Unconjugated bilirubin (indirect) is normal or elevated.
    c. Total bilirubin is elevated.

       d. Urine bilirubin is absent or elevated.

       e. Urine urobilinogen may be decreased or increased.

       f. Fecal urobilinogen may be elevated, decreased, or absent.

       g. Aspartate aminotransferase is normal or elevated.

       h. Alanine aminotransferase is normal or elevated.

       i. Partial thromboplastin time is normal or prolonged.

E. **Nursing management (See section II.D.)**

1. **Assess and document degree of jaundice** of skin and sclera.
2. **Intervene to reduce anxiety.** Reinforce the health care provider's explanations about the cause and expected outcome of jaundice, and encourage the client to express feelings and concerns about body-image changes.
3. **Promote adequate nutrition.** Assess dietary intake and nutritional status. Encourage the client to adhere to a high-carbohydrate diet, with protein intake consistent with that recommended for hepatic encephalopathy.
4. **Provide a referral** to the American Liver Foundation. (See appendix A.)

V. PORTAL HYPERTENSION

A. **Description.** Portal hypertension is elevated pressure in the portal vein associated with increased resistance to blood flow through the portal venous system. Incidence is similar to that for cirrhosis.

B. **Etiology**

1. Cirrhosis
2. Mechanical obstruction (e.g., thrombosis, tumor)

C. **Pathophysiology**

1. Obstruction of portal venous flow through the liver leads to:
   a. formation of esophageal, gastric, and hemorrhoidal varicosities due to increased venous pressure
   b. accumulation of fluid in the abdominal cavity (i.e., ascites).
2. The spleen and other organs that empty into the portal system also undergo the effects of congestion.

D. **Assessment findings**

1. Ascites
2. Shifting dullness or fluid wave on abdominal percussion
3. Dilated abdominal vessels radiating from the umbilicus (e.g., caput medusae)
4. Enlarged, palpable spleen
5. Bruits detected over the upper abdominal area because of esophageal and gastric varicosities

E. **Nursing management (See section II.D.)**

1. **Administer medications,** which may include diuretics. (See *Drug chart 16-1.*)
2. **Measure and record abdominal girth and body weight daily;** assess for abdominal fluid wave. (See *Figure 16-2,* page 442.)
3. **Promote measures to prevent or reduce edema.**
   a. Encourage the client to elevate the lower extremities and wear support hose to prevent lower-extremity edema.

DRUG CHART 16-1

Medications for liver, biliary, and pancreatic disorders

Classifications	Indications	Selected interventions
Antacids aluminum hydroxide calcium carbonate dihydroxyaluminum sodium carbonate magaldrate magnesium hydroxide	Neutralize the hydrochloric acid secreted by the stomach	▪ Instruct the client to take 1 and 3 hours after meals and at bedtime; tell him to not take antacids with other medications. ▪ Instruct the client to chew antacid tablets and shake liquids before taking.
Antibiotics neomycin sulfasuxidine sulfathalidine	Inhibit ammonia-forming bacteria in the GI tract, thereby reducing ammonia and improving neurologic status	▪ Administer orally or as a retention enema. ▪ Before administering the first dose, assess the client for allergies and determine whether culture has been obtained. ▪ After multiple doses, assess the client for superinfection (thrush, yeast infection, diarrhea); notify the health care provider if these occur. ▪ Monitor the client's neurologic status. ▪ To assess effectiveness, monitor the client's ammonia level.
Antidiuretic hormone vasopressin	Constrict the splanchnic arterial bed and reduce portal pressure	▪ Administer I.V. or intra-arterially. ▪ Closely monitor the client for vasoconstrictive effects, such as angina or bowel ischemia.

Diuretics
Thiazide diuretic —
  chlorothiazide
Loop diuretic —
  furosemide
Potassium-sparing diuretic —
  spironolactone
	Decrease blood volume, which decreases the workload of the heart	▪ Monitor potassium level; do not administer if hypokalemic or hyperkalemic.
		▪ Monitor intake and output; increase fluid intake if necessary.
		▪ Hold and question the order if the client's blood pressure is < 90/60 mm Hg; teach the client about orthostatic hypotension.
		▪ Teach the client to weigh himself daily and to report weight gain of more than 2 lb in 1 day.

Histamine receptor antagonists cimetidine famotidine ranitidine	Block receptors that control secretion of hydrochloric acid by the parietal cells	▪ Instruct the client to continue taking the medication regularly, even after pain subsides. ▪ When administering I.V., dilute and monitor closely. ▪ Emphasize the importance of adhering to all aspects of therapy.
Immunoglobulin gamma globulin	Provide passive immunity through immunoglobulin G antibodies to protect against infection	▪ Before administering, obtain the client's allergy and immunization response history. ▪ After administering, monitor the client closely for signs and symptoms of allergic reaction.
Laxatives lactulose	Reduce serum ammonia levels by inducing catharsis, which decreases colonic pH and inhibits fecal flora from producing ammonia from urea	▪ Advise the client to expect two or three soft stools daily (ammonia is removed along with the stool), and explain that watery diarrhea indicates overdose. ▪ Dilute the medication with fruit juice to modify sweetness.

(continued)

DRUG CHART 16-1
Medications for liver, biliary, and pancreatic disorders *(continued)*

Classifications	Indications	Selected interventions
Opioid and nonopioid analgesics codeine hydrocodone hydromophone morphine propoxyphene	Relieve moderate to severe pain by reducing pain sensation, producing sedation, and decreasing the emotional upset often associated with pain; most often schedule II drugs	■ Assess the pain for location, type, intensity, and what increases or decreases it; rate pain on a scale of 1 (no pain) to 10 (worst pain). ■ Rule out any complications. Is this pain routine or expected? Is this a complication that needs immediate intervention? ■ Medicate according to pain scale findings. ■ Institute safety measures — bed in low position, side rails up, and call light within reach. ■ Evaluate effectiveness of pain medication in 30 minutes.
Pancreatic enzymes pancrelipase	Replace the enzymes necessary to digest protein, starches, and fats	■ Administer dose just before or during the meal. ■ Do not crush (or have the client chew) the medication, which has an enteric coating to protect it from gastric juices.
Proton-pump inhibitor omeprazole	Prevent the final transport of hydrogen ions into the gastric lumen by binding to an enzyme on gastric parietal cells	■ Instruct the client to take regularly as prescribed by the health care provider. ■ Instruct the client to avoid any products that may cause GI irritation.
Vitamin K AquaMEPHYTON	Promote clotting by providing fat-soluble vitamin necessary for clotting mechanism	■ Vitamin K may be administered I.M., subcutaneously, or I.V., however, I.V. administration is dangerous and should only be used as a last resort. ■ Explain to the client that green, leafy vegetables are high in vitamin K.

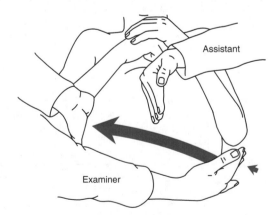

FIGURE 16-2
When assessing for abdominal fluid wave, the examiner places his hands along the client's flank, then strikes one flank sharply, detecting any fluid wave with the other hand. An assistant's hand is placed (ulnar side down) along the client's midline to prevent the fluid wave from being transmitted through the tissues of the abdominal wall.

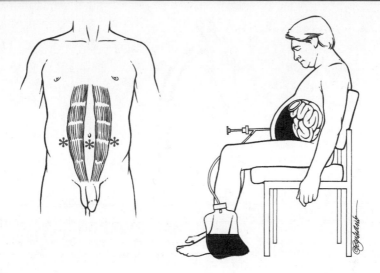

FIGURE 16-3
When the client with ascites undergoes paracentesis (aspiration of fluid for testing or drainage), the trocar is inserted to avoid the musculature (see stars above). To prevent hypotension, oliguria, hyponatremia, and possible shock, no more than 3 L of fluid should be aspirated.

Source: Smeltzer, S.C., and Bare, B.G. *Brunner and Suddarth's Textbook of Medical-surgical Nursing*, 10th ed. Philadelphia: Lippincott Williams & Wilkins, 2003.

       b. Administer salt-poor albumin, which temporarily elevates the serum albumin level. This increases serum osmotic pressure, helping to reduce edema by causing ascitic fluid to be drawn back into the bloodstream and eliminated by the kidneys.

    4. Assist the health care provider with paracentesis, which removes the fluid (e.g., ascites) from the peritoneal cavity; the volume usually is limited to 2 to 3 L of fluid, but it may be more. Observe the client closely for signs and symptoms of vascular collapse. (See *Figure 16-3*.)

    5. Prepare the client for peritoneojugular (LeVeen) shunting, if indicated, to shunt ascitic fluid to the venous system (not used often because of a high complication rate).

    6. Provide health education as detailed in *Client and family teaching 16-1*, page 437.

    7. Provide a referral to the American Liver Foundation. (See appendix A.)

VI. HEPATIC ENCEPHALOPATHY

  A. Description. Hepatic encephalopathy is a neurologic syndrome that develops as a complication of liver disease. It may be acute and self-limiting or chronic and progressive. Incidence is similar to that for cirrhosis.

  B. Etiology

    1. Severe liver injury

    2. Hepatocellular failure

    3. Portal shunting directly from the portal system to systemic venous circulation

    4. Increased serum ammonia levels from GI bleeding, a high-protein diet, or bacterial growth in the intestine and uremia

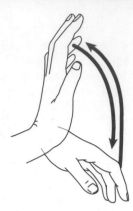

FIGURE 16-4
Asterixis or "liver flap" may occur in hepatic encephalopathy. The client is asked to hold his arm out with the hand held forward (dorsiflexed). Within a few seconds, the hand falls forward involuntarily and then quickly returns to the dorsiflexed position.

C. Pathophysiology. Hepatic encephalopathy results from accumulation of ammonia and other identified toxic metabolites in blood because of the liver cells' inability to convert ammonia to urea. Increased blood ammonia concentration leads to neurologic dysfunction and possible brain damage. Hepatic coma is the most advanced stage of hepatic encephalopathy.

D. Assessment findings
  1. **Clinical manifestations**
     a. Neurologic dysfunction progressing from minor mental aberrations and motor disturbances to coma
     b. Asterixis or flapping tremors of the hands (See *Figure 16-4.*)
  2. **Laboratory and diagnostic study findings**
     a. Serum ammonia level is elevated.
     b. Serum bilirubin level is elevated.
     c. Prothrombin time is prolonged.

E. Nursing management (See section II.D.)
  1. **Administer prescribed medications,** which may include antibiotics and laxatives. (See *Drug chart 16-1,* pages 441 and 442.)
  2. **Administer a high cleansing enema** to reduce ammonia absorption from the GI tract.
  3. **Closely monitor neurologic status for any changes.**
     a. Assess level of consciousness.
     b. Monitor for restlessness and agitation.
     c. Monitor handwriting daily; it becomes worse with increasing ammonia levels.
     d. Assess deep tendon reflexes.
  4. **Provide ongoing assessment.**
     a. Evaluate serum ammonia values daily.
     b. Monitor for signs of impending coma. Reduce or eliminate the client's dietary protein intake if you detect evidence of impending coma.
     c. Monitor electrolyte status and intervene as indicated to correct any imbalances.

🖐 *d.* Monitor the client closely, and administer a conservative dose of prescribed sedative or analgesic medication, because liver damage alters drug metabolism.

5. **Provide health education** as detailed in *Client and family teaching 16-1,* page 437.

6. **Provide a referral** to the American Liver Foundation. (See appendix A.)

VII. BLEEDING ESOPHAGEAL VARICES

A. **Description.** Bleeding esophageal varices are hemorrhagic processes involving dilated,
tortuous veins in the submucosa of the lower esophagus. Incidence is similar to that for cirrhosis.

B. **Etiology.** The most common cause is portal hypertension resulting from obstructed portal venous circulation.

C. **Pathophysiology**

1. In portal hypertension, collateral circulation develops in the lower esophagus as venous
blood, which is diverted from the GI tract and spleen because of portal obstruction,
seeks an outlet.

2. Because of excessive intraluminal pressure, these collateral veins become tortuous, dilated, and fragile. They are particularly prone to ulceration and hemorrhage. Rupture of
esophageal varices is the most common cause of death of clients with hepatic cirrhosis.

D. **Assessment findings**

1. **Clinical manifestations**

   a. Hematemesis and melena, if ulcerated massive hemorrhage occurs

   b. Signs of hepatic encephalopathy

   c. Dilated abdominal veins

   d. Ascites

2. **Laboratory and diagnostic study findings**

   a. Endoscopy identifies the cause and site of bleeding.

   b. Ultrasound and computed tomography assist in identifying the site of bleeding.

🔲 E. **Nursing management (See section II.D.)**

1. **Administer prescribed medication,** which may include vasopressin and vitamin K.
(See *Drug chart 16-1,* pages 441 and 442.)

2. **Provide ongoing assessment.**

   a. Assess for ecchymosis, epistaxis, petechiae, and bleeding gums.

   b. Monitor level of consciousness, vital signs, and urinary output to evaluate fluid balance.

   c. Monitor the client during blood transfusion administration if prescribed.

🖐 3. **Institute measures to address bleeding.** Use small-gauge needles, and apply pressure or cold for bleeding.

4. **Provide nursing care for the client undergoing a prescribed balloon tamponade
to control bleeding.** (See *Figure 16-5,* page 446.)

   a. Explain the procedure to the client to reduce fear and enhance cooperation with insertion and maintenance of the esophageal tamponade tube.

   b. Monitor the client closely to prevent accidental removal or displacement of the tube
   with resultant airway obstruction.

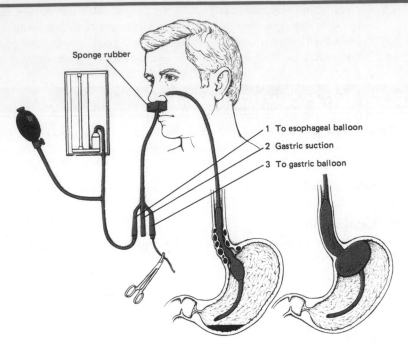

Sponge rubber

1 To esophageal balloon
2 Gastric suction
3 To gastric balloon

FIGURE 16-5
To stop variceal bleeding, an esophageal tamponade tube (also called a *compression balloon tube*) may be advanced and secured so that the compression balloon can be inflated against the bleeding. The various lumens permit inflation, deflation, suction, and other procedures.

Source: Nettina, S.M., ed. *The Lippincott Manual of Nursing Practice,* 8th ed. Philadelphia: Lippincott Williams & Wilkins, 2005.

5. **Provide nursing intervention for the client undergoing a prescribed iced saline lavage.**
    a. Ensure nasogastric tube patency to prevent aspiration.
    b. Observe gastric aspirate for evidence of bleeding.
    c. Protect the client from chilling.
6. **After injection sclerotherapy** (see *Figure 16-6*), assess for:
    a. aspiration
    b. esophageal perforation
    c. continued bleeding.
7. **After portal-systemic surgical intervention, monitor for complications.**
    a. Development of systemic encephalopathy
    b. Liver failure
    c. Continued bleeding
8. **Provide health education** as detailed in *Client and family teaching 16-1,* page 437.
9. **Provide a referral** to the American Liver Foundation. (See appendix A.).

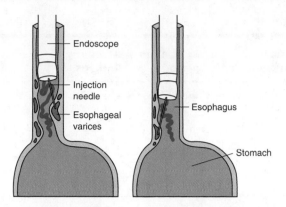

FIGURE 16-6
Injection of sclerosing agent into esophageal varices through an endoscope promotes thrombosis and eventual sclerosis, thereby obliterating the varices.

VIII. HEPATITIS

A. Description. Hepatitis is an inflammatory disorder of the liver parenchyma occurring in hepatitis A, hepatitis B, hepatitis C, hepatitis D, hepatitis E, and toxic or drug-induced hepatitis.

B. Etiology
1. Hepatitis A through E, which is usually linked to unidentifiable viral infection, can result from transfusion of contaminated blood products, exposure to infected persons in renal transplant and dialysis units, or parenteral drug abuse. (See *Table 16-1*, page 448.)
2. Toxic or drug-induced hepatitis results from chemicals or medications that damage the parenchyma (e.g., carbon tetrachloride, halothane, acetaminophen).

C. Pathophysiology
1. Hepatocellular damage results from the body's immune response to the virus or toxin and is characterized by diffuse inflammatory infiltration with local necrosis. Bile flow is interrupted, antigen-antibody complexes activate the complement system, bilirubin diffuses into tissues, bile salts accumulate, and hepatomegaly and splenomegaly occur. In uncomplicated cases, hepatocellular repair usually is completed within 3 to 4 months of onset.
2. Possible complications include fulminating hepatitis (a rare but life-threatening condition), chronic hepatitis, a chronic carrier state for hepatitis B surface antigen, cholestatic hepatitis, aplastic anemia, and pancreatitis.

D. Assessment findings
1. **Clinical manifestations.** The clinical findings produced by the various types of viral hepatitis have similarities and differences. (See *Table 16-1*, page 448.) Similar symptoms are classified into three stages.
   a. In the **preicteric stage,** the earliest symptoms are nonspecific, flulike symptoms that may include malaise, fatigue, headache, myalgias, anorexia, nausea, vomiting, and diarrhea.

TABLE 16-1
Viral hepatitis

Type	Modes of transmission	Incubation period	Assessment findings	Prevention
Type A	■ Fecal-oral route ■ Poor sanitation ■ Contaminated food and water ■ Person-to-person contact ■ Endemic in some parts of the world	15 to 50 days	■ May occur with or without symptoms ■ Preicteric phase: headache, malaise, fatigue, anorexia, fever ■ Icteric phase: dark urine, jaundice, tender liver	■ Careful handwashing, especially after bowel movement ■ Safe food and water supply ■ Effective sewage disposal ■ Hepatitis A vaccine ■ Administration of globulin within 2 weeks of exposure
Type B	■ Parenteral transmission ■ Sexual contact with carriers ■ Perinatal transmission ■ Contaminated instruments (e.g., syringes)	25 to 160 days	■ Same as hepatitis A ■ Fever and respiratory problems rare ■ Possibly arthralgias and rashes ■ Possibly jaundice ■ Light-colored stools and dark urine	■ Continued screening of potential blood donors ■ Disposable syringes, needles, and lancets ■ Needleless I.V. delivery systems ■ Adherence to standard precautions ■ Administration of specific hepatitis B immune globulin ■ Hepatitis B vaccine
Type C	■ Transfusion of blood and blood products ■ Exposure to contaminated blood through equipment or drug paraphernalia (formerly known as non-A, non-B hepatitis)	15 to 160 days	■ Similar to hepatitis B but less severe and anicteric ■ Increased risk of chronic liver disease	■ Screening of blood transfusions ■ Adherence to standard precautions ■ Instruction to I.V. drug users to not share needles
Type D	■ Requires hepatitis B surface antigen for replication, so only clients with hepatitis B at risk for hepatitis D ■ Parenteral transmission ■ Sexual contact with carriers ■ Perinatal transmission ■ Contaminated instruments (e.g., syringes)	21 to 140 days	■ Similar to hepatitis B except client is more likely to have chronic active hepatitis and cirrhosis	■ Same as hepatitis B ■ Type D common among I.V. drug abusers, clients undergoing hemodialysis, and clients with multiple blood transfusions ■ Safe sex practices ■ Adherence to standard precautions
Type E	■ Fecal-oral route ■ Person-to-person contact	15 to 65 days	■ Similar to hepatitis A ■ Very severe in pregnant women	■ Avoiding close contact with persons with hepatitis E ■ Careful handwashing

    b. In the **icteric stage,** which occurs a few days to weeks after the preicteric stage, symptoms include jaundice, dark-colored urine, light-colored stool, steatorrhea, and an enlarged liver.

    c. In the **posticteric stage,** a convalescent stage lasting a few weeks, fatigue decreases, jaundice resolves, and appetite returns.

  2. Laboratory and diagnostic study findings

    a. Serum liver function test results are elevated.

b. Serum bilirubin level is increased.

c. Serum antibody markers identify specific type of hepatitis.

d. Urinalysis reveals increased bilirubin levels.

e. Prothrombin time or partial thromboplastin time may be prolonged.

E. Nursing management (See section II.D.)

1. **Administer prescribed medications,** which may include immunoglobulins and immunizations. (See *Drug chart 16-1,* pages 441 and 442; also see *Table 16-1.*)

2. **Prevent the transmission of infection.**

   a. Institute enteric and blood and body secretion standard precautions.

   b. Ensure proper hand washing after caring for the client, especially after handling soiled clothing and linens, after using the restroom, and before eating or handing food.

3. **Promote adequate rest without complications.**

   a. Encourage the client to decrease activities and stay on bed rest until enlarged liver and liver enzymes return to normal. Convalescence may be 2 to 4 months; gradually increase activity.

   b. Institute measures to prevent complications of prolonged bed rest, such as pressure ulcers, pneumonia, constipation, and deep vein thrombosis.

4. **Encourage proper nutrition.** Proteins are restricted when the liver is unable to metabolize proteins. Provide a high-calorie, low-fat diet in small, frequent feedings.

5. **Intervene to provide symptomatic relief as appropriate** (e.g., antacids, antiemetics).

6. **Promote client and family coping.** Address the client and family's psychosocial concerns, especially when lifestyle must be altered because of the disease process.

7. **Provide health education** concerning the mechanism of disease transmission, methods for maintaining adequate environmental hygiene, prophylactic immunizations, and avoidance of blood donations by infected persons.

IX. CHOLELITHIASIS AND CHOLECYSTITIS

A. Description

1. **Cholelithiasis** refers to formation of calculi (e.g., gallstones) in the gallbladder. The condition affects approximately 20% of the population in the United States, is the fifth leading cause of hospitalization of adults, and is associated with about 90% of all gallbladder disease in the United States. Incidence is greater among women than men before age 50 but is approximately equal after age 50.

2. **Cholecystitis** is acute or chronic inflammation of the gallbladder.

   a. **Acute cholecystitis** may be calculous (with gallstones) or acalculous (without gallstones). It is most common in middle-aged persons. The incidence is greater in women than in men (about 3:1).

   b. **Chronic cholecystitis** may follow acute cholecystitis, although it often occurs independently. It is usually associated with gallstone formation. The chronic form usually affects the elderly. The incidence is greater in women than in men (about 3:1).

B. Etiology

1. **Cholelithiasis** results from changes in bile components or bile stasis, which may be associated with such factors as infection, cirrhosis, pancreatitis, celiac disease, diabetes mellitus, pregnancy, and hormonal contraceptive use.

2. **Cholecystitis** can result from:

   a. obstruction of the cystic duct by an impacted gallstone (90% to 95% of cases)

   b. tissue damage due to trauma, massive burns, or surgery

     c. gram-negative septicemia

     d. multiple blood transfusions

     e. prolonged fasting

     f. hypertension

     g. overuse of opioid analgesics.

C. Pathophysiology

1. **Cholelithiasis**

    a. Calculi usually form from solid constituents of bile; the three major types are:

      – **cholesterol gallstones,** the most common type, thought to form in supersaturated bile

      – **pigment gallstones,** formed mainly of unconjugated pigments in bile precipitate

      – **mixed types,** with characteristics of pigment and cholesterol stones.

    b. Gallstones can obstruct the cystic duct, causing cholecystitis, or the common bile duct, which is called choledocholithiasis.

2. **Cholecystitis**

    a. In acute and chronic cholecystitis, inflammation causes the gallbladder wall to become thickened and edematous and causes the cystic lumen to increase in diameter. Submucosal hemorrhage, mucosal ulceration, and polymorphonuclear infiltration follow.

    b. If inflammation spreads to the common bile duct, obstruction of bile drainage can lead to jaundice. Other possible complications include:

      – empyema (i.e., pus-filled gallbladder)

      – perforation

      – emphysematous cholecystitis.

D. Assessment findings

1. **Clinical manifestations**

    a. **Cholelithiasis.** Up to one half of persons with gallstones are asymptomatic; however, possible clinical manifestations include:

      – episodic (commonly after a high-fat meal), cramping pain in the right upper abdominal quadrant or the epigastrium, possibly radiating to the back near the right scapular tip (i.e., biliary colic)

      – nausea and vomiting

      – fat intolerance

      – fever and leukocytosis

      – signs and symptoms of jaundice.

    b. **Acute cholecystitis** is commonly marked by:

      – biliary colic

      – tenderness and rigidity in the right upper quadrant elicited on palpation (i.e., Murphy's sign)

      – fever

      – nausea and vomiting

      – fat intolerance

      – signs and symptoms of jaundice.

    c. **Chronic cholecystitis** is commonly marked by:

      – pain, which is less severe than in the acute form

      – fever, which is less severe than in the acute form

      – fat intolerance

      – heartburn

      – flatulence.

2. **Laboratory and diagnostic study findings**

   a. **Cholelithiasis.** Biliary ultrasonography (i.e., cholecystosonography) can detect gallstones in most cases.

   b. **Cholecystitis**
   - White blood cell count reveals leukocytosis.
   - Serum alkaline phosphatase is elevated.
   - Ultrasonography detects gallstones.
   - Oral cholecystography cannot visualize the gallbladder.
   - Endoscopic retrograde cholangiopancreatography may reveal inflamed common bile ducts, gallbladder, and gallstones.
   - Percutaneous transhepatic cholangiography can identify gallstones within the bile ducts.

E. Nursing management (See section II.D.)

1. **Administer prescribed medications,** which include analgesics and antacids. (See *Drug chart 16-1,* pages 441 and 442.)

2. **Provide nursing interventions** during an acute gallbladder attack.
   a. Intervene to relieve pain; give prescribed analgesics.
   b. Promote adequate rest.
   c. Administer I.V. fluids, and monitor intake and output.
   d. Monitor nasogastric tube and suctioning.
   e. Administer antibiotics if prescribed.

3. **Promote adequate nutrition.** Assess nutritional status. Encourage a high-protein, high-carbohydrate, low-fat diet.

4. **Monitor for signs and symptoms of possible complications.**

5. **Teach the client about planned treatments.**
   a. Chenodeoxycholic acid is administered to dissolve gallstones. It is effective in dissolving about 60% of radiolucent gallstones. Pigment gallstones cannot be dissolved and must be excised.
   b. Nonsurgical removal, such as lithotripsy or extracorporeal shock wave therapy, may be implemented.
   c. Surgical treatment may be ordered.
      - Laparoscopic cholecystectomy (usually outpatient surgery) is performed through a small incision made through the abdominal wall in the umbilicus. Assess incision sites for infection. Instruct the client to notify the health care provider if loss of appetite, vomiting, pain, abdominal distention, or fever occur. Advise the client that he will need assistance at home for 2 to 3 days.
      - Cholecystectomy is removal of the gallbladder after ligation of the cystic duct and artery. Inform the client that a T-tube will be inserted to drain blood, serosanguineous fluids, and bile and that the T-tube must be taped below the incision.
      - Choledochostomy is an incision into the common bile duct for calculi removal.
      - Cholecystomy is the surgical opening of the gallbladder for removal of stones, bile, or pus, after which a drainage tube is placed.

X. ACUTE PANCREATITIS

A. Description. Acute pancreatitis is inflammation of the pancreas ranging from a relatively mild, self-limiting disorder to rapidly fatal, acute hemorrhagic pancreatitis.

B. Etiology

1. The major causes of acute pancreatitis are:
   a. alcoholism
   b. cholecystitis
   c. surgery involving or near the pancreas.
2. Other possible predisposing factors include:
   a. viral hepatitis, mumps, peptic ulcer disease, periarteritis, hyperlipidemia, hypercalcemia, anorexia nervosa, shock with ischemia, trauma to the pancreas, and endoscopic retrograde cholangiopancreatography
   b. use of medications, such as thiazide diuretics, furosemide, valproic acid, estrogens, tetracycline, azathioprine, mercaptopurine, sulfonamides, and glucocorticoids.

C. Pathophysiology.

Acute pancreatitis involves various pathologic changes, ranging from edema and inflammation to necrosis and hemorrhage. Because of abnormal pancreatic enzyme activation in the pancreas (instead of in the GI tract), the pancreas begins to digest itself. Kinin activation alters cell membrane permeability, causing a loss of protein-rich fluid into the tissues and peritoneal cavity and producing hypovolemia.

D. Assessment findings

1. **Clinical manifestations**
   a. Abdominal tenderness with back pain
   b. GI problems, such as nausea, vomiting, diarrhea, and steatorrhea
   c. Fever
   d. Jaundice
   e. Mental confusion
   f. Flank or umbilical bruising
   g. Hypotension
   h. Signs of hypovolemia
   i. Possibly, respiratory distress
2. **Laboratory studies and diagnostic study findings.** Blood studies may reveal elevated amylase, lipase, and white blood cell count levels.

E. Nursing management (See section II.D.)

1. **Administer prescribed medications,** which include opioid or nonopioid analgesics, histamine receptor antagonists, and proton-pump inhibitors. (See *Drug chart 16-1,* pages 441 and 442.)
2. **The client should avoid oral intake** to inhibit pancreatic stimulation and secretion of pancreatic enzymes. Total parenteral nutrition is administered to assist with metabolic stress.
3. **Maintain patent nasogastric suctioning** to relieve nausea and vomiting, decrease painful abdominal distention, and remove hydrochloric acid.
4. **Maintain fluid and electrolyte balance.** Assess fluid and electrolyte status (e.g., skin turgor, mucous membranes, intake and output), and provide replacement therapy as indicated.
5. **Promote adequate nutrition.** Assess nutritional status; monitor glucose levels; monitor I.V. therapy; provide a high-carbohydrate, low-protein, low-fat diet when tolerated; and instruct the client to avoid spicy foods.
6. **Maintain optimal respiratory status.** Place the client in semi-Fowler's position to decrease pressure on the diaphragm. Teach the client coughing and deep-breathing techniques.

7. **Institute measures to prevent complications of immobility,** such as impaired skin integrity, constipation, and deep vein thrombosis.

8. **Monitor for complications,** which may include fluid and electrolyte disturbances, pancreatic necrosis, shock and multiple organ failure.

9. **Provide a referral** to Alcoholics Anonymous, if indicated. (See appendix A.)

XI. CHRONIC PANCREATITIS

A. **Description.** Chronic pancreatitis is progressive pancreatic inflammation resulting in permanent structural damage to pancreatic tissue.

B. **Etiology**
   1. Chronic pancreatitis typically results from repeated episodes of acute pancreatitis.
   2. More than half of chronic pancreatitis cases are associated with alcoholism.

C. **Pathophysiology.** With repeated attacks of pancreatitis, pancreatic cells are progressively replaced with fibrous tissue, causing increased pressure within the pancreas. Eventually, this results in mechanical obstruction of the pancreatic duct, common bile duct, and duodenum. Other effects include atrophy of the ductal epithelium, inflammation, and destruction of pancreatic cells.

D. **Assessment findings**
   1. **Clinical manifestations** of chronic pancreatitis commonly include pain, weight loss, steatorrhea, and anorexia.
   2. **Laboratory and diagnostic study findings**
      a. Serum amylase and lipase levels are elevated.
      b. White blood cell count is elevated.
      c. Endoscopic retrograde cholangiopancreatography detects pancreatic calcification.
      d. Glucose tolerance test values are abnormal.

E. **Nursing management (See section II.D.)**
   1. **Administer prescribed medications,** which include pancreatic enzymes, nonopioid pain medications, antacids, histamine receptor antagonists, and proton-pump inhibitors. (See *Drug chart 16-1,* pages 441 and 442.)
   2. **Promote measures to provide comfort.**
      a. Provide symptomatic treatment, focusing on relieving pain, promoting comfort, and treating new attacks.
      b. Emphasize the importance of avoiding alcohol, caffeine, and foods that tend to cause abdominal discomfort.
      c. See section X for the nursing care for a client with an acute exacerbation of chronic pancreatitis.
   3. **Prepare the client for surgery** to relieve pain and drain cysts, if indicated.
   4. **Manage any endocrine insufficiency,** such as diabetes mellitus, by initiating dietary and insulin or oral hypoglycemic therapy.
   5. **Provide a referral** to Alcoholics Anonymous, if indicated. (See appendix A.)

Study questions

1. Which assessment finding indicates that lactulose is effective in decreasing the ammonia level in the client with hepatic encephalopathy?
   1. Passage of two or three soft stools daily
   2. Evidence of watery diarrhea
   3. Daily deterioration in the client's handwriting
   4. Appearance of frothy, foul-smelling stools

2. For the client with jaundice, which statement indicates that the nurse understands the rationale for instituting skin care measures?
   1. "Jaundice is associated with pressure ulcer formation."
   2. "Jaundice impairs urea production, which produces pruritus."
   3. "Jaundice produces pruritus due to impaired bile acid excretion."
   4. "Jaundice leads to decreased tissue perfusion and subsequent breakdown."

3. Which rationale supports explaining the placement of an esophageal tamponade tube in a client who is hemorrhaging?
   1. Obtaining cooperation and reducing fear
   2. Beginning teaching for home care
   3. Allowing the client to help insert the tube
   4. Maintaining the client's level of anxiety and alertness

4. Which nursing intervention would be *most* helpful for a client with chronic pancreatitis?
   1. Modifying dietary protein
   2. Encouraging daily exercise
   3. Allowing liberalized fluid intake
   4. Counseling to stop alcohol consumption

5. A client is in end-stage liver failure. Which interventions should the nurse implement when addressing hepatic encephalopathy? (Select all that apply.)
   1. Assessing the client's neurologic status every 2 hours
   2. Monitoring the client's hemoglobin and hematocrit levels
   3. Evaluating the client's serum ammonia level
   4. Monitoring the client's handwriting daily
   5. Preparing to insert an esophageal tamponade tube
   6. Making sure the client's fingernails are short

6. Which instruction would be included in the teaching plan for the client taking antacids?
   1. "Take the antacid with 8 oz of water."
   2. "Avoid taking other medications within 2 hours of this one."
   3. "Continue taking antacids even when pain subsides."
   4. "Weigh yourself daily when taking this medication."

7. Which clinical manifestations would the nurse expect a client diagnosed with acute cholecystitis to exhibit?
   1. Nausea, vomiting, and anorexia
   2. Ecchymosis, petechiae, and coffee-ground emesis
   3. Jaundice, dark urine, and steatorrhea
   4. Acute right lower quadrant (RLQ) pain, diarrhea, and dehydration

8. Which intervention should the nurse include in the care plan for a client with acute pancreatitis?
   1. Administration of vasopressin and insertion of a balloon tamponade
   2. Preparation for a paracentesis and administration of diuretics

3. Maintenance of nothing-by-mouth status and insertion of a nasogastric (NG) tube with low intermittent suction
4. Dietary plan of a low-fat diet and increased fluid intake to 2,000 ml/day

9. When teaching a client about pancreatic function, the nurse understands that pancreatic lipase performs which function?
1. Breaks down fat into fatty acids and glycerol
2. Transports fatty acids into the brush border
3. Triggers cholecystokinin to contract the gallbladder
4. Breaks down protein into dipeptides and amino acids

10. After administering diuretic therapy to a client with ascites, which nursing action would be most effective in ensuring safe care?
1. Measuring serum potassium for hyperkalemia
2. Assessing the client for hypervolemia
3. Measuring the client's weight weekly
4. Documenting precise intake and output

11. Which outcome would be most appropriate for the client in hepatic coma?
1. The client is oriented to time, place, and person.
2. The client exhibits no ecchymotic areas.
3. The client increases oral intake to 2,000 calories/day.
4. The client exhibits increased serum albumin level.

12. Which nursing intervention would be included in the care plan for the client with jaundice who is experiencing pruritus?
1. Keeping the client's fingernails short and smooth
2. Applying pressure when giving I.M. injections

3. Decreasing the client's dietary protein intake
4. Administering vitamin K subcutaneously

13. Which diet, when selected by the client with cholecystitis, indicates that the nurse's teaching has been successful?
1. Six small meals of low-carbohydrate foods daily
2. High-fat, high-carbohydrate meals
3. Low-fat, high-carbohydrate meals
4. High-fat, low-protein meals

14. Which assessment finding indicates a complication after percutaneous transhepatic cholangiography?
1. Fever and chills
2. Hypertension
3. Bradycardia
4. Nausea and diarrhea

15. When planning home care for a client with hepatitis A, which preventive measure should be emphasized to protect the client's family?
1. Keeping the client in complete isolation
2. Using good sanitation with dishes and shared bathrooms
3. Avoiding contact with blood-soiled clothing or dressings
4. Forbidding the sharing of needles or syringes

16. Which intervention would be *most* important for the client with hepatic cirrhosis who has altered clotting mechanisms?
1. Allowing complete independence of mobility
2. Applying pressure to injection sites
3. Administering antibiotics as prescribed
4. Increasing nutritional intake

Answer key

1. The answer is **1.**
Lactulose reduces serum ammonia levels by inducing catharsis, subsequently decreasing colonic pH and inhibiting fecal flora from producing ammonia from urea. Ammonia is removed with the stool. Two or three soft stools daily indicate effectiveness of the drug. Watery diarrhea indicates overdose. Daily deterioration in the client's handwriting indicates an increase in the ammonia level and worsening of hepatic encephalopathy. Frothy, foul-smelling stools indicate steatorrhea, caused by impaired fat digestion.

2. The answer is **3.**
Jaundice is a symptom characterized by increased bilirubin concentration in the blood. Bile acid excretion is impaired, increasing the bile acids in the skin and causing pruritus. Jaundice is not associated with pressure ulcer formation. However, edema and hypoalbuminemia are. Jaundice itself does not impair urea production or lead to decreased tissue perfusion.

3. The answer is **1.**
An esophageal tamponade tube would be inserted in critical situations. Typically, the client is fearful and highly anxious. The nurse therefore explains about the placement to help obtain the client's cooperation and reduce his fear. This type of tube is used only short term and is not indicated for home use. The tube is large and uncomfortable. The client would not be helping to insert the tube. A client's anxiety should be decreased, not maintained, and depending on the degree of hemorrhage, the client may not be alert.

4. The answer is **4.**
Chronic pancreatitis typically results from repeated episodes of acute pancreatitis. More than half of chronic pancreatitis cases are associated with alcoholism. Counseling to stop alcohol consumption would be the most helpful for the client. Dietary protein modification is not necessary for chronic pancreatitis. Daily exercise and liberalizing fluid intake would be helpful but not the most beneficial intervention.

5. The answers are **1, 3, 4.**
Hepatic encephalopathy results from an increased ammonia level due to the liver's inability to covert ammonia to urea, which leads to neurologic dysfunction and possible brain damage. The nurse should monitor the client's neurologic status, serum ammonia level, and handwriting. Monitoring the client's hemoglobin and hematocrit levels and insertion of an esophageal tamponade tube address esophageal bleeding. Keeping fingernails short addresses jaundice.

6. The answer is **2.**
Antacids neutralize gastric acid and decrease the absorption of other medications. The client should be instructed to avoid taking other medications within 2 hours of the antacid. Water, which dilutes the antacid, should not be taken with antacid. A histamine receptor antagonist should be taken even when pain subsides. Daily weights are indicated if the client is taking a diuretic, not an antacid.

7. The answer is **1.**
Acute cholecystitis is an acute inflammation of the gallbladder commonly manifested by the following: anorexia, nausea, and vomiting; biliary colic; tenderness and rigidity in the right upper quadrant (RUQ) elicited on palpation (e.g., Murphy's sign); fever; fat intolerance; and signs and symptoms of jaundice. Ecchymosis, petechiae, and coffee-ground emesis are clinical manifestations of esophageal bleeding. The coffee-ground appearance indicates old bleeding. Jaundice, dark urine, and steatorrhea are clinical manifestations of the icteric phase of hepatitis.

Pain of cholecystitis is typically located in the RUQ, not the RLQ. RLQ pain is commonly present with appendicitis. Diarrhea and dehydration are not common with acute cholecystitis.

8. The answer is **3.**
With acute pancreatitis, the client is kept on nothing-by-mouth status to inhibit pancreatic stimulation and secretion of pancreatic enzymes. NG intubation with low intermittent suction is used to relieve nausea and vomiting, decrease painful abdominal distention, and remove hydrochloric acid. Vasopressin would be appropriate for a client diagnosed with bleeding esophageal varices. Paracentesis and diuretics would be appropriate for a client diagnosed with portal hypertension and ascites. A low-fat diet and increased fluid intake would further aggravate the pancreatitis.

9. The answer is **1.**
Lipase hydrolyzes or breaks down fat into fatty acids and glycerol. Lipase is not involved with the transport of fatty acids into the brush border. Fat itself triggers cholecystokinin release. Protein breakdown into dipeptides and amino acids is the function of trypsin, not lipase.

10. The answer is **4.**
For the client with ascites receiving diuretic therapy, careful intake and output measurement is essential for safe diuretic therapy. Diuretics lead to fluid losses, which if not monitored closely and documented, could place the client at risk for serious fluid and electrolyte imbalances. Hypokalemia, not hyperkalemia, commonly occurs with diuretic therapy. Because urine output increases, a client should be assessed for hypovolemia, not hypervolemia. Weights are also an accurate indicator of fluid balance. However, for this client, weights should be obtained daily, not weekly.

11. The answer is **1.**
Hepatic coma is the most advanced stage of hepatic encephalopathy. As hepatic coma resolves, improvement in the client's level of consciousness occurs. The client should be able to express orientation to time, place, and person. Ecchymotic areas are related to decreased synthesis of clotting factors. Although oral intake may be related to level of consciousness, it is more closely related to anorexia. The serum albumin level reflects hepatic synthetic ability, not level of consciousness.

12. The answer is **1.**
The client with pruritus experiences itching, which may lead to skin breakdown and possibly infection from scratching. Keeping his fingernails short and smooth helps prevent skin breakdown and infection from scratching. Applying pressure when giving I.M. injections and administering vitamin K subcutaneously are important if the client develops bleeding problems. Decreasing the client's dietary protein intake is appropriate if the client's ammonia levels are increased.

13. The answer is **3.**
For the client with cholecystitis, fat intake should be reduced. The calories from fat should be substituted with carbohydrates. Reducing carbohydrate intake would be contraindicated. Any diet high in fat may lead to another attack of cholecystitis.

14. The answer is **1.**
Septicemia is a common complication after a percutaneous transhepatic cholangiography. Evidence of fever and chills, possibly indicative of septicemia, is important. Hypotension, not hypertension, is associated with septicemia. Tachycardia, not bradycardia, is most likely to occur. Nausea and diarrhea may occur but are not classic signs of sepsis.

15. The answer is **2.**
Hepatitis A is transmitted through the fecal-oral route or from contaminated water or

food. Measures to protect the family include good handwashing, personal hygiene and sanitation, and use of standard precautions. Complete isolation is not required. Avoiding contact with blood-soiled clothing or dressings or avoiding the sharing of needles or syringes are precautions needed to prevent transmission of hepatitis B.

16. The answer is **2**.

The client with cirrhosis who has altered clotting is at high risk for hemorrhage. Prolonged application of pressure to injection or bleeding sites is important. Complete independence may increase the client's potential for injury, because an unsupervised client may injure himself and bleed excessively. Antibiotics and good nutrition are important to promote liver regeneration. However, they are not most important for a client at high risk for hemorrhage.

17 *Urinary and renal disorders*

I. STRUCTURE AND FUNCTION OF THE URINARY AND RENAL SYSTEM

A. Structure

1. **Urinary system**

   a. Ureters are slender tubes that extend behind the peritoneum from the hilus of the kidney to enter the bladder.

   b. The bladder is a smooth, collapsible, muscular sac located retroperitoneally in the pelvis that has openings to the ureters and urethra.

   c. The urethra extends from the base of the bladder to the urinary meatus.

   d. The urinary meatus is the external opening of the urethra.

2. The **kidneys** are paired organs located on either side of the vertebral column. They are between the 12th thoracic and 3rd lumbar vertebrae in the posterior abdomen behind the peritoneum.

   a. **External structures**

      – **Hilum.** The medial border of the kidney is indented by the hilum, the area where nerves, blood vessels, and the ureter enter the kidney. The hilum gives the kidney its bean-shaped appearance.

      – The **renal capsule** is the fibrous, transparent outer covering of the kidneys (excluding the hilum) that gives the kidney a glistening appearance. A layer of adipose tissue surrounds the kidney.

   b. **Internal structures** (See *Figure 17-1*.)

      – The **cortex** is the outer portion containing the glomerules, tubules, and part of the Henle's loop.

      – The **medulla** is the middle portion containing part of Henle's loop and the collecting ducts.

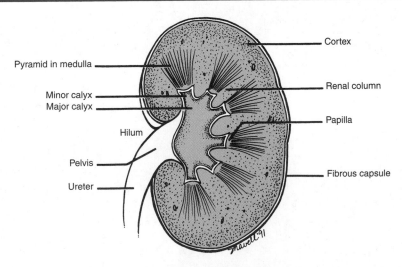

FIGURE 17-1
Gross structure of a bisected kidney

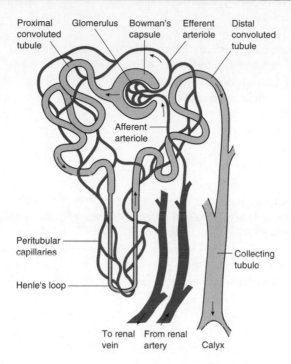

FIGURE 17-2
Structure of the nephron and glomerulus

- The **renal pyramids** are collecting ducts with bases on the border between the cortex and medulla. They are separated by the renal columns, which are extensions of the cortex tissue.
- **Papillae** are apices of pyramids, which extend toward the renal pelvis. Urine travels through the papillae to the renal pelvis.
- The **renal pelvis** is the inner portion where urine is collected.
  - The **narrowed portion** becomes the proximal aspect of the ureter as it approaches the hilum.
  - **Minor** and **major calyces** are recesses of the pelvis that receive urine from papillae of collecting ducts.
- The **nephron,** the functional unit of the kidney, contains the glomerulus, tubules, and collecting ducts. (See *Figure 17-2*.)
  - The **glomerulus** is the beginning of the nephron. It is a tuft of capillaries supplied by afferent arterioles and drained by efferent arterioles within Bowman's capsule.
  - The **proximal tubule** is the convoluted portion with a border of microvilli lining the lumen.
  - **Henle's loop** has two major portions, the descending and ascending limbs. The descending loop narrows as it dips from the cortex to the medulla.
  - The **distal tubule** passes between afferent and efferent arterioles of glomerulus as it moves back into the cortex.

- The **collecting duct** passes through the cortex and medulla, receiving the terminal end of several nephrons.
  c. **Renal circulation**
    - The **renal artery** branches from the abdominal aorta.
    - **Subdivisions of interlobular arteries** carry blood into the corticomedullary zone.
    - **Arcuate arteries** form arches around bases of pyramids.
    - **Interlobular arteries,** subdivisions of the arcuate arteries, supply the renal capsule.
  d. **Neurologic control.** Renal innervation is supplied through sympathetic and parasympathetic nerves. Adrenergic fibers also are in proximity to juxtaglomerular apparatus.

B. **Function**
  1. **The urinary system**
    a. **Ureters** transport urine to the bladder by peristaltic waves of smooth muscle. The ureterovesical junction prevents backflow of urine (i.e., reflux).
    b. The **bladder** serves as a reservoir for urine until it is excreted from the body.
    c. The **urethra** carries urine by peristalsis from the bladder to the outside of the body.
    d. **Urine formation** is a result of three processes: filtration, reabsorption, and secretion.
      - The glomerulus filters the blood, which results in a filtrate that includes waste products and such useful substances as water, glucose, ions, and amino acids.
      - The useful substances in the filtrate are reabsorbed into the blood by the proximal and distal convoluted tubules.
      - Tubular secretion is reabsorption in reverse. The waste products are secreted into the filtrate in the tubules and excreted in the urine.
    e. **Micturition** (e.g., voiding) is under voluntary and involuntary control. The urge to void normally occurs when 150 to 300 ml urine has accumulated. The bladder normally contains no residual urine after voiding.
  2. **Kidneys.** *Table 17-1* gives a summary of major nephron component functions. Overall functions of the renal system include:
    a. blood pressure regulation by renin secretion
    b. red blood cell production regulation by erythropoietin secretion
    c. metabolism of vitamin D.

NURSING PROCESS OVERVIEW

 II. THE URINARY AND RENAL SYSTEM

A. **Assessment**
  1. **Health history**
    a. **Explore the client's health history for risk factors** associated with renal and urinary disorders, including:
      - exposure to certain nephrotoxins (e.g., chemicals, tar, plastics)
      - history of smoking
      - multiple pregnancies
      - history of diabetes mellitus or hypertension.
    b. **Elicit a description of the client's present illness and chief complaint,** including onset, course, duration, location, and precipitating and alleviating factors. Cardinal signs and symptoms indicating altered urinary and renal function include:

TABLE 17-1
Major functions of nephron components

Nephron component	Major functions
Glomerulus	■ Filtration
Proximal tubule	■ 65% sodium (Na) and water (H_2O) reabsorbed (antidiuretic hormone [ADH] not required) ■ Glucose, potassium (K), amino acids reabsorbed ■ Bicarbonate (HCO_3^-) reabsorbed ■ Hydrogen (H^+) secreted ■ Urea reabsorbed ■ Filtrate leaves isotonic
Henle's loop	■ Countercurrent multiplying and exchange mechanisms established between long, thin loops of Henle of juxtamedullary nephrons and adjacent vasa recta ■ Filtrate leaves hypotonic
Distal tubule	■ Na^+ reabsorbed and K^+ secreted in presence of aldosterone; opposite occurs in absence of aldosterone ■ H_2O reabsorbed with Na^+; ADH also influences water reabsorption ■ Filtrate leaves hypotonic or isotonic
Collecting duct	■ Na^+ reabsorbed and K^+ regulated by aldosterone ■ Acid-base regulation; H^+ secretion, HCO_3^- reabsorption, ammonia secretion, ammonium excretion ■ ADH determines final urine volume

- dysuria
- hesitancy
- flank pain
- urinary frequency
- urethral discharge
- hematuria
- incontinence
- nocturia.

2. **Physical examination**
   a. **Inspection**
   - Inspect the masses in the upper abdomen and flank area.
   - Inspect the external meatus for signs of discharge, cleanliness, location, and size.
   b. **Palpation.** Palpate for the lower poles of the right and left kidney, noting enlargement.
   c. **Percussion.** Percuss above the symphysis pubis for a distended bladder.
   d. **Auscultation.** Auscultate for bruits over the renal arteries.
3. **Laboratory and diagnostic studies**
   a. **Urinalysis** involves assessment of urine color, opacity, odor, specific gravity, osmolality, and pH. It also identifies the presence of glucose, ketones, proteins, red and white blood cells, sediment, and bacteria.
   b. **Urine culture and sensitivity,** which requires a midstream clean-catch urine specimen, detects infective microorganisms.

    c. **Blood analysis**
- **Plasma creatinine** analysis provides an excellent indication of renal function.
- **Blood urea nitrogen** analysis evaluates renal function.

    d. **Creatinine clearance** evaluates glomerular filtration rate (GFR). Creatinine clearance levels increase as renal function diminishes.

    e. **Vascular studies**
- **Radionuclide tests**
  - Renal scan provides anatomic information.
  - Renogram provides information about renal blood flow, GFR, and tubular secretion.
- **Renal arteriography** outlines renal vasculature.
- **Renal venography** outlines renal veins.

    f. **Radiographs** of kidneys, ureters, and bladder visualize the size, shape, and position of urinary structures.

    g. **Ultrasound studies** identify gross renal anatomy.

    h. **Computed tomography** detects renal masses, vascular disorders, and filling defects of the collecting system.

    i. **I.V. and retrograde pyelography** and **cystourethrography** provide information about the size, shape, and position of urinary-tract structures and evaluate renal excretory function.

    j. **Hemodynamic studies** evaluate motor and sensory function of the bladder and micturition process.

    k. **Cystoscopic examination** allows direct endoscopic visualization of the entire urinary tract.

    l. **Bladder and kidney biopsy** determines the nature and extent of disease.

B. Nursing diagnoses
1. Acute pain
2. Risk for infection
3. Impaired urinary elimination
4. Deficient or excess fluid volume
5. Imbalanced nutrition: less than body requirements
6. Impaired skin integrity
7. Activity intolerance
8. Deficient knowledge
9. Ineffective coping

C. Planning and outcome identification. The major goals for the client diagnosed with a urinary or renal disorder may include relief of pain and discomfort, prevention of infection, return to normal elimination patterns, maintenance of fluid and nutritional intake, intact skin integrity, participation in activity within tolerance, increased knowledge of prevention and treatment, and effective coping with disorder.

D. Implementation
1. **Provide pain relief.** Assess the client's level of pain, rule out complications, administer pain medications as prescribed, and evaluate effectiveness of pain medication.
2. **Promote measures to prevent infection.** Monitor the client's vital signs, assess for signs and symptoms of infection, and monitor the white blood cell count.
3. **Promote measures to ensure adequate urinary elimination** to include ensuring the client voids clear and odor-free urine at least every 2 to 3 hours.
4. **Promote measures to maintain fluid and electrolyte balance.**

a. Assess the client's fluid status, including intake and output, skin turgor, presence of edema, and jugular vein distention.

b. Weigh the client daily at the same time and in the same clothes.

c. Encourage the client to drink at least 2 L of fluid daily (water is preferable), if not contraindicated.

5. **Promote measures to ensure adequate nutrition.** Encourage the client to adhere to the prescribed diet, explain the rationale for the diet, and monitor for weight loss or gain.

6. **Maintain skin integrity.** Turn the client every 2 hours, and assess skin for any redness or breakdown.

7. **Enhance activity tolerance.** Encourage the client to alternate activity with rest.

8. **Provide client and family teaching.** Provide explanations for the cause, treatment, and expected course of renal or urinary disorder.

9. **Promote client and family coping.** Encourage the client to verbalize feelings and assist coping with the discomforts, treatment regimen, and changes in lifestyle.

E. Evaluation

1. The client reports pain relief.

2. The client displays no evidence of urinary tract infection or kidney infection.

3. The client demonstrates a normal voiding pattern without pain or discomfort.

4. The client exhibits adequate intake and output, no weight gain, or no peripheral edema.

5. The client maintains an adequate nutritional intake.

6. The client's skin remains intact.

7. The client expresses the intention to increase activity as tolerated.

8. The client verbalizes knowledge about the course of illness, need to drink 2 L of fluid daily, and required follow-up care.

9. The client and family exhibit effective coping strategies during the illness.

III. URINARY RETENTION

A. Description. Urinary retention is urine retained in the bladder in the presence of normal urine production, with an inability to release it even when the micturition reflex is activated.

B. Etiology

1. **Male factors**

   a. Benign prostatic hypertrophy

   b. Urethral stricture

   c. Calculi or foreign body in the urethra

   d. Urethritis

   e. Tumor

   f. Phimosis

2. **Female factors**

   a. Urethral obstruction secondary to stricture, calculi, vaginal cysts, tumor, or edema

   b. Retroverted gravid uterus

3. **Male and female factors**

   a. Reflex spasm of sphincters after surgery or invasive procedures

   b. Trauma

   c. Neurogenic bladder dysfunction

CLIENT AND FAMILY TEACHING 17-1
Prevention of urinary tract infections

- Instruct the client on hygienic measures, including showering rather than bathing, wiping from front to back after a bowel movement, and wearing cotton underwear.
- Encourage the client to drink at least 2 L of water each day; instruct the client to fill a 2-L bottle of water each night and drink it before the next night.
- Instruct the client to avoid alcohol and caffeinated coffee, tea, and soft drinks.

- Encourage the client to void every 2 to 3 hours during the day, making sure the bladder is completely emptied.
- Instruct the client to void immediately after sexual intercourse.
- Teach the client to take the medication exactly as prescribed and not to save any pills.
- Discuss the importance of follow-up visits with the health care provider to obtain urine culture and sensitivity after antibiotic therapy.

> *d.* Medications (e.g., anticholinergics, antihistamines)
> *e.* Fecal impaction
> *f.* Psychogenic retention

C. Pathophysiology

1. Decreased nerve innervation of the bladder muscle causes the urge to void to be suppressed.
2. Retention may be acute or chronic. Chronic retention can lead to overflow incontinence or residual urine. Other possible complications of chronic urinary retention include urinary tract infection (UTI), bladder distention and damage, and hydronephrosis.

D. Assessment findings

1. **Clinical manifestations**
   a. Inability to void, urinary urgency, urinary hesitancy, and dribbling
   b. Lower abdominal pain or discomfort
   c. Restlessness and diaphoresis
   d. Visible or palpable bladder distention
   e. Dullness on bladder percussion
   f. Possibly signs and symptoms of lower UTI
2. **Laboratory and diagnostic study findings.** Bladder catheterization commonly reveals residual urine.

E. Nursing management (See section II.D.)

1. **Facilitate bladder emptying.**
   a. Provide privacy, run water, have the client assume a normal voiding position, and provide pain relief.
   b. Promote relaxation of the sphincter by providing sitz baths, warm showers, and hot tea to drink.
2. **Obtain and record strict urinary output every time the client voids.**
3. **If the client cannot void, perform intermittent catheterization** to prevent overdistention of the bladder.
4. **Prepare the client for surgical intervention** (e.g., dilation of urethra, cystoplasty), if indicated.
5. **Provide health education** on measures to prevent UTIs as detailed in *Client and family teaching 17-1.*
6. **Provide a referral** to the National Kidney Foundation. (See appendix A.)

IV. URINARY INCONTINENCE

A. Description. Urinary incontinence refers to the inability of the urinary sphincters to control the release of urine. The incidence of urinary incontinence increases with age.

1. **Enuresis,** or *bedwetting,* is usually a childhood problem.
2. **Stress incontinence** is dribbling resulting from any kind of physical stress (e.g., coughing, sneezing, laughing). It most commonly affects women.
3. **Urgency incontinence** is the inability to hold back urine flow when feeling the urge to void.
4. **Overflow incontinence** is frequent, sometimes almost constant, loss of urine from the bladder. The bladder cannot empty normally and becomes overdistended.
5. **Continuous incontinence** is completely uninhibited micturition reflex, with an unpredictable voiding pattern.
6. **Functional incontinence** occurs when the function of the lower urinary tract is intact but other factors (e.g., physical impairments, mental impairment) make it difficult for the client to identify the need to void.

B. Etiology

1. **Temporary episodes** of incontinence can result from:
   a. inflammation
   b. stress
   c. certain medications (e.g., opioids, tranquilizers, sedatives, diuretics, antihistamines, antihypertensive medications, atropine-like medications).
2. **Persistent or permanent incontinence** may result from neuromuscular dysfunction associated with such disorders as:
   a. bladder lesions
   b. spinal cord injury
   c. multiple sclerosis
   d. spinal cord tumor
   e. complications of pelvic surgery
   f. stroke
   g. large bowel disease (e.g., spastic colon, diverticular disease).
3. **Anatomic causes** of incontinence include:
   a. weak abdominal and perineal muscle tone due to obesity and a sedentary lifestyle
   b. sphincter weakness or damage from obstetric trauma, surgery, or congenital conditions
   c. urethral deformity due to recurrent urinary tract infections (UTIs), trauma, surgery, or estrogen-deficiency vulvitis
   d. altered urethrovesical angle in women linked to previous pregnancies and perineal muscle weakness.
4. **Psychosocial factors** (e.g., rebellion, dependence, regression, anxiety, attention-getting behavior) cause incontinence in some people.

C. Pathophysiology. The exact pathogenesis of urinary incontinence is unknown, but one or more of the following may be responsible: decreased urethral resistance, dysfunction of the urinary sphincter, instability of the motor or sensory nerve stimulation, severe central nervous system disorders and, occasionally, severe psychologic dysfunction.

DRUG CHART 17-1
Medications for renal and urinary disorders

Classifications	Indications	Selected interventions
Alkalinizing agents bicitra Shohl's solution sodium bicarbonate	Elevate the plasma pH, thereby causing potassium to move into the cells and lower the serum potassium levels	▪ Monitor arterial blood gases for signs of metabolic acidosis or alkalosis.
Antibiotics ciprofloxacin nitrofurantoin sulfisoxazole trimethoprim-sulfamethoxazole	Prevent bacterial growth in the kidneys and bladder.	▪ Before administering the first dose, assess the client for allergies and determine whether culture has been obtained. ▪ After multiple doses, assess the client for superinfection (thrush, yeast infection, diarrhea); notify the health care provider if these occur. ▪ Assess the insertion site for phlebitis if antibiotics are being administered I.V. ▪ To assess the effectiveness of antibiotic therapy, monitor urinalysis.
Antiemetics benzquinamide dimenhydrinate promethazine scopolamine trimethobenzamide hydrochloride	Relieve nausea and vomiting by inhibiting medullary chemoreceptor triggers; drug choice depends on the cause of vomiting	▪ Advise the client that this medication may cause drowsiness. ▪ Because the medication may cause chemical irritation, administer by deep I.M. injection into a large muscle mass. ▪ Measure emesis and maintain accurate intake and output; monitor for dehydration.
Calcium supplements parenteral calcium salts (e.g., calcium gluconate, chloride, gluceptate) Os-Cal	Strengthen skeletal system by supplementing calcium intake	▪ Assess for hypocalcemia by checking for Chvostek's and Trousseau's signs. ▪ Explain to the client that vitamin D increases calcium absorption in the GI tract. ▪ Increase dietary intake of calcium (milk products, green leafy vegetables).
Erythropoietin epogen epoetin alfa	Aid in the production of red blood cells	▪ May be administered I.V. or subcutaneously in clients not receiving dialysis. ▪ Monitor blood pressure, complete blood count with differential blood urea nitrogen, and platelet counts.
Folic acid supplement apo-folic folvite	Supplement folic acid intake; minimum daily requirement is 50 g (Folic acid is found in most meats, fresh vegetables, and fresh fruits but is destroyed when cooked more than 15 minutes.)	▪ May be given orally, I.M., I.V., or subcutaneously.
Histamine receptor antagonists cimetidine famotidine ranitidine	Block receptors that control the secretion of hydrochloric acid by the parietal cells	▪ Instruct the client to continue taking the medication regularly, even after pain subsides. ▪ When administering I.V., dilute and monitor closely and watch the site for infiltration. ▪ Emphasize the importance of adhering to all aspects of therapy.

DRUG CHART 17-1
Medications for renal and urinary disorders *(continued)*

Classifications	Indications	Selected interventions
Ion exchange resins sodium polystyrene sulfonate	Exchange a sodium ion for a potassium ion in the intestinal tract	▪ If administered by retention enema, the client should retain for 30 minutes. ▪ Sorbitol is often administered with medication to induce a diarrhea-type effect. ▪ Monitor serum potassium level.
Iron supplements ferrous sulfate iron-dextran injection	Supplement daily iron, an essential component of proteins that carry or use oxygen; most part of hemoglobin	▪ Administer I.M. medications by Z-track and in large muscle mass; liquid preparation can stain teeth, so administer through a straw; parenteral doses may cause anaphylactic reactions. ▪ Instruct the client to take iron with food to decrease stomach irritation; vitamin C increases absorption of iron. ▪ Inform the client that feces turn dark black and tarry; instruct on ways to prevent constipation.
Opioid analgesics hydrocodone hydromophone meperidine morphine propoxyphene	Relieve moderate to severe pain by reducing pain sensation, producing sedation, and decreasing the emotional upset often associated with pain; most often schedule II drugs	▪ Assess the pain for location, type, intensity, what increases or decreases it; rate pain on a scale of 1 (no pain) to 10 (worst pain). ▪ Rule out any complications. Is this pain routine or expected pain? Is this a complication that needs immediate intervention? ▪ Medicate according to pain scale findings. ▪ Institute safety measures — bed in low position, side rails up, and call light within reach. ▪ Evaluate effectiveness of pain medication in 30 minutes.
Phosphate-binding agents aluminum hydroxide	Decrease absorption of phosphate from the intestines, thereby decreasing serum phosphate levels	▪ Instruct client to restrict sodium intake, drink plenty of fluids, and follow a low-phosphate diet.
Proton pump inhibitor omeprazole	Prevent the final transport of hydrogen ions into the gastric lumen by binding to an enzyme on parietal cells	▪ Instruct the client to take the medication regularly as prescribed by the health care provider. ▪ Instruct the client to avoid any products that may cause GI irritation.

D. Assessment findings

1. **Associated findings.** The client may exhibit or express anxiety, frustration, depression, poor self-esteem, or other psychological distress. Incontinence is commonly viewed as an infantile behavior and may provoke feelings of helplessness, hopelessness, and frustration.

2. **Clinical manifestations**

    a. Clothing or bedding wet with urine

    b. Reports of dribbling, urgency, hesitancy, or inability to get to the bathroom before voiding starts

E. Nursing management

1. **Administer prescribed medications,** which may include antibiotics for treatment of infection. (See *Drug chart 17-1.*)

2. **Provide pain relief.** (See section II.D.1.)
3. **Promote measures to decrease physiologic and psychologic complications of urinary incontinence.**
   a. Maintain skin integrity. Protect the client's skin by keeping the perineal area dry. Change clothing and bed linens as necessary. (See section II.D.6.)
   b. Promote measures to maintain fluid and electrolyte balance. (See section II.D.4.)
   c. Promote measures to ensure adequate nutrition. (See section II.D.5.)
   d. Provide an environment that promotes easy access to the bathroom, supply a bedpan or urinal within easy reach, and advise the client to select clothing that is easy to remove when using the toilet.
   e. Promote client and family coping. (See section II.D.9.)
   f. Refer the client for psychological evaluation as appropriate.
4. **Provide bladder training,** if indicated. Teach the client to do perineal and Kegel exercises to help improve muscular control, as appropriate. The exercises can be done lying, sitting, or standing as follows:
   a. Contract the perineal muscles as though stopping urination.
   b. Sustain contraction for 5 to 10 seconds and release.
   c. Perform 10 to 15 sets of 10 repetitions each daily.
5. **Assess the client's medication regimen** for any drugs that could cause or contribute to incontinence.
6. **Discuss and prepare the client for surgical correction for stress incontinence** if indicated (e.g., vaginal repair, abdominal suspension of the bladder).
7. **Provide health education** on measures to prevent UTIs as detailed in *Client and family teaching 17-1,* page 466.
8. **Provide a referral** to the National Kidney Foundation. (See appendix A.)

V. NEUROGENIC BLADDER DYSFUNCTION

A. Description. This condition is dysfunction of the bladder resulting from impaired neurologic control caused by central or peripheral nervous system lesions.
   1. A **spastic (hypertonic) bladder** is characterized by automatic, reflex, or uncontrolled expulsion of urine from the bladder without complete emptying.
   2. A **flaccid bladder** has loss of sensation of bladder fullness, which results in overfilling and distention of the bladder.

B. Etiology
   1. Major causes of neurogenic bladder include:
      a. spinal cord injury or tumor
      b. herniated intervertebral disk
      c. stroke and other cerebral disorders
      d. neurologic disorders (e.g., multiple sclerosis, diabetes mellitus, and syphilis)
      e. congenital anomalies (e.g., spina bifida and myelomeningocele)
      f. infection.
   2. Spastic neurogenic bladder is caused by an upper motor neuron lesion. Flaccid neurogenic bladder is caused by lower motor neuron lesion.

C. Pathophysiology
   1. **Spastic (reflex or autonomic) neurogenic bladder,** the most common type, follows this course:

      a. Loss of conscious sensations and cerebral motor control

      b. Reduced bladder capacity and marked bladder-wall hypertrophy

      c. A pattern of spontaneous, uncontrolled voiding

  2. Flaccid (atonic, nonreflex, areflexic, or autonomous) neurogenic bladder follows this course:

      a. Inability of bladder musculature to contract allows the bladder to fill until it becomes grossly distended.

      b. When intrabladder pressure reaches a certain point, small amounts of urine dribble from the urethra.

      c. Sensory loss may make the client unaware of incontinence.

      d. Extreme, prolonged bladder distention can result in damage to bladder musculature, urinary stasis and infection, and renal infection.

  3. Mixed neurogenic bladder, which is usually associated with lesions at the conus-cauda equina junctions, involves a combination of spastic and flaccid dysfunction.

  4. Possible long-term complications of neurogenic bladder include urinary tract infections, hydronephrosis, urolithiasis, and renal failure.

D. Assessment findings

  1. Clinical manifestations of neurogenic bladder depend on the type and degree of neurologic damage. Common signs and symptoms include:

      a. residual urine detected on bladder catheterization

      b. some degree of incontinence

      c. bladder distention

      d. restlessness.

  2. Laboratory and diagnostic study findings

      a. Blood urea nitrogen, creatinine clearance, and serum creatinine levels are elevated.

      b. Cystography detects vesicoureteral reflux.

      c. Urethrography detects urethral complications.

      d. Urine pressure and flow studies reveal abnormal pressures.

      e. Cystoscopy may reveal a loss of muscle fibers and elastic tissues and provide opportunity for tissue biopsy.

▓ E. Nursing management (See section II.D.)

  1. Discuss and provide assistive techniques to empty bladder.

      a. Perform intermittent catheterization usually every 4 to 6 hours. This is a normal urination pattern and avoids the complications of an indwelling Foley catheter.

      b. Instruct the client and his family on self-catheterization.

      c. Instruct the male client on the care of a three-way catheter with closed drainage, which may be inserted to avoid overdistention. Instruct him on taping the drainage tube laterally to the thigh.

      d. Instruct the client on the proper way to apply and use an external collecting device (e.g., condom catheter).

  2. Provide bladder training, if appropriate.

  3. Prevent calculi. Encourage a diet low in calcium.

  4. Encourage activity with a wheelchair or tilt-table.

  5. Provide health education on measures to prevent UTIs as detailed in *Client and family teaching 17-1,* page 466.

  6. Provide referrals to the American Association of Kidney Patients and the National Kidney Foundation. (See appendix A.)

VI. URINARY TRACT INFECTION

A. Description

1. Inflammation and infection of urinary tract structures are classified as upper urinary tract infections (UTIs) or lower UTIs.

   a. **Upper UTIs** are known as pyelonephritis (e.g., inflammation of the kidney).

   b. **Lower UTIs** include:
   - cystitis (e.g., inflammation of the bladder wall), the most common type
   - ureteritis (e.g., inflammation of the ureter)
   - urethritis (e.g., inflammation of the urethra).

2. Women develop UTI more frequently than men because of their shorter urethras. Approximately 25% of all women experience UTIs at some time. Incidence among women increases with aging. Incidence among men peaks after age 50.

B. Etiology

1. UTIs result from pathogenic microorganisms in the urinary tract (e.g., *Escherichia coli, Proteus, Klebsiella, Enterobacter*).

2. Predisposing factors include:

   a. loss of resistance to invading microorganisms

   b. sexual intercourse

   c. indwelling catheterization

   d. urine stasis

   e. urinary tract instrumentation

   f. residual urine

   g. urinary reflux

   h. bladder overdistention

   i. loss of intact mucosal lining

   j. metabolic disorders.

C. Pathophysiology

1. An upper UTI is a bacterial infection of the renal pelvis, tubules, and interstitial tissue of one or both kidneys that occurs because of reflux of urine into the ureters.

2. A lower UTI is an infection that typically ascends from the urethra to the bladder and possibly to the ureter.

3. Other pathways of upper and lower UTIs include blood and lymph.

D. Assessment findings

1. **Clinical manifestations**

   a. **Upper UTI**
   - Flank pain
   - Costovertebral angle tenderness
   - Fever and chills
   - Dysuria
   - Frequency and urgency
   - Malaise
   - Possibly bloody or cloudy urine

   b. **Lower UTI**
   - Frequency and urgency
   - Burning on urination
   - Nocturia

– Inflamed, edematous meatus in urethritis
2. **Laboratory and diagnostic study findings**
   a. **Upper UTI.** Urinalysis findings reveal elevated white blood cell count, white cell casts, and bacteria.
   b. **Lower UTI**
      – Urinalysis reveals bacteriuria and red blood cells in urine.
      – Urine culture identifies the causative microorganism.

E. Nursing management (See section II.D.)
1. **Administer prescribed medication,** which includes antibiotics. (See *Drug chart 17-1*, pages 468 and 469.)
2. **Provide pain relief.** Apply heat to the perineum and encourage hot tub baths.
3. **Promote measures to prevent infection.**
4. **Promote measures to maintain fluid and electrolyte balance.**
5. **Provide client and family teaching.** Provide health education on measures to prevent UTIs as detailed in *Client and family teaching 17-1*, page 460.
6. **Promote client and family coping.**

VII. UROLITHIASIS

A. Description. Urolithiasis (i.e., renal calculi) is described as calculi in the urinary tract — the bladder, the ureters and, most commonly, the kidneys. (See *Figure 17-3*, page 474.) Incidence peaks between ages 30 and 50 years and is higher among men than women.

B. Etiology. Predisposing factors in calculi formation include:
1. immobility
2. hypercalcemia
3. urinary tract infection (UTI)
4. urine stasis
5. high urine specific gravity
6. genetic predisposition.

C. Pathophysiology
1. Calculi are formed by deposition of crystalline substances, including calcium oxalate, calcium phosphate, and uric acid. Most calculi contain calcium or magnesium in combination with phosphorus or oxalate.
2. Calculi may pass through the urinary tract, or they may lodge, causing obstruction leading to infection and possibly hydronephrosis.

D. Assessment findings
1. **Clinical manifestations** vary with the location, size, and cause of calculi and may include:
   a. acute, sharp, intermittent pain (i.e., ureteral colic)
   b. dull, tender ache in the flank (i.e., renal colic)
   c. nausea and vomiting accompanying severe pain
   d. fever and chills
   e. hematuria
   f. abdominal distention
   g. pyuria
   h. rarely, oliguria or anuria.

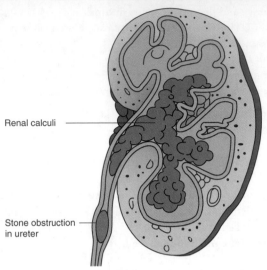

FIGURE 17-3
Renal calculi obstructing the entire renal pelvis

2. **Laboratory and diagnostic study findings**
    a. Kidneys, ureters, and bladder radiograph reveals visible calculi.
    b. Stone analysis detects mineral content of calculi.
    c. I.V. pyelography determines size and location of calculi.
    d. Renal ultrasonography reveals obstructive changes, such as hydronephrosis.

E. Nursing management (See section II.D.)
    1. **Provide pharmacologic therapy.**
        a. Administer prescribed medication, which may include I.V. opioid medications, pro-
        phylactic antibiotics, and antiemetics. (See *Drug chart 17-1*, pages 468 and 469.)
        b. Medicate the client for pain around the clock with morphine or meperidine. Shock
        and syncope can occur from the excruciating pain.
    2. **Provide comfort measures.**
        a. Encourage bed rest.
        b. Teach relaxation techniques.
        c. Provide hot baths or moist heat to the flank areas.
    3. **Encourage around-the-clock, high-fluid intake** if the client is not nauseated or vom-
    iting.
    4. **Prepare the client who cannot pass the calculus spontaneously for one of the fol-
    lowing nonsurgical procedures:**
        a. Extracorporeal shock wave lithotripsy, which is used to break up calculus so that the
        client can pass the particles during urination.
        b. Ureteroscopy, which involves insertion of instruments through a cystoscope to vi-
        sualize and access the calculus and then remove or fragment it with laser energy or
        ultrasound.
        c. Stone dissolution, which involves infusion of chemolytic solutions (i.e., alkylating or
        acidifying agents) through a percutaneous nephrostomy tube. This procedure is used
        for clients who are poor risks for other treatments.

    d. Endourologic procedures, which integrate the skills of the radiologist and urologist to extract renal calculi without major surgery. An endoscopic instrument is introduced through a percutaneous nephrostomy. Forceps or a basketlike device on the instrument extracts the calculus.

  5. Prepare the client for nephrolithotomy (incision into the kidney for removal of the calculus) if nonsurgical methods fail.

    a. Monitor for signs and symptoms of dehydration resulting from postobstructive diuresis.

    b. Intervene as necessary to restore fluid balance.

  6. Inform the client that chemical analysis of the calculus is performed to determine the composition (i.e., calcium oxalate, calcium phosphate, or irate). The composition guides further diet therapy.

  7. Institute measures to help prevent calculi recurrence.

    a. Encourage dietary modifications based on the calculi composition. Those with calcium calculi should avoid dietary calcium and phosphorus; those with uric calculi should avoid foods high in purine, such as shellfish, anchovies, asparagus, and organ meats; and those with oxalate calculi should avoid green leafy vegetables, beans, celery, beets, tea, and coffee.

    b. Increase fluid intake to 3 to 4 L per day.

    c. Instruct the client to drink fluids in the late evening to prevent stasis of urine in kidneys and bladder.

    d. Promote increased physical activity.

    e. Monitor urine pH.

    f. Administer prescribed medications such as:

      – aluminum hydroxide, which binds with excess phosphorus, causing it to be excreted through the intestinal tract

      – sodium cellulose phosphate, which helps prevent calcium stones

      – allopurinol, which reduces serum uric acid levels and urinary uric acid excretion.

  8 Instruct the client to avoid sudden increases in environmental temperatures, which may cause a fall in urinary volume.

  9. Provide health education on measures to prevent UTIs as detailed in *Client and family teaching 17-1*, page 466.

VIII. ACUTE RENAL FAILURE

  A. Description. Acute renal failure is defined as sudden, rapid, potentially reversible deterioration of renal function. It can be classified according to underlying cause as:

    1. prerenal azotemia, stemming from decreased blood flow to kidneys

    2. postrenal obstruction, involving obstruction of urine outflow

    3. intrarenal acute failure, involving intrinsic damage to renal structures.

  B. Etiology

    1. Prerenal azotemia is caused by factors that interfere with renal perfusion, such as:

      a. hypovolemia (e.g., from hemorrhage, shock, burns)

      b. increased intravascular capacity (e.g., from sepsis, neurogenic shock)

      c. cardiac disorders (e.g., myocardial infarction, arrhythmias)

      d. renal artery obstruction

      e. hepatorenal syndrome.

2. **Postrenal obstruction** may result from:
   a. ureteral obstruction due to calculi, strictures, trauma, or pregnancy
   b. bladder obstruction (e.g., cancer, prostatic hypertrophy).
3. **Intrarenal acute failure** may result from:
   a. acute tubular necrosis, which accounts for about 75% of all cases of acute renal failure
   b. acute glomerulonephritis
   c. acute pyelonephritis.

C. **Pathophysiology**
   1. The exact pathogenesis of acute renal failure is not always known, but it is associated with a severe reduction in the glomerular filtration rate. This may be caused by decreased renal blood flow that leads to increased renal-vascular resistance, increased hydrostatic pressure in Bowman's capsule, or a disruption of tubular epithelium. There are four clinical phases of acute renal failure:
      a. The **onset phase** extends from the time of the precipitating event to the beginning of the oliguric-anuric phase.
      b. The **oliguric-anuric phase** is marked by urine output of less than 400 ml/day, volume overload, elevated blood urea nitrogen (BUN) and creatinine levels, electrolyte abnormalities, metabolic acidosis, and uremia.
      c. The **diuretic phase** extends from the time that output becomes more than 400 ml/day to the time the BUN stops rising and stabilizes in normal range. During this phase, electrolyte and acid-base problems begin to normalize.
      d. The **convalescent phase** extends from the time the BUN stabilizes until the client returns to normal activity. The client may take up to 2 years to regain 70% to 80% of normal function.
   2. Systemic effects of acute renal failure are widespread and may include:
      a. fluid and electrolyte imbalances
      b. acidosis
      c. increased susceptibility to infection
      d. anemia
      e. platelet dysfunction
      f. GI disturbances (e.g., anorexia, nausea, vomiting, diarrhea or constipation, stomatitis)
      g. pericarditis
      h. uremic encephalopathy.

D. **Assessment findings**
   1. **Clinical manifestations** depend on the underlying condition. Some of the most common include:
      a. altered urine output; may be oliguria, anuria, or (rarely) polyuria
      b. hypertension or hypotension
      c. tachypnea
      d. signs of fluid overload or extracellular fluid depletion.
   2. **Laboratory and diagnostic study findings**
      a. **Urinalysis**
         – **Urine osmolality**
            - In prerenal azotemia, values are higher than 900 mOsm/kg.
            - In postrenal obstruction, values may be normal.
            - In intrarenal parenchymal failure, values are less than 250 mOsm/kg.

- **Urine sodium**
  - In prerenal azotemia, values are less than 20 mEq/L.
  - In postrenal obstruction, values may be normal.
  - In intrarenal failure, values are more than 27 mEq/L.
- *b.* **Blood analysis**
  - BUN, serum creatinine, and potassium levels are elevated.
  - Blood pH, bicarbonate, hemoglobin, and hematocrit values are decreased.

E. Nursing management (See section II.D.)

1. **Administer prescribed medication,** which may include alkalizing agents, antibiotics, phosphate-binding agents, ion exchange resins, calcium supplements, histamine receptor antagonists, and proton-pump inhibitors. (See *Drug chart 17 1,* pages 468 and 469.)
2. **Provide prompt, aggressive interventions** to manage the underlying problem.
3. **Promote measures to ensure normal potassium levels.**
   a. Monitor potassium level and assess for effects of hyperkalemia.
   b. Restrict dietary potassium as necessary.
   c. Monitor cardiac telemetry for electrocardiographic changes.
   d. Prepare to administer insulin and glucose, which drives potassium back into the cell.
4. **Promote measures to maintain fluid balance.** Assess fluid balance, and restrict intake to 24-hour urine output plus 500 ml/day.
5. **Promote measures to maintain acid-base balance.**
   a. Monitor for acidosis.
   b. Administer an alkalinizing agent.
   c. Monitor arterial blood gas values for signs of metabolic acidosis or alkalosis.
   d. Be prepared to institute ventilatory measures if respiratory problems develop.
6. **Promote measures to assess and prevent infection.**
   a. Assess for infection, especially of the respiratory and urinary tracts.
   b. Do not leave the urinary catheter in place.
   c. Administer prophylactic antibiotics as prescribed.
   d. Monitor for hyperphosphatemia.
   e. Administer phosphate-binding agents.
   f. Monitor serum phosphorus level.
7. **Promote measures to ensure normal sodium and phosphate levels.** Instruct the client to restrict sodium intake, drink plenty of fluids, and follow a low-phosphate diet.
8. **Promote measures to ensure normal calcium levels.**
   a. Monitor for hypocalcemia.
   b. Administer calcium supplements.
   c. Assess for hypercalcemia by checking for Chvostek's and Trousseau's signs.
9. **Prevent GI bleeding** by administering histamine receptor antagonists and proton pump inhibitors.
10. **Promote comfort and encourage bed rest** to reduce exertion and metabolic rate. As prescribed, administer short-acting barbiturates to control pain, and assess for central nervous system complications, such as drowsiness, confusion, delirium, coma, and convulsions.
11. **Provide a high-calorie and low-protein diet,** with hyperalimentation if the client cannot eat.
12. **If indicated, prepare the client for dialysis** to correct hyperkalemia, fluid overload, acidosis, or severe uremia.
13. **Adjust dosages of drugs secreted by the kidney as necessary.**

14. **Provide referrals** to the National Kidney Foundation and American Association of Kidney Patients. (See appendix A.)

IX. CHRONIC RENAL FAILURE

A. **Description.** Chronic renal failure is the end result of progressive, irreversible loss of functioning renal tissue. It usually develops gradually, possibly taking up to several years to develop. In some cases, it may occur rapidly because of an acute disorder (e.g., unresolved acute renal failure).

B. **Etiology**
   1. Hypertensive nephropathy
   2. Diabetic nephropathy
   3. Chronic glomerulonephritis
   4. Chronic pyelonephritis
   5. Lupus nephritis
   6. Polycystic kidney disease
   7. Chronic hydronephrosis

C. **Pathophysiology.** Decreased renal function results in an accumulation of waste products (i.e., uremia) in the bloodstream. Uremia develops and adversely affects every system in the body.
   1. Three basic stages of chronic renal failure have been identified:
      a. **Decreased renal reserve.** During this stage, renal function is 40% to 50% of normal and homeostasis is maintained.
      b. **Renal insufficiency.** During this stage, renal function is 20% to 40% of normal; glomerular filtration rate (GFR), clearance, and urine concentration are decreased; and homeostasis is altered.
      c. **End-stage renal disease.** During this stage, renal function is less than 10% to 15% of normal; all renal functions are severely decreased; and homeostasis is significantly altered.
   2. In chronic renal failure, retention of sodium and water leads to edema, heart failure, and hypertension. Conversely, episodes of diarrhea and vomiting may lead to sodium and water depletion, which can exacerbate uremia and produce hypotension and hypovolemia.
   3. Metabolic acidosis occurs, interfering with the kidney's ability to excrete hydrogen ions, produce ammonia, and conserve bicarbonate.
   4. Decreased GFR results in:
      a. increased serum phosphate
      b. decreased serum calcium
      c. increased parathormone but depleted bone calcium, leading to bone changes (e.g., uremic bone disease, osteomalacia)
      d. increased serum magnesium.
   5. Erythropoietin production decreases, resulting in anemia.
   6. Neurologic complications develop, such as:
      a. altered mental function
      b. personality and behavioral changes
      c. convulsions
      d. coma.

7. *Table 17-2,* pages 480 to 482, gives more information on the widespread pathologic effects of chronic renal failure.

D. Assessment findings

1. **Clinical manifestations** of chronic renal failure depend on the stage of the disorder:
    a. In **decreased renal reserve,** the client is asymptomatic as long as there is no exposure to severe physiologic or psychologic stress.
    b. In **renal insufficiency,** clinical manifestations include polyuria, nocturia, and signs and symptoms of mild anemia.
    c. In **end-stage renal disease,** widespread systemic manifestations are evident. (See *Table 17-2,* pages 480 to 482.)
2. **Laboratory and diagnostic study findings.** Blood analysis reveals
    a. anemia
    b. elevated blood urea nitrogen (BUN) and serum creatinine levels
    c. elevated serum phosphorus level
    d. decreased serum calcium level
    e. decreased serum protein (particularly albumin) levels
    f. low blood pH.

E. Nursing management (See section II.D.)

1. **Administer prescribed medication,** which may include ion exchange resin, alkalizing agents, antibiotics, erythropoietin, folic acid supplements, iron supplements, phosphate-binding agents, calcium supplements, histamine receptor antagonists, and proton pump inhibitors. (See *Drug chart 17-1,* pages 468 and 469.)
2. **Provide conservative therapy,** as indicated.
    a. Maintain strict fluid control; daily fluid intake should equal 500 ml (insensible loss) plus the amount of the previous 24 hours' urinary output; daily weight; and strict intake and output
    b. Encourage intake of high biologic value protein foods, such as eggs, diary products, and meats (causes positive nitrogen balance needed for growth and healing).
    c. Encourage high-calorie, low-protein, low sodium, and low potassium snacks between meals.
    d. Encourage alternating activity with rest. Encourage independence as much as possible.
    e. Assess the client and family's response to chronic illness. Encourage therapeutic conversations to help cope with chronic illness.
    f. Provide symptomatic treatment. (See *Table 17-2,* pages 480 to 482.)
    g. Be prepared to identify and treat complications, which include hyperkalemia, pericarditis, pericardial effusion, pericardial tamponade, hypertension, anemia, and bone disease.
3. **Prepare the client for peritoneal dialysis,** if indicated. Assist with the procedure as instructed, maintaining septic technique and monitoring for signs and symptoms of peritonitis (e.g., rigid, boardlike abdomen; fever; cloudy peritoneal fluid).
4. **Prepare the client for and assist with hemodialysis,** if indicated. Provide proper shunt care, and assess for possible complications (e.g., bleeding due to heparinization; hypovolemia and hypotension due to excessive water removal; dialysis disequilibrium syndrome [headache, confusion, and seizures] due to rapid removal of urea from plasma).

(Text continues on page 482.)

TABLE 17-2

Systemic manifestations of chronic renal failure and management

System	Manifestations	Pathophysiologic basis	Management
Cardiovascular	Fluid overload; edema	■ Decreased excretion of water ■ Fluid overload	■ Dietary fluid restriction ■ Dietary sodium restriction ■ Dietary potassium restriction ■ Alkaline medications (e.g., Shohl's solution, Bicitra, sodium bicarbonate) ■ Antihypertensive medications ■ Correction of electrolyte imbalance ■ Dialysis
	Congestive heart failure	■ Hypertension	
	Electrolyte imbalance	■ Decreased excretion of electrolytes	
	Metabolic acidosis	■ Decreased hydrogen ion secretion ■ Decreased bicarbonate ion reabsorption and generation ■ Retention of acid end products of metabolism	
	Hypertension	■ Decreased ammonia synthesis and ammonium excretion ■ Fluid overload ■ Increased sodium retention	
	Arrhythmias	■ Inappropriate activation of the renin angiotensin system ■ Electrolyte imbalances, especially hyperkalemia, hypocalcemia, and variations in sodium levels	
	Pericarditis, effusion, and tamponade	■ Uremic toxins ■ Increased pericardial membrane permeability	
Gastrointestinal	Anorexia, nausea, and emesis	■ Uremic toxins ■ Decomposition of urea in the GI tract, releasing ammonia, which irritates the GI mucosa and produces small ulcerations	■ Dialysis ■ Oral hygiene ■ Oral assessment ■ Hemoglobin and hematocrit monitoring ■ Diarrhea or constipation control ■ Increased dietary bulk ■ Exercise regimen ■ Self-care instruction
	Stomatitis and uremic halitosis	■ Uremic toxins ■ Decomposition of the urea in the oral cavity, releasing ammonia	
	Gastritis and bleeding	■ Uremic toxins ■ Decomposition of urea in the GI tract, releasing ammonia, which irritates the GI mucosa and produces small ulcerations ■ Increased capillary fragility	
	Bowel problems: diarrhea	■ Uremic toxins ■ Hypermotility due to electrolyte imbalances, especially hyperkalemia	
	Constipation	■ Hypomotility due to electrolyte imbalances, decreased fluid intake, decreased activity, and decreased bulk in the diet	

TABLE 17-2

Systemic manifestations of chronic renal failure and management *(continued)*

System	Manifestations	Pathophysiologic basis	Management
Hematopoietic	Anemia	■ Decreased erythropoietin secretion by kidneys ■ Loss of red blood cells through the GI tract, mucous membranes, or dialysis ■ Decreased red blood cell survival time due to uremic toxins ■ Uremic toxins interfering with folic acid action	■ Iron supplements ■ Folic acid supplements ■ Androgens ■ Blood transfusions ■ Dialysis ■ Epogen
	Alterations in coagulation	■ Platelet dysfunction due to uremic toxins	
	Increased susceptibility to infection	■ Decreased neutrophil phagocytosis and chemotaxis due to uremic toxins	
Integumentary	Pallor	■ Uremic anemia	■ Bath oils and lotions ■ Dialysis ■ Correct hyperphosphatemia ■ Self-care instruction
	Yellowness	■ Retained urochrome pigment excreted through the skin	
	Dryness	■ Decreased secretions from oil and sweat glands due to uremic toxins	
	Pruritus	■ Dry skin ■ Calcium or phosphate deposits in the skin ■ Uremic toxins' effect on nerve endings	
	Purpura and ecchymosis	■ Increased capillary fragility ■ Platelet dysfunction	
	Uremic frost (seen only in terminal or severely critically ill clients)	■ Urea or urate crystals excreted through the skin	
Neuromuscular	Drowsiness, confusion, coma, and irritability	■ Uremic toxins producing a uremic encephalopathy ■ Metabolic acidosis	■ Dialysis ■ Seizure precautions ■ Safety precautions during ambulation, exercise, and activities of daily living
	Tremors, twitching, and convulsions	■ Electrolyte imbalances ■ Uremic toxins producing a uremic encephalopathy	
	Peripheral neuropathy – Stage 1: restless leg syndrome and paresthesias – Stage 2: motor involvement leading to footdrop – Stage 3: paraplegia	■ Decreased motor and sensory nerve conduction due to uremic toxins	

(continued)

TABLE 17-2
Systemic manifestations of chronic renal failure and management *(continued)*

System	Manifestations	Pathophysiologic basis	Management
Psychosocial	Decreased mentation, decreased concentration, and altered perceptions (even to the point of frank psychoses)	▪ Uremic toxins producing uremic encephalopathy ▪ Electrolyte imbalances ▪ Metabolic acidosis ▪ Tendency to develop cerebral edema	▪ Dialysis ▪ Psychosocial counseling ▪ Client and family education
Respiratory	Pulmonary edema	▪ Fluid overload ▪ Increased pulmonary capillary permeability ▪ Left ventricular dysfunction	▪ Fluid restriction ▪ Dialysis ▪ Cardiovascular treatments ▪ Antibiotics ▪ Pulmonary hygiene (coughing and deep-breathing exercises, oral care) ▪ Acidosis treatment
	Pneumonia or pneumonitis	▪ Thick tenacious oral secretions due to decreased fluid intake	
	Kussmaul's respirations	▪ A weak, lethargic client with a depressed cough reflex due to uremia ▪ Decreased pulmonary macrophage activity ▪ Fluid overload ▪ An increase in the rate and depth of respirations to decrease the amount of carbon dioxide in the body to compensate for the metabolic acidosis	
Skeletal	Hypocalcemia and hyperphosphatemia	▪ Hyperphosphatemia due to decreased renal excretion ▪ Decreased GI absorption of calcium due to decreased renal conversion of vitamin D	▪ Dialysis ▪ Calcium supplements ▪ Vitamin D supplements ▪ Self-care instruction ▪ Phosphate-binding medications given with meals—Amphojel, Basaljel
	Osteodystrophy	▪ Increased osteoclastic activity in response to an increased secretion of parathyroid hormone	
	Metastatic calcifications	▪ Deposition of calcium phosphate crystals in soft tissue and other structures	

5. **Prepare the client for kidney transplantation,** if indicated.
   a. Provide postoperative care for any client who has undergone major surgery (see chapter 21), with special attention to catheter patency and adequacy, intake and output, fluid replacement, and protection from infection.
   b. Monitor for signs and symptoms of complications, such as graft rejection (e.g., fever, elevated white blood cell count, electrolyte abnormalities, abnormal renogram) and infection stemming from immunosuppressive therapy (e.g., sepsis pneumonia, wound infection, and urinary tract infection).
6. **Provide referrals** to the National Kidney Foundation and American Association of Kidney Patients. (See appendix A.)

Study questions

1. Which laboratory test result would the nurse expect in a client whose renal function is deteriorating?
   1. Increase in blood urea nitrogen
   2. Decease in serum creatinine levels
   3. Increase in urine creatinine clearance
   4. Decrease in serum potassium levels

2. The nurse is aware that acute tubular necrosis (ATN) is characterized by which client condition?
   1. Oliguria (usually)
   2. Gradual onset
   3. Irreversibility
   4. Glucosuria

3. Which intervention would be most appropriate in a client diagnosed with chronic renal failure who is attempting to manage fluid intake at home?
   1. Subtracting the previous day's urine output from 500 ml and limiting intake to milk
   2. Adding 500 ml to the previous day's urine output and dividing that amount over the next 24 hours
   3. Consuming all of the fluid allowance during the day to prevent nighttime bladder distention
   4. Weighing self before each meal and drinking 500 ml of fluid four times each day

4. After the health care provider orders a culture and sensitivity test, why would the nurse instruct the client to obtain a clean-catch midstream urine specimen?
   1. The urinary tract normally harbors some microorganisms.
   2. Microorganisms on the client's external genitalia may contaminate the specimen.
   3. The nurse does not want to catheterize the client.

4. A midstream specimen obtains the largest number of microorganisms in the lower urinary tract.

5. Which medical condition would the nurse suspect in a client complaining of dribbling, urgency, and an inability to get to the bathroom before urinating starts?
   1. Urinary tract infection (UTI)
   2. Renal calculi
   3. Acute renal failure
   4. Urinary incontinence

6. Which intervention is important for the nurse to implement for a client who has undergone a kidney biopsy?
   1. Decreasing fluid intake to less than 100 ml/day
   2. Instructing the client to ambulate as soon as possible after the procedure
   3. Monitoring vital signs closely
   4. Performing neurologic checks every 3 to 4 hours for the first 24 hours

7. Which medical condition could cause the client to experience acute tubular necrosis (ATN)?
   1. Prolonged ischemia
   2. Goodpasture's syndrome
   3. Ureteral calculi
   4. Prostatic hypertrophy

8. The nursing diagnosis deficient knowledge related to the need for teaching to prevent pyelonephritis would least likely apply to which client?
   1. A 25-year-old, sexually active man
   2. A bedridden, elderly client with an indwelling (Foley) catheter
   3. An 18-month-old infant with a history of vesicoureteral reflux
   4. A 55-year-old woman who has been treated for urinary retention

9. Which scientific rationale supports the nursing intervention to address malnutrition for a client with renal failure?
1. Anemia causes increased absorption of water-soluble vitamins.
2. The client requires increased carbohydrate intake.
3. Increased anabolism occurs in renal failure.
4. Anemia often causes anorexia, nausea, and vomiting.

10. After dietary instruction, evaluation of effective learning for a client with chronic renal failure would reveal the client's understanding of which fact about high biologic value proteins?
1. They contain the five essential amino acids in each food.
2. They are found in fish, poultry, and eggs.
3. They should compose only a small portion of a dialysis client's total protein intake.
4. They are found in legumes, breads, and cereals.

11. A client with chronic renal failure often experiences pruritus. To intervene effectively, the nurse should teach the client to perform which self-care measure at home?
1. Increasing dietary intake of phosphate
2. Increasing dietary intake of protein
3. Applying glycerin to the skin
4. Using superfatted soaps and lotions

12. Which clinical manifestations and assessment findings support a diagnosis of acute pyelonephritis?
1. Urinary stress incontinence and abdominal pain
2. Flank pain, fever, and dysuria
3. Burning on urination and inflamed urinary meatus
4. Acute, sharp, intermittent pain and anuria

13. Which statement by the client indicates that he understands how to do Kegel exercises correctly?

1. "I should pretend like I am starting and stopping my urine stream."
2. "I should do exercises three times a week."
3. "I can only do the exercises while lying down."
4. "This will prevent urinary retention."

14. On auscultating over the precordium of a client with chronic renal failure, the nurse hears a pericardial friction rub. Which medical condition does this finding indicate?
1. Pleural effusion
2. Cardiac tamponade
3. Ventricular arrhythmias
4. Pericarditis

15. An 18-year-old client who has had renal transplantation has expressed frustration about feeling alone in the hospital room. "I wish I could be out in the waiting room visiting with my friends." Which response would be most appropriate by the nurse?
1. Allowing the client to go the waiting room for 5 minutes only
2. Allowing the client's friends to come into the room for a short visit
3. Allowing the client to verbalize feelings of isolation
4. Discussing activities that the client can do to combat isolation

16. Which nursing interventions should be included in the care plan for the client diagnosed with renal calculi who is attempting to pass the calculi? (Select all that apply.)
1. Increasing fluid intake to more than 3,000 ml/day
2. Encouraging the client to ambulate as much as possible
3. Medicating the client with I.V. meperidine as needed
4. Straining all urine and putting any material in a sterile container
5. Instructing the client to wipe front to back after a bowel movement
6. Encouraging the client to eat a low-fat, low-cholesterol diet

Answer key

1. The answer is **1.**
Because decreased amounts of urea nitrogen are filtered in renal failure, the plasma level increases. The level of serum creatinine increases, creatinine clearance decreases, and serum potassium increases in renal failure.

2. The answer is **1.**
Urine output is usually decreased in ATN. ATN has sudden onset and is usually reversible with treatment. Glucosuria is not commonly associated with ATN.

3. The answer is **2.**
Insensible losses (500 ml) plus urine output determine intake in renal failure. The first directive is an incorrect formulation. Fluid intake should be divided over a 24-hour period. Drinking 500 ml of fluid four times each day far exceeds the recommended allotment.

4. The answer is **2.**
External genitalia normally harbor microorganisms. The urinary tract is considered sterile. Catheterization is unnecessary for a culture and sensitivity specimen. A midstream specimen does not obtain the largest number of microorganisms in the lower urinary tract.

5. The answer is **4.**
Bed wetting, dribbling, urgency, hesitancy, or an inability to get to the bathroom are clinical manifestations of incontinence. Clinical manifestations of UTI include flank pain, fever, chills, and dysuria. Clinical manifestations of renal calculi are acute, sharp, and intermittent pain along with nausea and vomiting. Clinical manifestations of urinary incontinence are altered urine output, hypertension, tachypnea.

6. The answer is **3.**
Vital-sign monitoring detects bleeding and shock. Fluid intake may be increased. The client remains on bed rest for 6 to 8 hours. Neurologic checks are unnecessary.

7. The answer is **1.**
Ischemia is a common cause of ATN. Goodpasture's syndrome is a glomerular disorder. Calculi and prostatic hypertrophy may cause hydronephrosis.

8. The answer is **1.**
Kidney infections are caused by immobility, reflux, stasis, and debilitation. Women are more prone to urinary tract infections (UTIs) than men. A bedridden, elderly client with an indwelling catheter, an 18-month-old toddler with a history of vesicoureteral reflux, and a 55-year-old woman who has been treated for urinary retention would be more prone to UTI than a young adult man.

9. The answer is **4.**
Anorexia, nausea, and vomiting may lead to decreased intake and poor absorption of nutrients. Anemia may lead to decreased absorption of vitamins. Increased carbohydrate intake is important to provide energy. Catabolism commonly occurs in renal failure.

10. The answer is **2.**
Fish, poultry, and eggs are good sources of high biologic value protein. High biologic value protein contains all essential amino acids and should compose the largest percentage of the total protein intake. Legumes, breads, and cereals contain low biologic value proteins.

11. The answer is **4.**
Superfatted soaps and lotion help keep skin moist and relieve pruritus. Excess phosphate in chronic renal failure contributes to skin problems. Dietary protein is decreased to help control the level of uremic toxins. Glycerin has a long-term drying effect.

12. The answer is **2.**

Common clinical manifestations of acute pyelonephritis include flank pain, fever, chills, dysuria, costovertebral angle tenderness, frequency and urgency, malaise and, possibly, bloody or cloudy urine. Urinary stress incontinence and abdominal pain; burning on urination and inflamed urinary meatus; and acute, sharp, intermittent pain and anuria are not signs and symptoms that support the diagnosis of acute pyelonephritis.

13. The answer is **1.**

Contracting the perineal muscles as though stopping urination is the correct way to perform Kegel exercises. The client should perform 10 sets of 10 to 15 repetitions each per day. These exercises can be done lying, sitting, or standing. Kegel exercises help prevent stress incontinence.

14. The answer is **4.**

Pericardial layers rub together because of inflammation from uremic toxins. Pleural effusion may lead to pleural friction rub. Pericardial friction rub disappears with tamponade. Arrhythmias are unrelated to pericardial friction rub.

15. The answer is **3.**

A posttransplantation client who is immunosuppressed is placed on mask isolation in a single room and protected from anyone with an infection. The nurse should allow the client to verbalize his feelings of isolation.

16. The answer are **1, 3, 4.**

Increasing fluid intake will help pass the calculi, I.V. pain medications are administered because shock or syncope may result from excruciating pain, and straining urine will determine when caculi is passed, enabling it to be sent to the laboratory for analysis. The client should be on bed rest because of the high doses of opioids administered for pain; wiping front to back helps prevent urinary tract infections not renal calculi; and a specific diet — such as a low-purine or low-calcium diet — may be ordered after calculi analysis, but a low-fat, low-cholesterol diet will not help calculi passing or prevention.

18 *Hematologic disorders*

I. STRUCTURE AND FUNCTION OF THE HEMATOLOGIC SYSTEM

A. **Structure.** Whole blood consists of formed elements (i.e., blood cells) suspended in a liquid component (i.e., plasma). In an adult, the total blood volume is approximately 5 L, constituting 7% to 8% of total body weight.

1. **Bone marrow,** accounting for 4% to 5% of total body weight, is contained within the spongy bones and central cavity of the long bones.

   a. **Red marrow** is the site of active cell formation and is the major blood-producing organ (i.e., hematopoiesis).

   b. **Yellow marrow** constitutes inactive areas composed mainly of fat.

   c. **Stem cells** are free, primitive cells present in bone marrow. They differentiate into mature blood cells.

2. **Blood cells.** Hematocrit refers to the percentage of total blood volume composed of cells. The normal value is approximately 45%. Whole blood contains three types of mature blood cells: erythrocytes, leukocytes, and thrombocytes (See *Figure 18-1.*)

   a. **Erythrocytes** (i.e., red blood cells [RBCs])
      - The average total RBC count is 5 million cells/mm³ of blood.
      - The major cellular element of circulating blood is the erythrocyte. These cells are biconcave disks that normally are about 7 mm in diameter and contain hemoglobin confined within a plasma membrane.
      - **Reticulocytes,** immature erythrocytes, may be released prematurely from marrow into the circulation under conditions necessitating rapid blood-cell production (i.e., compensatory mechanism).
      - **Hemoglobin,** consisting of an iron-containing pigment and a simple protein, makes up about 95% of the erythrocyte mass. Hemoglobin has the ability to bind oxygen loosely and reversibly; when combined with oxygen, it is called oxyhemoglobin. Whole blood normally contains about 15 g of hemoglobin per 100 ml of blood.

   b. **Leukocytes** (i.e., white blood cells [WBCs]). The average total WBC count is 5,000 to 10,000 cells per cubic millimeter of blood. The two major types of leukocytes are based on cell structure.
      - **Granular leukocytes** (i.e., granulocytes or polymorphonuclear leukocytes)
        - Produced in bone marrow, **granulocytes** normally make up 70% of all WBCs.
        - Granulocytes are subdivided into three types based on staining properties: **neutrophils** (stain a dull violet hue), **eosinophils** (stain bright red), and **basophils** (stain deep blue).
      - **Mononuclear leukocytes** (i.e., agranular leukocytes) are subdivided into two groups.
        - **Lymphocytes** are produced in bone marrow and undergo differentiation in lymph tissue. These comprise 30% of total leukocytes.
        - **Monocytes** are produced in bone marrow and transform into macrophages on release into tissues. They make up 5% of total leukocytes.

   c. **Thrombocytes** (i.e., platelets)
      - Normal platelet count is 150,000 to 450,000/mm³.
      - Thrombocytes are formed from fragments of membrane and cytoplasm from very large cells in bone marrow, lung, and spleen called megakaryocytes. The normal life span of thrombocytes is 7 to 14 days.

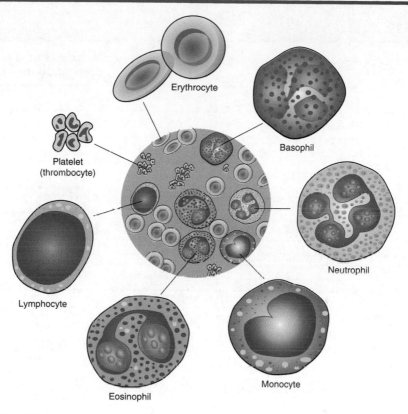

FIGURE 18-1
Types of blood cells

3. **Plasma**

   a. Plasma, the liquid portion of whole blood remaining after blood cells are removed, constitutes 55% of blood volume and contains large quantities of organic and inorganic substances.

   b. Serum is the fluid remaining when plasma is allowed to clot (i.e., plasma minus fibrinogen and several clotting factors).

   c. Plasma proteins

   – **Albumin,** largest of the plasma proteins, is produced in the liver.
   – **Globulins** are subdivided into two types.
     - **Gamma globulins** consist mainly of antibodies known as immunoglobulins.
     - **Alpha and beta fractions** include coagulation (clotting) factors, which are produced in the liver, and transport proteins. (See *Table 18-1,* page 490.)
   – **Fibrinogen** is a high-molecular-weight protein that is important in blood clotting.

B. Function

1. **General blood functions** include:

   a. transporting oxygen absorbed from lungs and nutrients absorbed from the GI tract to body cells for cellular metabolism

TABLE 18-1
Blood coagulation proteins

Factor	Synonyms	Normal plasma concentrations (mg/dl)
I	Fibrinogen	200 to 400
II	Prothrombin	10
III	Tissue thromboplastin, tissue factor	0
IV	Calcium ion	4 to 5
V	Proaccelerin factor, labile factor	1
VII	Serum prothrombin conversion accelerator, stable factor	0.05
VIII	Antihemophilic factor	1 to 2
IX	Christmas factor	0.3
X	Stuart-Power factor	1
XI	Plasma thromboplastin antecedent	0.5
XII	Hageman factor	3
XIII	Fibrin stabilizing factor	1 to 2
Prekallikrein	Fletcher factor	5
High-molecular-weight kininogen	Fitzgerald factor, Flaujeac factor, Williams factor, contact activation cofactor	6

b. transporting waste products from tissues to excretory organs

c. aiding in chemical, acid-base, and thermal regulation of the body

d. transporting hormones and other substances internally secreted to their tissue sites of action

e. aiding in defense against infection through the actions of antibodies and phagocytes

f. aiding in regulation of extracellular fluid volume

g. promoting hemostasis through the arrest of bleeding by blood clot formation, followed by clot dissolution.

2. **Bone marrow**

a. All blood cells are produced in bone marrow, although some cells (e.g., lymphocytes, monocytes) differentiate and mature in various tissues. This process of hematopoiesis is dynamic and constant, because the body needs to turn over blood cells rapidly and continually produce new cells.

b. During the process of hematopoiesis, stem cells in the bone marrow divide into the myelocyte stem cell line and the lymphoid stem cell line, transform into committed precursors, and eventually differentiate into mature blood cells.

3. **Blood cells**
    a. **Erythrocytes**
       - Normal erythrocyte production (i.e., erythropoiesis), occurring in the bone marrow, is stimulated by erythropoietin (i.e., substance produced primarily by the kidneys) and requires several nutrients, notably iron, folic acid and pyridoxine (i.e., vitamin B complex), and ascorbic acid (i.e., vitamin C).
       - Erythrocytes transport oxygen from lungs to tissues. In active tissues, oxygen readily dissociates from hemoglobin. In venous blood, hemoglobin combines with hydrogen ions produced by cellular metabolism, buffering excess acid.
       - The average life span of a circulating erythrocyte is 120 days. Erythrocytes are removed by phagocytosis in the reticuloendothelial system, particularly the liver and spleen. Reticuloendothelial cells produce bilirubin, a pigment from hemoglobin released from destroyed erythrocytes excreted in bile.
    b. **Leukocytes** defend the body against invasion by infectious and parasitic organisms through the processes of phagocytosis (i.e., ingestion and destruction of invading organisms and foreign particles) and antibody production.
       - **Neutrophils** are phagocytic cells that arrive early at the site of inflammatory reaction but have a relatively short life span of several days. Increased numbers (i.e., neutrophilia) occur with the onset of infection, especially with pyogenic bacteria that augment the body's resistance. Infection also may produce a "shift to the left," which is the appearance of more immature forms of neutrophils in circulation, such as bands and metamyelocytes.
       - **Eosinophils** and **basophils** contain and release potent biologic materials (e.g., histamine, serotonin, heparin), which alter blood supply to tissues and help mobilize the body's defense mechanisms.
       - **Monocytes,** the largest nongranular leukocytes, can phagocytize large foreign particles, cell fragments, and necrotic tissue.
       - **Lymphocytes** produce substances that aid in attacking foreign cells and substances.
          - **B lymphocytes** produce antibodies.
          - **T lymphocytes** kill foreign cells directly or release lymphokines, substances that enhance activity of phagocytic cells.
          - **Natural killer cells** defend against microorganisms and some types of malignant cells.
    c. **Thrombocytes** (i.e., platelets) help control bleeding by:
       - physically aggregating and adhering to sites of vascular injury, forming a patch or plug that temporarily stops bleeding; approximately 10% to 15% of circulating platelets are continually being consumed in normal, ongoing, intravascular clot formation during the repair of small vascular injuries
       - releasing biochemical substances that activate coagulation factors in plasma to form a stable fibrin clot.
4. **Plasma** is part of the extracellular fluid of the body and provides a medium for circulation of blood cells.
    a. **Plasma proteins** are mostly located in the circulatory system; the plasma protein concentration is approximately 3.5 times that of the fluid outside the capillaries.
       - Albumin primarily causes osmotic pressure at the capillary membrane, which prevents plasma from leaking out of the capillaries into the interstitial spaces; this pressure is called colloid osmotic pressure.
       - Globulins

- **Alpha and beta globulins** perform diverse functions in the circulation, such as transport of other substances by combining with them (e.g., thyroid-binding globulin carries thyroxine, transferrin carries iron), acting as substrates for formation of other substances, and transporting proteins from one part of the body to another.
- **Gamma globulins** protect the body against infections (i.e., immunity); these are mainly antibodies that resist infection and toxicity.
- **Fibrinogen,** a high-molecular-weight protein, is one of the essential factors in the coagulation process; thrombin acts on fibrinogen to form the reticulum of the clot.

  b. **Constituent substances in plasma** provide for the following functions:
    - **Blood coagulation** (i.e., clotting and hemostasis)
      - In the **vascular phase,** the injured vessel immediately constricts. This vessel spasm is sufficient to stop capillary bleeding.
      - In the **platelet phase,** platelets aggregate at the bleeding site. Tiny cells are rapidly attracted to the damaged endothelium and form loose plugs. This platelet plug effectively stops bleeding and provides temporary protection in larger injuries.
      - In the **coagulation phase,** which can be initiated through the extrinsic pathway (i.e., trauma to the vascular wall) or intrinsic pathway (i.e., in the blood itself), the prothrombin activator forms. This causes conversion of prothrombin to thrombin; the thrombin acts as an enzyme to convert fibrinogen into fibrin threads that enmesh platelets, blood cells, and plasma to form the clot.
    - **Maintenance of acid-base balance.** Protein buffers are located within the cells. These proteins are composed of amino acids, some of which have free acidic radicals that can dissociate into a base plus hydrogen ions.
    - **Clot lysis**
      - The **fibrinolytic system** is a plasma enzyme system responsible for blood-clot removal after blood-vessel integrity is restored.
      - **Plasminogen** is activated into the enzyme plasmin, which digests fibrinogen and fibrin in a process called fibrinolysis.
      - **Fibrinolysis** produces fibrin split products, also known as *fibrin degradation products,* which are removed from circulation by the reticuloendothelial system and liver and spleen. Fibrin split products normally are not present in circulation.
    - **Transportation of nutritional and hormonal substances.** Albumin has the ability to bind several plasma substances, such as fatty acids, drugs, metals, and bilirubin, for transport.

NURSING PROCESS OVERVIEW

 II. THE HEMATOLOGIC SYSTEM

A. **Assessment**
  1. **Health history**
     a. **Elicit a description of the client's present illness and chief complaint,** including onset, course, duration, location, and precipitating and alleviating factors. Cardinal signs and symptoms indicating altered hematologic function include:
     - weakness, fatigue, and general malaise

- hemorrhagic tendencies
- dyspnea
- pallor and ulcerations of mucous membranes
- pallor and dryness of skin
- anxiety.

   b. **Explore the client's health history for risk factors** associated with hematologic disease, including poor nutritional intake of vitamins and genetic tendencies.

2. **Physical examination**
   a. **Inspection.** Observe skin and mucous membranes for color changes, which are best assessed where capillary beds are superficial and pigmentation minimal (e.g., nail beds, hard palate, lips, palms, soles, conjunctivae). Color changes should be noted.
   - Pallor (i.e., paleness) occurs with decreased hemoglobin or decreased blood flow.
   - Cyanosis (i.e., bluish discoloration) occurs with increased circulating unoxygenated hemoglobin due to hypoxia (e.g., buccal, peripheral).
   - Rubor (i.e., redness) occurs with increased visibility of normal oxyhemoglobin because of dilation of superficial blood vessels (e.g., fever) or increased blood flow (e.g., inflammation).
   - Jaundice (i.e., yellowish discoloration) results from increased bilirubin levels due to red blood cell (RBC) hemolysis and appears first in the sclera, then the mucous membranes, and then becomes generalized.
   - Petechiae are pinpoint hemorrhages on skin or mucous membranes that most commonly occur with quantitative or qualitative platelet disorders; they are generally more numerous over bony prominences (i.e., increased trauma) or dependent areas (i.e., increased venous pressure).
   - Ecchymoses (i.e., bluish-black maculae) result from seepage of blood into skin or mucous membranes and are often caused by trauma.
   - Pruritus and malignant infiltrative skin lesions occur with certain hematologic malignancies (e.g., leukemias, lymphomas).
   - Glossitis (i.e., inflammation of the tongue) and ulcerative lesions of the oral cavity occur with certain anemias.
   - Gingival hypertrophy (i.e., enlargement of gums) is common in monocytic leukemia and is caused by leukemic cell infiltration.
   b. **Palpation.** Palpate the thorax and abdomen for signs of:
   - splenomegaly (i.e., enlarged spleen), which occurs in various hematologic disorders, including several anemias and hematologic malignancies
   - hepatomegaly (i.e., enlarged liver), possibly indicating inflammation (e.g., hepatitis), venous congestion, or a hematologic malignancy
   - lymphadenopathy (i.e., enlarged lymph nodes), which may point to regional or systemic infection or a hematologic malignancy.

3. **Laboratory and diagnostic studies**
   a. **Bone marrow aspiration and biopsy** evaluate specimens of bone marrow and bone, which are obtained by introducing a needle with stylet into the iliac crest (the sternum may be used for aspiration in adults). The purposes of these studies include:
   - diagnosing hematologic disorders by evaluating precursors of peripheral blood cells or iron content
   - evaluating the effectiveness of treatment
   - diagnosing nonhematologic diseases (e.g., infectious diseases, certain granulomas) or staging solid tumor malignancies.

b. **Complete blood cell count** includes:
  - **enumeration of the number of RBCs, white blood cells (WBCs), and platelets** per milliliter of venous blood
  - **differential WBC count,** or respective percentages of neutrophils, eosinophils, basophils, lymphocytes, and monocytes contributing to the total WBC count.

c. **Reticulocyte count** detects the percentage of young (1- to 2-day-old) nonnucleated erythrocytes in peripheral blood.

d. **RBC indices** involve three calculated measurements of average RBC size and the hematocrit and hemoglobin content. These values are helpful in diagnosing and evaluating the severity of anemic disorders. Specific indices include:
  - **mean corpuscular hemoglobin,** which is the average amount of hemoglobin contained within RBCs
  - **mean corpuscular hemoglobin concentration,** which is the percentage representing the ratio of the weight of hemoglobin to the volume of an average RBC
  - **mean corpuscular volume,** which is the value for average RBC size.

e. **Hemoglobin electrophoresis** provides a means for identifying different hemoglobins (e.g., A, A_2, F, S) by the speed at which they travel when exposed to electrical current.

f. **The sickling test** detects characteristic sickling of RBCs occurring with sickle-cell trait or disease by exposing blood to a reducing agent, depriving cells of oxygen.

g. **Coombs' test** detects immune globulin plasma (i.e., indirect Coombs' test). This test is used in diagnosing various hemolytic anemias.

h. **Leukocyte alkaline phosphatase testing** estimates the amount of this enzyme (normally present in high concentrations in neutrophils) through a special stain of peripheral blood.

i. **Bleeding time** involves measuring in minutes the time it takes for bleeding to stop after a standardized skin puncture, usually on the forearm. This measurement helps detect disorders of platelet function.

j. **Platelet aggregation** measures the time and completeness of platelet aggregate formation in a plasma sample after addition of a triggering agent.

k. **Prothrombin time (PT)** measures coagulation through extrinsic and common pathways. A serious problem with this form of reporting is that test results can vary widely among laboratories, which is why international normalized ratio (INR) is now being used to measure coagulation. The purposes of PT include:
  - monitoring warfarin therapy
  - providing a screening test for liver disease and coagulation-factor deficiencies.

l. **INR** measures coagulation time but ensures that test results from various laboratories are comparable. The purpose of INR is to monitor warfarin therapy. INR is determined by multiplying the observed PT ratio by a correction factor specific to the particular thromboplastin preparation employed by the test.

m. **Partial thromboplastin time (PTT)** evaluates coagulation through intrinsic and common pathways. The purposes of PTT include:
  - monitoring heparin therapy
  - screening for coagulation-factor deficiencies.

n. **Thrombin clotting time** measures thrombin-induced conversion of fibrinogen to fibrin in the coagulation cascade. This measurement is used to monitor heparin therapy.

o. **Coagulation factor assay** provides the definitive test for quantitative deficiency of coagulation factor. In this test, a sample of the client's plasma is added to a sample of factor-deficient plasma, and the amount of correction in PT and PTT values is compared with correction by normal plasma (arbitrarily defined as 100% activity).

B. Nursing diagnoses
1. Activity intolerance
2. Imbalanced nutrition: less than body requirements
3. Ineffective tissue perfusion
4. Ineffective breathing pattern
5. Decreased cardiac output
6. Acute or chronic pain
7. Risk for injury
8. Deficient knowledge
9. Ineffective coping

C. Planning and outcome identification. The major goals of the client experiencing hematologic disorders are tolerance of normal activity, maintenance of adequate nutrition, improvement of tissue perfusion and breathing patterns, increased cardiac output, pain relief, compliance with measures to prevent bleeding, and increased knowledge of and ability to cope with chronic condition.

D. Implementation
1. **Provide ongoing assessment.**
   a. Assess the pallor of skin and mucous membranes and the jaundice and dryness of skin and hair.
   b. Assess vital signs, cardiovascular status, neurologic status, and GI status.
   c. Assess stool and vomitus for frank and occult blood.
   d. Assess nutritional status, activity level, and current weight (loss or gain).
2. **Promote activity tolerance and rest.**
   a. Assist with activities of daily living that may be beyond the client's tolerance or require exertion.
   b. Provide diversionary activities that promote rest and quiet, but prevent boredom and withdrawal.
   c. Plan nursing activities to provide sufficient rest.
3. **Promote nutritional balance.**
   a. Provide sufficient oral intake (2 to 3 L) to prevent dehydration.
   b. Collaborate with a registered dietitian and provide appropriate diet and supplements.
4. **Promote measures to maintain tissue perfusion.**
   a. Turn the client every 2 hours.
   b. Assess bony prominences.
   c. Provide good skin care. Keep the skin dry. Apply lotion to dry skin.
5. **Promote adequate airway exchange.**
   a. Position the client for optimal air exchange; elevate the head of the bed.
   b. Collaborate with the respiratory therapist when administering supplemental oxygen.
6. **Promote measures to increase cardiac output.** Explain steps to prevent orthostatic hypotension (i.e., rise slowly and wait a few minutes before rising from lying to standing position).
7. **Provide pain relief.**
   a. Assess the client for pain. Rule out complications that may require medical attention.
   b. Administer pain medications as prescribed. Evaluate the effectiveness of medications.

8. **Prevent injury.** Discuss safety issues with the client and family, such as using hand rails in bath areas and near steps and equipment to prevent fatigue.
9. **Provide client and family teaching.** Provide explanations for the cause, treatment, and expected course for the client with a hematologic disorder.
10. **Promote coping.** Encourage the client to verbalize feelings and assist with coping with the discomforts, treatment regimen, and changes in lifestyle.

E. Outcome evaluation

1. The client demonstrates normal activity tolerance.
2. The client maintains adequate nutritional status.
3. The client regains or maintains adequate tissue perfusion.
4. The client maintains normal breathing pattern.
5. The client demonstrates adequate cardiac output.
6. The client reports minimal or no pain and an acceptable comfort level.
7. The client remains free from injury.
8. The client verbalizes understanding of the cause and treatment of the blood disorder.
9. The client demonstrates effective coping with diagnosis and effects of treatment.
10. The client identifies strengths that can enhance coping skills and empower the client.

III. ANEMIAS: GENERAL CONSIDERATIONS

A. Description

1. **Anemia** is a clinical condition (not a laboratory result) defined as a decrease in hemoglobin content or red cell mass that impairs oxygen transport. It is one of the most common problems in clinical practice.
2. **Classification** of anemia is based on morphologic characteristics of erythrocytes or etiologic mechanisms resulting in decreased hemoglobin or red blood cell (RBC) mass. Morphologic characteristics refer to average RBC size and hemoglobin content. Average RBC size may be:
   a. normal (i.e., normocytic)
   b. smaller than normal (i.e., microcytic)
   c. larger than normal (i.e., hypochromic).

B. Etiology

1. **Anemias can result from:**
   a. inadequate production of RBCs
   b. premature or excessive destruction of RBCs
   c. blood loss
   d. deficits in nutrients
   e. hereditary factors
   f. chronic diseases.
2. **Types of anemias** (based on cause)
   a. Aplastic anemia
   b. Iron deficiency anemia
   c. Megaloblastic anemia
      - Vitamin B_{12} deficiency anemia
      - Folic acid deficiency anemia
   d. Hemolytic anemia

  - Inherited
    - Hereditary spherocytosis
    - Sickle cell anemia
    - Thalassemia
    - Glucose-6-phosphate dehydrogenase deficiency
  - Immune hemolytic anemia, which is acquired
  e. Blood loss anemia
  f. Anemia of renal disease
  g. Anemia in chronic disease

C. Pathophysiology

1. Anemia is not a disease but an indication of some disease process or alteration in body function.
2. The oxygen-carrying capacity of hemoglobin is reduced, causing tissue hypoxia. Excessive loss of red cells from blood loss or destruction, or impaired production from lack of nutritional elements or bone-marrow failure causes the clinical manifestations of anemia.

D. Assessment findings

1. **Clinical manifestations**
   a. Signs and symptoms reflect deficient oxygenation of tissues and compensatory cardiopulmonary mechanisms, regardless of the cause of anemia, and include:
      - pallor
      - susceptibility to fatigue
      - central nervous system manifestations, including headache, dizziness, lightheadedness, slowing of thought processes, irritability, restlessness, and depression
      - effects of increased cardiac workload, including tachycardia, palpitations, and angina pectoris or heart failure in susceptible persons
      - tachycardia and dyspnea progressing from exertional to at rest
      - complaints of feeling cold because of blood being shunted to areas of greater need.
   b. Severity of symptoms depends on:
      - speed of onset (Generally, the more rapidly anemia develops, the more severe are the symptoms.)
      - cardiopulmonary reserve
      - metabolic requirements
      - other medical disorders
      - specific complications and features associated with the cause of anemia.
2. **Laboratory and diagnostic study findings.** See specific anemias for pertinent laboratory and diagnostic studies.

E. Nursing management (See section II.D.)

1. **Direct general management toward addressing the cause of anemia and replacing blood loss as needed** to sustain adequate oxygenation.
2. **Promote optimal activity and protect the client from injury.**
   a. Encourage ambulation and participation in activities of daily living as tolerated; emphasize hazards of immobility (e.g., hypotension, muscle wasting).
   b. Assess the client's subjective response to activity (e.g., complaints of fatigue, weakness, lightheadedness, breathlessness).
   c. Observe for dizziness or unsteady gait, and provide support as necessary.

CLIENT AND FAMILY TEACHING 18-1
Prevention and management of anemias

- Encourage the client to organize activity with rest periods to prevent physical exhaustion.
- Assist the client to identify situations that precipitate palpitations and dyspnea and avoid them.
- Explain the need to ensure adequate oxygenation. Tell him to avoid cold environments, activities that cause exertion, and high altitudes.
- Encourage the client to drink 2 to 3 L of water to prevent dehydration.
- Instruct the client to report signs of fluid retention (peripheral edema, decreased urinary output), paresthesias, poor coordination, ataxia, and confusion.

- Collaborate with a registered dietitian and discuss dietary requirements for the specific anemia.
- In general, encourage a well-balanced diet high in protein and high-calorie foods, fruits, and vegetables.
- Advise the client to avoid alcoholic beverages (alcohol interferes with the use of essential nutrients) and spicy foods (causes gastric irritation).
- Explain and prepare the client for a wide variety of blood tests that must be done on a continuing basis.
- Explain the purpose of blood components and initiation of blood transfusions.

---

   3. **Reduce activities and stimuli that cause tachycardia and increase cardiac output.**
      a. Encourage the client to report palpitations, chest pain, or dyspnea experienced with activity or psychological stress.
      b. For a client experiencing dyspnea, elevate the head of the bed; avoid gas-forming foods (abdominal distention may aggravate dyspnea); and administer oxygen therapy if necessary.
      c. Observe and report signs of fluid retention (e.g., peripheral edema, neck vein distention, decreased urinary output).
   4. **Provide teaching** as described in *Client and family teaching 18-1*.
   5. **Provide for nutritional needs.**
      a. Provide high-protein and high-calorie foods and sufficient fruits and vegetables to ensure essential nutrients for erythropoiesis.
      b. Administer any prescribed nutritional supplements (e.g., iron, vitamin B_{12}, and folic acid). (See *Drug chart 18-1*.) See specific anemias for nursing interventions.
      c. Promote small, frequent meals to help cope with problems of fatigue and anorexia.

IV. IRON DEFICIENCY ANEMIA

   A. **Description.** Iron deficiency anemia is marked by below-normal total body iron and inadequate hemoglobin production for body requirements. It is the most common type of anemia in all age groups, affecting 10% to 30% of adults in the United States.

   B. **Etiology**
      1. Chronic blood loss from GI bleeding (e.g., ulceration, tumor, hemorrhoids, hookworm infestation), excessive menstrual bleeding, or multiple pregnancies
      2. Insufficient dietary iron intake
      3. Impaired GI absorption of iron because of gastrectomy or prolonged, severe diarrhea
      4. Increased iron requirements during periods of rapid body growth, pregnancy, or menstruation

   C. **Pathophysiology.** In iron deficiency anemia, body stores of iron decrease, as do stores of transferrin, which binds with and transports iron. This leads to depletion of red blood cells (RBCs), resulting in decreased hemoglobin concentration and decreased oxygen-carrying capacity of the blood.

DRUG CHART 18-1
Medications for hematologic disorders

Classifications	Indications	Selected interventions
Antibiotics aminoglycosides (gentamicin, tobramycin) amoxicillin erythromycin penicillin tetracycline	Prevent or treat infections caused by pathogenic microorganisms	▪ Before administering first dose, assess the client for allergies and determine whether culture has been obtained. ▪ After multiple doses, assess the client for superinfection (thrush, yeast infection, diarrhea); notify the health care provider if these occur. ▪ Assess the insertion site for phlebitis if antibiotics are being administered I.V. ▪ To assess the effectiveness of antibiotic therapy, monitor white blood cell count. ▪ Monitor peaks and troughs for aminoglycosides.
Antipyretic agents acetaminophen aspirin	Produce diaphoresis and vasodilation by acting on the brain's thermoregulatory center	▪ Do not give aspirin to children because of its association with Reye's syndrome. ▪ Watch for GI distress and possible bleeding from aspirin. ▪ Report any tinnitus (ringing in ears), a sign of aspirin toxicity.
Corticosteroids — oral hydrocortisone methylprednisolone prednisone	Strengthen biologic membrane, which inhibits capillary permeability and prevents leakage of fluid into the injured area and development of edema (exact mechanism unknown)	▪ Instruct the client to take the medication exactly as directed and to taper discontinuation rather than stop it abruptly, which could cause serious withdrawal symptoms leading to adrenal insufficiency, shock, and death. ▪ Forewarn the client that the medication may cause reportable cushingoid effects (weight gain, moon face, buffalo hump, and hirsutism) and may mask signs and symptoms of infection.
Epinephrine adrenalin	Cause bronchodilation and vasoconstriction to relieve bronchial edema	▪ Administered subcutaneously with a TB syringe, rotate vial to mix suspension. ▪ Common adverse effects are increased heart rate, muscle tremors, anxiety, and nervousness; large doses can produce an acute hypertensive episode and cardiac arrhythmias.
Folic acid supplements apo-folic folvite	Supplement folic acid intake; minimum daily requirement is 50 g (Folic acid is found in most meats, fresh vegetables, and fresh fruits but is destroyed when cooked more than 15 minutes.)	▪ May be given orally, I.M., I.V., or subcutaneously.
Histamine (H_1)-receptor antagonist diphenhydramine	Inhibit H_1 release by selectively binding to H_1-receptors	▪ Teach the client to avoid alcohol, driving, or engaging in hazardous activities because medication causes drowsiness, which may subside with continued use. ▪ Encourage sucking on hard candy or ice chips for relief of dry mouth.

(continued)

DRUG CHART 18-1

Medications for hematologic disorders (continued)

Classifications	Indications	Selected interventions
Immunoglobulin gamma globulin	Provide passive immunity by immunoglobin G antibodies to protect against infection	■ Before administering, obtain allergy and immunization history. ■ After administering, monitor the client closely for signs and symptoms of allergic reaction.
Iron supplements Oral— ferrous sulfate	Synthesize heme, the essential protein of hemoglobin	■ Inform the client that his stool will be dark and tarry; instruct him on ways to prevent constipation. ■ Tell the client to notify his health care provider of adverse effects, such as diarrhea, constipation, GI upset, or nausea and vomiting that become severe or intolerable. ■ Tell the client to store iron safely out of reach of children (in whom iron poisoning may be fatal).
Parenteral— dextran	Synthesize heme, the essential protein of hemoglobin	■ Administer using Z-track technique to avoid leakage into subcutaneous tissues. ■ Caution the client that preparation may discolor skin and cause local pain. ■ Be alert for possible anaphylactic reaction.
liquid iron	Synthesize heme, the essential protein of hemoglobin	■ Forewarn the client that liquid iron may stain teeth. ■ Suggest diluting the iron and administering it through a straw or dropper placed at the back of the tongue.
Opioid analgesics codeine hydrocodone hydromorphone morphine propoxyphene	Relieve moderate to severe pain by reducing pain sensation, producing sedation, and decreasing the emotional upset often associated with pain; most often schedule II drugs	■ Assess the pain for location, type, intensity, what increases or decreases it; rate pain on a scale of 1 (no pain) to 10 (worst pain). ■ Rule out any complications. Is this pain routine or expected? Is this a complication that needs immediate intervention? ■ Medicate according to pain-scale findings. ■ Institute safety measures—bed in low position, side rails up, and call light within reach. ■ Evaluate effectiveness of pain medication in 30 minutes.
Vasopressors metaraminol norepinephrine	Rapidly restore blood pressure in anaphylaxis by producing vasoconstriction and stimulating the heart	■ Monitor the client's vital signs, intake and output, mental status, peripheral pulses, and skin color. ■ The client should be on telemetry and monitored continuously.
Vitamin B$_{12}$ Vitamin B$_{12}$ injection	Stimulate a key reaction in the synthesis of thymidylate, a component of deoxyribonucleic acid; deficiency results in the release of too few blood cells	■ Must be given I.M. to bypass the intestine for systemic absorption. ■ Vitamin B$_{12}$ injections are virtually free of adverse effects; initially taken by daily injections and then monthly throughout life.

D. Assessment findings

1. **Clinical manifestations**
   a. Iron deficiency anemia presents primarily with general manifestations of anemia. (See section III.D.1.)
   b. Skin and mucous membrane manifestations may include fissuring at angles of mouth; smooth, sore tongue; and spoon-shaped, brittle nails.
   c. Some clients may exhibit pica (i.e., craving to eat unusual substances such as clay or laundry starch) or an extreme craving for ice.

2. **Laboratory and diagnostic study findings**
   a. Microcytic hypochromia reveals small RBCs, which are relatively devoid of pigment.
   b. The hemoglobin count is proportionally lower than the hematocrit and RBC count.
   c. Measurement of iron stores indicates a low serum iron concentration, high total iron-binding capacity, and low serum ferritin.
   d. The reticulocyte count is decreased.

E. Nursing management (See section II.D.)

1. **Administer prescribed medications,** which may include iron supplements. (See *Drug chart 18-1*, pages 499 and 500.)
2. **Treat the underlying cause of anemia and correct the iron deficit** through diet and supplemental iron preparations.
3. **Provide information on preventive measures.**
   a. Counsel and instruct high-risk clients (e.g., menstruating and pregnant women) about preventive education.
   b. Review foods high in iron (e.g., organ and other meats, cooked white beans, leafy vegetables, raisins, molasses).
   c. Encourage the client to take a source of vitamin C with iron-rich foods to enhance absorption.
   d. Advise the client that tannates (in tea) and carbonates hinder iron absorption.
4. **Provide teaching** as described in *Client and family teaching 18-1*, page 498.

V. MEGALOBLASTIC ANEMIA

A **Description.** Megaloblastic anemias are hematologic disorders characterized by the production and peripheral proliferation of large, immature, and dysfunctional red blood cells (RBCs). Types include:

1. vitamin B_{12} deficiency anemia (under which pernicious anemia is categorized)
2. folic acid deficiency anemia.

B. Etiology

1. **Vitamin B_{12} deficiency anemia**
   a. Inadequate dietary intake of vitamin B_{12} is rare, except in strict vegetarians.
   b. Faulty absorption of vitamin B_{12} from the GI tract occurs because of a lack of secretion of intrinsic factor, normally produced by gastric mucosal cells.
   c. Certain small-intestine disorders impair absorption of vitamin B_{12}. This is referred to as pernicious anemia.

2. **Folic acid deficiency anemia**
   a. Inadequate dietary intake of uncooked vegetables, fruits, and other sources of folic acid (This may occur in clients on prolonged I.V. hyperalimentation.)

b. Impaired absorption of folic acid in the upper jejunum

c. Increased requirements for folic acid, common in alcoholism, pregnancy, and chronic hemolytic anemias

C. Pathophysiology

1. Vitamin B_{12} and folic acid are essential for normal deoxyribonucleic acid (DNA) synthesis and hematopoiesis. In deficiency, RBCs cannot produce DNA, and normal nuclear maturation is arrested.

2. Cytoplasmic maturation proceeds, however, resulting in abnormally large cells with increased membrane surface area.

3. Because DNA metabolism is essential to formation of all cellular elements in bone marrow, white blood cells and platelets are diminished.

D. Assessment findings

1. **Clinical manifestations.** Both types of megaloblastic anemia manifest with common general signs and symptoms of anemia. (See section III.D.1.) Additional manifestations may include:

   a. smooth, sore tongue

   b. diarrhea

   c. paresthesias

   d. impaired coordination and position sense

   e. confusion, behavioral changes.

2. **Laboratory and diagnostic study findings**

   a. Serum folate level is decreased.

   b. Serum vitamin B_{12} level is low.

   c. Blood smear shows marked variation in size and shape of cells and a variable number of abnormally large cells with a normal hemoglobin concentration.

   d. Schilling test reveals impaired vitamin B_{12} absorption.

E. Nursing management (See section II.D.)

1. **Provide nursing care for the client with vitamin B_{12} deficiency anemia.**

   a. Administer prescribed medications, which may include vitamin B_{12}. (See *Drug chart 18-1*, pages 499 and 500.) For pernicious anemia, lifelong vitamin B_{12} therapy is required.

   b. Advise the client to consume foods high in vitamin B complex, which include organ meats, legumes, nuts, enriched or whole-grain products, and wheat germ.

2. **Provide nursing care for the client with folic acid deficiency anemia**

   a. Administer prescribed medications, which include folic acid supplements. (See *Drug chart 18-1*, pages 499 and 500.) Reassure the client that folic acid supplement therapy can cease when the hemoglobin level returns to normal.

   b. Advise the client to consume foods high in folic acid, which include green leafy vegetables, orange juice, liver, peanuts, legumes, whole-grain products, and wheat germ.

   c. Provide client and family teaching. Inform the client that chronic alcohol ingestion, anticonvulsant medications, and hormonal contraceptives will alter folic acid absorption.

3. **Provide teaching** as described in *Client and family teaching 18-1*, page 498.

VI. SICKLE CELL ANEMIA AND SICKLE CELL CRISIS

A. Description

1. **Sickle cell anemia**

    a. Sickle cell anemia is a severe, chronic, incurable hemolytic anemia resulting from an inherited defective hemoglobin molecule (i.e., hemoglobin S [Hb_S]) and marked by episodic painful crises.

    b. The incidence of sickle cell anemia is highest among persons of tropical African descent. About 10% of blacks carry the abnormal gene (i.e., sickle cell trait), and 1 of 600 black neonates are born with the disease. Significant incidence of sickle cell anemia is also found in the Middle East, the Mediterranean, India, South America, and the Caribbean islands.

2. **Sickle cell crisis**

    a. Sickle cell crisis occurs when the client experiences decreased oxygen resulting in the entanglement of rigid sickle-shaped cells with one another, causing increased blood viscosity; this results in blood stasis with enlargement and engorgement of organs, infarction with ischemia and destruction of red blood cells (RBCs), and replacement fibrous tissue.

    b. Various types of crises include vaso-occlusive crises, aplastic crises, hyperhemolytic crises, and sequestration crises. These crises often occur in combination rather than as isolated events.

    c. Crises typically become less frequent and severe with aging. The risk of death from crisis is greatest in children younger than age 5.

B. Etiology

1. **Sickle cell anemia** results from homozygous inheritance of the Hb_S-producing gene. An individual has the sickle cell trait when the heterozygous person has normal hemoglobin A and abnormal Hb_S.

2. **Sickle cell crisis**

    a. **Vaso-occlusive crises** may be caused by dehydration, infection, fatigue, menstruation, alcohol use, and emotional stress.

    b. **Aplastic crises** are associated with infection and decreased RBC numbers.

    c. **Hyperhemolytic crises** (i.e., increased hemolysis) can occur with infection.

    d. **Sequestration crises** (most common in infants) is of unknown origin.

C. Pathophysiology

1. **Sickle cell anemia**

    a. The Hb_S molecule acquires its characteristic sickle shape when exposed to low oxygen tension. Hb_S is significantly less soluble than normal hemoglobin when it gives up its oxygen. Deoxygenated Hb_S turns into a firm gel, deforming RBC shape. Hb_S-containing RBCs have a decreased survival time and adhere to vascular endothelium, causing anemia and vascular occlusion.

    b. In clients with sickle cell anemia, premature death commonly results from infection or from the effects of recurrent occlusion of microcirculation (e.g., stroke).

2. **Sickle cell crisis**

    a. When the sickle hemoglobin is deprived of oxygen, it becomes sickled. Sickling occurs when one Hb_S molecule interacts with another, causing a semisolid polymer that changes the RBC shape and deforms the cell.

b. A high concentration of misshaped cells during sickling crises makes blood abnormally viscous, resulting in sluggish circulation and sludging of sickled cells, especially within microcirculation. Occlusion in microcirculation increases hypoxia, which triggers sickling in other RBCs, perpetuating the cycle.

– **Vaso-occlusive** crises may be experienced if ischemia or infarction occurs. The organs most vulnerable to infarction include the brain, kidneys, bone marrow, and spleen.

– **Aplastic crises** can cause a precipitous, life-threatening drop in hemoglobin; diminished RBC production results in profound anemia.

– **Hyperhemolytic crises** (i.e., increased hemolysis) lead to increased bilirubin levels, predisposing the client to gallstone formation (i.e., bilirubin stones).

– **Sequestration crises** lead to a rapid onset of splenomegaly (from blood pooling) and a precipitous drop in hemoglobin.

D. Assessment findings

1. **Clinical manifestations**

   a. **Sickle cell anemia**
   - Jaundice
   - Progressively impaired kidney function
   - Signs and symptoms secondary to hemolysis and thrombosis
   - Enlarged facial and skull bones
   - Susceptibility to infections, especially osteomyelitis and pneumonia
   - Leg ulcers, usually caused by trauma
   - Gallstones
   - Splenomegaly
   - Cardiomegaly
   - Tachycardia, flow murmurs
   - Growth retardation
   - Delayed puberty
   - In adulthood, characteristic spiderlike body habitus (e.g., elongated extremities, narrow shoulders and hips, barrel chest, curved spine, elongated skull)

   b. **Sickle cell crisis**
   - **Vaso-occlusive crisis**
     - Severe abdominal, chest, back, muscle, or bone pain
     - Increased jaundice
     - Dark urine
     - Low-grade fever
     - Possibly edema
   - **Aplastic crisis**
     - Pallor
     - Dyspnea
     - Lethargy, stupor, possibly coma
   - **Hyperhemolytic crisis**
     - Pallor
     - Jaundice
     - Hemoglobinuria
   - **Sequestration crisis**
     - Pooling of large amounts of blood in liver and spleen
     - Pallor

- Lethargy
- If untreated, signs and symptoms of hypovolemic shock

2. Laboratory and diagnostic study findings

   a. Stained blood smear exhibits sickle cells.

   b. Serum electrophoresis shows Hb$_S$ and distinguishes between trait and disease.

   c. Reticulocyte count is increased.

   d. The sickle-turbidity test is commonly used for screening purposes; a positive result requires serum electrophoresis.

E. Nursing management (See section II.D.)

1. Provide nursing care for the client with sickle cell anemia.

   a. Instruct the client in measures to prevent crises, such as avoiding infections, dehydration, strenuous physical activity, emotional stress, tight or restrictive clothing, and high altitudes. Institute infection-prevention measures, which include:
   - encouraging appropriate dental care and prompt treatment for breaks in skin integrity
   - reviewing immunization schedule with client and family
       advising the client and family to observe for fever, cough, tachypnea, urinary symptoms, and any reddened, painful, or open areas. Instruct the client to seek prompt medical attention if they develop.

   b. Administer folic acid replacement, if indicated, to support erythropoiesis.

   c. Provide support for the client and family.
   - Review genetic implications, and refer for counseling as necessary.
   - Encourage participation in support groups.
   - Encourage verbalization from the client and family. Assist with developing coping skills in identifying strengths.

   d. Manage priapism (i.e., persistent penile erection), which male clients may develop. Instruct the client to empty his bladder at onset of attack, exercise, and take a warm bath. If it persists more than 4 hours, the client should notify the health care provider.

   e. Inform the client about experimental medications (i.e., hydroxyurea, cetiedil citrate, and pentoxifylline) and food additives (i.e., vanilla), which are being evaluated in treating sickle cell anemia.

   f. Provide teaching as detailed in *Client and family teaching 18-1,* page 498.

2. Provide nursing care for the client in sickle cell crisis.

   a. Administer prescribed medications, which may include around-the-clock opioid analgesics. (See *Drug chart 18-1,* pages 499 and 500.) Use patient-controlled analgesia. Do not administer meperidine because of the potential for meperidine-induced seizure.

   b. Increase oral or I.V. fluid intake (3 to 5 L/day), which helps dilute blood and reverse sludging of cells. Monitor intake and output.

   c. Use small-gauge needles or catheters to prevent trauma.

   d. Administer blood transfusions if prescribed. Simple RBC or exchange transfusion may be indicated for aplastic crisis; for severe, painful crisis unresponsive to other therapies; preoperatively to dilute the amount of sickled blood; during the final trimester of pregnancy to prevent crisis; or to treat leg ulcers unresponsive to therapy.

   e. Encourage the client to rest and support affected joints as indicated.

VII. LEUKEMIAS

A. Description

1. Leukemias are malignant disorders of blood-forming tissues characterized by uncontrolled proliferation of white blood cells (WBCs) in the bone marrow (replacing normal marrow elements), liver, spleen, lymph nodes, and nonhematologic organ systems (i.e., skin, kidney, GI tract, and central nervous system).

2. Classification of leukemias are based on:
   a. specific cell lines involved, such as lymphocytic, myelocytic, and monocytic
   b. maturity of malignant cells, such as acute (i.e., immature cells) and chronic (i.e., differentiated cells).

3. Types of leukemias include:
   a. acute myelogenous leukemia (AML), also known as *acute nonlymphocytic leukemia*
   b. acute lymphocytic leukemia (ALL)
   c. chronic myelogenous leukemia (CML)
   d. chronic lymphocytic leukemia (CLL).

4. Incidence varies with type.
   a. AML is most common in adults. The incidence increases with age.
   b. ALL is most common in children.
   c. CML is uncommon before age 20. The incidence rises with age.
   d. CLL is the most common type of leukemia in persons age 50 and older.

B. Etiology.

The cause is unknown, but certain factors are associated with increased incidence, including:

1. exposure to radiation
2. chemical agents (e.g., benzene, alkylating chemotherapeutic agents)
3. infectious agents (Viruses have been implicated in animal models.)
4. genetic variables. (An increased incidence is reported in clients with Down syndrome, and there are reports of increased familial incidence.)

C. Pathophysiology

1. **Acute leukemias** are rapidly progressive diseases usually characterized by uncontrolled proliferation of very immature cells (i.e., blasts) in bone marrow and peripheral tissue. Leukemic blast cells in marrow suppress differentiation and proliferation of normal hemopoietic cells, predisposing to severe anemia, thrombocytopenia (i.e., hemorrhage), and granulocytopenia (i.e., infection). Acute leukemias typically prove rapidly fatal if untreated.
   a. **AML** affects cells committed to granulocytic, monocytic, megakaryocytic, and erythrocytic stem cell lines. Typically, aberration in the growth of one cell type predominates. The most common types of AML involve maturational arrest and proliferation of cells in myeloblastic and monoblastic stages of development.
   b. **ALL** affects lymphoid-committed stem cell lines and is characterized by proliferation of immature lymphoid cells (i.e., lymphoblasts) in bone marrow.

2. **Chronic leukemias** are milder and have more normal cells than acute cells. They are characterized by proliferation of differentiated cells.
   a. **CML** involves malignancy of myeloid stem cells, with more mature cells present than in acute forms and symptoms generally not as severe as in acute forms (i.e., terminal phase of disease involves progression to less differentiated, or blastic, phase). Onset typically is gradual and insidious.

b. **CLL** is characterized by a marked increase in mature lymphocytes in circulation and lymphoid tissue. The disease may be relatively asymptomatic over many years; progressive anemia and thrombocytopenia may result from bone marrow infiltration, immune destruction, or hypersplenism.

D. Assessment findings

1. Clinical manifestations

a. AML
- Pallor, fatigue, dyspnea secondary to anemia
- Bleeding tendencies, such as petechiae, ecchymoses, epistaxis, gingival bleeding, and retinal hemorrhages due to thrombocytopenia
- Gingival hypertrophy
- Lymphadenopathy, splenomegaly, or hepatomegaly due to tissue invasion
- Bone pain and arthralgias due to pressure from rapidly proliferating cells in marrow

b. ALL
- Splenomegaly and hepatomegaly due to tissue invasion
- Headache and vomiting due to meningeal involvement
- Bone pain due to pressure from rapidly proliferating cells in marrow
- Fever and signs and symptoms of infection due to neutropenia

c. CML
- Similar to AML, but signs and symptoms are less severe
- Many clients without symptoms for years
- Splenomegaly (often occurs)

d. CLL
- Asymptomatic
- Usually diagnosed during physical examination or treatment for another cause
- Anemia, infection, or enlargement of lymph nodes or abdominal organs (may occur)

2. Laboratory and diagnostic study findings

a. AML and ALL
- Peripheral WBC count varies widely (1,000 to >100,000/mm³) but always includes immature cells.
- Bone marrow specimen reveals a large percentage (60% to 90%) of bone marrow's nucleated cells identified as blasts (which normally make up 5% or less of normal marrow elements), with reduced erythroid precursors, mature cells, and megakaryocytes.
- Erythrocyte and platelet counts are decreased.

b. CML
- Leukocyte count is elevated.
- Leukocyte alkaline phosphatase is low.
- Genetic testing reveals Philadelphia chromosome present in bone marrow cells in more than 90% of clients.

c. CLL
- Leukocyte count is elevated, possibly exceeding 100,000/mm³.
- Red blood cell count shows decreased erythrocytes, granulocytes, and platelets.

E. Nursing management (See section II.D.)

1. Manage and prevent infection.
a. Monitor temperature, and report elevation.

    b. Assess for and report other signs and symptoms of infection. Be aware that classic signs of infection may not be apparent in a client with leukemia.

    c. Teach the client and family signs and symptoms of infection and preventive techniques.

    d. Maintain a protective environment, as indicated, until the infection subsides.

    e. Recognize that the client is at high risk for infection when the absolute neutrophil count falls below 1,000 cells/mm³ and at grave risk when the count is 500 cells/mm³ or less.

    f. Obtain cultures and initiate I.V. antibiotic therapy, as prescribed. (See *Drug chart 18-1,* pages 499 and 500.)

2. **Maintain integrity of skin and mucous membranes.**
3. **Promote positive coping mechanisms** to help the client and family deal with stressors related to the disease and its treatment.
4. **Institute measures to prevent bleeding, and monitor for bleeding.**
5. **Provide pain relief as needed and as prescribed.**
6. **Provide information on scheduled treatments** (see chapter 20) and discuss with the client as appropriate.

    a. For **AML** and **ALL,** treatment includes initial combination chemotherapy, allogenic bone marrow transplantation, consolidation therapy, and intermittent long-term maintenance chemotherapy for several years.

    b. For **CML,** treatment includes initial single-agent chemotherapy, followed by long-term, low-dose maintenance therapy. In the acute exacerbation phase (i.e., blast crisis), the client may undergo bone marrow transplantation.

    c. For **CLL,** no treatment may be indicated when the client is asymptomatic. For symptomatic clients, treatment may initially include single-agent chemotherapy, followed by combination chemotherapy and possibly splenectomy for refractory thrombocytopenia.

VIII. LYMPHOMAS

A. **Description.** Lymphomas are neoplastic diseases of cells of the lymphoreticular system: lymphocytes and histiocytes (i.e., fixed, nonmotile macrophages).

1. **Classification of lymphomas** is based on:

    a. predominant malignant cell type (i.e., lymphocytic lymphomas, histiocytic lymphomas, or Hodgkin's disease)

    b. degree of malignant cell differentiation (i.e., well-differentiated, poorly differentiated, or undifferentiated).

2. **Types of lymphomas**

    a. Lymphomas are usually divided into three subgroups based on morphologic appearance of involved lymph nodes:

      – Hodgkin's disease

      – Non-Hodgkin's lymphomas

      – Mycosis fungoides (a rare, chronic, cutaneous T-cell lymphoma producing skin lesions closely resembling those of Hodgkin's disease in lymph nodes and viscera)

3. **Incidence**

    a. **Hodgkin's disease** most commonly affects young adults. The incidence is higher among males than females and peaks in two age groups: ages 15 to 38 and in people older than age 50.

TABLE 18-2
Ann Arbor Staging System for Hodgkin's lymphoma

Stage*	Description
I	Involvement of a single lymph node region (I) or of a single extralymphatic organ or site (IE)
II	Involvement of two or more lymph node regions on the same side of the diaphragm (II) or localized involvement of extralymphatic organ or site and of one or more lymph node regions on the same side of the diaphragm (IIE)
III	Involvement of lymph node regions on both sides of the diaphragm (III), which may also be accompanied by localized involvement of extralymphatic organ or site (IIIE), the spleen (IIIS), or both (IIISE)
IV	Diffuse or disseminated involvement of one or more extralymphatic organs or tissues, with or without associated lymph node enlargement. The reason for stage IV classification should be identified further by site-defining symbols.

*Systemic symptoms: Each stage is subdivided into A and B categories. A is for clients without defined symptoms; B is for those with defined symptoms. The B classification applies to a client with unexplained weight loss of more than 10% of body weight in the 6 months before diagnosis, unexplained fever exceeding 100.4°F (38° C), and night sweats.

    b. **Non-Hodgkin's lymphomas** are two to three times more common among men than women and affect all age groups; the incidence increases with age.

    c. **Mycosis fungoides** is rare; peak incidence is between ages 40 and 60.

B. Etiology. The cause of lymphomas is unknown.

C. Pathophysiology. Lymphomas usually originate in lymph nodes and may originate in or involve lymphoid tissue throughout the body (e.g., spleen, tonsils, stomach wall, liver, bone marrow). They commonly spread to extralymphatic tissue (e.g., lungs, kidneys).

   1. **Hodgkin's disease**

     a. The key cell of Hodgkin's disease is the Reed-Sternberg cell, a gigantic, atypical tumor cell of unique morphology and uncertain origin.

     b. Hodgkin's disease usually shows a highly predictable pattern of spread through lymphatic channels to contiguous nodes. It also may spread by a hematogenous route to extranodal sites (e.g., GI tract, bone marrow, skin).

     c. The clinical pattern at presentation determines the all-important stage (extent) of disease (see *Table 18-2*) and strongly correlates with histologic subtype.

     d. Different histopathologic subtypes are associated with various prognoses:

      – **Lymphocyte predominant** has the most favorable prognosis.

      – **Nodular sclerosing** has the next best prognosis.

      – **Mixed cellularity** is characteristically more aggressive than nodular sclerosing or lymphocyte-predominant subtypes.

      Lymphocyte depleted has the most unfavorable prognosis.

   2. **Non-Hodgkin's lymphomas**

     a. Non-Hodgkin's lymphomas are more likely than Hodgkin's disease to involve generalized lymph node disease or extranodal disease at the time of diagnosis. Bone marrow invasion, with associated anemia and thrombocytopenia, and immune dysfunction, with associated infections, are evident with these lymphomas.

  b. In non-Hodgkin's lymphomas, the major determinants of clinical patterns of disease and of prognosis are:
- cell type of origin (state of differentiation)
- pattern of growth within involved lymph nodes (i.e., follicular or diffuse).

  c. Diagnostic terminology has been clarified in a major comparative study. According to the working formulation, three broad groups may be defined:
- **low-grade or favorable group,** which has less aggressive cell types or possesses a follicular (i.e., nodular) growth pattern
- **intermediate-grade group,** which has aggressive cell types in follicular patterns or diffuse patterns of cells, many or all of which appear aggressive
- **high-grade or unfavorable group,** which has a diffuse pattern of growth and highly malignant appearing cell type.

 3. Mycosis fungoides commonly begins in skin as a pruritic, red rash, and months or years later manifests with mushroomlike growths (i.e., lymphoma) that are 1 to 5 cm in diameter. The disease eventually spreads to lymph nodes, spleen, liver, and lungs.

D. Assessment findings

 1. Clinical manifestations

  a. Palpable lymph nodes, especially cervical, axillae, or groin

  b. Fatigue

  c. Weight loss

  d. Mild to high fever, often exhibiting Pel-Ebstein fever pattern

  e. Chills, night sweats

  f. Pruritus

  g. Signs and symptoms secondary to encroachment of enlarged mediastinal and retroperitoneal lymph nodes, including:
- dyspnea from pressure against the trachea
- dysphagia from pressure against the esophagus
- laryngeal paralysis and brachial, lumbar, or sacral neuralgias from pressure on nerves
- edema in extremities or effusions into pleura or peritoneum due to pressure on veins
- signs of obstructive jaundice from pressure on the common bile duct
- splenomegaly
- hepatomegaly.

 2. Laboratory and diagnostic study findings

  a. **Hodgkin's disease**
- Lymph node biopsy reveals the presence of Reed-Sternberg cells.
- Chest radiograph shows mediastinal, hilar, or intrapulmonary metastatic disease.
- Computed tomography (CT) scan reveals lymph node involvement.
- Bone marrow biopsy reveals metastasis to the bone.
- Liver function tests and liver scan reveal metastasis to the liver.
- Lymphangiography reveals abdominal lymph node involvement.

  b. **Non-Hodgkin's lymphomas**
- Lymph node biopsy reveals malignant lymphomas with absence of Reed-Sternberg cells.
- Bone marrow aspirate and biopsy reveals metastasis to bone.
- Liver and renal function tests reveal any metastasis to liver or kidney.
- CT scan reveals lymphoma in lymph nodes and organs.

    c. **Mycosis fungoides**
- Biopsies of skin lesions reveal a widened, fibrotic papillary dermis.
- Biopsies of lymph nodes, bone marrow, and liver reveal malignant proliferation of helper T cells.

E. **Nursing management (See section II.D.)**
1. **Administer analgesics as needed** to relieve painful encroachment of enlarged lymph nodes. (See *Drug chart 18-1,* pages 499 and 500.)
2. **Maintain skin integrity.**
   a. Maintain optimal skin hydration and protection to decrease pruritus.
   b. Care for skin reactions in radiation treatment fields as prescribed by the radiation oncology center.
3. **Treat fever symptomatically** with antipyretics after infection is ruled out.
4. **Protect the client from infection.**
5. **Promote coping.** Provide emotional and psychological support during extensive diagnostic testing and treatments.
6. **Instruct the client and family about treatment protocols.** (See chapter 20.)
7. **Discuss and prepare the client for treatment as needed.**
   a. **Hodgkin's disease.** Depending on stage, symptoms, and cell type, radiation therapy and combination chemotherapy may be indicated. In disease resistant to conventional chemotherapy or in relapse, intensive therapy with autologous bone marrow transplant rescue may be indicated.
   b. **Non-Hodgkin's lymphomas.** Depending on staging and histopathologic classification, radiation therapy (possibly curative with localized disease) or combination chemotherapy (for widespread disease) may be indicated. In clients with relapsed or refractory disease after initial intensive therapy, autologous (or less commonly, allogeneic) bone marrow transplantation may be indicated.
   c. **Mycosis fungoides.** Based on clinical staging, topical chemotherapy (e.g., nitrogen mustard) or corticosteroids for skin manifestations; radiation therapy; systemic chemotherapy; or a combination of topical chemotherapy, radiation therapy, and systemic chemotherapy may be indicated.

IX. BLEEDING DISORDERS

A. **Description.** Bleeding disorders refer to various disorders of impaired hemostasis, which is the physiologic process involved in terminating abnormal bleeding. Specific disorders include:
1. **thrombocytopenia,** a quantitative platelet disorder, which is the most common cause of generalized bleeding
2. **idiopathic thrombocytopenic purpura (ITP),** a group of bleeding disorders of unknown origin that affects people of all ages but is more common among children and young women (Viral infections sometimes precede the disease.)
3. **clotting factor defects,** which include hemophilia A and B (Hemophilia A is the most common inherited disorder of coagulation, affecting approximately 1 of 10,000 males. The incidence of hemophilia B is 5 to 10 times lower than that of hemophilia A.)
4. **Von Willebrand's disease,** a platelet function disorder, which is caused by a mild deficiency of factor VIII

5. **disseminated intravascular coagulation (DIC),** which is a bleeding disorder that uses up all the clotting factors and platelets

6. **vascular disorders,** which may cause bleeding from small blood vessels because of structurally weak vessels that have been damaged by inflammation or an immune response.

B. Etiology

1. **Thrombocytopenia** can result from:
   a. decreased production of platelets by marrow (e.g., infiltrative diseases of marrow, such as leukemia, myelosuppressive therapy, myelofibrosis)
   b. increased platelet destruction (e.g., infection, immune disorders)
   c. abnormal distribution or sequestration (e.g., hypersplenism)
   d. loss of platelets from blood stream (e.g., excessive bleeding without replacement, extracorporeal circulation).

2. **ITP** is of unknown origin.

3. **Clotting factor** defects result from inherited (sex-linked recessive) deficiency of individual coagulation factors.
   a. **Hemophilia A** involves deficiency of factor VIII (i.e., antihemophilic factor).
   b. **Hemophilia B** involves deficiency of factor IX (i.e., Christmas factor).

4. **Von Willebrand's disease** is a common bleeding disorder with an autosomal dominant or recessive inheritance pattern.

5. **DIC** always results from an underlying disease or condition, including:
   a. septicemia
   b. obstetric complications
   c. disseminated malignancies
   d. massive tissue injury (burns and trauma)
   e. hemolytic transfusion reaction
   f. shock
   g. anaphylaxis.

6. **Vascular disorders** may be localized or widespread and result from:
   a. vascular injury due to drug reactions, allergic disorders, collagen-vascular diseases, and bacterial infections
   b. alteration in the connective tissue framework supporting blood vessels due to vitamin C deficiency, adrenocortical hormone, and senile purpura.

7. **Other causes of coagulation defects**
   a. **Warfarin drug toxicity** can interfere with the synthesis of vitamin K-dependent coagulation factors by the liver. Excessive doses or administration with other medication that interfere with metabolism can produce prothrombin deficiency.
   b. **Heparin administration** can interfere with thrombin-induced conversion of fibrinogen to fibrin.
   c. **Clotting factor deficiencies** can result from impaired synthesis by the liver.
   d. **Massive transfusion** may create a dilutional clotting factor deficiency, unless all coagulation factors included in blood components are transfused.

C. Pathophysiology

1. **Bleeding disorders** can result from defects in vessels, platelets, coagulation factors, or the fibrinolytic system. When tissue repair of the vessel endothelium has occurred, the fibrin clot is lysed or dissolved by the fibrinolytic system, a plasma protein system.

  a. **Thrombocytopenia** is marked by a deficient number of circulating platelets. Because platelets play a vital role in coagulation, thrombocytopenia poses a serious threat to hemostasis.

  b. **ITP** involves immune destruction of platelets and production of antiplatelet antibodies, which markedly shorten platelet life span.

  c. **Clotting factor defects** involve a deficiency of one of the factors necessary for coagulation of the blood. This characteristically manifests with large, spreading bruises and bleeding into muscles and joints with even minor trauma. Recurrent joint hemorrhages can result in such severe damage that chronic pain or ankylosis (i.e., fixation) of the joint occurs. The risk of bleeding correlates with coagulation factor assay results in:

  - severe bleeding diathesis (i.e., high risk of spontaneous bleeding), with 5% or less of circulating factor VIII or IX
  - moderate bleeding diathesis (i.e., minimal to moderate risk of spontaneous bleeding but high risk of profuse bleeding with surgery or trauma), with 5% to 25% circulating factor VIII or IX
  - mild bleeding diathesis (i.e., rare spontaneous bleeding, abnormal bleeding with surgery or trauma), with 25% to 40% circulating factor VIII or IX.

  d. **Von Willebrand's disease** is characterized by mild deficiency of factor VIII (15% to 50% of normal), producing impaired platelet function. This results in such manifestations as nosebleeds, menorrhagia, prolonged bleeding from cuts, and postoperative bleeding. Massive soft tissue and joint hemorrhages are absent.

  e. **DIC** is characterized by widespread clotting in microcirculation, leading to consumption of coagulation factors and platelets and ultimately resulting in bleeding. Bleeding can range from minimal occult internal bleeding to profuse hemorrhaging from all orifices. The clinical picture is a complex combination of thrombosis and bleeding. Acute renal failure may result from fibrin deposition in the renal microcirculation.

  f. **Vascular disorders** are spontaneous ruptures of small vessels that are injured, resulting in blood leaking into the skin and mucous membranes; the smallest hemorrhages are called petechiae, and larger lesions are called ecchymoses or bruises.

  2. **Internal hemorrhaging** is a complication of bleeding disorders that may result in massive blood loss leading to hypovolemic shock, which necessitates immediate emergency intervention.

D. Assessment findings

  1. **Clinical manifestations.** Signs and symptoms of bleeding disorders vary with the particular defect. (See *Table 18-3,* page 514.)

  a. **Platelet defects,** such as thrombocytopenia and ITP, usually produce:
  - petechiae
  - easy bruising
  - bleeding that generally stops with local pressure and does not recur when pressure is released.

  b. **Coagulation factor defects,** such as clotting factor defects (hemophilia) and von Willebrand's disease, usually manifest with:
  - deep tissue bleeding after minor trauma, such as I.M. hematomas and hemarthroses (i.e., bleeding into joint spaces)
  - usually, no petechiae or superficial hemorrhages
  - recurrence of external bleeding several hours after pressure is removed.

TABLE 18-3

Clinical distinction among blood vessel, platelet, and coagulation disorders

Findings	Disorders of coagulation	Disorders of platelets or vessels ("purpuric disorders")
Bleeding from superficial cuts and scratches	Minimal	Persistent, often profuse
Deep dissecting hematomas	Characteristic	Rare
Delayed bleeding	Common	Rare
Hemarthrosis	Characteristic	Rare
Petechiae	Rare	Characteristic
Positive family history	Common	Rare
Sex of patient	80% to 90% of hereditary forms occur only in males	Relatively more common in females
Superficial ecchymoses	Common, usually large and solitary	Characteristic, usually small and multiple

     c. **DIC**
- Bleeding from mucous membranes and venipuncture sites
- Bleeding from GI and urinary tracts
- Bleeding from all orifices, ranging from minimal bleeding to profuse hemorrhaging

     d. **Vascular abnormalities** usually manifest as local bleeding into the skin. Purpura refers to extravasation of blood into skin and mucous membranes.

     e. **Internal bleeding and hemorrhage,** potential complications of bleeding disorders, may have the following manifestations:
- abdominal, flank, or joint pain resulting from internal bleeding
- hypotension; tachycardia; chest pain; pallor; cool, clammy skin; tachypnea; or altered responsiveness resulting from internal bleeding associated with hypovolemia
- headache and altered neurologic signs and symptoms resulting from cerebral hemorrhage
- vision changes resulting from retinal hemorrhage
- dyspnea, respiratory distress, hemoptysis, cyanosis, or rales resulting from interstitial hemorrhage in lungs

  2. **Laboratory and diagnostic study findings**

     a. **Thrombocytopenia**
- Bone marrow biopsy reveals increased megakaryocytes (i.e., stem cells from which platelets come) when the cause of thrombocytopenia is platelet destruction.
- Platelet count is less than 20,000 cells/mm^3 (i.e., petechiae appear, nosebleeds), or the platelet count is less than 5,000 cells/mm^3 (i.e., fatal).

     b. **ITP**
- Platelet count is less than 20,000/mm^3.
- Bleeding time is prolonged.
- Bone marrow biopsy reveals abundant megakaryocytes.

  c. **Clotting factor defects**
  - Coagulation factor assay is abnormal.
  - Partial thromboplastin time (PTT) is prolonged.

  d. **Von Willebrand's disease**
  - Coagulation factor assay is abnormal.
  - Platelet count is normal.
  - Bleeding time is prolonged.
  - PTT is slightly prolonged.

  e. **DIC**
  - Platelet count is decreased.
  - Serum fibrinogen is decreased.
  - Prothrombin time and PTT are prolonged.
    Fibrin split product level is increased.
  - Peripheral smear reveals schistocytes (i.e., red cell fragments).

  f. **Vascular disorders**
  - Platelet count is usually normal.
  - Coagulation test results are usually normal.

E. Nursing management (See section II.D.)

  1. **Provide ongoing assessment.**
     a. Observe location of petechiae and ecchymoses (e.g., petechiae in the conjunctiva of the eye may be a clinical indication of spontaneous bleeding as opposed to petechiae over bony prominences or areas subjected to trauma).
     b. Note color of ecchymoses to distinguish between old and new bleeding (i.e., purple or purplish blue, fading to green, yellow, and brown with time).
     c. Observe for frank bleeding from any orifice, including the mouth (gums), nose, vagina, rectum, and urethra, and look for bleeding from suture lines and venous access sites.
     d. Test all drainage and excreta for occult blood (e.g., feces, urine, emesis, gastric drainage).
     e. Assess joints for edema, mobility limitation, and pain.
     f. Assess color and temperature of skin (e.g., pale, cool, clammy). Note tachypnea, hypotension, tachycardia, palpitations, altered responsiveness, or decreased urine output; these findings may indicate inadequate tissue oxygenation or decreased blood volume.
     g. Measure blood loss; weigh linens, bandages, and the like.
     h. Monitor for orthostatic changes in blood pressure and pulse.
  2. **Minimize invasive procedures.** Avoid injections, or if injection is essential, use small-gauge needles with Z-track technique, and apply firm pressure for up to 5 minutes.
  3. **Avoid increasing intracranial pressure.** Avoid Valsalva's maneuver in a client with a platelet count of less than 20,000/mm^3, which poses a risk of cerebral bleeding. Symptomatically treat cough, constipation, chills, nausea, and vomiting, and instruct the client to avoid strenuous activity, forceful nose blowing, and like actions to help avoid increasing intracranial pressure.
  4. **Intervene to control bleeding,** as indicated.
     a. For **thrombocytopenia,** administer prophylactic platelet transfusions, corticosteriods, or other immune modulation and hormonal control of menstrual periods. (See *Drug chart 18-1,* pages 499 and 500.)

   b. For **ITP,** administer corticosteroids and gamma globulin (see *Drug chart 18-1,* pages 499 and 500), and prepare the client for splenectomy or immunosuppression therapy (e.g., vincristine, cyclophosphamide, azathioprine).

   c. For **clotting factor defects,** administer appropriate replacement therapy (factor VIII or IX concentrates) to prevent or treat bleeding.

   d. For **von Willebrand's disease,** administer cryoprecipitate, which contains factor VIII, fibrinogen, and factor XIII.

   e. For **DIC,** provide transfusion of red cells, platelets, or cryoprecipitate. Administer I.V. heparin to slow the coagulation process.

   f. For **warfarin toxicity,** administer oral or parenteral vitamin K to correct the prothrombin deficiency. If urgent replacement is needed, provide transfusion of single-donor plasma or prothrombin complex concentrates.

   g. To correct **excess heparin dosage,** administer protamine sulfate.

   h. For **factor deficiencies** from liver disease, provide transfusion of fresh frozen plasma, fresh whole blood, or factor IX concentrate.

5. **Promote comfort** with analgesics, orthopedic devices, and a bed cradle as indicated.

6. **Promote client and family coping.** Provide psychological support to the client and his family. Assess their anxiety level and understanding of the disorder and its treatment. Encourage verbalization of questions and fears.

7. **Provide client and family teaching.**
   a. Instruct the client in general preventive measures, including:
      – using an electric razor
      – using a soft or sponge-tipped toothbrush
      – maintaining rigorous dental prophylaxis
      – avoiding contact sports
      – avoiding the use of rectal thermometers, suppositories, enemas, and vaginal tampons
      – warning the client to avoid alcohol and medication containing aspirin, which interfere with platelet function.

   b. **Provide information to facilitate the client's participation and control in the preventive and therapeutic regimens.** Emphasize safe physical activities along with realistic restrictions.

   c. **Provide information to assist the client and his family with the adjustment to the disease process,** including:
      – signs and symptoms in relation to disease pathophysiology
      – rationale for interventions
      – measures to prevent and control bleeding
      – rehabilitative measures (e.g., mobilization and physiotherapy subsequent to hemarthrosis)
      – genetic implications of the bleeding disorder, as appropriate.

   d. **Provide a referral** to the National Hemophilia Foundation. (See appendix A.) Refer the client and his family to counseling or support groups as indicated.

X. BLOOD TRANSFUSION THERAPY

A. Types of blood transfusion therapies

1. **Whole blood transfusion**
   a. One unit of whole blood consists of 450 ml of blood collected into 60 to 70 ml of preservative or anticoagulant. Whole blood stored for more than 6 hours does not pro-

vide a therapeutic platelet transfusion, nor does it contain therapeutic amounts of labile coagulation factors (i.e., factors V and VIII).

b. Generally, whole blood transfusion is indicated only for clients who need increased oxygen-carrying capacity and restored blood volume when there is no time to prepare or obtain needed, specific blood components.

2. **Blood component therapy** involves transfusion of a specific portion or fraction of blood lacking in a client. A summary of blood components is provided in *Table 18-4,* pages 518 and 519. Advantages of blood component therapy include:

   a. avoiding the risk of sensitizing the client to other blood components

   b. providing optimal therapeutic benefit while reducing the risk of volume overload

   c. increasing availability of needed blood products to larger a population.

B. **Resources for blood transfusions.** Whole blood or blood components may be obtained from donors or acquired through autologous transfusions, which avoid viral infections from another person's blood. Autologous transfusions may be collected preoperatively or intraoperatively.

   1. **Preoperative donations** are best collected 2 to 6 weeks before surgery. Iron supplements may be prescribed during this time.

   2. **Intraoperative donations** are salvaged from the operative site and reinfused into the client immediately.

   3. **Potential donors** must be in good health and are disqualified if any of the following is true:

      a. history of viral hepatitis

      b. history or evidence of drug abuse

      c. history or possible exposure to acquired immunodeficiency syndrome (AIDS)

      d. history of a blood transfusion or blood products in the last 6 months

      e. history of recent asthma, urticaria, or allergy to medications

      f. history of recent tattoos (risk of hepatitis)

      g. history of exposure to infectious disease within the last month

      h. any person younger than age 17 or older than age 65

      i. history of living in countries with mad cow disease.

C. **Complications of blood transfusion.** Various complications may result from blood transfusion therapy. Clinical manifestations of these complications vary depending on the precipitating factor. (See *Table 18-5,* page 520.)

   1. **Hemolytic transfusion reaction** is a life-threatening complication occurring from transfusion of donor blood that is incompatible with the recipient's blood.

      a. In a hemolytic transfusion reaction, antibodies in the recipient's plasma combine with antigens on donor erythrocytes, causing agglutination and hemolysis in circulation or in the reticuloendothelial system. Similarly, antibodies in donor plasma combine with antigen on the recipient's erythrocytes; however, complications from infusion of incompatible plasma are less severe than those associated with infusion of incompatible erythrocytes. The most rapid hemolysis occurs in ABO incompatibility; Rh incompatibility is usually less severe.

      b. A delayed hemolytic transfusion reaction occurs 1 to 2 weeks after transfusion; erythrocytes hemolyzed by antibodies are not detectable during crossmatch but are formed rapidly after transfusion. A delayed hemolytic transfusion reaction generally is not dangerous, but subsequent transfusions may be associated with acute hemolytic reaction.

TABLE 18-4
Summary of blood components

Component	Major indications	Action	Not indicated for
Whole blood	▪ Symptomatic anemia with large volume deficit	Restoration of oxygen-carrying capacity, restoration of blood volume	▪ Condition responsive to specific component ▪ Volume expansion
Red blood cells	▪ Symptomatic anemia	Restoration of oxygen-carrying capacity	▪ Pharmacologically treatable anemia ▪ Coagulation deficiency
Red blood cells, leukocytes removed	▪ Symptomatic anemia, febrile reactions from leukocyte antibodies	Restoration of oxygen-carrying capacity	▪ Pharmacologically treatable anemia ▪ Coagulation deficiency
Red blood cells, adenine-saline added	▪ Symptomatic anemia with volume deficit	Restoration of oxygen-carrying capacity	▪ Pharmacologically treatable anemia ▪ Coagulation deficiency
Fresh frozen plasma	▪ Deficit of labile and stable plasma coagulation factors and thymidine triphosphate	Source of labile and non-labile plasma factors	▪ Condition responsive to volume replacement
Liquid plasma and plasma	▪ Deficit of stable coagulation factors	Source of nonlabile factors	▪ Deficit or labile coagulation factors, or volume replacement
Cryoprecipitated antihemophilic factor	▪ Hemophilia A ▪ Von Willebrand's disease ▪ Hypofibrinogenemia ▪ Factor XIII deficiency	Provides factor VIII, fibrinogen, von Willebrand's factor, factor XIII	▪ Conditions not deficient in contained factors
Platelets; platelets, pheresis	▪ Bleeding from thrombocytopenia or platelet function abnormality	Improves hemostasis	▪ Plasma coagulation deficits and some conditions with rapid platelet destruction (e.g., idiopathic thrombocytopenic purpura)
Granulocytes	▪ Neutropenia with infection	Provides granulocytes	▪ Infection responsive to antibiotics

   c. In hemolytic reaction, the severity of complications correlates with the amount of incompatible blood transfused; chances of fatal reaction decrease if less than 100 ml of incompatible blood is infused.

2. Febrile, nonhemolytic transfusion reaction, the most common type of reaction, usually is caused by sensitivity to leukocyte or platelet antigens.

3. Septic reaction is a serious complication resulting from transfusion of a blood product contaminated with bacteria.

4. Allergic reactions may result from sensitivity to plasma protein or donor antibody, which reacts with recipient antigen.

Special precautions	Hazards	Rates of infusion
■ Must be ABO identical ■ Labile coagulation factors deteriorate within 24 hours after collection	Infectious diseases, septic/toxic, allergic, febrile reactions; circulatory overload; graft-versus-host disease (GVHD)	For massive loss, fast as client can tolerate; must be infused in less than 4 hours
■ Must be ABO compatible	Infectious diseases, septic/toxic, allergic, febrile reactions; GVHD	As patient can tolerate but less than 4 hours
■ Must be ABO compatible	Infectious diseases, septic/toxic, allergic reaction unless plasma also removed (e.g., by washing)	As patient can tolerate but less than 4 hours
■ Must be ABO compatible	Infectious diseases, septic/toxic, allergic, febrile reactions, circulatory overload	As patient can tolerate but less than 4 hours
■ Should be ABO compatible	Infectious diseases, allergic reactions, circulatory overload	Less than 4 hours
■ Should be ABO compatible	Infectious diseases, allergic reactions	Less than 4 hours
■ Frequent repeat doses may be necessary	Infectious diseases, allergic reactions	Less than 4 hours
■ Should not use some microaggregate filters (check manufacturer's instructions)	Infectious diseases; septic/toxic, allergic reactions	Less than 4 hours
■ Must be ABO compatible; do not use depth-type microaggregate filters	Infections diseases, allergic reactions, febrile reactions	One pheresis unit over 2 to 4 hour period — closely observe for reactions

Adapted with permission from: American Association of Blood Banks. *Circular of Information for the Use of Human Blood and Blood Components.* July 2002. Available at: www.aabb.org/All_About_Blood/COI/aabb_coi.htm.

5. **Circulatory overload** results from administration at a rate or volume greater than can be accommodated by the circulatory system, precipitating heart failure or pulmonary edema.

6. **Infectious diseases** can be transmitted through blood transfusion, although this is rare. Several infectious diseases that may be transmitted include:

   a. hepatitis B and hepatitis C

   b. malaria

   c. syphilis

   d. AIDS.

TABLE 18-5
Assessment findings in transfusion complications

Complication	Assessment findings
Hemolytic transfusion reaction	Fever, chills, low back pain, flank pain, headache, nausea, flushing, tachycardia, tachypnea, hypotension, hemoglobinuria (cola-colored urine)
Delayed hemolytic reaction	Fever, mild jaundice, gradual drop in hemoglobin level, positive Coombs' test
Febrile nonhemolytic reaction	Temperature rise during or soon after transfusion, chills, headache, flushing, anxiety
Allergic reaction	Hives, generalized pruritus, wheezing, anaphylaxis (rare)
Circulatory overload	Dyspnea, orthopnea, tachycardia, sudden anxiety, jugular vein distention, crackles in base of lungs, rise in central venous pressure
Infectious disease transmission	Rapid or insidious onset of symptoms, depending on specific disease
Graft-versus-host disease	Skin changes (reddening, ulcerations), edema, hair loss, hemolytic anemia, positive Coombs' test result
Massive transfusion	Vary according to specific condition

7. **Graft-versus-host (GVH) disease** results from engraftment of immunocompetent lymphocytes in the bone marrow of immunosuppressed recipients, which triggers an immune response of the graft against the host.

8. **Reactions associated with massive transfusions** (>10 units of packed red blood cells [RBCs] in 1 to 6 hours) include:

    a. **hypocalcemia,** resulting from binding of recipient's circulating calcium to anticoagulant (i.e., citrate) in packed RBCs

    b. **citrate intoxication** due to accumulation of citrate

    c. **hyperkalemia** because stored RBCs progressively increase extracellular potassium concentration

    d. **exacerbation of liver disease** due to increased ammonia levels in stored blood

    e. **hypothermia,** in which transfusion of cold blood (< 98.6° F [37° C]) at rates higher than 100 ml/minute may produce arrhythmias and cardiac arrest.

9. **Aggregates of leukocytes and platelets in the lungs** result from accumulation of the aggregates during blood storage.

10. **Hemorrhage** results from excessive dilution of the recipient's platelets and clotting factors.

D. **Nursing management**

1. **Help prevent transfusion reaction.**

    🖐 *a.* Meticulously verify client identification, beginning with type and crossmatch sample collection and labeling to double-check blood product before the transfusion. Verify information with licensed personnel only.

    b. Inspect the blood product for gas bubbles, clotting, or abnormal color before administration.

    c. Begin transfusion slowly (10 drops/minute) and observe the client closely, particularly during the first 15 minutes. Severe reactions usually manifest within 15 minutes after the start of transfusion. Take vital signs every 5 minutes for the first 15 minutes.

d. Transfuse blood within 4 hours (usually over 2 hours if no signs of fluid overload), changing tubing (Y-tubing) every 2 units to minimize the risk of bacterial growth at warm room temperatures.

e. Prevent infectious disease transmission through careful donor screening or performing pretests available to identify selected infectious agents.

f. Prevent graft-versus-host disease (GVHD) by ensuring irradiation of blood products containing viable white blood cells (i.e., whole blood, platelets, packed red blood cells [RBCs], and granulocytes) before transfusion; irradiation alters the ability of donor lymphocytes to engraft and divide.

g. Prevent hypothermia by warming blood unit to 98.6° F (37° C) before transfusion.

h. Remove leukocyte and platelet aggregates from donor blood by installing a microaggregate filter (20- or 40-mm pore size) in the blood line to remove these aggregates during transfusion.

2. **Take action after detecting any signs or symptoms of reaction.**

a. Stop the transfusion immediately, and notify the health care provider.

b. Disconnect the transfusion set, but keep the I.V. line open with 0.9% saline solution to provide access for possible I.V. drug infusion.

c. Send the blood bag and tubing to the blood bank for repeat typing and culture.

d. Draw another blood sample for plasma hemoglobin, culture, and retyping.

e. Collect a urine sample as soon as possible for hemoglobin determination.

3. **Address symptoms of the specific reaction.**

a. Manage **hemolytic reaction** by correcting hypotension, disseminated intravascular coagulation (DIC), and renal failure associated with RBC hemolysis and hemoglobinuria.

b. Treat **febrile, nonhemolytic transfusion** reactions symptomatically with prescribed antipyretics. (See *Drug chart 18-1,* pages 499 and 500.) Provide leukocyte-poor blood products for subsequent transfusions.

c. Manage **septic reaction** with antibiotics, steroids, and vasopressors (see *Drug chart 18-1,* pages 499 and 500) and increased hydration as prescribed.

d. Manage **allergic reaction** by administering histamine-1-receptor antagonist (antihistamines), steroids, and epinephrine as indicated by the severity of the reaction. (See *Drug chart 18-1,* pages 499 and 500.) If hives are the only manifestation, transfusion can sometimes continue, but at a slower rate.

e. Manage **circulatory overload** initially by positioning the client upright with feet dependent, discontinuing blood, and providing prescribed diuretics, oxygen, and aminophylline.

f. Manage **infectious diseases** by treating the acquired disease. Notify the blood bank of tainted blood, which warrants further investigation of blood. Interventions are aimed at prevention by safe screening of all potential donors.

g. Manage **GVHD** by supporting nursing and medical interventions aimed at such signs and symptoms as high fever, skin rash, nausea, vomiting, and diarrhea.

h. Manage **massive transfusions** by supportive nursing and medical interventions, such as monitoring serum calcium, potassium, and liver function tests; monitoring for and treating circulatory overload; and aiming treatment at the client's signs and symptoms.

Study questions

1. Which assessment data would the nurse identify as the *most* characteristic sign of thrombocytopenia?
1. Petechiae
2. Hemostasis
3. Melena
4. Hemarthrosis

2. Which blood component would the nurse expect to administer to therapeutically provide all of the coagulation factors?
1. Cryoprecipitate
2. Random donor platelets
3. Fresh frozen plasma
4. Stored whole blood

3. Which clinical sign would suggest anemia secondary to vitamin B_{12} deficiency rather than folic acid deficiency?
1. Smooth, sore tongue
2. Palpitations
3. Paresthesias
4. Dizziness

4. Which nursing intervention should be implemented when caring for a client diagnosed with idiopathic thrombocytopenic purpura whose complete blood count (CBC) reveals a white blood cell count of 5,000 cells/mm³, hemoglobin concentration of 12.9 g/dl, and platelet count of 7,000/mm³?
1. Coughing and deep breathing every 4 hours to prevent infection
2. Platelet transfusions to maintain platelet count above 20,000/mm³
3. Aspirin as needed to control temperature or chills
4. Stool softeners as needed to prevent constipation

5. Which instruction would be included in a client teaching plan about self-management of fatigue associated with anemia?
1. "Continue bed rest to conserve energy."
2. "Participate in all usual activities of daily living."

3. "Follow a progressive ambulatory program."
4. "Exercise to increase cardiopulmonary function."

6. Which statement by the client indicates the need for additional instruction about prescribed ferrous sulfate therapy?
1. "I take my iron supplements with food to enhance their absorption."
2. "I know that the gastrointestinal side effects that I'm experiencing are common."
3. "I eat organ meats weekly because they are a good dietary source of iron."
4. "I take vitamin C tablets to enhance iron absorption."

7. The client receiving a unit of packed red blood cells has these baseline vital signs: temperature of 98° F (36.7° C), blood pressure of 136/72 mm Hg, pulse rate of 100, and respiratory rate of 22. Fifteen minutes later, the client's temperature is 101° F (38.3° C), blood pressure is 140/76 mm Hg, pulse is 104, and respiratory rate is 24. Which intervention should the nurse implement *first*?
1. Continuing the transfusion, monitoring every 15 minutes for further findings
2. Stopping the transfusion immediately, and notifying the health care provider
3. Continuing the transfusion, and administering aspirin for the client's fever
4. Slowing the rate of transfusion, and continuing to monitor the client

8. Which action by the parents indicates ineffective adjustment to their infant son's diagnosis of hemophilia?
1. Requesting family planning and counseling information
2. Demonstrating I.V. administration of factor VIII
3. Verbalizing feelings about shame and guilt

4. Discouraging the child's participation in sports

9. Which sign and symptom would lead the nurse to suspect that the client who is receiving a blood transfusion was experiencing circulatory overload?
1. Anxiety and complaints of shortness of breath
2. Fever and complaints of low back pain
3. Red splotches on the face with complaints of itching
4. Complaints of severe abdominal pain and dark urine

10. Which clinical manifestations support the client's diagnosis of Hodgkin's disease?
1. Palpable lymph nodes, fatigue, and weight loss
2. Petechiae, easy bruising, and stoppage of bleeding with pressure
3. Pallor, headache, and tachycardia
4. Severe abdominal pain, increased jaundice, and dark urine

11. Which nursing intervention should be included in the care plan for a client experiencing a sickle cell crisis?
1. Administering vitamin B_{12} I.V.
2. Applying cold compresses to joints
3. Encouraging active range-of-motion exercises
4. Administering round-the-clock analgesics

12. Which assessment finding indicates a positive response to heparin therapy in the client diagnosed with disseminated intravascular coagulation?
1. Increased platelet count
2. Increased fibrinogen
3. Decreased fibrin split products
4. Reduced bleeding

13. Which nursing intervention would be included in the care plan for the client diagnosed with a bleeding disorder?

1. Administering enteric-coated aspirin
2. Inspecting for petechiae and ecchymoses
3. Assessing for jugular vein distention (JVD)
4. Administering ferrous sulfate daily

14. Which interventions should the nurse implement when administering the first unit of packed red blood cells to a client? (*Select all that apply.*)
1. Taking the client's vital signs every 30 minutes after starting the transfusion
2. Meticulously verifying the client's identification blood transfusion band with the unit of blood
3. Beginning the transfusion rate at 125/ml an hour so that the blood can infuse in two hours.
4. Administering the unit of blood via Y-tubing with 250 ml of dextrose 5% in water (D_5W)
5. Completing the pretransfusion assessment prior to obtaining the blood from the laboratory
6. Ensuring that an 18-gauge needle is patent prior to starting the blood transfusion

15. Which statement by the client indicates a successful teaching plan about the disease process for the client diagnosed with pernicious anemia?
1. "I should eat lots of iron-rich foods and take my iron supplement."
2. "The nurse has to give my folic-acid injection by the Z-track method."
3. "I will have to take vitamin B_{12} replacement therapy for the rest of my life."
4. "When my hemoglobin returns to normal, I can stop my folic acid."

16. Which type of leukemia would the nurse expect to find most commonly in a child?
1. Acute myelogenous leukemia (AML)
2. Acute lymphocytic leukemia (ALL)
3. Chronic myelogenous leukemia (CML)
4. Chronic lymphocytic leukemia (CLL)

Answer key

1. The answer is **1.**
Petechiae are characteristic of quantitative or qualitative platelet defects, because platelets are primarily responsible for cessation of bleeding in small vessels. Although hemostasis and melena may occur with thrombocytopenia, they are not the most characteristic. Hemarthrosis is characteristic of coagulation-factor deficiencies.

2. The answer is **3.**
Fresh frozen plasma contains all the coagulation factors, including the labile factors. Cryoprecipitate contains factor VIII, fibrinogen, and factor XIII. Random donor platelets contain large amounts of platelets in a minimum (nontherapeutic) amount of plasma. Stored whole blood does not include the labile coagulation factors.

3. The answer is **3.**
Vitamin B_{12} is essential for nervous system function. Neurologic manifestations of B_{12} deficiency, such as paresthesias, are not seen with folic acid deficiency. A smooth, sore tongue may be seen with B_{12} or folic acid deficiency. Palpitations and dizziness are general manifestations of anemia and can be observed with either deficiency.

4. The answer is **4.**
Based on the client's CBC results, the platelet count is severely decreased. The client is at risk of spontaneous bleeding. Preventing constipation decreases the risk of intracerebral bleeding secondary to increased intracranial pressure with Valsalva's maneuver. Coughing increases intracranial pressure and should be avoided. Platelets are not transfused prophylactically in clients with idiopathic thrombocytopenic purpura because the cells are destroyed, producing little therapeutic benefit. Aspirin is contraindicated in bleeding disorders because it interferes with platelet function. Nonaspirin antipyretics should be used instead.

5. The answer is **3.**
The client should gradually increase activity and subsequently promote endurance by alternating periods of rest with periods of activity to conserve energy. Immobility is associated with muscle wasting and hypotension. The client should participate in the usual activities of daily living as tolerated, with activities causing undue fatigue replanned or deferred. Care should be directed toward decreasing activities that necessitate increased cardiac output, such as exercise until the anemia improves.

6. The answer is **1.**
Adequate iron absorption requires an acidic environment. Supplements should be taken between meals or after a meal if severe GI upset occurs. Various GI adverse effects, such as nausea, heartburn, and abdominal cramping, are common with iron therapy. Organ meats are one of the best food sources of iron. Vitamin C, an acid, enhances iron absorption and is included in several iron preparations.

7. The answer is **2.**
Temperature elevation may indicate a hemolytic transfusion reaction. The transfusion must be stopped, and the health care provider and blood bank must be notified. Whenever there is a possibility or suspicion of a hemolytic transfusion reaction, the transfusion must be stopped immediately. Antipyretics may be administered after a health care provider's order only if the medical diagnosis is febrile, nonhemolytic transfusion reaction. Continuing the transfusion or slowing the rate is inappropriate, because

the transfusion must be stopped to enable the health care provider to rule out hemolytic or nonhemolytic transfusion reaction (due to leukocyte or platelet antigens).

8. The answer is **4.**
For the child with hemophilia, contact sports should be avoided. However, noncontact sports such as swimming are acceptable activities and can contribute to the child's independence and self-esteem. Preventing the child from engaging in safe physical activity may indicate overprotective behavior. Seeking information about family planning and counseling is a positive coping strategy, indicating an understanding of the genetic implications of the disease. Demonstrating the I.V. administration technique provides evidence of the parent's interest and participation in the therapeutic regimen, which is essential in adjusting to illness. Guilt is a common parental reaction to genetically based illnesses. Verbalizing identified feelings facilitates coping.

9. The answer is **1.**
Signs of circulatory overload include dyspnea, orthopnea, tachycardia, or sudden anxiety and jugular vein distention, crackles in lung bases, and a rise in central venous pressure. Fever and complaints of low back pain are associated with a hemolytic transfusion reaction. Red splotches on the face with itching indicate an allergic reaction. Complaints of severe abdominal pain and dark urine are associated with sickle cell crisis.

10. The answer is **1.**
Hodgkin's disease usually shows a predictable pattern of spread through lymphatic channels to nodes and results in palpable lymph nodes, fatigue, and weight loss. Petechiae, easy bruising, and stoppage of bleeding with pressure support the diagnosis of thrombocytopenia. Pallor, headache, and tachycardia are associated with anemia. Severe abdominal pain, increased jaundice, and dark urine

are associated with sickle cell crisis.

11. The answer is **4.**
The client in sickle cell crisis is in severe pain. A round-the-clock schedule for analgesic medications can help keep pain at a tolerable level and decrease anxiety about needing, asking for, or receiving pain medication. Increasing fluid intake can dilute the blood and reverse sludging of cells. Vitamin B_{12} is administered to persons with megaloblastic anemia. Cold compresses cause vasoconstriction, which increases pain. During the crisis, the client needs rest and support of the affected joints. Exercise increases pain.

12. The answer is **2.**
Effective heparin therapy should stop the process of intravascular coagulation, which should result in increased fibrinogen. Heparin has no effect on the platelet count or fibrin split products. Bleeding should cease due to the increased availability of platelets and coagulation factors.

13. The answer is **2.**
Bleeding disorders involve impaired hemostasis. The nurse would inspect the client for petechiae and ecchymoses. Petechiae are pinpoint hemorrhages on the skin or mucous membranes that occur with quantitative or qualitative platelet disorders; ecchymoses are bluish-black maculae resulting from seepage of blood into skin or mucous membranes, usually after trauma. Aspirin is contraindicated in clients with bleeding disorders. JVD is a sign of fluid volume overload, not a bleeding disorder. Iron (ferrous sulfate) is used to treat anemias, not bleeding disorders.

14. The answers are **2, 5, 6.**
The nurse must verify that the correct unit of blood is being administered to the correct client, the pretransfusion assessment should be completed because the unit of blood must be hung within 20 to 30 minutes after taking it from the laboratory, and an 18-gauge nee-

dle (20-gauge needle, if necessary) must be patent prior to starting the blood transfusion. The unit of blood should be infused slowly (20 gtt/min) at first. Vital signs should be taken every 5 minutes to detect a possible blood transfusion reaction. The blood is administered via Y-tubing with normal saline only; D_5W will cause lysis of the blood.

15. The answer is **3.**

Vitamin B_{12} and folic acid are essential for normal deoxyribonucleic acid synthesis and hematopoiesis; therefore, the client must take replacement therapy for life. Eating iron-rich foods and using an iron supplement is ap-

propriate for iron deficiency anemia. Iron dextran must be given with the Z-track technique. Stopping folic acid when hemoglobin returns to normal is appropriate for folic acid deficiency anemia.

16. The answer is **2.**

ALL is the most common type of leukemia in children. It accounts for approximately 85% of all leukemia cases and 90% of leukemias in children. AML is most common in adults; incidence increases with age. CML is uncommon before age 20; incidence rises with age. CLL is the most common type of leukemia in persons age 50 and older.

19

Infectious disorders

I. ESSENTIAL CONCEPTS OF INFECTIOUS DISORDERS

A. Pathogenesis of infectious disorders

1. **Types of infectious agents,** which are organisms capable of causing disease, include:
   a. bacteria
   b. viruses
   c. rickettsiae
   d. protozoa
   e. fungi
   f. helminths.

2. **Types of infections**
   a. **Communicable diseases** are infectious diseases that can be transmitted from an infected person, animal, or object to an uninfected person.
   b. **Nosocomial infections** are infections acquired within a health care facility.
   c. **Opportunistic infections** are infections that occur in immunocompromised hosts (e.g., elderly persons, organ-transplant recipients) by microbes that rarely cause infection in hosts with healthy immune systems or organisms that normally inhibit homeostasis (i.e., normal flora).

3. **A reservoir** is any person, plant, animal, substance, or location that provides nourishment for a microorganism and enables further dispersal of the organism. The most common reservoirs of infection include:
   a. urinary tract
   b. surgical wounds
   c. respiratory tract.

4. **Modes of transmission**
   a. Contact (e.g., sexually transmitted diseases [STDs])
   b. Common source of transmission (e.g., shared foods or drinks)
   c. Airborne (e.g., droplet nuclei resulting in tuberculosis, histoplasmosis)
   d. Vector borne (e.g., mosquitoes carrying malaria)

5. **Portals of entry**
   a. **Skin.** Infectious organisms burrow into the skin (e.g., hookworm larvae), are injected by insect bite (e.g., malaria), or enter the host through a break in skin integrity (e.g., surgical wound, pressure sore).
   b. **GI tract.** Typically, contaminated foods and drinks (e.g., food with cholera) carry infectious organisms through the GI tract.
   c. **Respiratory tract.** Airborne droplet nuclei (e.g., tuberculosis, influenza) enter the host through the respiratory tract.
   d. **Genitourinary tract.** STDs and sometimes contamination from the GI tract infect the host by way of the genitourinary tract.
   e. **Placenta.** Although the placenta is rarely a portal, syphilis spirochete can pass through.
   f. **Blood.** Invasive procedures (e.g., venipuncture) or insect bites can transport infectious organisms through the blood.

6. **Portals of exit**
   a. Routes by which infectious agents leave the host body include the skin, GI tract, respiratory tract, genitourinary tract, placenta, and blood.

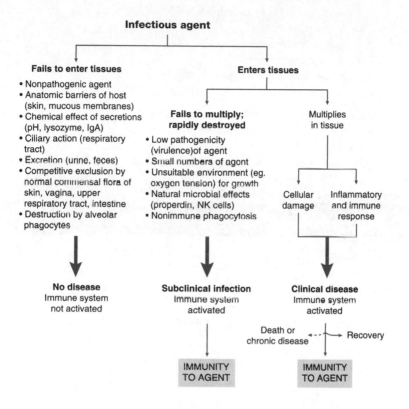

FIGURE 19-1
Possible results of an encounter with an infectious agent

Adapted with permission from Chandrasoma, P., and Taylor, C.R. *Concise Pathology*, 3rd ed. Stamford, Conn.: Appleton & Lange, 1998.

b. Identifying the portal of exit for a specific microorganism guides interventions to prevent disease transmission (e.g., wearing gown and gloves when bathing, changing bed linen for a client with hepatitis A because the virus leaves the host by way of the feces).

7. **Severity** depends on organism factors (e.g., virulence) and host factors (e.g., susceptibility, amount of exposure). (See *Figure 19-1*.)

   a. **Virulence** refers to an organism's degree of pathogenicity (i.e., ability to cause disease). Not all infections (i.e., presence of organisms within a host) cause a pathologic process or disease. Opportunistic pathogens are less virulent and only cause disease when the host's defense mechanisms are impaired.

   b. Factors that increase a host's **susceptibility to infection** include:
   - damaged or inadequate defense mechanisms
   - debilitation and stress (e.g., hospitalized clients)

- invasive procedures that provide a route of access for microorganisms (e.g., urinary catheterization)
- therapies that cause immunosuppression (e.g., corticosteroids, chemotherapy).

c. **Exposure** can result in one of four conditions:
- exposure with no infection
- subclinical infection
- disease limited by host responses (resolves without treatment)
- severe disease requiring treatment.

B. **Trends in infectious disorders.** Deaths from infectious disorders have declined greatly in industrialized nations. However, infectious disorders continue to be a major cause of death in developing countries. Infectious disorders, such as acquired immunodeficiency syndrome, hepatitis B, and tuberculosis, plague industrialized and developing nations.

NURSING PROCESS OVERVIEW

 ## II. INFECTIOUS DISORDERS

A. **Assessment**
1. **Health history**
   a. **Explore the client's health history** for risk factors associated with infectious disorders, including:
   - exposure to person with known or possible infectious disease
   - travel to places where certain infections are endemic
   - unsafe sexual practices
   - noncompliance with recommended immunizations
   - conditions that may compromise defenses (e.g., cancer, diabetes mellitus, chemotherapy, corticosteroid therapy).
   b. **Elicit a description of the client's present illness and chief complaint,** including onset, course, duration, location, and precipitating and alleviating factors. Cardinal signs and symptoms indicating an infectious process include:
   - systemic symptoms, such as fever and chills, dysuria, arthralgias, myalgias, generalized weakness, and anorexia
   - signs and symptoms of local infection, such as redness, edema, pain, and warmth.
2. **Physical examination**
   a. **Inspection**
   - Inspect lesions on the skin or mucous membranes.
   - Assess the skin for rashes or reddened areas.
   - Assess any abnormal drainage from open lesions or body orifices.
   - Assess sputum for color, consistency, and odor.
   - Assess core temperature and skin temperature.
   b. **Palpation.** Palpate lymph nodes for enlargement.
   c. **Auscultation**
   - Auscultate lung sounds.
   - Auscultate blood pressure.
   - Auscultate heart sounds.
3. **Laboratory and diagnostic studies**
   a. **Microbiologic specimens**—including urine, blood, sputum, wound exudate, feces, and mucous-membrane secretions—are used to identify causative organisms.

    b. **White blood cell (WBC) count** determines presence of infection; the WBC count is elevated in infection.

    c. **Serologic studies** detect presence of antigens or antibodies to specific diseases.

    d. **Tuberculin skin test** reveals individuals exposed to tuberculosis.

    e. **Chest X-ray** is used to evaluate suspected pulmonary disease and to follow progress of the disease.

    f. **Culture and sensitivity tests** identify causative organisms.

B. Nursing diagnoses

1. Risk for imbalanced body temperature
2. Impaired gas exchange
3. Excess or deficient fluid volume
4. Acute pain
5. Impaired skin integrity
6. Social isolation
7. Activity intolerance
8. Deficient knowledge

C. Planning and outcome identification.
The major goals for a client diagnosed with an infectious disease include prevention of spread of infection, maintenance of normothermia, improved breathing patterns, maintenance of adequate fluid volume status, absence of pain, skin integrity, improved social interaction and activity tolerance, and knowledge about the infection and its treatment.

D. Implementation

1. **Carefully implement measures to treat infection, minimize risk for further infection, and prevent the spread of infection.**

    a. Administer prescribed medications, which may include opioid or nonopioid analgesics, antipyretics, antibiotics, aerosol treatments, and topical ointments. (See *Drug chart 19-1,* pages 532 and 533.)

    b. Implement measures to prevent the spread of infection in health care facilities and the community. (See *Box 19-1,* page 534. See also *Box 19-2,* page 535.)

2. **Reduce elevated body temperature.**

    a. Assess vital signs frequently to monitor the pattern and severity of febrile episodes.

    b. Keep in mind that not every infection is accompanied by fever and, conversely, that fever does not always indicate infection. In some clients, fever may be an adaptive response; antipyretic measures are not always indicated.

    c. In cases where antipyretic measures are indicated, provide appropriate interventions.
- Sponge the client's body with tepid water; avoid cold water or direct application of ice.
- Remove heavy or restrictive garments and excess bed linens.
- Apply cool compresses to areas of increased blood supply (i.e., axilla, groin, and face).
- Use a hypothermia blanket if indicated.

    d. Encourage increased fluid intake to replace losses from sweating.

    e. Promote rest and comfort.

3. **Improve gas exchange.**

    a. Assess for signs and symptoms of impaired gas exchange:
- dyspnea
- increased respiratory rate and depth
- signs of hypoxia and hypercapnia

DRUG CHART 19-1
Infectious disorder medications

Classifications	Indications	Selected interventions
Antibiotics aminoglycosides (gentam- icin, tobramycin) amoxicillin carbenicillin cefazolin chloramphenicol erythromycin nafcillin penicillin tetracycline	Prevent or treat infections caused by pathogenic microorganisms	■ Before administering the first dose, assess the client for allergies and determine whether culture has been obtained. ■ After multiple doses, assess the client for super-infection (thrush, yeast infection, diarrhea); notify the health care provider if these occur. ■ Assess the insertion site for phlebitis if antibiotics are being administered I.V. ■ To assess the effectiveness of antibiotic therapy, monitor white blood cell count. ■ Monitor peaks and troughs for aminoglycosides. ■ Instruct the client to not eat or drink dairy products when taking tetracycline. ■ Intruct the client to notify his health care provider if bleeding, sore throat, oral mucosal lesions, or pallor occurs (bone marrow depression) when taking chloramphenicol. ■ When administering topical ointments, clean the area with warm water and dry thoroughly before applying, and wash hands before and after application.
Antifungal medications amphotericin B	Treat systemic fungal infections or superficial fungal infections	■ Monitor I.V. administration closely. ■ Be alert for signs and symptoms of renal damage. ■ Monitor the client's potassium, calcium, magnesium, and liver enzyme levels regularly.
ketoconazole	Treat systemic fungal infections or deep organ candidiasis	■ Teach the client who is taking oral medication to clean his mouth before taking the medication and to swish and swallow.
miconazole nystatin	Treat superficial candidiasis	■ Instruct the client to wash her hands before and after applying vaginal medication. ■ Tell the client to continue the medication as prescribed to prevent infection (usually for 1 to 2 weeks after symptoms subside).
Antihelmintic drugs	Fight against helminths; helminthiasis (worm infestation) occurs frequently in intestines but can occur in liver, blood, and lymphatics	■ Instruct the client that the tablet form may be chewed, swallowed whole, or crushed and mixed with food. ■ Instruct the client to take medications with milk, fruit juice, or food. ■ Instruct the client that the entire prescribed dose should be taken at one time.
mebendazole	Deplete the glycogen that the parasites need for survival	
pyrantel	Paralyze the worms	
Antipruritic diphenhydramine	Prevent initiation and transmission of nerve impulses, thereby decreasing itching	■ Advise the client that drowsiness may occur initially but usually subsides with continued use.

DRUG CHART 19-1
Infectious disorder medications (continued)

Classifications	Indications	Selected interventions
Antipyretic acetaminophen aspirin	Act on the thermoregulatory center of the brain to produce diaphoresis and vasodilation	■ Do not give aspirin to children because of its association with Reye's syndrome. ■ Watch for GI distress and possible bleeding from aspirin. ■ Report tinnitus (ringing in ears), a sign of aspirin toxicity.
Antituberculin agents ethambutol	Act against tubercle bacilli that are resistant to isoniazid and rifampin	■ Medications are administered alone or in combination for a 9- to 18-month course ■ Instruct the client to notify the health care provider if changes in visual acuity, perception, and color interpretation occur (signs of optic neuritis).
isoniazid	Treat tuberculosis by inhibiting bacterial wall synthesis	■ Instruct the client to take the medication on an empty stomach. ■ Instruct the client to notify the health care provider if tingling, numbness, or pain of the hands and feet occur (sign of peripheral neuropathy).
rifampin	Inhibit RNA synthesis; always administered with other antitubercular agents; a broad-spectrum antibiotic	■ Inform the client that urine, feces, sputum, tears, and sweat will turn red-orange. ■ Instruct the client to notify the health care provider if jaundice, anorexia, malaise, fatigue, or nausea occur (signs of hepatotoxicity).
streptomycin	Treat suspected resistant or severe tuberculosis	■ Explain to the client that I.M. injection two to three times each week will be prescribed. ■ Be aware of injury to the eighth cranial nerve (hearing loss and disturbance in balance) and nephrotoxicity. ■ Monitor peak and trough levels.
Antiviral drug amantadine (Symmetrel)	Suppress viral growth (exact mechanism not clearly understood); also used for prophylaxis and treatment of infections caused by influenza type A	■ Instruct the client on how to prevent orthostatic hypotension. ■ Instruct the client to notify the health care provider if shortness of breath and edema in extremities occur.
Vasopressors metaraminol norepinephrine	Rapidly restore blood pressure in anaphylaxis by producing vasoconstriction and heart stimulation	■ Monitor the client's vital signs, intake and output, mental status, peripheral pulses, and skin color. ■ The Client should be on telemetry and monitored continuously.

- restlessness, confusion, and somnolence
- decreased lung sounds, rales, rhonchi, and expiratory wheezes.
b. Administer oxygen therapy for hypoxia; monitor with pulse oximeter.
c. Reposition the client to increase lung expansion, perfusion, and ventilation.
d. Encourage good pulmonary hygiene, including:
- coughing and deep-breathing exercises
- diaphragmatic breathing
- cessation of smoking and a smoke-free environment.

BOX 19-1

Interventions to prevent infectious disorders in health care facilities (nosocomial infections)

- **Reduce host susceptibility.**
  - Improve host nutritional and fluid status.
  - Administer prescribed medical therapy to treat immunodeficiencies.
  - Teach the client about the importance of immunizations and about immunization methods.
  - Prevent damage to host defenses (e.g., avoid invasive procedures when possible).
- **Prevent urinary tract infections.**
  - Avoid urinary catheterization when possible.
  - Use aseptic technique during catheterization.
  - Maintain asepsis of urinary drainage systems.
  - Remove urinary catheters as soon as possible, and avoid irrigating catheters.
- **Prevent surgical wound infections.**
  - Maintain asepsis intraoperatively.
  - Use aseptic technique during dressing changes.
  - Avoid preoperative hair removal when possible; if hair removal is necessary, use clippers or depilatories instead of razors, and remove hair immediately before surgery.
  - Limit personnel movement into and out of the operating room during surgical procedures. Change dressings over closed wounds only when wet or if signs and symptoms of infection develop.
- **Prevent respiratory tract infections.**
  - Use only properly disinfected and sterilized respiratory equipment.
  - Perform respiratory therapies (e.g., tracheal suctioning) using aseptic technique.
  - Assist the client in maintaining respiratory hygiene through deep breathing and coughing exercises.
- **Prevent bacteremias.**
  - Limit invasive procedures when possible.
  - Maintain aseptic technique during invasive procedures.
  - Change I.V. and intraarterial fluids and tubing at recommended intervals.
  - Assess I.V. catheter sites for signs of infection.
  - Alternate I.V. catheter sites at recommended intervals.
  - Prevent and treat infections at other body sites; microbes from other sites can gain access to vasculature.
- **Practice proper handwashing procedures.**
  - Thorough handwashing is the most important nursing action to decrease spread of infection. To wash hands: remove jewelry; use regular soap for routine client care; wash for 10 to 15 seconds under briskly running water for routine client care; keep nails short, and always

scrub around and under them; and use an antimicrobial product to kill organisms when working with immunocompromised clients or before invasive procedures.
  - Be sure to wash hands after intense, prolonged client contact; before any invasive procedure; before and after caring for susceptible clients (e.g., neonates, elderly persons); before and after touching mucous membranes, body fluids, secretions, or excretions — even if gloves were worn; after contact with objects that likely are contaminated (e.g., urine measuring devices); before entering high-risk units (e.g., intensive care nursery); and between direct contacts with different clients.
  - Adhere to Centers for Disease Control and Prevention standard precautions in accordance with institution policies.
  - Standard precautions are used by all health care workers who have direct contact with client or body fluids or indirect contact through emptying trash, changing linens, or cleaning patient rooms. These precautions apply to all clients whether they are known to have an infectious disease or not.
  - Wear gloves and other barriers (e.g., mask, face shield, impermeable gown) when in contact with or at risk of contact with blood or other body fluids and substances.
  - Ensure a private room for clients with highly communicable or virulent infections and clients with poor personal hygiene who are likely to contaminate the environment.
  - Wear barrier garments to prevent transmitting infection to a client (e.g., an immunosuppressed client at risk for infection).
  - Strictly adhere to Occupational Safety and Health Administration (OSHA) guidelines, whose goal is the reduction of risk exposure; by law, OSHA must protect health care providers from known industry hazards.
- **Maintain isolation precautions as indicated to prevent the transmission of microorganisms.**
  - *Contact isolation* requires a private room with a closed door; gowns, masks, and gloves are indicated for all persons entering the room.
  - *Droplet (respiratory) isolation* requires a private room; masks are indicated for all persons entering the room; a room with individualized ventilation may be required.
  - *Reverse isolation* is required when the client is immunocompromised and the individuals entering the room are a risk to the client. Individuals should wear a mask when in the room.

   e. Facilitate mobilization of secretions by:
  - ensuring adequate hydration
  - promoting rest and comfort
  - splinting the client's chest during coughing to minimize discomfort

BOX 19-2

Interventions to prevent the spread of infectious disease in communities

- Perform case finding and reporting.
- Provide individual and community teaching.
  - Teach about methods to improve host defenses, including maintaining adequate nutrition and keeping immunizations current.
  - Teach the importance of chemoprophylaxis (e.g., taking chloroquine when traveling in malaria-infested regions).
  - Teach ways to maintain good hygiene, proper sanitation, safe meal preparation, and proper food storage.
  - Teach guidelines for "safe sex" to prevent sexually transmitted diseases.
  - Encourage the client with an infection to remain at home to decrease the chance of transmitting the virus.
- Participate in community immunization programs as possible.

- encouraging ambulation as tolerated.

4. **Resolve any fluid volume deficit.**
   a. Assess for signs and symptoms of fluid volume deficit, including:
      postural hypotension
      - tented skin turgor
      - tachycardia
      - weight loss
      - oliguria
      - weakness
      - decreased urine specific gravity
      - flat neck veins.
   b. Encourage oral fluid intake.
   c. Administer I.V. fluids if indicated.
   d. Monitor intake and output and vital signs.

5. **Promote comfort.**
   a. Reposition the client as needed.
   b. Use nonpharmacologic pain-control methods when appropriate, which include guided imagery, distraction, relaxation techniques, hypnosis, and massage.
   c. Provide prompt treatment for infection.

6. **Resolve impairment in skin integrity.**
   a. Monitor for changes in skin color (e.g., blanched or reddened), changes in turgor suggesting dehydration or edema, and open lesions.
   b. Maintain optimal nutrition.
   c. Maintain appropriate personal hygiene.
   d. Obtain culture and sensitivity of any draining lesions.
   e. Change dressings as appropriate.

7. **Minimize social isolation.**
   a. Explain the rationale for isolation procedures to the client and support persons.
   b. Encourage the maximum social contact possible while under isolation.
   c. Schedule regular periods to talk with the client.
   d. Interact with the client in a caring, nonjudgmental manner.
   e. Encourage the client to express anxieties and emotions.
   f. Discontinue isolation as soon as possible.
   g. Work with the client to devise means of reducing boredom.
   h. Teach the client stress-reduction techniques.

CLIENT AND FAMILY TEACHING 19-1
Prevention and treatment of infection

- Assess what the client and family already know; listen carefully to what the client says about the illness and treatment.
- Provide brief explanations about the organism and route of transmission, treatment goals, follow-up, and prevention of transmissions to others; clarify when necessary.
- Provide written materials and audiovisual aids when available; allow opportunities for questions and discussions.
- Instruct the client to cover the mouth and nose when coughing and sneezing; teach him to dispose of tissues in separate sacks and to not throw tissues on floors or counter tops.

- Instruct the client on the importance of handwashing techniques.
- Instruct the client to take all doses of antibiotics and not to save antibiotics.
- Instruct the client to keep all immunizations current.
- Instruct the client on disinfection, asepsis, and disposal of health care equipment in the home.
- Instruct the client on the signs and symptoms of complications that should be reported to the health care provider.
- Discuss community resources that are available, if necessary.

---

8. **Promote measures that help increase activity level.**
   a. Provide rest periods during the day, especially before and after priority activities.
   b. Help the client rearrange the daily schedule and organize activities to conserve energy.
   c. Instruct the client to increase activity gradually when resuming normal activity level.
   d. Assist and instruct the client to obtain assistance when ambulating and transferring from the bed to a chair or from the bathtub because of fatigue from the infectious process.

9. **Instruct the client and his family about the disease process, treatments, and necessity for self care.**
   a. Explain to the client that noncompliance with the medication and treatment regimen is a primary reason for recurrent infection and more serious complications of infections.
   b. Provide health education as detailed in *Client and family teaching 19-1*.

10. **Provide referrals** to the Centers for Disease Control and Prevention and the National Foundation for Infectious Diseases. (See appendix A.)

E. Outcome evaluation

1. The client and his family use appropriate methods to prevent the spread of infection and the client avoids reinfection.
2. The client maintains temperature within normal range without complications.
3. The client maintains adequate gas exchange, as evidenced by clear lungs, no dyspnea, arterial blood gases within normal limits, and a pulse oximeter reading above 93%.
4. The client maintains normal fluid balance, as evidenced by elastic skin turgor, normal blood pressure and heart rate, absence of venous distention and edema, and maintenance of a normal elimination pattern.
5. The client maintains or regains integrity of skin and mucous membranes.
6. The client verbalizes feelings about social isolation and finds appropriate activities to address boredom.
7. The client regains normal activity tolerance.
8. The client reports no or minimal pain and discomfort.

9. The client and family members verbalize measures to help prevent disease transmission, maintain the medical regimen, prevent disease spread, and recognize possible complications.

III. SEPTICEMIA AND SEPTIC SHOCK

A. Description

1. **Septicemia,** or *sepsis,* is a systemic infection of the bloodstream producing clinically apparent manifestations.
2. **Septic shock** is a life-threatening form of shock resulting from uncontrolled septicemia. Approximately 40% of septicemia cases lead to septic shock.

B. Etiology

1. **Septicemia** most commonly results from gram-negative bacteria, including *Escherichia coli, Klebsiella, Enterobacter, Pseudomonas aeruginosa, Proteus, Neisseria meningitidis,* and *Bacteroides fragilis.* Gram-positive bacteria (i.e., *Staphylococcus aureus* and *Streptococcus pneumoniae*) have been implicated in some cases.
2. **Septic shock** results from septicemia in persons with compromised defenses. Risk factors include:
   a. hospitalization
   b. invasive procedures especially indwelling Foley catheters
   c. immunodeficiency
   d. advanced age
   e. trauma
   f. burns
   g. disorders that result in debilitation.

C. Pathophysiology

1. **Septicemia.** Infectious organisms or pyrogenic substances from any part of the body that enter the circulating bloodstream may cause this systemic infection.
2. **Septic shock**
   a. The pathophysiology of septic shock is incompletely understood. It is thought to result from a reaction to an endotoxin that triggers the release of chemical mediators and hormones. These mediators and hormones cause cardiovascular changes and cellular injury.
      – Arteriolar and venous spasms cause pooling of blood in pulmonary, renal, splanchnic, and peripheral tissues, leading to tissue anoxia and acidosis.
      – Intense vasoconstriction increases peripheral resistance, decreases cardiac output, and diminishes blood flow to major organs.
      – Activation of factor XII of the intrinsic coagulation system can produce intravascular coagulation and fibrinolysis.
      – Death may occur from vascular collapse.
   b. Septic shock typically occurs in two phases: hyperdynamic and hypodynamic.
      – The hyperdynamic phase is the predominant physiologic feature characterized by high cardiac output, which is attributable to an intact and functional compensatory sympathetic response to decreased peripheral resistance.
      – The hypodynamic phase can be equated with the irreversible stage of hemorrhagic shock with effects of myocardial depression and low cardiac output. Once septic shock has progressed to this state, survival is doubtful, and therapeutic measures are usually futile.

c. The sooner the disorder is detected and treated, the better the outcome.

D. Assessment findings

1. **Clinical manifestations**

   a. **Septicemia** commonly produces fever, chills, prostration, pain, headache, nausea, and diarrhea. Confusion may be the first sign of infection and sepsis in elderly patients.

   b. **Septic shock.** Clinical manifestations depend on the stage of shock, causative organism, and the client's condition.

   – In the hyperdynamic phase, common findings include:
   - warm, flushed skin
   - normal or high urine output
   - mild hypotension
   - tachycardia
   - edema (due to capillary leakage).

   – In the hypodynamic phase, manifestations include:
   - marked hypotension
   - cold, dry skin
   - oliguria or anuria
   - edema
   - respiratory abnormalities (e.g., apnea, tachypnea)
   - restlessness, confusion secondary to hypoxia
   - altered level of consciousness.

2. **Laboratory and diagnostic study findings**

   a. Blood cultures can detect the causative organism.

   b. Arterial blood gases reveal metabolic acidosis, indicated by decreased partial pressure of carbon dioxide, partial pressure of oxygen, bicarbonate, and pH levels.

   c. Serum clotting studies reveal clotting abnormalities.

   d. Complete blood cell counts reveal anemia.

E. Nursing management (See section II.D.)

1. **Administer prescribed medications,** which may include vasopressors and antibiotics. (See *Drug chart 19-1,* pages 532 and 533.)

2. **Administer I.V. fluid replacement, packed red blood cells, and platelets if prescribed.**

3. **Provide ongoing assessment.** Monitor vital signs, intake and output, daily weights, and for signs of dehydration. Monitor and report abnormal laboratory findings (i.e., abnormal levels of blood urea nitrogen, creatinine, white blood cells, and serum albumin) to the health care provider.

4. **Promote measures to enhance the client's nutritional status.** Encourage nutritional supplements high in protein; enteral feedings may be administered.

5. **Minimize anxiety.** Explain all procedures to the client and family to help relieve anxiety.

6. **Intervene as indicated to limit blood loss due to clotting abnormalities.**

   a. Protect the client from trauma that could cause hemorrhage (e.g., bumps, falls).

   b. Avoid venipuncture and other invasive procedures when possible.

   c. Use small-gauge needles when injections and venipuncture are unavoidable.

   d. Apply firm pressure to venipuncture sites for 3 to 7 minutes; for prolonged bleeding, apply sandbags.

   e. Prevent the client from coughing, vomiting, or straining with bowel movements.

f. Provide assistance with activities of daily living; teach the client to avoid shaving, brushing with a hard-bristled toothbrush, and flossing.

7. **Help the client maintain as normal a sleep pattern as possible.** Keep the room quiet and dimly lit; promote rest and relaxation; and cluster necessary procedures to minimize disturbances.

8. **Provide health education** as detailed in *Client and family teaching 19-1,* page 536.

IV. STAPHYLOCOCCAL INFECTIONS: SPECIFIC BACTERIAL INFECTION

A. **Description.** Staphylococcal infections are caused by pathogenic species of *Staphylococcus,* a gram-positive bacteria. Types include bacteremia, pneumonia, enterocolitis, osteomyelitis, food poisoning, skin infections, invasive infections, and toxic shock syndrome. Chapter 10 offers more extensive discussion of toxic shock syndrome.

B. **Etiology**
1. The most common causative bacteria are *S. aureus* and *S. epidermidis.*
2. Modes of transmission include direct contact, common source, and animal.
3. Persons at greatest risk include neonates and those with impaired skin integrity and prosthetic heart valves or joints.

C. **Pathophysiology**
1. Bacteria are free-living organisms that use the nutrients of the body as a food source and a favorable environment for growth. Unlike viruses, bacteria do not require living cells for growth.
2. Pathogenic effects of bacterial infections usually result from substances, such as enzymes or toxins produced by the bacteria, or from injury caused by the inflammatory response of the body to the bacteria.
3. Staphylococci are part of normal flora of the skin and mucous membranes. They are also widely distributed in air, dust, and fomites.
4. Staphylococci are a common cause of nosocomial infections. *Staphylococcus epidermidis* is a common cause of infection in clients with intravascular devices.

D. **Assessment findings**
1. Clinical manifestations
   a. **Bacteremia**
   - Fever
   - Tachycardia
   - Abscesses throughout the body
   b. **Pneumonia**
   - Fever
   - Tachycardia
   - Pulmonary infiltrates
   c. **Osteomyelitis**
   - High fever
   - Bone pain
   d. **Food poisoning**
   - Nausea and vomiting
   - Abdominal cramps

 – Diarrhea
 – Anorexia
  e. **Skin infection**
 – Cellulitis
 – Painful abscesses
 – Boils
 – Other skin lesions
  f. **Invasive infection** (may produce signs and symptoms of systemic infections).
 – Endocarditis
 – Meningitis
 – Arthritis
 – Urinary tract infections.
 2. **Laboratory and diagnostic study findings.** Culture and Gram stain studies reveal the causative organism.

E. Nursing management (See section II.D.)
 1. Administer prescribed medications, which include antipyretics and antibiotics. (See *Drug chart 19-1,* pages 532 and 533.)
 2. Provide health education as detailed in *Client and family teaching 19-1,* page 536.

V. TUBERCULOSIS: SPECIFIC BACTERIAL INFECTION

A. Description. Tuberculosis is a chronic granulomatous infection that usually affects the pulmonary system but may also invade other organs and tissues. The incidence is highest in crowded, poverty-stricken settings.

B. Etiology
 1. Infectious agents include:
  a. Mycobacterium tuberculosis
  b. Mycobacterium bovis (rarely).
 2. Transmission occurs through inhalation or ingestion of infected droplets from a person with active disease.
 3. Those at greatest risk include persons who are immunocompromised or debilitated and persons with a history of previous infection.

C. Pathophysiology
 1. Infected droplets travel to the pulmonary alveoli, where the bacilli form lesions known as tubercles. Tubercles may heal, leaving scar tissue, or may continue as granuloma, which may heal and be reactivated later. Granulomas may produce necrosis, liquefaction, sloughing, and cavitation of lung tissue.
 2. The initial lesion may disseminate bacilli to other tissues (e.g., kidneys, bones, lymph nodes).

D. Assessment findings
 1. **Clinical manifestations.** In early stages, tuberculosis often produces no symptoms. Manifestations of advancing tuberculosis include:
  a. fatigue and weight loss
  b. cough that is initially dry but later productive of mucopurulent sputum
  c. hemoptysis
  d. fever and chills.
 2. **Laboratory and diagnostic study findings**

     a. Tuberculin skin test can detect infection (purified protein derivative [PPD]). The test is read at 48 and 72 hours.

     b. Chest radiograph and sputum sample analyses identify active disease. Follow-up sputum cultures are performed every 2 to 4 weeks to determine effectiveness of medication therapy.

E. Nursing management (See section II.D.)

  1. Provide drug therapy.

     a. Administer prescribed medications, which include the antituberculosis drugs isoniazid, rifampin, streptomycin, pyrazinamide, and ethambutol (See *Drug chart 19-1,* pages 532 and 533.)

     b. Instruct the client that the multidrug regimen must be adhered to for 6 to 12 months; a client is considered noninfectious after 2 to 3 weeks of continuous medication therapy.

  2. Encourage the client to increase fluid intake to liquefy secretions.

  3. Carefully implement measures to treat infection and prevent the spread of infection in health care facilities and the community.

  4. Address the client's nutritional needs. Offer small frequent nutritional meals and liquid nutritional supplements if needed.

  5. Instruct the client to avoid factors that may exacerbate symptoms, such as smoking, asbestos, and secondhand smoke.

  6. Consult social services to investigate insurance coverage and proper follow-up care.

  7. Schedule follow-up appointments at convenient times and places.

  8. Treat the client with dignity and respect. Remain nonjudgmental when caring for the client.

  9. Reduce elevated body temperature.

  10. Improve gas exchange.

  11. Minimize social isolation.

  12. Provide client and family teaching.

  13. Provide referrals.

VI. INFLUENZA: SPECIFIC VIRAL INFECTION

A. Description. Influenza is an acute, highly contagious respiratory tract infection. It usually occurs seasonally in epidemics.

B. Etiology

  1. Influenza results from one of three types of myxovirus influenzae: type A, type B, or type C.

  2. Persons at high risk include young children, elderly people, people with chronic diseases, and health care workers.

C. Pathophysiology

  1. Infection occurs by droplet transmission from an infected person or by indirect contact (e.g., sharing a contaminated cup). The infection invades the respiratory tract epithelium, causing inflammation and desquamation; symptoms typically appear after an incubation period of 24 to 72 hours.

  2. Usually a self-limiting disorder, influenza can cause life-threatening complications (e.g., pneumonia) in people who are at high risk.

D. Assessment findings

1. Respiratory manifestations of influenza may include:
   a. sinusitis
   b. dyspnea
   c. sore throat
   d. nasal stuffiness
   e. nasal discharge
   f. dry cough.
2. Other common signs and symptoms include fever, chills, malaise, headache, and myalgias.

E. Nursing management (See section II.D.)

1. **Administer prescribed medications,** such as the antiviral medication amantadine for influenza A. (See *Drug chart 19-1,* pages 532 and 533.)
2. **Encourage annual vaccination for people high risk.**
3. **Promote measures to enhance comfort and rest.**
4. **Provide health education** as detailed in *Client and family teaching 19-1,* page 536.

VII. ROCKY MOUNTAIN SPOTTED FEVER: SPECIFIC RICKETTSIAL INFECTION

A. Description. Rocky Mountain spotted fever is a potentially fatal, tick-borne infectious disease marked by fever and skin rash. It may lead to shock and renal failure. The incidence is highest in the south central and south Atlantic regions of the United States, and the number of cases peaks in early summer.

B. Etiology

1. The infectious agent, *Rickettsia rickettsii,* is transmitted by the dog tick *(Dermacentor variabilis),* wood tick *(Dermacentor andersoni),* and other tick species in the United States.
2. Common reservoirs include dogs, rodents, and wild animals.

C. Pathophysiology. The infectious agent reproduces in the endothelium of small and medium-sized blood vessels, causing widespread edema and degeneration. This generalized vasculitis produces disease symptoms, which may involve multiple body organs and systems.

D. Assessment findings

1. **Clinical manifestations**
   a. Malaise, lethargy, and stupor
   b. Severe headache
   c. Photophobia
   d. Anorexia
   e. High, continuous fever with chills
   f. Rash on extremities, spreading medially (usually occurring on the third to fifth day after onset)
   g. Possible skin necrosis, especially of the ear lobes, scrotum, toes, and fingers
   h. Generalized edema
   i. Myalgia, arthralgia, and abdominal pain
   j. Splenomegaly

2. **Laboratory and diagnostic study findings.** Blood studies reveal thrombocytopenia, coagulation defects, and serologic confirmation of infection.

E. Nursing management (See section II.D.)

1. **Administer prescribed medications,** which include the antibiotics tetracycline and doxycycline. (See *Drug Chart 19-1,* pages 532 and 533.)
2. **Determine the extent of edema** by measuring the circumferences of arms, legs, and abdomen.
3. **Resolve impairment in skin integrity.**
4. **Reduce elevated body temperature.**
5. **Promote comfort.**
6. **Monitor intake and output** because the client is at risk for developing renal failure.
7. **Teach preventive measures.**
    a. Advise the client to inspect the skin frequently for ticks when in endemic areas.
    b. Teach tick removal techniques, such as flicking an unattached tick off the skin and removing an attached tick with tweezers by grasping it close to the attachment point.
    c. Instruct the client to wash his hands and the attachment site immediately after tick removal.
    d. Advise the client to wear protective clothing and tick repellent when in endemic areas.

VIII. CANDIDIASIS: SPECIFIC FUNGAL INFECTION

A. Description. Candidiasis a variable fungal infection producing superficial mucocutaneous and, less commonly, serious systemic manifestations.

B. Etiology

1. Infectious agents are those of the *Candida* genus (e.g., *Candida albicans, Candida tropicalis*), which are commonly part of the normal flora of the mouth, GI tract, vagina, and skin.
2. They can cause infection when some change in the body triggers proliferation or systemic invasion; such factors may include:
    a. immunosuppression
    b. invasive procedures
    c. use of broad-spectrum antibiotics
    d. hyperglycemia
    e. debilitation.
3. A woman with vaginal candidiasis can pass the infection on to the neonate during vaginal delivery.

C. Pathophysiology

1. Candidiasis usually is a mild, superficial infection affecting the skin, mucous membranes, or nails.
2. Rarely, organisms enter the bloodstream and invade deep organs (e.g., meninges, lungs, endocardium), causing serious infection that can lead to shock and death.

D. Assessment findings

1. **Clinical manifestations**
    a. **Oral candidiasis (thrush)**
        – Creamy, white, curdlike patches on the tongue and oral mucosa
        – Painful, bleeding lesions, especially if patches are scraped

b. *Candida* esophagitis
- Painful swallowing; feeling of obstruction with swallowing
  - Substernal chest discomfort
  - Nausea and vomiting
c. *Candida* vaginitis
- A scanty to moderate amount of thick, white, curdlike discharge
- Severe vulvar pruritus
- Vaginal and labial erythema
- Symptoms of secondary urethral infection
d. Disseminated candidiasis is commonly marked by high fever, chills, hypotension, prostration and, possibly, rash. Other signs and symptoms depend on the site of infection:
- In the pulmonary system, manifestations include hemoptysis and cough.
- In the renal system, manifestations include flank pain, dysuria, hematuria, and pyuria.
- In the brain, manifestations include headache, nuchal rigidity, seizures, and focal neurologic deficits.
- In the endocardium, manifestations include heart murmur and chest pain.
- In the eyes, manifestations include blurred vision, pain, scotoma, and exudate.

2. **Laboratory and diagnostic study findings**
   a. The *Candida* antibody test detects the presence of the antibody and is helpful in the diagnosis of systemic *Candida* infection.
   b. Tissue culture reveals *Candida albicans*.
   c. Histologic examination of biopsy specimen reveals *Candida albicans*.

E. Nursing management (See section II.D.)
1. **Administer prescribed medications,** which may include antipruritics, topical antifungal agents, and systemic antifungal medications. (See *Drug chart 19-1,* pages 532 and 533.)
2. **Promote comfort.** Instruct the client to apply cool compresses to affected areas.
3. **Teach the client to prevent oral, esophageal, and disseminated candidiasis.** Teach the client proper oral care methods.
4. **Teach the client to prevent vaginal candidiasis.**
   a. Encourage the client to have sex partners checked for infection and to use condoms to prevent transmission.
   b. Advise the client to avoid tight-fitting underwear and pants.
   c. Instruct the client to avoid synthetic underwear. Encourage cotton underwear instead.
   d. Encourage the client to practice good perineal hygiene.
5. **Promote good nutrition.**
   a. Assess for signs and symptoms of undernutrition, such as malaise, fatigue, nausea, and vomiting. Assess for physical and biochemical indices of malnutrition.
   b. Observe for a decrease in intake or a loss of interest in food.
   c. Encourage a high-calorie, high-protein diet.
   d. Monitor the client's weight.
   e. Encourage small, frequent meals, especially if the client is fatigued or nauseated.
   f. Administer total parenteral nutrition or tube feedings, if indicated.
6. **Help the client maintain oral mucosal integrity.**
   a. Promote frequent, thorough mouth care.

b. Instruct the client to avoid alcohol-containing mouthwashes, which dry the mucosa and can cause pain.

c. Observe for signs of disseminated infection.

7. **Resolve impairment in skin integrity.**

a. Apply topical antifungal agents as prescribed.

b. Keep affected areas clean, dry, and open to air.

c. Observe for signs of disseminated infection.

8. **Intervene as necessary to maintain adequate cardiac output and tissue perfusion.**

IX. ASCARIASIS: SPECIFIC HELMINTHIC INFECTION

A. Description. Ascariasis is a parasitic infection caused by roundworm infestation. Ascariasis occurs worldwide but is most common in tropical regions with poor sanitation and in Asia, where many farmers use human feces for crop fertilization.

B. Etiology

1. The infectious organism is *Ascaris lumbricoides,* a large roundworm (15 to 35 cm long).

2. Ingesting ova contained in contaminated food, water, or soil transmits infection. Direct person-to-person transmission does not occur.

C. Pathophysiology

1. After ingestion, *A. lumbricoides* ova hatch and release larvae, which penetrate the intestinal wall and travel through the bloodstream to the lungs and heart. In the lungs, larvae penetrate alveoli and move up the respiratory tree to the pharynx. From the pharynx, larvae are swallowed; they then travel through the GI tract back to the small intestine, where they mature into worms. This entire process takes about 3 months.

2. The life span of *A. lumbricoides* is approximately 18 months.

3. Heavy infestation can cause obstruction of the trachea, intestine, bile duct, pancreatic duct, or appendix, producing severe pain and other symptoms.

D. Assessment findings

1. **Clinical manifestations**

a. Some infections are asymptomatic.

b. Large numbers of worms in the intestine may produce severe cramping pain and nausea and vomiting.

c. Dyspnea, fever and chills, cough, and pneumonia commonly mark invasion of the lungs.

d. Eosinophilia commonly occurs during the larval stage.

2. **Laboratory and diagnostic study findings.** Ova or adult worms in stool confirm ascariasis.

E. Nursing management

1. **Administer medications,** which may include antihelmintic drugs. (See *Drug chart 19-1,* pages 532 and 533.)

2. **Teach preventive measures to people traveling to endemic areas.**

a. Instruct the client to practice good personal hygiene.

b. Advise the client to avoid ingestion of contaminated food or water.

3. **Improve gas exchange.** (See section II.D.3.)

4. **Promote comfort.** (See section II.D.5.)

Study questions

1. Which is *most* appropriate action for the nurse to do on discovering a sputum sample at a client's bedside that is dated with today's date, labeled with the client's name and identification number, but has no time marked on it?
1. Sending the sample to the clinical laboratory immediately for analysis
2. Discarding the sample, and collecting another one as soon as possible
3. Sending the sample immediately, but informing the laboratory of the unknown collection time
4. Refrigerating the sample and calling the clinical laboratory to pick it up as soon as possible

2. Which client would the health care provider strongly encourage to take the influenza vaccine?
1. A 45-year-old man who is admitted for an appendectomy
2. A 13-year-old boy with recurrent tonsillitis
3. A 35-year-old man who is going to travel to Mexico
4. A 68-year-old female who lives in a long-term care facility

3. Which statement accurately reflects the nurse's understanding about nosocomial infections when planning care for a client in a health care facility?
1. "Nosocomial infections occur primarily in immunocompromised hosts."
2. "Nosocomial infections occur in at least 30% of clients in a given hospital."
3. "Nosocomial infections, present in the community, are not always clinically apparent."
4. "Nosocomial infections are those infections acquired in a health care facility."

4. When administering the fourth dose of an aminoglycoside antibiotic to a female client with an infection, which interventions should the nurse implement? (Select all that apply.)
1. Determining if the client has any allergies to antibiotics
2. Assessing the client for thrush, diarrhea, and vaginal itching
3. Checking to see if the health care provider has ordered a peak and trough
4. Administering the antibiotic over 20 minutes
5. Assessing the client's I.V. site for redness and irritation
6. Assessing the client's hemoglobin and hematocrit levels prior to administering

5. Which intervention should the nurse include when caring for a client with elevated body temperature secondary to an infectious process?
1. Sponging the client's body with ice water
2. Encouraging limited fluid intake
3. Administering antipyretic medications
4. Applying heavy, restrictive clothing

6. Which intervention is recommended to prevent nosocomial wound infections?
1. Shaving body hair 24 hours before surgery
2. Changing closed wound dressings every 6 hours
3. Catheterizing clients whenever possible
4. Maintaining asepsis during surgery

7. In an intensive care unit, which intervention should the nurse perform before caring for clients?
1. Washing hands using a new bar of soap
2. Soaking all rings in isopropyl alcohol for 5 minutes
3. Donning sterile gloves instead of washing hands
4. Scrubbing around and under nails

8. Which nursing intervention would be appropriate to prevent the spread of infectious diseases in communities?
1. Teaching about ways to maintain proper sanitation and safe meal preparation
2. Advising individuals to wear gloves when in contact with their own blood
3. Discouraging clients from keeping immunizations up to date
4. Encouraging persons to adhere to Occupational Safety and Health Administration (OSHA) standard precautions in the home

9. Which indicator would lead the nurse to suspect minimal blood loss in a client with septicemia at risk for coagulation defects?
1. Blood pressure of 102/64 mm Hg
2. Hematocrit level of 44%
3. Tented skin turgor
4. Apical heart rate of 135 beats/minute

10. Which behavior indicates that a client understands measures that may prevent acquiring influenza?
1. The client covers his nose and mouth when sneezing or coughing.
2. The client routinely takes prophylactic antibiotics.
3. The client receives the appropriate flu vaccine each year.
4. The client asks to have a throat culture done to detect infection.

11. Which instruction should the nurse give to a person planning a backpacking trip in an area known to have ticks that carry organisms causing Rocky Mountain spotted fever?
1. "Inspect your face and hands frequently for ticks."
2. "Flick unattached ticks off the skin."
3. "Crush an attached tick between your fingernails."
4. "Rub an attached tick with soap to remove it."

12. Which statement would indicate that a client requires additional teaching about measures to prevent recurrent vaginal candidiasis?
1. "I douche regularly with a vinegar preparation."
2. "I now wear only cotton underwear."
3. "I have stopped using hormonal contraceptives."
4. "My boyfriend now wears a condom with vaginal intercourse."

13. Which nursing intervention would be included in the care plan for a client diagnosed with an infection and experiencing a fluid volume deficit?
1. Monitoring intake, output, and vital signs
2. Evaluating arterial blood gases (ABGs) and pulse oximeter reading
3. Repositioning the client and encouraging guided imagery
4. Applying cool compresses and a hypothermia blanket

14. For an elderly client just admitted with uncontrolled diabetes and heart failure, which intervention would be most important to reduce the client's risk of nosocomial infection?
1. Inserting a urinary catheter as soon as possible
2. Monitoring arterial blood gas (ABG) values every 30 minutes
3. Changing I.V. catheter sites every 4 hours
4. Encouraging frequent coughing and deep breathing

15. Which statement would be the nurse's *best* response to the client who asks, "How does someone get tuberculosis?"
1. "You inhale infected air droplets from a person with active tuberculosis."
2. "You can only get tuberculosis through blood transfusions."

3. "Tuberculosis can be transmitted through sexual intercourse."
4. "Frequent handwashing can prevent the spread of tuberculosis."

16. When assessing a person with suspected ascariasis, which assessment data would the nurse expect to find?

1. Severe headache and photophobia
2. Creamy, white, curdlike patches on the tongue
3. History of exposure to animal bites
4. Abdominal cramping, nausea and vomiting

Answer key

1. The answer is **2.**
Prompt delivery and analysis of microbiologic specimens is essential for accurate results. Because the specimen had set for an unknown period, it must be discarded and another sample must be obtained. Sending the sample to the laboratory immediately, even with informing the laboratory of the unknown collection time, and refrigerating the sample are inappropriate.

2. The answer is **4.**
The influenza vaccine is recommended for people older than age 65, residents in extended-care facilities, those with chronic pulmonary or cardiovascular diseases, and health care providers. The 45-year-old client scheduled for an appendectomy, the adolescent with recurrent tonsillitis, and the 35-year-old man traveling to Mexico are not considered at high risk for influenza.

3. The answer is **4.**
Nosocomial infections are those that are acquired during hospitalization or treatment within a health care facility. They can occur in persons who are immunocompromised and in persons with normal immune systems. Although there can be multiple cases of nosocomial infections within an institution, they can also occur in a single client. An endemic infection is one that is usually present within a community but is not always clinically apparent.

4. The answers are **2, 3, 5.**
Aminoglycoside antibiotics are nephrotoxic and ototoxic. The health care provider will order peak and troughs to determine serum blood levels. The nurse should assess the client's I.V. site as to not administer antibiotics through an irritated vein. The nurse should also assess for signs of thrush, diarrhea, and vaginal itching (i.e., signs of superinfection), which occur when antibiotics destroy normal body flora. This is the client's fourth dose, so the client is not allergic to this antibiotic. The antibiotic should be administered over 1 hour (not 20 minutes), and the white blood cell count and blood urea nitrogen and creatinine levels should be assessed. Assessment of hemoglobin and hematocrit levels is performed for blood loss.

5. The answer is **3.**
Antipyretic agents affect the thermoregulatory center of the brain, resulting in diaphoresis and vasodilation, thereby decreasing temperature. The body should be sponged with tepid water, fluid intake should be increased, and heavy or restrictive clothing should be removed.

6. The answer is **4.**
Maintaining asepsis during surgery, such as by limiting personnel movement in and out of the operating room, helps to prevent surgical wound infection. Preoperative hair removal should be avoided when possible. However, if necessary, it should be done immediately before surgery using clippers or depilatories. Dressings over closed wounds should be changed only when wet or if signs and symptoms of infection develop. Catheterizing clients should be avoided whenever possible.

7. The answer is **4.**
Proper handwashing includes scrubbing the nails thoroughly. In special care units, an antimicrobial cleanser should be used instead of plain soap. Jewelry should be removed before washing hands. However, it does not need to be soaked in isopropyl alcohol. Wearing gloves is not a substitute for handwashing.

8. The answer is **1.**
Teaching ways to maintain good hygiene, proper sanitation, safe meal preparation, and proper food storage can prevent spread of infection in communities. Individuals do not need to be protected from their own blood. Gloves are unnecessary. Clients should be encouraged to keep immunizations current. OSHA standard precautions protect health care providers from known industry hazards. They are not indicated for use in the home.

9. The answer is **2.**
The hematocrit level indicates the percentage of total blood volume comprised of cells. The normal value is approximately 45%. The client with a hematocrit level of 44% would be experiencing only a minimal loss of blood. A blood pressure of 102/64 mm Hg, tented skin turgor, and an apical heart rate of 135 beats/minute represent abnormal values indicative of a more serious problem. The blood pressure should be above 110/70 mm Hg, the skin turgor should be elastic, and heart rate should be between 80 and 100 beats/minute.

10. The answer is **3.**
Vaccination is the best method of protecting against influenza infection. Covering the nose and mouth when sneezing or coughing protects others but cannot protect the client from getting the flu. Antibiotics, which work against bacteria, are not effective against the influenza virus. Submitting to diagnostic procedures cannot prevent the client from contracting influenza.

11. The answer is **2.**
Unattached ticks should be removed by flicking them off the skin. Ticks are most likely to burrow into skin in warm, moist areas of the body, including the scalp. The face and hands are less likely areas of burrowing. Attached ticks should never be crushed, because crushing may expose broken skin to contaminated tick secretions. Rather, they should be removed with tweezers. Rubbing soap on an attached tick does not help remove it.

12. The answer is **1.**
Douching, which alters the normal flora of the vagina, has not been shown to be effective against recurrent vaginitis. Douching may predispose the client to infection. Cotton underwear is recommended because cotton is more absorbent than synthetic fabrics and keeps the perineal area drier. Because hormonal contraceptive use is associated with increased incidence of recurrent candidiasis, many practitioners recommend alternative birth-control measures. Condom use lessens the chance of transmitting the fungus between sexual partners.

13. The answer is **1.**
Interventions to address a fluid volume deficit include monitoring intake, output, and vital signs in conjunction with encouraging fluid intake and monitoring I.V. fluid therapy. The client is assessed for signs and symptoms of dehydration and fluid overload. Evaluating ABG and pulse oximeter readings is appropriate for improving gas exchange. Repositioning the client and encouraging guided imaging aid in promoting comfort. Using cool compresses and a hypothermia blanket help to reduce elevated body temperature.

14. The answer is **4.**
Frequent coughing and deep breathing, a noninvasive respiratory hygiene measure, helps to prevent nosocomial pneumonias. For any client, urinary catheterization should be avoided whenever possible. Frequent invasive procedures such as repetitive ABG de-

terminations increase the risk of nosocomial bacteremias. I.V. sites should be changed at regular intervals according to established protocols and when signs of infection occur. However, changing I.V. sites every 4 hours is too frequent, exposing the client to multiple invasive procedures, increasing his risk of infection.

15. The answer is **1.**

Transmission of tuberculosis occurs through inhalation or ingestion of infected droplets from a person with active disease. Tuberculosis is not transmitted through blood transfusions or sexual intercourse. Handwashing cannot prevent the spread of tuberculosis.

16. The answer is **4.**

Ascariasis refers to a parasitic infection caused by roundworm infestation. Although some cases of ascariasis are asymptomatic, worms in the intestines usually cause severe abdominal cramping and nausea and vomiting. Invasion of the lungs results in dyspnea, fever, chills, and cough. Severe headache and photophobia are signs and symptoms of Rocky Mountain spotted fever. Creamy, white, curdlike patches on the tongue are signs oral candidiasis (i.e., thrush). Animal bites do not transmit ascariasis.

20 *Cancer nursing*

I. ESSENTIAL CONCEPTS OF CANCER

A. Description

1. Cancer is the general name given to a large group of diseases characterized by:
   a. uncontrolled growth and spread of abnormal cells
   b. proliferation (i.e., rapid reproduction by cell division)
   c. metastasis (i.e., spread or transfer of cancer cells from one organ or part to another not directly connected).
2. Specific types of cancer are detailed in *Table 20-1*.
3. Cancer is second only to cardiovascular disease as the leading cause of death in the United States.
4. Cure is considered to be achieved when the client exhibits no evidence of disease; reference points of 5- and 10-year survival rates are used. After cure, the client would have the same expected life span as age- and sex-matched persons without cancer.

B. Etiology

1. Healthy cells are transformed by unknown mechanisms or exposure to certain etiologic agents, including:
   a. viruses (e.g., Epstein-Barr, herpes simplex type II, cytomegalovirus, papillomavirus, hepatitis B)
   b. chemical carcinogens (e.g., chromium, cobalt, tar, soot, asphalt, nitrogen mustards, certain plastics, aniline dyes, hydrocarbons in cigarette smoke, air pollutants from industry, crude paraffin oil, fuel oils, nickel, asbestos, arsenicals)
   c. physical stressors (e.g., excessive exposure to sunlight or radiation, chronic irritation)
   d. hormonal factors (e.g., imbalance of endogenous or exogenous hormones, such as estrogen or diethylstilbestrol)
   e. genetic factors (e.g., abnormal chromosome patterns, such as in Burkitt's lymphoma, chronic myelogenous or acute leukemia, and skin cancers; familial predisposition, such as in breast, endometrial, colorectal, stomach, lung, colon, and kidney cancers).
2. The causes for specific types of cancer are detailed in *Table 20-1*.

C. Pathophysiology

1. **Cancer development** is closely linked to immune-system failure, as evidenced by:
   a. increased incidence of malignancy in organ-transplant recipients who receive immunosuppressive therapy
   b. increased risk for developing secondary cancers in clients receiving long-term chemotherapy to treat a primary malignancy
   c. increased incidence of lymphoma in clients diagnosed with acquired immunodeficiency syndrome
   d. increased incidence of cancers early in life in clients with an immature immune system or later in life in clients with a failing immune system.
2. **Proliferation.** Neoplasms have several proliferative patterns.
   a. **Benign** (i.e., usually harmless, does not infiltrate other tissues) and **malignant** (i.e., always harmful; may spread or metastasize to tissues far from the original site) cells display different characteristics of cellular growth; the degree of differentiation (i.e., anaplasia) determines the potential for malignancy.
   b. **Hyperplasia** involves an increase in the number of cells in a tissue; it may be a normal or an abnormal cellular response.

(Text continues on page 556.)

TABLE 20-1
Cancer types: Characteristics and treatments

Type	Etiology and risk factors	Clinical manifestations	Treatment
Bladder cancer	■ Carcinogens in the workplace, such as dyes, rubber, leather, ink, or paint ■ Recurrent bacterial infection of urinary tract ■ Smoking	■ Gross, painless hematuria ■ Urinary frequency ■ Urgency ■ Dysuria ■ Pelvic or back pain with metastasis	■ Intravesical (into bladder) chemotherapy ■ Chemotherapy ■ Radiation therapy ■ Uretoroenterocutaneous diversions (intestines used) or cutaneous (opening onto abdominal walls)
Bone tumors	■ Unclear ■ Osteogenic sarcoma: < 20 years old ■ Chondrosarcoma: adult males ■ Multiple myeloma: 50 to 70 years old	■ Bone pain (mild to severe) ■ Movement limitation ■ Palpable fixed mass on bone ■ Pathological bone fractures	■ Surgery (amputation) ■ Chemotherapy ■ Radiation therapy
Brain cancer (gliomas, meningiomas, pituitary adenomas, neurinomas)	■ Unknown, but areas under investigation include genetic changes, hereditary, ionizing radiation, environmental hazards, viruses, and injury	■ Depend on tumor type, location, rate of growth ■ General manifestations: increased intracranial pressure (headache, vomiting, papilledema, and altered sensorium)	■ Surgery ■ Chemotherapy ■ Radiation therapy
Breast cancer	■ Exact cause unknown ■ Familial history ■ Early menarche, late menopause, nulliparous or first child after age 34 ■ High-fat diet ■ Hormonal contraceptive use	■ A nontender lump, usually in an upper outer quadrant ■ Axillary lymphadenopathy (late) ■ Fixed nodular breast mass (late) ■ Pain (late)	■ Chemotherapy ■ Radiation therapy ■ Mastectomy
Cervical cancer	■ Unknown ■ Associated factors are multiple sex partners, early sexual activity, and viral infections of the cervix	■ Abnormal Papanicolaou (Pap) smear findings ■ Vaginal discharge (early) ■ Spotting (early) ■ Chronic erosion of cervix (early) ■ Pain in back and legs (late)	■ Radiation implant ■ Chemotherapy ■ Hysterectomy
Colon cancer	■ Familial history ■ Chronic inflammatory bowel disease ■ Polyps ■ Low-fiber diet	■ Change in bowel habits ■ Passage of blood in stools ■ Unexplained anemia, anorexia, weight loss, and fatigue ■ Right sided: abdominal pain, melena ■ Left sided: abdominal pain, cramping, narrowing stools, constipation, distention	■ Chemotherapy ■ Radiation therapy ■ Segmental resection with anastomosis ■ Abdominoperineal reaction with sigmoid colostomy ■ Temporary colostomy ■ Permanent colostomy or ileostomy

(continued)

TABLE 20-1

Cancer types: Characteristics and treatments *(continued)*

Type	Etiology and risk factors	Clinical manifestations	Treatment
Esophageal cancer	■ Chronic irritation ■ Ingestion of alcohol and tobacco use	■ Disease usually advanced when symptoms occur ■ Dysphagia with solid foods ■ Feeling of a mass in the throat ■ Painful swallowing	■ Radiation therapy ■ Chemotherapy ■ Esophagectomy
Gastric cancer	■ Diet high in smoked foods ■ Lack of fruits and vegetables ■ Chronic stomach inflammation ■ Pernicious anemia ■ Achlorhydria (absence of hydrochlroic acid) ■ Gastric ulcers ■ *Helicobacter pylori* bacteria	■ Early signs may be absent, leading to indigestion ■ Anorexia ■ Dyspepsia ■ Weight loss ■ Abdominal pain ■ Constipation	■ Radical surgery ■ Subtotal gastrectomy ■ Total gastrectomy ■ Chemotherapy
Kidney cancer	■ Tobacco use ■ Occupational exposure to industrial chemicals	■ Most produce no symptoms and are discovered on routine physical examination ■ Classic triad hematuria, pain, mass in flank	■ Radical nephrectomy along with radiation therapy ■ Hormone therapy ■ Chemotherapy
Laryngeal cancer	■ Familial tendency ■ Cigarette smoking ■ Chronic vocal straining ■ Prolonged alcohol ingestion	■ Intrinsic; persistent hoarseness ■ Extrinsic; no early hoarseness, throat pain and burning when drinking hot or acidic liquids; pain possibly radiating to ear ■ Late symptoms of both: dysphagia, hoarseness, dyspnea, cough, hemoptysis, foul-smelling breath, weight loss	■ Partial laryngectomy ■ Total laryngectomy ■ Radial neck dissection ■ Chemotherapy ■ Radiation therapy
Liver cancer	■ Factors include hepatitis B infection ■ Chronic liver disease ■ Anabolic steroid use ■ Long-term androgen therapy, primarily for metastatic sites	■ Recent weight loss ■ Weakness ■ Fatigue ■ Hepatomegaly ■ Jaundice ■ Ascites ■ Liver mass detected on palpation	■ Malignant liver cancer almost always fatal ■ Chemotherapy ■ Surgery ■ Transplantation
Lung cancer	■ Smoking ■ Occupational exposure to carcinogenic substances (asbestos, coal dust)	■ Persistent cough ■ Hemoptysis ■ Dyspnea ■ Hoarseness ■ Chest pain ■ Recurrent pleural effusion or pneumonia ■ Weight loss and fatigue	■ Chemotherapy ■ Radiation therapy ■ Lobectomy ■ Pneumectomy

TABLE 20-1

Cancer types: Characteristics and treatments *(continued)*

Type	Etiology and risk factors	Clinical manifestations	Treatment
Multiple myeloma	▪ Unclear	▪ Severe bone pain ▪ Signs or symptoms of anemia secondary to bone-marrow replacement with plasma cells ▪ Weight loss	▪ Combination chemotherapy ▪ Radiation therapy ▪ Protect from pathologic fractures
Oral cancer	▪ Associated with use of alcohol and tobacco, including smokeless tobacco	▪ No symptoms in early stages ▪ Painless sore or mass that does not heal, painless indurated (hardened) ulcer with raised lesions ▪ With progression, difficulty chewing, swallowing, or speaking	▪ Varies with nature of lesion ▪ Resectional surgery ▪ Radiation therapy ▪ Chemotherapy
Ovarian cancer	▪ Familial history ▪ Diethylstilbestrol (DES) therapy for pregnant woman ▪ DES in utero	▪ Pelvic pain or backache (early) ▪ Irregular menses ▪ Premenstrual tension ▪ Postmenstrual bleeding ▪ Dyspepsia ▪ Breast tenderness ▪ Silent onset	▪ Radiation therapy ▪ Chemotherapy ▪ Total abdominal hysterectomy with removal of fallopian tubes, ovaries, and omentum
Pancreatic cancer	▪ Exposure to chemicals ▪ High-fat diet ▪ Cigarette smoking ▪ Chronic pancreatitis	▪ May be initial or when cancer is in advanced stage ▪ Anorexia, weight loss ▪ Abdominal pain ▪ Jaundice ▪ Diarrhea or steatorrhea ▪ Palpable epigastric mass	▪ Chemotherapy ▪ Radiation therapy for palliation ▪ Pancreaticoduodenectomy ▪ Surgery for palliation
Penile cancer	▪ Males who are uncircumcised	▪ Painless ▪ Wartlike growth of ulcer on the glans or coronal sulcas	▪ Chemotherapy ▪ Radical prostatectomy ▪ Orchiectomy
Prostate cancer	▪ Age, race, familial history, alcohol intake, fat intake ▪ Exposure to fertilizer and occupation in tire and rubber industry	▪ Hematuria ▪ A hard, fixed nodule or asymptomatic	▪ Radiation therapy ▪ Hormonal therapy ▪ Chemotherapy ▪ May not be treated if life expectancy is <10 years
Skin cancer	▪ Sun exposure	▪ Small, elevated, multicolored nodules with irregular markings ▪ Large, flat, darkly pigmented area with irregular margins and scattered black margin	▪ Surgical excision ▪ Cryotherapy ▪ Curettage and electrodesiccation ▪ Radiation therapy ▪ Chemotherapy

(continued)

TABLE 20-1

Cancer types: Characteristics and treatments *(continued)*

Type	Etiology and risk factors	Clinical manifestations	Treatment
Spinal cord cancer	■ Unknown, but may develop as a consequence to metastatic tumors from lungs, breasts, the kidney, and GI tract	■ Pain ■ Motor dysfunction (muscle weakness, spasticity, decreased muscle tone, hyperreflexia, positive Babinski's sign) ■ Sensory deficits (loss of pain, temperature, and touch sensation) ■ Urinary retention ■ Constipation	■ Surgery ■ Radiation therapy ■ Chemotherapy
Testicular cancer	■ Cryptorchidism ■ Systemic infections ■ Epididymitis ■ Endocrine factors ■ Local trauma plays a role in development	■ Painless enlargement of the scrotum ■ Feeling of heaviness in the scrotum ■ Backache ■ Abdominal pain ■ Weight loss ■ Weakness ■ Palpable, firm, smooth testicular mass ■ Elevated alpha-fetoprotein and human chorionic gonadotropin levels	■ Orchiectomy ■ Radiation therapy ■ Chemotherapy
Thyroid cancer	■ Associated with exposure to external head and neck irradiation	■ Respiratory distress ■ Sensation of lump in throat ■ Dysphagia ■ Palpable, hard, painless nodule in the thyroid	■ Surgery (thyroidectomy) ■ Chemotherapy ■ Radiation therapy
Uterine (endometrial) cancer	■ Obesity, diabetes mellitus, hypertension, nulliparity, polycystic ovary disease, history of uterine polyps, history of infertility	■ Irregular vaginal bleeding ■ Postmenopausal bleeding ■ Abnormal Pap smears (25%)	■ Chemotherapy ■ Total hysterectomy ■ Bilateral salpingoophorectomy ■ External radiation therapy ■ Brachytherapy
Vulvular cancer	■ Unknown, but strong relationship with herpes simplex II and human papillomavirus infection	■ Pruritus (early) ■ Vulvar bleeding ■ Foul-smelling discharge ■ Pain ■ Vulvar mass or ulceration	■ Radiation therapy ■ Radial vulvectomy ■ Chemotherapy ■ Laser therapy

c. **Metaplasia** refers to the conversion of one type of cell in a tissue to another type not normal for that tissue. It results from an outside stimulus affecting parent stem cells and may be reversible. It could also progress to dysplasia.

d. **Dysplasia** refers to a change in size, shape, or arrangement of normal cells into bizarre cells; it may precede an irreversible neoplastic change.

e. **Anaplasia** involves a change in the DNA cell structure and in their orientation to one another, characterized by a loss of differentiation and a return to a more primitive form. The resulting poorly differentiated, irregularly shaped cells usually are malignant.

CLIENT AND FAMILY TEACHING 20-1
Ways to prevent cancer

- Explain to the client that risk reduction involves specific actions aimed at decreasing (but not eliminating) the risk of cancer development.
- Discuss with the client the American Cancer Society's nutritional guidelines to reduce the risk of many types of cancer:
  - Avoid obesity.
  - Decrease total dietary fat intake.
  - Eat more high-fiber foods, such as whole-grain cereals, fruits, and vegetables.
  - Include foods rich in vitamins A and C in the daily diet.
  - Include cruciferous vegetables (e.g., cabbage, broccoli, brussels sprouts, kohlrabi, cauliflower) in the diet.
  - Consume alcoholic beverages only in moderation.
  - Consume salt-cured, smoked, and nitrite-cured foods only in moderation.
- Strongly encourage the client to avoid tobacco use in all forms (e.g., cigarettes, cigars, smokeless tobacco).
- Encourage the client to avoid excessive sun exposure, particularly between 10 a.m. and 3 p.m. Instruct the client to use sunscreen with a sun-protection factor of 30 or greater and to wear large hats and long-sleeved clothing.
- Discuss with the client the importance of avoiding exposure to industrial agents known to increase cancer risk (e.g., nickel, asbestos, coal tar, rubber manufacture).

3. **Metastasis.** The metastatic process may be divided into three stages:
   a. **Invasion.** Neoplastic cells from primary tumor invade into surrounding tissue with penetration of blood or lymph; this occurs because cells are not encapsulated.
   b. **Spread.** Tumor cells spread through lymph or circulation or by direct expansion.
   c. **Establishment and growth.** Tumor cells are established and grow at secondary site: in lymph filter (lymph nodes) or in organs from venous circulation.

D. Prevention and detection

1. **Primary prevention**
   a. Cancer prevention focuses on reducing modifiable risk factors (see *Table 20-1*) in the external and internal environment that increase a person's susceptibility to cancer development. (See *Client and family teaching 20-1*.)
   b. General factors that influence cancer incidence and mortality include sex, age, geographic location, socioeconomic status, ethnic or cultural background, personal habits, occupation, and personal and family health histories.
2. **Secondary prevention** involves detection and case-finding efforts to achieve early diagnosis. (See *Table 20-2, page 558*.)
   a. Recognizing early signs and symptoms and seeking prompt treatment can significantly reduce morbidity and mortality of several types of cancer.
   b. After early detection, prompt intervention may halt the cancerous process in some cases.

E. Cancer management (See Table 20-1 for types of cancer treatment.)

1. **Surgery** is the surgical removal of tumors, the most commonly used treatment modality for cancer.
   a. **Preventive** or **prophylactic surgery** involves removing precancerous lesions (e.g., unusual skin growth, colorectal polyps, cervical cancer in situ).
   b. **Diagnostic surgery** is done to confirm or rule out malignancy from analysis of tissue samples obtained from incisional, excisional, or needle biopsies.
   c. **Curative surgery,** the most widely used cancer treatment, is a localized intervention aimed at removing all tumor tissue while limiting structural and functional impairment.

TABLE 20-2

Summary of American Cancer Society recommendations for the early detection of cancer in asymptomatic people

Test	Gender	Age	Frequency
Sigmoidoscopy, preferably flexible	Males and females	50 and older	Every 5 years
Fecal occult blood test	Males and females	50 and older	Every year
Colonoscopy	Males and females	50 and older	Every 10 years
Digital rectal examination	Males and females	50 and older	Every year
Prostate examination*	Males	50 and older	Every year
Papanicolaou (Pap) test	Females	All women who are or who have been sexually active, or who have reached 18 years of age, should have an annual Pap test and pelvic examination. After a woman has had three or more consecutive satisfactory normal annual examinations, the Pap test may be performed less frequently at the discretion of her physician.	
Breast self-examination	Females	20 and older	Every month (optional)
Breast clinical examination	Females	20 to 40	Every 3 years
		Older than 40	Every year
Mammography	Females	40 and over	Every year

*Men age 50 years and older should have an annual digital rectal examination and prostate-specific antigen (PSA) analysis. If the result of either test is abnormal, further evaluation should be considered.

Adapted with permission from *Cancer Facts and Figures—2004*. Atlanta: American Cancer Society, 2004.

   d. **Reconstructive surgery** aims to improve the client's quality of life by restoring maximal function and appearance; best outcomes depend on the cancer site and extent of surgery.
   e. **Palliative surgery** is done to:
   – retard tumor growth
   – decrease tumor size
   – relieve distressing manifestations of cancer when cure is no longer possible.
2. **Radiation therapy** involves directing high-energy ionizing radiation to destroy malignant tumor cells without harming surrounding tissues.
   a. **Curative radiation therapy**
   – Curative radiation therapy is used as localized treatment for solid tumors; approximately 50% of cancer clients receive radiation therapy at some point during the course of disease.
   – Curative radiation therapy aims to eradicate all disease and give the client the same life expectancy as a person who never had cancer.

      b. **Control radiation therapy** also may be used as an adjunct to other therapy, with the goal of prolonged and improved survival without disease eradication (e.g., preoperative radiation therapy to shrink a tumor, postoperative radiation therapy to eradicate microscopic disease, in conjunction with chemotherapy).

      c. **Palliative radiation therapy** may be used in advanced cancer to relieve symptoms of metastatic disease (e.g., pain, obstruction, bleeding, pathologic fractures).

  3. **Chemotherapy** involves administering antineoplastic drugs to promote tumor cell death by interfering with cellular functions and reproduction.

      a. **Curative therapy** involves early, aggressive treatment aimed at eradicating disease.

      b. **Salvage therapy** is a second attempt at curative intervention when disease recurs.

      c. **Control therapy** (consolidation therapy) aims to cause or sustain tumor regression and diminish symptoms to extend and improve the client's quality of life when cure is no longer possible.

      d. **Palliative treatment** is given to relieve or diminish distressing symptoms, such as pain, obstruction, pleural effusions, or hypercalcemia.

  4. **Bone marrow peripheral stem cell transplantation** involves aspirating bone marrow cells from a compatible donor and infusing them into the recipient. Bone marrow transplantation is a complex therapy with a high risk of complications. Objectives of bone marrow transplant include:

      a. cure

      b. complete marrow recovery within 6 to 8 weeks

      c. proliferation of donor cells in marrow, leading to release of functional blood cells into circulation.

  5. **Immunotherapy** uses the body's own immune mechanisms to combat and overcome cancer. Through the administration of chemical or microbial agents, immunotherapy aims to challenge and induce mobilization of immune defenses. The resultant delayed hypersensitivity response can be directed against cancer cells.

  6. **Biologic response modifiers (BRMs)** involve agents or treatment methods that have the ability to alter the immunologic relationship between tumor and host in a therapeutically beneficial way. The objective of BRM therapy is the destruction or cessation of malignant growth.

  7. **Gene therapy** treats the disease by the transfer of genetic material into the deoxyribonucleic acid of the client's cells, which involves removal of cells, culturing the cells in a specific medium, altering the cells using a vector containing the desired gene, and reintroducing the cells into the client. Gene therapy is used as adjunctive therapy. Research shows that altered cells have remained active for 2 to 11 months.

NURSING PROCESS OVERVIEW

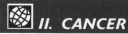 *II. CANCER*

A. Assessment

  1. **Health history**

      a. **Elicit a description of the client's present illness and chief complaint,** including onset, course, duration, location, and precipitating and alleviating factors.

        – Clinical manifestations vary with the type of cancer. (See *Table 20-1,* pages 553 to 556.)

- 🖐 – Cancer's seven early warning signals (remember the acronym CAUTION):
  - **C**hange in bowel or bladder habits
  - **A** sore that does not heal
  - **U**nusual bleeding or discharge
  - **T**hickening of lump in breast or elsewhere
  - **I**ndigestion or difficulty in swallowing
  - **O**bvious change in wart or mole
  - **N**agging cough or hoarseness
  - *b.* **Explore the client's health history for risk factors** associated with oncology disorders. Specific risk factors vary with the type of cancer. (See *Table 20-1*, pages 553 to 556.)
2. **Physical examination.** *Table 20-1,* pages 553 to 556, shows types of cancer and clinical manifestations found on physical examination.
   - *a.* **Inspection**
     - Assess the skin and mucous membranes for lesions, bleeding, petechiae, and irritation.
     - Assess stools, urine, sputum, and vomitus for acute or occult bleeding.
     - Inspect the scalp, noting hair texture and hair loss.
   - *b.* **Palpation**
     - Palpate the abdomen for any masses, bulges, or abnormalities.
     - Palpate lymph nodes for enlargement.
   - *c.* **Auscultation**
     - Auscultate lung sounds.
     - Auscultate heart sounds.
     - Auscultate bowel sounds.
3. **Laboratory and diagnostic studies**
   - *a.* **Complete blood cell count** identifies abnormalities in platelet count ($<100,000/mm^3$) and white blood cell (WBC) count (normal, $10,000/mm^3$).
   - *b.* **Tumor markers** are used to identify substances in the blood that are made by the tumor.
   - *c.* **Magnetic resonance imaging** creates sectional images of various body structures.
   - *d.* **Endoscopy** allows direct visualization of a body cavity.
   - *e.* **Nuclear medicine imaging** reveals images of tissues that have concentrated radioisotope substances.
   - *f.* **Biopsy** is performed to obtain tissue and cells for analysis of cancer, including its stage and grade.
     - Staging determines the size of the tumor and the existence of metastasis. The tumor, node, and metastasis system is frequently used in describing malignancies. (See *Table 20-3*.)
     - Grading refers to the classification of tumor cells. Low numeric grades (e.g., grade I) reflect well-differentiated tumors that deviate minimally from normal cells. High numeric grades (e.g., grade IV) reflect poorly differentiated tumors.

B. Nursing diagnoses
1. Acute or chronic pain
2. Impaired skin integrity
3. Impaired oral mucous membrane
4. Risk for injury
5. Risk for infection

TABLE 20-3
TNM classification system

T subclasses

Tx	Tumor cannot be adequately assessed
T0	No evidence of primary tumor
T1S	Carcinoma *in situ*
T1, T2, T3, T4	Progressive increase in tumor size and involvement

N subclasses

Nx	Regional lymph nodes cannot be assessed clinically
N0	Regional lymph nodes demonstrably normal
N1, N2, N3, N4	Increasing degrees of demonstrable abnormalities of regional lymph nodes

M subclasses

Mx	Not assessed
M0	No (known) distant metastasis
M1	Distant metastasis present, specify site(s)

Histopathology

G1	Well-differentiated grade
G2	Moderately well-differentiated grade
G3, G4	Poorly to very poorly differentiated grade

T—Primary tumor; N—Regional lymph nodes; M—Distant metastasis

Adapted from National Cancer Institute. "Staging: Questions and Answers." Available at: *http://cis.nci.nih.gov/fact/5_32.htm.* Last accessed: August 24, 2004

6. Fatigue
7. Imbalanced nutrition: less than body requirements
8. Risk for imbalanced fluid volume
9. Disturbed body image
10. Deficient knowledge
11. Ineffective coping
12. Social isolation

C. **Planning and outcome identification.** The major goals of the client diagnosed with cancer include pain relief, integrity of skin and oral mucosa, absence of injury and infection, fatigue relief, maintenance of nutritional intake and fluid and electrolyte balance, improved body image, absence of complications, knowledge of prevention and cancer treatment, effective coping through the recovery and grieving process, and optimal social interaction.

D. Implementation

1. **Promote measures that relieve pain and discomfort.**

    ✋ *a.* Assess the client's pain, rule out any complications of treatment therapy or disease process, provide pain management as needed, and evaluate the effectiveness of pain medication.

    b. Use distraction, relaxation techniques, and imagery before, during, and after chemotherapy.

    ✋ *c.* Always believe the client, and do not be judgmental about pain tolerance.

2. **Promote measures that maintain intact skin integrity.**

    a. Keep the radiated treatment area dry.

    b. Wash with water only, patting skin dry.

    ✋ *c.* Never apply ointment, powder, lotion, heat, ice, or other substances to the treatment field unless prescribed by the radiotherapist.

    d. Avoid washing off target marks made by the radiation therapist.

    e. Shave with an electric razor only in the treatment area.

    f. Instruct the client to avoid clothes that rub or bind.

    g. Teach the client to avoid sun exposure to the treatment site.

    h. If the client suffers hair loss from therapy, instruct him to cover his head when outdoors to prevent body heat loss or sunburn.

3. **Promote measures that maintain the oral mucosa.**

    a. Assess the oral cavity daily for signs of stomatitis and report changes in sensation, appearance, or taste.

    ✋ *b.* Encourage oral hygiene only as prescribed by the radiation therapist; warn the client to avoid commercial mouthwashes and lemon and glycerin products, as these promote drying and irritation.

    c. Offer artificial saliva or sugarless candy to increase salivation if xerostomia (i.e., dryness due to salivary changes) occurs.

    d. Instruct the client to swish and swallow with 1 to $1^1/_2$ teaspoons of antacid before meals.

    e. Teach the client to gargle with a solution of baking soda and water (1 teaspoon in 500 ml) or salt (0.5 teaspoon), baking soda (1 teaspoon), and water (1,000 ml) or hydrogen peroxide with water (1:4 ratio).

    f. Recommend the use of a soft toothbrush or "toothette."

    g. Instruct the client to remove dentures except for eating.

    h. Advise the client to avoid extremely hot or cold foods, spices, and citrus juices.

    i. Advise the client to avoid smoking and alcohol intake.

    j. Teach the client to keep his lips moist with a water-based lip balm.

    ✋ *k.* Instruct the client to report any redness, open lesions, decreased tolerance to temperature of food, and discomfort that interferes with nutritional intake and lasts more than 2 days.

4. **Promote measures to prevent injury from abnormal bleeding.**

    ✋ *a.* Monitor platelet count, and notify the health care provider if it drops below 100,000/mm³.

    b. Teach the client to avoid aspirin products.

    c. Instruct the client on the signs and symptoms of hemorrhage.

    d. Assess for pallor, dizziness, rapid pulse, tinnitus, and anginal pain.

    e. Observe the client's skin frequently for ecchymoses and petechiae.

    f. Instruct the client to avoid cuts, bruises, or other trauma; instruct the client to shave with an electric razor and keep nails short.

    g. Avoid administering parenteral injections; if they are unavoidable, apply pressure to the injection site after administration for at least 5 minutes.

    h. Administer blood products as prescribed.

    i. Administer oprelvekin, which stimulates platelet production.

5. **Promote measures to identify and prevent infection.**

    a. Monitor WBC count, and notify the health care provider if it drops below 2,000/mm³.

    b. Teach the client with a depressed WBC count the signs and symptoms of infection to watch for and report.

    c. Explain the client's increased vulnerability to infection; caution against exposure to upper respiratory and other infections.

    d. Encourage frequent handwashing and overall cleanliness.

    e. Institute standard precautions at all times. Maintain the client in reverse isolation, if needed.

    f. Administer filgrastim to stimulate WBC production.

6. **Promote measures to help decrease the client's fatigue and increase his activity level.**

    a. Reassure the client that fatigue commonly results from radiation therapy, chemotherapy, bone marrow transplant, and blood transfusions and is not an indicator of worsening disease.

    b. Provide for rest periods during the day, especially before and after priority activities.

    c. Help the client rearrange daily schedule and organize activities to conserve energy.

    d. Encourage the client to ask for assistance with necessary chores.

    e. Administer erythropoietin, which stimulates red blood cell production.

7. **Promote measures that ensure adequate nutritional intake.**

    a. Promote a high-protein, high-calorie diet (if the client is not diabetic).

    b. Provide a bland diet as indicated.

    c. Adjust the client's diet before and after treatment according to food preferences. Experiment with sour foods; avoid sweet, fatty, or spicy foods.

    d. Provide cold or room-temperature foods to minimize food odors, which can trigger nausea.

    e. Offer clear liquids to be sipped slowly.

    f. Eliminate unpleasant sights, odors, and sounds from the client's environment.

    g. Provide refreshing mouth care before meals.

    h. Make provisions for calorie counting and diet history.

    i. Present small portions attractively in a pleasant setting, ensure physical comfort, and encourage mealtime company.

    j. Keep in mind that cancer or cancer treatment may contribute to altered taste and food preferences.

8. **Promote measures that ensure adequate fluid and electrolyte balance.**

    a. Promote increased fluid intake (up to 3,000 ml/day) if not contraindicated.

    b. Monitor frequency of vomiting and the amount and character of emesis.

    c. Weigh the client daily, noting any weight loss.

    d. Assess for dehydration, checking skin turgor and the oral mucosa.

    e. Maintain accurate intake and output records.

    f. Monitor stools for diarrhea; if indicated, reinforce a low-residue diet and high-fluid intake, and administer antidiarrheal medication as prescribed.

    g. If the client complains of nausea, administer antiemetics before meals or as needed, and plan rest periods before and after meals.

9. **Promote measures to enhance body image.**

✋ *a.* Take an honest, gentle, caring approach, encouraging the client to express fears and feelings of loss.

b. Encourage the client to verbalize feelings concerning change in body image.

c. Encourage the client and significant others to share concerns about altered body image regarding sexuality or sexual concerns and to explore alternatives to usual sexual expression.

d. Encourage the client with mastectomy to use community resources available to cope with body-image changes, including advocacy groups and spiritual advisors.

e. Discuss the possibility of reconstructive surgery, which provides psychologic benefit for altered body image, and encourage the client to discuss this option with support groups that provide education and peer support.

f. If the client has an amputation, encourage the client to look at, feel, and care for the residual limb. Help him to regain his previous level of independent functioning.

g. Inform the client if hair loss is expected.

h. Explain that the hair that regrows may differ in color or texture. If hair loss is the result of radiation therapy to the head, prepare the client to understand that the alopecia may be permanent.

i. Suggest that occasional wig wearing before hair loss may ease the adjustment process, and help the client obtain a hairpiece before hair loss begins.

j. Arrange for contact with another person who has experienced hair regrowth after chemotherapy.

✋ *k.* Never communicate that hair loss is an insignificant problem compared with life-threatening alternatives; the client's emotional needs may be as great as physical needs.

l. Instruct the client to use a mild, protein-based shampoo every 3 to 5 days, avoid excessive shampooing, rinse thoroughly, and gently pat the hair dry.

m. Advise the client to avoid using hair dryers, electric curlers, curling irons, hair clips, elastic bands, barrettes, bobby pins, hair spray, dye, and permanents — all of which may increase the fragility of hair.

n. Suggest that the client sleep on a satin pillowcase to decrease hair trauma and tangles.

o. Advise the client to avoid excessive brushing and combing of hair; comb only with a wide-tooth comb.

p. Encourage the client to wear a cap or scarf at night to prevent heat loss through the scalp.

10. **Promote measures that address preventing complications of cancer therapy.**

a. Assess for central nervous system (CNS) changes; report any significant findings.

b. Assess the client's compliance with the prescribed medication regimen (e.g., steroids).

c. Monitor for urinary-system complications (e.g., hematuria, dysuria, frequency).

d. Reinforce radiation safety precautions.

e. Monitor laboratory results for reduced leukocytes, erythrocytes, and platelets, and report abnormal findings.

f. Observe for evidence of infection and bleeding; during menses, record pad count, and note the amount of saturation.

g. Instruct the client to avoid using enemas and straining during bowel movements.

h. Institute measures to prevent complications from immobility.

11. **Instruct the client and his family about the disease process and treatments, and provide necessary information for self-care.**
    a. Provide oral instructions and written materials.
    b. Encourage return demonstration of all teaching when applicable.
    c. Instruct the client to report signs and symptoms of complications to the health care provider.
12. **Promote measures that help the client and his family cope effectively with the disease process and the grieving process.**
    a. Allow and encourage verbalization of anger, sadness, or resentment by the client and significant others.
    b. Assess for signs and symptoms of depression, which include irritability, withdrawal, apathy, tearfulness, decreased ability to make decisions, impaired concentration or memory, increasing insomnia, and suicidal ideas.
    c. Assess the client's stressors, and evaluate the client's perception of stressors and beliefs about their causes.
    d. Determine available resources and support systems.
    e. Design strategies; gather agency support to address concerns about equipment, prostheses, home care, and hospice.
    f. Identify unsuccessful coping behaviors, and make referrals to mental health professionals or clergy as indicated.
    g. Encourage the client and his family to discuss advance directives, durable power of attorney for health care, last will and testament, and the funeral plan.
    h. Refer the client to the American Cancer Society. (See appendix A.)
13. **Promote measures to reduce social isolation.**
    a. Encourage frequent telephone calls to friends and relatives.
    b. Promote diversionary activities, such as television, radio, puzzles, and hobbies, depending on mobility.
    c. Provide frequent staff checks on the client, with time to talk whenever possible.
14. **Provide nursing interventions for the client undergoing surgery for cancer** following the basic principles of preoperative and postoperative nursing care. (See chapter 21.) Selected nursing interventions for some types of cancer have been included in this section.
    a. Provide nursing interventions for the client with laryngeal cancer undergoing a total laryngectomy (i.e., total removal of the larynx).
       – Monitor nasogastric tube feedings.
       – Offer thick liquids after the laryngectomy tube is removed (3 to 6 weeks postoperatively) because they prevent choking and aspiration.
       – Instruct the client to cleanse around the stoma site twice each day.
       – Instruct the client to not allow water into the stoma.
       – Instruct the client to avoid hair spray, powders, and tissues around the stoma or getting small hairs in the stoma when shaving.
       – Discuss alternate forms of communication (e.g., esophageal speech, electronic larynx, transesophageal speech).
    b. Provide nursing interventions for the client with colon cancer undergoing a colostomy (ascending, transverse, descending, sigmoid).
       – Assess the abdominal stoma for edema, pink color, small amount of mucus drainage, and no excessive bleeding.

- Assess rectoperineal dressing with a Penrose drain; assist with mechanical irrigation and sitz baths.
- Apply a protective skin barrier around the stoma.
- Demonstrate and discuss colostomy irrigation and care (e.g., skin care; applying, managing, and removing drainage pouch; irrigating the colostomy).
- Discuss nutritional status.
- Discuss sexuality issues.

c. Provide nursing interventions for the client with breast cancer who has had a mastectomy.
  - Assess the surgical drain from the mastectomy, and instruct the client on care of the surgical site.
  - Teach and have a return demonstration of postmastectomy exercises.
  - Instruct the client to avoid restrictive clothing on the affected side, with no blood draws or heavy objects on the affected side.
  - Instruct the client to avoid injuries (e.g., sunburn, cuts, burns) on the affected side and to notify a health care provider about complications.
  - Discuss sexuality issues.
  - Discuss the importance of self-examination and mammograms of the remaining breast.

15. **Provide nursing interventions for the client undergoing radiation therapy.**
    a. Explain to the client that external radiation therapy usually is applied by high-energy radiograph machines (e.g., betatron, linear accelerator) or machines containing a radioisotope (e.g., cobalt 60). Clients receiving external radiation therapy do not retain radioactivity after therapy.
    b. Explain that internal radiation therapy involves placing specially prepared radioisotopes directly into or near the tumor itself or into systemic circulation. Sources include:
      - sealed source, involving isotopes placed in applicators, needles, seeds, ribbons, or catheters before placement into malignant tumor or cavities; removed when exposure time is adequate or may be left in tumor permanently (depends on half-life of the source)
      - unsealed source, used in systemic therapy and administered I.V. or orally (e.g., phosphorus 32).
    c. Discuss with the client the special precautions that must be adhered to during radiation therapy.
      - Discuss that the nurse must follow calculated safe time (less time, less exposure) and distance parameters (greater the distance, less exposure) specified by the radiation physicist when caring for the client.
      - Discuss the need for customized blocks and shields, which are used to protect normal tissues. Using lead or other materials to absorb energy helps reduce exposure in some cases. The type of rays emitted determines the radioactive precautions specified by the radiation safety officer.
    d. When counseling a client about possible adverse effects, be sure to emphasize the benefits of therapy. The severity of adverse effects depends on radiation dosage, type of radiation, proximity of tumor to skin surface, and size of treatment field.

16. **Provide nursing interventions for the client undergoing chemotherapy.**
    a. Discuss combination chemotherapy, which consists of two or more drugs (used effectively as single agents) administered simultaneously or in sequence to treat specific cancer and reduce the likelihood of drug resistance.

    b. Discuss adjuvant chemotherapy, which involves administering chemotherapeutic agents in combination with surgery or radiation therapy. This therapy may eradicate possible micrometastasis before it becomes clinically apparent.

    c. Provide anticancer drugs directly or indirectly to disrupt reproduction of cells by altering essential biochemical processes. Agents are classified according to their mechanism of action.

- Antimetabolites inhibit cell reproduction by interfering with manufacture of protein.
- Alkylating agents interfere with deoxyribonucleic acid (DNA) replication.
- Antineoplastic antibiotics interfere with or inhibit DNA or ribonucleic acid (RNA) synthesis.
- Vinca alkaloids inhibit cell division at metaphase.
- Various hormones and steroidal agents may influence processes related to RNA-to protein synthesis.
- Chemoprotective agents protect normal cells from damage.

    d. Provide nursing care during the administration of chemotherapy.

- Special care must be taken during administration of vesicant agents, because extravasation can cause tissue necrosis and damage to underlying tendons, nerves, and blood vessels. Only specially trained health care providers and nurses should administer vesicants.
- Provide nursing care for a long-term central venous catheter or implantable infusion device, which may be necessary if frequent, prolonged administration of vesicants is anticipated.
- Provide regional administration of chemotherapy, which allows high concentrations of drugs to be directed to a localized tumor. The types include:
  - topical
  - intrathecal (instillation into the CNS using lumbar puncture or an Ommaya reservoir placed in a ventricle)
  - intracavitary, in which medication is instilled directly into such areas as the abdomen, bladder, or pleural space
  - intraarterial, which allows major organs or tumor sites to receive maximal exposure with limited serum levels of drugs, reducing systemic adverse effects
  - intraperitoneal chemotherapy, used to treat colorectal and ovarian cancers.
- Take special precautions during chemotherapy.
- Never use chemotherapeutic agents to test vein patency.
- Stop the infusion any time vein patency is in question.
- Anticipate possible extravasation and hypersensitivity and review management procedures before administration (some medications have antidotes).
- Anticipate anaphylactic reactions as for any drug; if generalized or local reactions occur, stop the infusion and maintain venous access with normal saline solution or sterile distilled water.
- Provide nursing care for activity intolerance because most anticancer agents depress bone-marrow function, resulting in decreased blood-cell production.
- Provide nursing care for risk for infection and abnormal bleeding because myelosuppression decreases WBC and platelet counts.

17. Provide nursing interventions for the client undergoing bone marrow transplantation.

    a. Explain the type of bone marrow transplantation.

- In autologous transplantation, the marrow donor is the recipient; marrow is harvested during a period of disease remission, treated, and stored for later infusion.
- In syngeneic transplantation, the marrow donor is the recipient's identical twin.
- In allogeneic transplantation, the marrow donor is a family member whose human leukocyte antigen (HLA) type matches that of the recipient.
- In matched unrelated donor transplantation, the marrow donor is a matched unrelated donor (MUD) whose HLA types match that of the recipient.

  b. Assess for signs and symptoms of graft-versus-host disease, a syndrome induced by donor T lymphocytes acting against host tissues.

18. **Provide nursing interventions for a client receiving immunotherapy.**
   a. Make sure the client understands the specific type of immunotherapy.
   - In active immunotherapy, the client is injected with an antigen that stimulates development of antibodies; it may be specific (i.e., client is vaccinated with tumor-associated antigen to stimulate immune response) or nonspecific (i.e., injected materials have no relation to the tumor but increase the client's overall immune capacity).
   - Passive immunotherapy involves direct transfer of antitumor antibodies, immunologically competent lymphocytes, or immune lymphoid cells from a donor (a person cured of cancer or in remission) to a client with an active neoplasm; it provides short-term immunity.
   - Adoptive immunotherapy involves transferring passive immunity to a client, who later develops and maintains active immunity. Cells with antitumor reactivity are administered to the client with cancer; the client adopts the immunity from the cells and then incorporates it into the client's own immune system.
   - Adjunctive immunotherapy is a combination of the described immunotherapeutic approaches with other cancer modalities (i.e., surgery, radiation therapy, and chemotherapy).
   b. Ensure that clients undergoing immunotherapy receive the same nursing care as any client undergoing cancer treatment.

19. **Provide nursing interventions for a client receiving immunotherapy with biologic response modifiers (BRMs).**
   a. When caring for a client receiving BRM therapy, be sure to gain familiarity with each agent given and its potential adverse effects.
   b. Carefully document all aspects of data collection and nursing care.
   c. Ensure that clients undergoing BRM therapy receive the same nursing care as any client undergoing cancer treatment.

20. **Provide nursing interventions for a client receiving gene therapy.**
   a. Ensure that clients undergoing gene therapy receive the same nursing care as any client undergoing cancer treatment.
   b. Fully inform the client about the experimental treatment.

E. Outcome evaluation
1. The client reports pain relief and a decrease in discomfort.
2. The client shows no evidence of altered skin integrity.
3. The client's oral mucosa remains intact.
4. The client shows no evidence of injury from abnormal bleeding.
5. The client shows no evidence of local or systemic infection.
6. The client expresses the intention to increase activity as tolerated.
7. The client maintains a dietary intake sufficient to meet nutritional needs.
8. The client maintains adequate intake and output and normal electrolyte levels.

9. The client demonstrates positive adaptation to body-image changes.
10. The client has no complications related to chemotherapy, radiation, surgery, or any type of treatment for cancer.
11. The client verbalizes knowledge about the course of illness, treatment regimen, and complications to report to a health care provider.
12. The client and family demonstrate appropriate coping mechanisms in adapting to disease.
13. The client interacts with others appropriately to reduce social isolation.

Study questions

1. Which treatment would the nurse expect as the *most frequent* major treatment modality for cancer?
   1. Bone marrow transplantation
   2. Chemotherapy
   3. Radiation therapy
   4. Surgery

2. A nurse is discussing ways to prevent cancer to a group of individuals with varying ages at a local health fair. What should the nurse include in the teaching? (Select all that apply.)
   1. Importance of women having mammograms every year after age 60
   2. Importance of wearing sunblock of at least sun-protection factor (SPF) 15 or below when out in the sun
   3. Importance of a low-fat, high-fiber diet and increased fluids
   4. Importance of performing self-breast exams monthly
   5. Importance of all men having a prostate examination every year after age 30
   6. Importance of sigmoidoscopy at age 50 and every 5 years after that

3. Which statement by the client indicates successful teaching for the client undergoing a total laryngectomy?
   1. "I'll be breathing and talking as usual after this surgery."
   2. "There is no reason why I cannot use hair sprays and powders."
   3. "I should not take tub baths or use hand-held shower heads."
   4. "I will be breathing through my neck and will have to talk in a new way."

4. Which statement would be the nurse's best response when a 28-year-old woman asks the nurse, "What can I do to make sure I don't get breast cancer like my mother and sister?"
   1. "There is nothing you can do to make sure you don't get breast cancer."
   2. "You can detect the cancer early with monthly self-breast examinations and yearly mammograms."
   3. "You're frightened that you may get breast cancer like your mother and sister."
   4. "You should get a digital rectal examination every year and a yearly pelvic examination with a Papanicolaou test."

5. Which statement by the client would indicate to the nurse that teaching about decreasing the risk of skin cancer has been effective?
   1. "It is all right for me to stay in the sun as long as I use a sun block with a sun-protection factor (SPF) of 15."
   2. "I should avoid excessive sun exposure between the hours of 10:00 and 3:00."
   3. "I should wear sleeveless shirts and caps when I am out in the sun."
   4. "Because I have no history of skin cancer in my family, I don't have to worry."

6. Which assessment finding would warrant immediate intervention for the client who has just undergone a sigmoid colostomy for rectal cancer?
   1. Moist stoma site with small streaks of bright red blood
   2. Hypoactive bowel sounds in all four

quadrants

3. Blood pressure of 110/70 mm Hg, a pulse of 90 beats/minute, and a temperature of 99.4° F (37.4° C)
4. Dark purple-colored stoma site

7. Which discharge instruction would be included in the care plan for a client receiving chemotherapy?
   1. "Do not remove target marks on the skin and decrease fluid intake during therapy."
   2. "Report any skin burns and apply lotion to burned areas."
   3. "Avoid cuts, bruises, and trauma and inspect the skin for bruises and tiny red spots."
   4. "Use a straight razor to shave and an 18-gauge needle for self-administration of I.M. injections."

8. Which statement by the client indicates to the nurse that discharge teaching about radiation therapy has been successful?
   1. "I should gargle with a commerical mouthwash every day."
   2. "I should have low-protein foods and cold drinks."
   3. "I'll use a hard-bristle toothbrush to brush my teeth."
   4. "I need to drink lots of fluids and avoid smoking."

9. When caring for a client receiving radiation therapy for a glioblastoma, the nurse should be alert for which adverse effects?
   1. Nausea and vomiting
   2. Diarrhea and stomatitis
   3. Constipation and headache
   4. Cystitis and hirtuism

10. Which statement would be *most* appropriate by the nurse in response to a client receiving radiation therapy for painful prostatic metastasis of the lumbosacral spine who states, "I am going to beat this disease"?
   1. "Once cancer gets into the bones, there is nothing to be done."

2. "Many cancers are curable with irradiation."
3. "Have you considered trying a macrobiotic diet?"
4. "You may obtain very good pain relief from the irradiation."

11. Which intervention is associated with the role of secondary cancer prevention?
   1. Prevention of second malignancies
   2. Detection and screening for early diagnosis
   3. Prevention of genetic cancer inheritance
   4. Avoidance of smoking and sun exposure

12. Which intervention is recommended by the American Cancer Society for early detection of colorectal cancer?
   1. Yearly digital rectal examinations after age 50 and stool examinations after age 50
   2. Monthly testicular self-examinations and yearly proctosigmoidoscopy after age 30
   3. Yearly physical examinations in conjunction with yearly kidney, ureter, and bladder radiographs
   4. Digital rectal examination yearly after age 25 and monitoring for changes in bladder habits

13. Which statement indicates accurate understanding by the nurse about bone marrow transplantation?
   1. It is performed when cure is impossible.
   2. It is fairly risk-free because of improved methods of marrow harvesting.
   3. Thorough assessment of donor and recipient is necessary.
   4. The donor is always a family member.

14. Which intervention would be included in the care plan for a patient receiving chemotherapy who develops thrombocytopenia?
   1. Instructing the client to use a mild, protein-based shampoo every 3 to 5 days
   2. Encouraging frequent handwashing and overall hygiene measures

3. Instructing the client to swish and swallow with an antacid before meals
4. Observing the client's skin frequently for ecchymoses and petechiae

15. Which intervention would be appropriate for the client with neutropenia secondary to chemotherapy?
1. Avoiding any clothes that rub or bind
2. Brushing teeth with a soft-bristle toothbrush
3. Minimizing exposure to other people with infections
4. Monitoring hemoglobin and hematocrit levels and platelet count

16. When discussing preventative dietary measures for cancer, which recommendation would be appropriate to include in the client teaching?
1. Eating foods low in vitamin A and C
2. Increasing total dietary fat intake
3. Eating a low-fiber diet
4. Eating cruciferous vegetables

Answer key

1. The answer is **4.**
Surgery is the most frequently used major modality in the treatment of cancer. Bone marrow transplantation, a complex therapy with a high risk of complications, is not a major cancer treatment modality. Chemotherapy and radiation therapy are major modalities, but they are not the most frequently used modalities.

2. The answers are **3, 4, 6.**
The American Cancer Society recommends a low-fat, high-fiber diet, sigmoidoscopy to prevent colon cancer, and self-breast exams monthly for early detection of breast cancer. Mammograms should be yearly after age 40 (not 60), sunblock with an SPF greater than 30 helps prevent skin cancer, and prostate exams should be yearly after age 50 (not 30). Younger men are at risk for testicular cancer, not prostate cancer.

3. The answer is **4.**
With a total laryngectomy, all airflow occurs through a permanent tracheostomy. No air passes over the vocal cords for speech. Speaking requires the use of esophageal speech or an electronic device. The client breathes through the tracheostomy and must learn how to use new speaking methods. Clients should avoid sprays and powders around the stoma site to prevent irritation

and subsequent inhalation. Clients should also use measures to prevent water from entering the stoma site to prevent aspiration.

4. The answer is **2.**
The American Cancer Society recommends monthly breast self-examinations and physical examinations every 3 years for women between ages 20 and 40. Mammograms are recommended yearly if there is a history of breast cancer in the family. Although it is true that nothing can prevent breast cancer, early detection provides an excellent chance of total recovery with no metastasis. Because the client is asking for specific information, therapeutic responses, typically appropriate in most situations, are not appropriate in this situation. An annual digital rectal examination and a yearly pelvic examination with a Papanicolaou test are recommended for early detection of colon cancer and cervical cancer, respectively.

5. The answer is **2.**
Avoiding exposure to sunlight during the hours of 10 a.m. and 3 p.m. is important, because it is during this time that the sun's ray are the strongest and most damaging. To reduce the risk of skin cancer, the American Cancer Society recommends the use of a sunscreen with an SPF of 30 or greater, long-sleeved shirts, and large hats when outdoors.

Overexposure to the sun is the most common reason for skin cancer, with or without family history.

6. The answer is **4.**
A stoma site that appears dark purple indicates that blood supply to the area is decreased. If left alone, a necrotic stoma could result. Immediate intervention is necessary to restore the blood supply. A moist stoma with small streaks of red blood; hypoactive bowel sounds in all four quadrants; and blood pressure of 110/70 mm Hg, a pulse of 90 beats/minute, and a temperature of 99.4° F are normal assessment findings for a postoperative client who has just undergone a colostomy.

7. The answer is **3.**
The client receiving chemotherapy is at risk for bleeding because of a decreased platelet count. The client should be instructed to avoid any activities that may cause bleeding. Ecchymoses (i.e., bruises) and petechiae (i.e., small red spots) are signs of bleeding. Target marks are made on the skin when the client is receiving radiation therapy, not chemotherapy. Fluid intake should be increased with chemotherapy. Areas of redness occur after radiation therapy, and lotion should not be applied. These reddened areas should not be referred to as burns. Because clients receiving chemotherapy are prone to bleeding, they should use only electric razors, and I.M. injections should be avoided. If an injection is necessary, a small-gauge needle (21 gauge) is recommended.

8. The answer is **4.**
For the client receiving radiation therapy, increased fluid intake helps soothe irritated tissue and moisturize mucous membranes. Because smoking is an irritant, it should be avoided. Commercial mouthwashes contain alcohol and promote further drying of mucous membranes. A high-protein, high-calorie diet is essential to facilitate healing of normal epithelial tissue. Radiation therapy may cause mouth ulcers. Gentle brushing with a soft toothbrush is recommended. Vigorous brushing is contraindicated.

9. The answer is **1.**
The adverse effects of radiation therapy are directly related to the body site being irradiated. When the brain is the site, nausea and vomiting are possible because of increased intracranial pressure resulting from brain irradiation. Headache is possible, and alopecia is to be expected. Brain irradiation does not result in diarrhea, stomatitis, or constipation. Diarrhea is common in clients receiving radiation to the abdomen or pelvis. Stomatitis is associated with head and neck irradiation. Hirtuism (abnormal hair growth) and cystitis (inflammation of the bladder) do not occur.

10. The answer is **4.**
The client is expressing hope. The nurse's best response would be to reinforce the positive effects of therapy for metastatic disease, such as pain relief, and avoid destroying hope with negative responses. Controlling the effects of metastatic disease is the goal of palliative, not curative, therapy. Asking the client about using a macrobiotic diet, an unproven treatment method, is inappropriate, possibly offering the client false hope.

11. The answer is **2.**
Secondary prevention involves detection and case-finding efforts to achieve early diagnosis. General cancer-prevention measures apply to any primary or secondary malignancy. There is no known way to prevent genetic tendencies. Avoiding smoking and sun exposure, modifiable risk factors, are primary prevention measures.

12. The answer is **1.**
For the prevention of colorectal cancer, the American Cancer Society recommends a digital rectal examination every year after age 50, stool examinations for occult blood every year after age 50, and proctosigmoidoscopy every 3 to 5 years after age 50 following two normal annual examination findings. Testic-

ular self-examinations are recommended to detect testicular abnormalities. Proctosigmoidoscopy is recommended regularly after age 50 to detect colon disease. The American Cancer Society recommends physical examinations every 3 years between the ages of 20 and 40. Radiographs of the kidney, ureter, and bladder are used to detect colorectal cancer. Any change in bowel (not bladder) habits may suggest colorectal cancer.

13. The answer is **3.**
With bone marrow transplantation, a thorough assessment of the recipient and donor is required to determine physical and psychosocial factors that may influence the outcome. Bone marrow transplantation is performed for curative purposes. It is a complex procedure with many risks. In autologous transplantations, the marrow donor is also the recipient.

14. The answer is **4.**
Thrombocytopenia, a reduction in the number of platelets, increases the client's risk for bleeding. Frequent observations of the client's skin for ecchymoses and petechiae, indicators of bleeding, are essential. Using a mild protein-based shampoo is appropriate for the client experiencing alopecia. Frequent handwashing and overall hygiene measures are important even if the client does not experi-

ence any effects associated with chemotherapy. However, these take on even greater importance if the client's white blood cell count decreases, increasing his risk for infection. Swishing and swallowing an antacid before meals is helpful if the client has developed stomatitis.

15. The answer is **3.**
Neutropenia refers to a decrease in the white blood cell count, placing the client at risk for infection. Exposing the client to possible sources of infection, such as other individuals with infection, should be avoided. Avoiding clothes that rub or bind is indicated if the client has impaired skin integrity. Using a soft-bristle toothbrush and monitoring the hemoglobin and hematocrit levels and platelet count can address abnormal bleeding tendencies.

16. The answer is **4.**
Dietary measures for cancer prevention include intake of cruciferous vegetables, such as cabbage, broccoli, and Brussels sprouts; high-fiber foods; and foods rich in vitamin A and vitamin C. Total dietary fat intake also should be decreased.

21 *Perioperative nursing*

I. PERIOPERATIVE NURSING OVERVIEW

A. Operative phases. The perioperative period encompasses a client's total surgical experience, including the preoperative, intraoperative, and postoperative phases. Perioperative nursing refers to activities performed by the professional nurse during these phases.

  1. The **preoperative phase** begins with the decision to perform surgery and ends with the client's transfer to the operating room table.

  2. The **intraoperative phase** begins when the client is received in the operating room and ends with his admission to the postanesthesia care unit (PACU).

  3. The **postoperative phase** begins when the client is admitted to the PACU and extends through follow-up home or clinic evaluation.

B. Categories of surgery

  1. **Optional surgery** is done totally at the client's discretion (e.g., cosmetic surgery).

  2. **Elective surgery** refers to procedures that are scheduled at the client's convenience (e.g., cyst removal, repair of scars, simple hernia or vaginal repair).

  3. **Required surgery** is warranted for conditions necessitating intervention within a few weeks (e.g., cataract surgery, thyroid disorders).

  4. **Urgent or imperative surgery** is indicated for a problem requiring intervention within 24 to 48 hours (e.g., acute gallbladder infection, appendicitis, kidney stones).

  5. **Emergency surgery** describes procedures that must be done immediately to sustain life or maintain function (e.g., repair of a ruptured aortic aneurysm, gunshot or knife wounds, extensive burns, fractured skull).

C. Types of anesthesia

  1. **General anesthesia** (inhaled or I.V.) refers to drug-induced depression of the central nervous system that produces analgesia, amnesia, and unconsciousness (affects whole body); stages include:

    a. stage I: beginning

    b. stage II: excitement

    c. stage III: surgical anesthesia

    d. stage IV: danger.

  2. **Regional anesthesia** is a form of local anesthesia that suspends sensation and motion in a body region or part; the client remains awake. Continuous monitoring is required in the event the block is not totally effective and the client experiences pain or reactions to blocking agents (e.g., nausea, cardiovascular collapse). Regional anesthesia differs in terms of location and size of the anatomic area anesthetized and the volume and type of anesthetic agent used.

  3. **Spinal anesthesia** is a local anesthetic injected into the subarachnoid space at the lumbar level to block nerves and suspend sensation and motion to the lower extremities, perineum, and lower abdomen.

  4. **Conduction blocks** sensation and motion on various groups of nerves, such as epidural block (i.e., anesthetic into space around the dura mater), brachial plexus block (i.e., produces anesthesia of the arm), paravertebral block (i.e., produces anesthesia of the chest, abdominal wall, and extremities), and transsacral (caudal) block (i.e., anesthesia of the perineum).

D. Perioperative team. The perioperative team generally includes the surgeon, anesthesiologist or nurse anesthetist, operating room nurse, the circulatory nurse, the scrub nurse, surgical technicians, radiographic or cardiovascular technicians, and the PACU nurse. Their roles are discussed with the client before surgery.

1. An **anesthesiologist or nurse anesthetist** makes a preoperative assessment to plan the type of anesthetic to be administered and to evaluate the client's physical status.

2. A **professional registered operating room nurse** makes preoperative nursing assessments and documents the intraoperative client care plan.

3. The **circulating nurse** manages the operating room and protects the safety and health needs of the client by monitoring the activities of the members of the surgical team and monitoring the conditions in the operating room.

4. The **scrub nurse** is responsible for scrubbing for surgery, including setting up sterile tables and equipment and assisting the surgeon and surgical technicians during the surgical procedure.

5. The **PACU nurse** is responsible for caring for the client until the client has recovered from the effects of anesthesia, is oriented, has stable vital signs, and shows no evidence of hemorrhage.

E. Principles of surgical asepsis

1. Operating-room personnel must practice strict standard precautions (i.e., blood and body substance isolation).

2. All items (e.g., instruments, needles, sutures, dressings, covers, solutions) used in the operating room must be sterile.

3. All operating-room personnel must perform a surgical scrub.

4. All operating-room personnel are required to wear specific, clean attire, with the goal of "shedding" the outside environment. Specific clothing requirements are prescribed and standardized for all operating rooms.

   a. Operating-room personnel must wear a sterile gown, gloves, and special shoe covers.

   b. Hair must be completely covered.

   c. Masks must be worn at all times in the operating room for the purpose of minimizing airborne contamination; they must be changed between operations or more often, if necessary.

5. Any personnel who harbor pathogenic organisms (e.g., those with colds or infections) must report themselves unable to be in the operating room to protect the client from outside pathogens.

6. Scrubbed personnel wearing sterile attire should touch only sterile items.

7. Sterile gowns and sterile drapes have defined borders of sterility. Sterile surfaces or articles may touch other sterile surfaces or articles and remain sterile; contact with unsterile objects at any point renders a sterile area contaminated.

8. The circulator and unsterile personnel must stay at the periphery of the sterile operating area to keep the sterile area free from contamination.

9. Sterile supplies are unwrapped and delivered by the circulator following specific standard protocol so as not to cause contamination.

10. The utmost caution and vigilance must be used when handling sterile fluids to prevent splashing or spillage.

11. Anything that is used for one client must be discarded or, in some cases, resterilized.

II. THE PERIOPERATIVE PERIOD

A. Assessment

1. **Identify any obvious risk factors for surgery-related complications.**
   a. The very young and old are at risk for increased stress from the surgical experience.
   b. Compromised nutritional status has a negative effect on recovery and wound healing.
   c. An obese client presents certain technical problems during surgery; is at greater risk for postoperative pulmonary complications, such as hypoventilation and hypoxia; and is more likely to have coexisting cardiac, hepatic, biliary, endocrine, or metabolic problems that could complicate surgery.
   d. Any possibility of pregnancy and any type of chronic illness or condition that may effect recovery from surgery must be identified.

2. **Assess respiratory status,** including history of pulmonary problems, to identify risk factors for postoperative complications, such as:
   a. dyspnea and complaints of shortness of breath
   b. upper respiratory infection
   c. cough and wheezing
   d. copious mucus or expectorate
   e. chest pain
   f. clubbed fingers
   g. history of smoking
   h. use of inhalants.

3. **Assess cardiovascular status,** noting:
   a. blood pressure
   b. apical pulse rate
   c. electrocardiographic tracings
   d. presence and amplitude of peripheral pulses.

4. **Assess for and report evidence of fluid and electrolyte imbalance,** including:
   a. dehydration
   b. hypovolemia
   c. prolonged vomiting, diarrhea, or bleeding
   d. abnormal serum potassium, sodium, magnesium, calcium, or pH level.

5. **Assess hepatic and renal function,** noting:
   a. history of liver disease (e.g., cirrhosis, chronic alcoholism)
   b. complaints of dysuria, oliguria or anuria, incontinence, or urinary tract infections
   c. urinalysis results.

6. **Examine the client's record for endocrine or metabolic problems** that could affect his response to surgery (e.g., poorly controlled diabetes mellitus).

7. **Assess immunologic and hematologic function,** noting:
   a. history of allergies
   b. previous reactions to blood transfusion
   c. immunosuppressed status
   d. history of substance abuse.

8. **Assess neurologic function,** noting:
   a. history of seizures or other neurologic disorders (e.g., Parkinson's disease, myasthenia gravis)

     b. level of consciousness, mental status and orientation

     c. unsteady gait

     d. unequal pupils.

  9. **Assess integumentary system,** noting:

     a. bleeding tendencies (e.g., ecchymosis, petechiae)

     b. contusions, abrasions, or skin breakdown.

  10. **Evaluate medication history** for drugs that could increase operative risk by affecting coagulation time or interacting with anesthetics, such as:

     a. steroids

     b. diuretics

     c. phenothiazines

     d. antidepressants

     e. antibiotics

     f. anticoagulants.

  11. **Assess the client for any type of prosthetic devices or metal implants** (e.g., false eye, hip or knee replacements, pacemakers).

  12. **Assess the client and his family's knowledge base** to guide the preoperative teaching program.

  13. **Consider psychosocial factors that could affect the client's response to surgery,** including:

     a. anxiety and fear

     b. defense mechanisms (e.g., regression, denial, intellectualization)

     c. self-esteem and body-image concerns.

B. Nursing diagnoses

  1. Anxiety

  2. Deficient knowledge

C. Planning and outcome identification. The major goals for the client during the preoperative period include decreased anxiety and increased knowledge of the surgical experience.

  1. **Promote measures that help decrease anxiety for the client and his family.**

     a. Assess the client and his family to identify concerns that can effect the surgical experience (e.g., fear of the unknown, fear of death, loss of work, loss of role).

     b. Encourage the client and his family to verbalize feelings. Listen attentively, and provide factual information that may allay concerns.

     c. Respect and support the spiritual beliefs of the client and his family and assist the client in obtaining the spiritual help that may be requested.

     d. Respect and support the cultural beliefs of the client and his family and allow any activities that do not directly effect the surgical experience.

  2. **Discuss the surgical experience with the client and his family to minimize anxiety and increase knowledge.**

     a. Provide a quiet, nonthreatening atmosphere when teaching the client and his family.

     b. Present information at the appropriate education level of the client, include any written or visual information, and allow time for questions and answers.

     c. Discuss exactly what will happen from the time the client is being prepared for surgery (e.g., no oral intake [NPO]; removing clothes, jewelry, prosthetics, or dentures), including when the client will be taken to the operating room by stretcher, how cold the operating room will be, the time waiting in the preoperative area, and waking up in the postanesthesia care unit.

    d. Discuss the approximate length of time of surgery and where family members should wait for the surgeon to discuss the client's surgery.

    e. Reiterate that the client will be able to have pain medication and should request it before pain is severe; discuss the use of patient-controlled analgesia (PCA) pumps, if appropriate.

    f. Discuss the equipment the client will have after surgery (e.g., I.V. line, Foley catheter).

    g. Discuss and identify the location of an advance directive, living will, and durable power of attorney for health care.

3. Provide client and family teaching. Instruct the client in:

    a. deep breathing and coughing exercises

    b. relaxation techniques

    c. postoperative exercises of extremities

    d. turning and moving techniques

    e. pain-control techniques

    f. incentive spirometry use.

4. Perform preoperative skin preparation as appropriate, which may include:

    a. shaving the skin in and around the surgical area (most often done in the operating room)

    b. using an electric razor or clippers

    c. applying antibiotic scrub to the surgical area.

5. Provide GI preparation as prescribed, which may include:

    a. restricting solid food and fluid for 8 to 10 hours before surgery (to reduce the risk of aspiration)

    b. posting an NPO sign at the client's bedside

    c. administering an enema and inserting a nasogastric tube as prescribed.

6. Make sure the client or a responsible family member has provided informed consent for surgery. Verify that an operative permit is signed and witnessed, with informed consent based on an understandable explanation from the surgeon about what will be done and the risks involved. The client must be a mentally competent adult or an emancipated minor to sign the consent form. If these requirements cannot be met, the responsible relative or guardian should sign for the client. State laws govern situations when a relative or guardian is not available.

7 Perform standard preoperative procedures. A preoperative checklist is completed before the client goes to the operating room. (See *Figure 21-1*, page 580.)

    a. Take and record vital signs.

    b. Verify any allergy, identification, or diabetic bands.

    c. Validate nothing-by-mouth status.

    d. Complete and record medical preoperative orders.

    e. Remove all jewelry, nail polish, acrylic nails, and hair pins.

    f. Have the client void and don a clean hospital gown.

    g. Remove dentures, eyeglasses, contacts, and hearing aids, or send labeled containers with the client to the operating room for safe placement in case removal becomes necessary.

    h. Administer preanesthetic medications, and instruct the client to stay in bed.

    i. Document any client condition requiring operating-room personnel attention (e.g., musculoskeletal or sensorineural problems).

8. Ensure safe transport of the client to the surgical suite (e.g., check for a stretcher with side rails, safety strap, and warm blankets).

FIGURE 21-1
Preoperative checklist

1. Patient's name: _____ Date: _____ Height: _____ Weight: _____
   Identification band present: _____
2. Informed consent signed: _____ Special permits signed: _____
3. History and physical examination report present: _____ Date: _____
4. Laboratory records present:
   CBC: _____ Hb: _____ Urinalysis: _____ Hct: _____

5. Item	PRESENT	REMOVED
a. Natural teeth		
Dentures: upper, lower, partial		
Bridge, fixed; crown		
b. Contact lenses		
c. Other prostheses — type: _____		
d. Jewelry:		
Wedding band (taped/tied)		
Rings		
Earrings: pierced, clip-on		
Neck chains		
e. Make-up		
Nail polish		
6. Clothing		
a. Clean patient gown		
b. Cap		
c. Sanitary pad, etc.		

7. Family instructed where to wait? _____
8. Valuables secured? _____
9. Blood available? _____ Ordered? _____ Where? _____
10. Preanesthetic medication given: _____ _____
    SIGNATURE TIME
11. Voided: _____ Amount: _____ Time: _____ Catheter: _____
    Mouth care given: _____
12. Vital signs: Temperature: _____ Pulse: _____ Resp: _____ Blood pressure: _____
13. Special problems/precautions (allergies, deafness, etc.): _____
14. Area of skin preparation: _____
15. _____ Date: _____ Time: _____
    SIGNATURE: NURSE RELEASING PATIENT

Source: Smeltzer, S.C., and Bare, B.G. *Brunner and Suddarth's Textbook of Medical-Surgical Nursing,* 10th ed. Philadelphia: Lippincott Williams & Wilkins, 2003.

D. Outcome evaluation
1. The client exhibits and reports decreased anxiety concerning the surgical experience.
2. The client's family reports decreased anxiety concerning the client's surgical experience.
3. The client is able to verbalize an understanding of the surgical procedure, the preoperative nursing care, and the expected postoperative course.

4. The client verbalizes understanding of postoperative pain relief, including how to use devices such as PCA pumps, if appropriate.

NURSING PROCESS OVERVIEW

 III. THE INTRAOPERATIVE PERIOD

A. Assessment

1. **Classify the client's physical status for anesthesia.**
   a. No organic or systemic disturbance
   b. Mild disturbance (e.g., mild cardiac disease, mild diabetes mellitus)
   c. Severe systemic disturbance (e.g., poorly controlled diabetes mellitus, pulmonary complications)
   d. Life-threatening systemic disease (e.g., severe renal or cardiac disease)
   e. Moribund, with little chance of survival (e.g., ruptured aortic aneurysm)
2. **Assess the client's record for appropriate documentation,** including:
   a. current signed consent form
   b. completed history and physical-assessment record
   c. recent laboratory and diagnostic reports
   d. evaluation of the client's overall physiologic, emotional, and psychologic status. (See *Figure 21-1.*)
3. **Ask the client about any known allergies.**
4. **Verify client identification and that the correct surgery is scheduled.**
5. **Assess for special surgical considerations and precautions.**
6. **Assess the client's risk for accidental hypothermia or malignant hyperthermia during anesthesia administration and surgery.** Be sure that antidotal supplies are readily available in an emergency.

B. Nursing diagnoses

1. Risk for fluid volume imbalance
2. Risk for imbalanced body temperature
3. Risk for infection
4. Ineffective cardiac, respiratory, and peripheral tissue perfusion
5. Risk for perioperative-positioning injury

C. Planning and outcome identification.

The major goals for the client during the intraoperative period include maintenance of fluid balance, maintenance of normothermia, prevention of infection, adequate tissue perfusion, and absence of injury.

D. Implementation

1. **Promote measures that maintain adequate fluid and electrolyte balance.**
   a. Monitor intake and output accurately; use a urometer if needed.
   b. Assess the client for dehydration to include skin turgor and mucous membranes.
   c. Assess the client for circulatory overload to include breath sounds, peripheral edema, and jugular vein distention.
   d. Monitor pertinent electrolyte values.
2. Promote measures that maintain the client's normal temperature of 98° to 99° F. (36.7° to 37.2° C)
   a. Ensure that the operating room temperature is between 78° to 80° F (25.6° to 26.7° C).
   b. Warm all I.V. and irrigating solutions.
   c. Monitor the client's temperature continuously.

d. Remove all wet gowns and drapes promptly and replace with dry ones to prevent heat loss.

3. **Promote measures that decrease the risk of infection.**
    a. Maintain sterile procedures and techniques during surgery.
    b. Apply sterile dressings to all wounds.
    c. Ensure nonscrubbed personnel refrain from touching or contaminating anything that is sterile.
4. **Promote measures that ensure adequate tissue perfusion in the client during surgery.**
    a. Assess the client's vital signs continuously.
    b. Assess the client's respiratory status, and assist with mechanical ventilation.
    c. Assess the client's cardiovascular status.
    d. Assess the client's peripheral vascular status.
5. **Ensure the client's safety in the operating room.**
    a. Set room temperature and humidity to prevent hypothermia.
    b. Remove any potential contaminants.
    c. Curtail unnecessary room traffic.
    d. Keep room noise and talk at a minimum.
    e. Recheck electrical equipment for proper operation.
    f. Make sure that necessary equipment and supplies are available.
    g. Ensure that instruments, sutures, and dressings are ready.
    h. Count and record sutures, needles, instruments, and sponges.
    i. Make sure that staff call the client by name and provide individualized attention.
    j. Assist in transferring the client to the operating room table.
    k. Cover the client with a warm blanket, and attach the safety strap.
    l. Remain at the client's side during anesthesia induction.
    m. Verify proper client positioning to protect nerves, circulation, respiration, and skin integrity. Always pad pressure areas.
    n. Ensure that newly requested items are quickly supplied to the anesthesia or scrub team by the circulating nurse.
6. **Perform other actions as appropriate.**
    a. Act in the role of client advocate, providing privacy and protection from harm.
    b. Follow established procedures and protocols.
    c. Document all operating room care.
    d. Help coordinate health team activities.
    e. Promote ethical behaviors (e.g., respect, confidentiality).
    f. Monitor blood, fluid, and other drainage output.
    g. Maintain a quiet, relaxing atmosphere. Remember, the client can hear.

E. Outcome evaluation
1. The client maintains adequate fluid balance as evidenced by elastic skin turgor, moist buccal mucosa, and no peripheral edema or jugular vein distention, and the electrolyte status remains within normal limits.
2. The client maintains satisfactory body temperature (96° to 100° F [35.6° to 37.8° C]) on completion of surgery.
3. The client shows no signs or symptoms of systemic or wound infection.
4. The client arrives safely in the postanesthesia care unit and exhibits adequate cardiac, respiratory, and peripheral circulation.
5. The client remains free of any operative injury from electrical, chemical, or physical hazards related to surgery.

6. The client remains free from injury linked to positioning during surgery, as evidenced by no complaints of numbness, paralysis, or abrasions.

NURSING PROCESS OVERVIEW

 ## IV. THE IMMEDIATE POSTOPERATIVE PERIOD

A. Assessment

✋ **1.** Perform assessment immediately on the client's admission to the postanesthesia care unit (PACU) to obtain baseline data. (See *Figure 21-2*, page 584.)

2. Position the client before assessment to ensure an adequate airway; most commonly, the lateral Sim's position is used for an unconscious client unless contraindicated.

3. Prioritize the assessment accordingly.

   a. Respiratory assessment, including airway patency and skin color

   b. Cardiovascular assessment, including vital signs

4. Obtain a verbal report from the operating room nurse and anesthesiologist or nurse-anesthetist. The verbal report should describe:

   a. client's age and general condition

   b. any intraoperative problems encountered

   c. medical diagnosis and pathology

   d. fluids administered, blood loss and replacement, tubings and drains present

   e. specific individual problems or deficits, including hearing, vision, and mental status and any symptoms that may need to be immediately reported to the surgeon.

B. Nursing diagnoses

1. Ineffective cardiac, respiratory, urinary, neurologic, and peripheral tissue perfusion

2. Ineffective airway clearance

3. Acute pain

4. Impaired bed mobility

5. Anxiety

C. Planning and outcome identification. The major goals for the client during the immediate postoperative period include adequate tissue perfusion, absence of postoperative complications, maintenance of airway patency and respiratory function, pain relief, prevention of complications of immobility, and decreased anxiety.

D. Implementation

1. Assess the client's cardiac, respiratory, urinary, neurologic, and neurovascular status, and document the client's condition on the recovery room scoring guide. (See *Figure 21-2*, page 584.) Seven points is the minimum score required for discharge from the PACU.

2. Promote measures that address potential complications.

✋   *a.* Assess the following at least every 15 minutes (or more frequently, depending on the client's status):

     – Airway

     – Vital signs (every 5 minutes X 3; then every 15 minutes)

     – General appearance

     – Level of consciousness and reflexes

     – Movement of extremities

     – Pain level

FIGURE 21-2
Postanesthesia care unit chart

Modified Aldrete score

Patient: _____ Final score: _____

Room: _____ Surgeon: _____

Date: _____ PACU nurse: _____

Area of assessment	Point score		After		
			1 h	2 h	3 h
Muscle activity Moves spontaneously or on command:					
▪ Ability to move all extremities	2				
▪ Ability to move 2 extremities	1				
▪ Unable to control any extremity	0				
Respiration ▪ Ability to breathe deeply and cough	2				
▪ Limited respiratory effect (dyspnea or splinting)	1				
▪ No spontaneous effort	0				
Circulation ▪ BP ± 20% of preanesthetic level	2				
▪ BP ± 20% to 49% of preanesthetic level	1				
▪ BP ± 50% of preanesthetic level	0				
Consciousness level ▪ Fully awake	2				
▪ Arousable on calling	1				
▪ Not responding	0				
O_2 Saturation ▪ Unable to maintain O_2 sat > 92% on room air	2				
▪ Needs O_2 inhalation to maintain O_2 sat > 90%	1				
▪ O_2 sat < 90% even with O_2 supplement	0				
Totals:					

Required for discharge from postanesthesia care unit: 7 points

_____ _____
Time of release   Signature of nurse

Source: Smeltzer, S.C., and Bare, B.G. *Brunner and Suddarth's Textbook of Medical-Surgical Nursing,* 10th ed. Philadelphia: Lippincott Williams & Wilkins, 2003.

DRUG CHART 21-1
Medications for perioperative clients

Classifications	Indications	Selected interventions
Antibiotics aminoglycosides (gentamicin, tobramycin) ampicillin cefazolin ceftazidime cephalothin	Prevent or treat infections caused by pathogenic organisms	■ Before administering the first dose, assess the client for allergies and determine whether culture has been obtained. ■ After multiple doses, assess the client for superinfection (thrush, yeast infection, diarrhea); notify the health care provider if these occur. ■ Assess the insertion site for phlebitis if antibiotics are being administered I.V. ■ To assess the effectiveness of antibiotic therapy, monitor white blood cell count. ■ Monitor peaks and troughs for aminoglycosides.
Antiemetics benzquinamide dimenhydrinate promethazine scopolamine trimethobenzamide hydrochloride	Relieve nausea and vomiting by inhibiting medullary chemoreceptor triggers; drug choice depends on the cause of vomiting	■ Advise the client that this medication may cause drowsiness. ■ Because the medication may cause chemical irritation, administer by deep I.M. injection into a large muscle mass. ■ Measure emesis and maintain accurate intake and output; monitor for dehydration.
Opioid analgesics codeine hydrocodone hydromorphone morphine propoxyphene	Relieve moderate to severe pain by reducing pain sensation, producing sedation, and decreasing the emotional upset often associated with pain; most often schedule II drugs	■ Assess the pain for location, type, intensity, what increases or decreases it; rate pain on scale of 1 (no pain) to 10 (worst pain). ■ Rule out any complications. Is this pain routine or expected? Is this a complication that needs immediate intervention? ■ Medicate according to pain scale findings. ■ Institute safety measures—bed in low position, side rails up, and call light within reach. ■ Evaluate effectiveness of pain medication in 30 minutes.

- Urine output
- I.V. or central line patency
- Drain or catheter patency
- Operative site and dressings for signs of hemorrhage or abnormal drainage
- Functioning of cardiac and oxygen monitors
- Signs and symptoms of hypovolemic shock, a potential postoperative complication stemming from loss of blood and plasma during surgery

    b. Administer prescribed medications, which may include opioid analgesics, prophylactic antibiotics, and antiemetics. (See *Drug chart 21-1.*)

3. **Maintain airway patency and optimal respiratory function.** Position the client on his side until awake, administer oxygen as necessary, and encourage him to turn, cough, and deep-breathe every 30 minutes until fully awake.

4. **Provide pain relief.** Assess the client's pain, rule out any complication that requires immediate intervention, medicate or intervene to decrease pain, and evaluate effectiveness of pain medication.

5. **Promote measures that prevent complications of immobility.**

a. Assess the client for signs and symptoms of skin breakdown, respiratory difficulties, deep vein thrombosis, and bladder or bowel problems.

b. Encourage the client to turn, cough, and deep-breathe frequently.

c. Encourage the client to perform passive and active range-of-motion exercises frequently.

6. **Offer emotional support and reassurance,** and allow the client to verbalize feelings of anxiety.

E. Outcome evaluation

1. The client has adequate tissue perfusion as evidenced by stable cardiovascular, respiratory, urinary, neurologic, and neurovascular status.

2. The client scores at least 7 of 10 possible points on a postanesthesia scoring chart by the time of discharge to a clinical unit.

3. The client performs deep breathing and coughing and exhibits clear lungs on auscultation.

4. The client reports pain relief with nursing interventions with adequate dosage of pain medication.

5. The client exhibits no complications from immobility as evidenced by intact skin, no respiratory complications, no deep vein thromboses, and no bowel or bladder problems.

6. The client reports a decreased anxiety level.

NURSING PROCESS OVERVIEW

V. THE INTERMEDIATE AND EXTENDED POSTOPERATIVE PERIODS

A. Assessment

1. **On the client's admission to the clinical unit, perform a head-to-toe physical assessment.**

 2. **Monitor the client's overall condition and blood pressure, pulse, and respirations** on arrival to the unit then every 15 minutes for the first hour, every 30 minutes for the next 2 hours and, if stable, every 4 hours thereafter.

3. **Assess respiratory status,** including:

a. airway patency

b. rate, depth, and pattern of respiration

c. character of breath sounds

d. signs of peripheral or buccal cyanosis

e. arterial blood oxygen level according to the pulse oximeter determination.

4. **Assess neurovascular status in extremities.**

5. **Observe level of consciousness and responsiveness.**

6. **Inspect surgical wounds, dressings, and drains.** Note signs of healing or infection, patency, and drainage characteristics.

7. **Assess the client's comfort level.**

a. Note:

– time of last pain medication

– current pain, including its location, nature, and intensity

– position of maximum comfort

– complaints of nausea or vomiting

– body temperature

– constrictive or irritating casts, dressings, and traction.

      b. Rule out any complications that require immediate intervention before adminis-
tering pain medication.
  8. Evaluate urinary status.
      a. Identify last voiding and amount.
      b. Note presence of indwelling catheter.
      c. Monitor and assess intake and output.
  9. Explore psychosocial concerns related to such factors as:
      a. the nature of the client's surgical diagnosis and prognosis
      b. available support systems
      c. the client's need for rest and quiet.
  10. Assess safety aspects, such as:
      a. the need for side rails on the bed
      b. correct I.V. infusion rate
      c. splinting of I.V. site
      d. call bell kept within easy reach
      e. ambulation status and the need for assistance
      f. condition of all equipment.

B. Nursing diagnoses
  1. Ineffective airway clearance
  2. Acute pain
  3. Risk for imbalanced fluid volume
  4. Constipation
  5. Risk for impaired skin integrity
  6. Deficient knowledge
  7. Ineffective coping

C. Planning and outcome identification. The major goals for the client during the in-
termediate and extended postoperative periods include maintenance of airway patency and
respiratory function, absence of postoperative complications, pain relief, maintenance of
fluid and nutritional intake, return to normal elimination patterns, prevention of wound infection and evisceration, increased knowledge of postoperative care, and effective coping
with surgical experience.

D. Implementation
  1. Promote lung expansion and help prevent atelectasis and pneumonia.
      a. Encourage coughing, deep breathing, and turning.
      b. Use an incentive spirometer, as indicated.
      c. Progress mobility from range-of-motion exercises to ambulation as tolerated.
      d. Monitor pulse oximeter as needed.
  2. Promote measures to address potential complications.
      a. Monitor for signs and symptoms of postoperative complications, including:
        – hypoxemia
        – hypovolemia
        – hemorrhage
        – pulmonary embolism
        – allergic drug reactions
        – cardiac arrhythmias.
      b. Encourage movement and ambulation, as indicated. Have the client gradually in-
crease exercise from lying, to sitting, to standing, and then to ambulating. Provide
assistance and encouragement; maintain safety precautions.

    c. Minimize the risk of deep vein thrombosis (DVT).

- Assess for early signs (e.g., redness, edema, tenderness along vein, positive Homans' sign).
- Apply elastic hose, a sequential compression device, or administer low-dose heparin, as prescribed.
- Teach measures to prevent vessel constriction.

    d. Intervene as appropriate to prevent postoperative depression, disorientation, or psychosis.

- Provide preoperative teaching and information to prevent these complications.
- Orient the client postoperatively.
- Provide prescribed medication, close supervision, and consultation with mental health personnel as required.

3. Provide appropriate pain-relief measures.

    a. Administer prescribed analgesics, and possibly, patient-controlled analgesia, as indicated.

    b. Implement nonpharmacologic pain-relief measures (e.g., relaxation, guided imagery).

    c. **Rule out any complications that require immediate intervention before administering pain medication.**

4. Promote optimal intake and output.

    a. Encourage adequate fluid intake, and monitor electrolyte balance.

    b. Monitor and assess fluid intake and output. Use a urometer if necessary.

    c. Assess for urinary retention after bladder catheter removal, particularly in clients who have undergone surgery involving the pelvic or rectal area.

    d. **Promote normal voiding patterns** through such measures as:

- providing privacy
- running tap water or providing other stimuli to induce urination
- increasing fluid intake
- relieving pain.

5. Promote return to normal GI function.

    a. Auscultate for bowel sounds to detect the return of peristalsis. (Paralytic ileus may occur after abdominal or bowel surgery.)

    b. As indicated, minimize abdominal distention resulting from decreased peristalsis (typically persisting 3 to 4 days postoperatively) through exercise, ambulation, decreased opioid dosage, or rectal tube placement.

    c. Assess for and report unrelieved nausea and vomiting. Administer antiemetics as prescribed (see *Drug chart 21-1,* page 585), and decrease the risk of aspirating vomitus through proper positioning.

6. Provide adequate nutrition. Resume oral feeding as soon as gastric and bowel function return, or provide total parenteral nutrition. (See *Box 21-1.*)

7. Promote wound healing.

    a. Assess the dressing or wound for signs and symptoms of infection, including redness, odor, drainage, and warmth.

    b. Monitor the client's temperature for elevation indicating systemic infection.

    c. Always use sterile technique when removing, irrigating, and changing surgical dressing.

    d. Document the surgical wound as specifically as possible: the length, width, and depth; what it looks like; and any bleeding or necrotic tissue.

BOX 21-1

Nursing care for a client on total parenteral nutrition

Nursing interventions before administering TPN
- Ensure that solutions are refrigerated until needed and then warmed to room temperature.
- Administer total parental nutrition (TPN) by performing the five rights of medication administration. Check each ingredient with the health care provider's order.
- Inspect TPN for particulate matter or discoloration.
- Inspect TPN for "cracking" that may occur with total nutrient admixture, which involves layering of the solution.
- Be sure to add any medication (e.g., insulin, heparin) ordered by the health care provider.
- Always use a pump or controller to ensure accurate infusion rates.
- Use appropriate I.V. tubing (may use filter).

Nursing interventions while administering TPN
- Weigh the client daily if he's in the facility (two or three times each week if at home).
- Measure accurate intake and output every 8 hours.
- Maintain accurate caloric count of any oral nutrients.
- Monitor electrolyte and protein levels.

- Monitor glucose levels every 6 hours per glucometer.
- Monitor vital signs every 6 hours.
- Assess renal function by watching blood urea nitrogen and creatinine levels.
- Assess liver function by monitoring liver enzymes, bilirubin, triglycerides, and cholesterol.
- Assess for signs of dehydration, hyperglycemia, and hypoglycemia.
- Change the I.V. administration tubing with every new bag; make sure all connections are secure to avoid breaks in the integrity of the system.
- Change subclavian dressing aseptically according to facility policy (usually two or three times weekly).
- Label dressing and tubing with date, time, and the initials of the nurse carrying out the procedure.
- Monitor for signs of inflammation, infection, and sepsis, the most common complications of TPN.
- If the TPN bag is not available, administer 10% dextrose solution at same rate as prescribed TPN.
- Always taper solution when removing the client from TPN.

---

   e. Reduce the risk of nosocomial infection by maintaining medical and surgical asepsis. Classify the original surgical wound as clean, clean-contaminated, contaminated, or infected. Observe for complications of a nonhealing wound.

   f. Respond quickly to evisceration (i.e., rupture of wound with coils of intestines pushed out, preceded by a gush of serosanguineous fluid) by:
   - staying with and attempting to calm the client
   - positioning the client to decrease abdominal strain
   - applying moist, sterile saline dressings to cover exposed intestine
   - notifying the surgeon, who will need to perform reclosure surgery as soon as possible.

8. **Provide client and family teaching.**
   a. Teach the client and his family to assess for and report signs or symptoms of complications, such as:
   - DVT
   - wound infection or systemic infection
   - wound dehiscence.
   b. Teach the client and his family about:
   - prescribed medications
   - treatments
   - diet
   - activity level
   - planned follow-up care.
   c. Provide health education as detailed in *Client and family teaching 21-1*, page 590.

9. **Provide client and family support, and promote coping.**
   a. Discuss postoperative depression and ineffective coping with the client and his family. Teach them about the grieving process and refer them to support groups as appropriate.

CLIENT AND FAMILY TEACHING 21-1
Guidelines for postoperative care

- Provide the client with verbal and written instructions concerning discharge instructions for home care.
- Instruct the client to inspect the incisional wound at least twice each day and to use a mirror if unable to view the wound completely.
- Instruct the client to notify the health care provider when the wound is reddened, irritated, or has any drainage or odor. Inspect the wound dressing for bleeding, drainage, or odor.
- Instruct the client to clean the wound with warm soap and water daily unless otherwise instructed by the health care provider. Be sure to dry thoroughly; pat dry, or use a hair dryer on the cold setting.
- Instruct the client to take his oral temperature twice daily and notify the health care provider if the temperature is greater than 101° F (38.3° C). Low-grade fever is not uncommon.
- Instruct the client not to put any increased strain on the incisional wound; no lifting is allowed for an abdominal wound and no walking for an incision on the leg.
- Instruct the client to take pain medications as prescribed and, if pain is not relieved, to notify the health care provider.
- Instruct the client on appropriate activity levels during the convalescent period.
- Instruct the client on dietary instructions appropriate during the convalescent period.
- Provide the client with follow-up visit information and the phone number of the health care provider.

   b. As necessary, refer the client and his family to social services to arrange for services such as:
   – home health care
   – meal delivery
   – transportation assistance
   – special equipment (e.g., wheelchair, walker, oxygen equipment).

E.   Outcome evaluation
   1. The client maintains optimal respiratory function, as evidenced by:
      a. the performance of deep-breathing exercises four times daily for the first 48 hours postoperatively
      b. demonstrating clear breath sounds on auscultation
      c. turning, exercising, and ambulating as instructed
      d. coughing effectively to expectorate secretions and sputum.
   2. The client has no postoperative complications, as evidenced by:
      a. no signs or symptoms of cardiac arrhythmias
      b. capillary refill time of less than 3 seconds and normal skin color
      c. normal body temperature and vital signs within acceptable ranges
      d. no signs of hemorrhage or hematoma
      e. absence of psychotic or disoriented behavior
      f. no evidence of DVT.
   3. The client reports adequate pain control.
   4. The client maintains optimal fluid and electrolyte status.
   5. The client maintains optimal nutritional status.
   6. The client demonstrates optimal bowel or bladder elimination pattern.
   7. The client displays optimal wound healing, as evidenced by:
      a. no abnormal wound drainage
      b. afebrile state with normal white blood cell count
      c. intact wound with no breakdown, redness, or signs of dehiscence or evisceration.

8. The client or his family verbalize understanding of prescribed medications, diet, activity, and other therapies.
9. The client or his family states that appropriate arrangements have been made for home care.
10. The client and his family cope effectively with the surgical experience.

Study questions

1. Which nursing intervention would be *most important* to assist in decreasing the anxiety of a client undergoing surgery?
   1. Discouraging the client from discussing the surgical procedure
   2. Verifying that the operative permit is signed and on the chart
   3. Ensuring the safety of the client while in surgery
   4. Assessing the client for concerns about the surgical experience

2. Which nursing diagnosis would the nurse identify for a 70-year-old client undergoing surgery with general anesthesia during which the ambient operating room temperature is 68° F (20° C)?
   1. Risk for injury
   2. Deficient fluid volume
   3. Hypothermia
   4. Risk for infection

3. Which intervention would be most effective in promoting adequate respiratory function in an unconscious client recently admitted to the postanesthesia care unit with no contraindications to movement?
   1. Performing the jaw thrust maneuver while the client is supine
   2. Turning the client from side to side at 10-minute intervals
   3. Extending the client's chin while on his side and a pillow at the back
   4. Placing the client prone to facilitate drainage of secretions

4. Which intervention would the nurse include when evaluating the client's urinary elimination status?

   1. Keeping the side rails up at all times
   2. Assessing the client's intake and output
   3. Monitoring the client's vital signs
   4. Inspecting the surgical wound for infection

5. Which intervention would be the nurse's best response to a female client scheduled for an emergency surgery who is crying and voicing that she is afraid of being put to sleep?
   1. Squeezing her hand and telling her, "There's nothing to be afraid of."
   2. Checking her name band, and asking the anesthesiologist to give her a sedative.
   3. Letting her cry, and telling others to leave her alone until she is anesthetized.
   4. Standing by her side, and quietly asking her to describe what she is feeling.

6. A client having excess fat suctioned from the thighs for cosmetic reasons is an example of which category of surgery?
   1. Optional
   2. Elective
   3. Required
   4. Urgent

7. A surgical client asks the nurse, "When will this hotel bring me some food?" after she has signed an informed consent form and the health care provider has left the room. After confirming that the client is confused, which intervention should the nurse implement first?
   1. Reporting that the consent has been obtained from a confused client
   2. Teaching preoperative moving, coughing, and deep-breathing exercises

3. Inserting a bladder catheter to evaluate urine output
4. Administering preoperative medication immediately

8. Which time schedule is most appropriate for assessing the vital signs of a client in the postanesthesia care unit (PACU)?
1. Every 5 minutes x 3; then every 15 minutes
2. Every 5 minutes for 1 hour; then every 15 minutes for 1 hour
3. Every 15 minutes x 4; then every hour
4. Every 30 minutes x 4; then every 2 hours

9. Which denotes the scientific rationale for operating-room personnel being required to cover hair and shoes and wear specific, clean operating-room attire?
1. Promotion of a totally sterile environment
2. Elimination of outside environmental hazards
3. The need for nonstatic uniforms
4. Isolation of the client's diseases from the operating staff

10. Which statement by the client indicates that the client understands the nurse's teaching about postoperative wounds?
1. "I should expect a slight odor from the surgical dressing."
2. "I should call my doctor if my wound is intact and has no drainage."
3. "I should not clean my surgical wound until I go back to my doctor in 2 weeks."
4. "I should call my doctor if I have a temperature of 102° F."

11. Which nursing intervention would be most appropriate to minimize the risk of deep vein thrombosis (DVT) in a postoperative client?
1. Applying a sequential compression device to the lower extremities
2. Encouraging the client to keep his legs immobile

3. Administering I.V. heparin immediately after surgery
4. Typing and crossmatching the client for whole blood administration

12. Two hours after surgery, a 60-year-old client's blood pressure drops from 126/78 mm Hg to 102/68 mm Hg, and his pulse rate increases from 80 to 106 beats/minute. His skin is cool and pale. Which intervention should the nurse implement first?
1. Continuing to monitor the client frequently every 4 hours
2. Increasing nasal cannula oxygen flow rate to 8 L
3. Placing the client in Trendelenburg's position
4. Alerting the surgeon, and ask for increased I.V. fluid rate

13. Which point score on the postanesthesia chart indicates that the client has fulfilled minimal criteria for discharge from the postanesthesia care unit (PACU)?
1. One point in each of the five areas for a total score of 5
2. One point in at least three areas — respiratory, circulatory, and consciousness — for a total score of 3
3. A total score for the five areas of 7 or more
4. Two points in each of the five areas for a total score of 10

14. Which intervention would be *priority* for a client who underwent abdominal surgery 36 hours earlier and is now exhibiting increased temperature and pulse rate; shallow, rapid breathing; and bilateral adventitious lung sounds?
1. Decreasing the client's I.V. fluid flow rate
2. Encouraging the client to turn, cough, deep-breathe
3. Calling the respiratory therapist to obtain immediate arterial blood gas (ABG) determinations
4. Keeping the client and the head of the bed flat

15. Which intervention should the nurse implement *first* for the client who develops an abdominal wound dehiscence after staple removal?
   1. Covering the wound with saline dressings, and calling the surgeon immediately
   2. Leaving the client, stating that you will be right back with help
   3. Completing a head-to-toe assessment before calling the surgeon
   4. Placing a sign on client's door to indicate the need for drainage precautions

16. The nurse is completing a client's postanesthesia scoring chart. The client has the ability to move all extremities, is able to cough and deep-breathe, has a blood pressure of 142/86 mm Hg, is fully awake, and has a pulse oximeter reading of 98%. What postanesthesia score should the nurse give this client?

_____

Answer key

1. The answer is 4.
Key to decreasing a client's anxiety is determining the underlying factors contributing to his anxiety. A client assessment of the concerns related to the surgery is crucial. During this assessment, the client may identify fear of the unknown, fear of death, or worry about loss of work or loss of role as concerns that could possibly affect the surgical experience. The nurse should encourage, not discourage, the client to discuss the surgical procedure. Verifying that the operative permit is signed and on the chart and ensuring the safety of the client while in surgery are appropriate interventions for surgery, but they have no effect on decreasing the client's anxiety.

2. The answer is 3.
Because of age-related changes and the lower environmental temperature of the operating room, this elderly client is very susceptible to accidental hypothermia from the environment. General anesthesia causes vasodilation, further aggravating this situation. Risk for injury and risk for infection are possible nursing diagnoses, but these would apply to any client undergoing surgery. Deficient fluid volume is a possible diagnosis, but this nursing diagnosis is related to the client's need to maintain nothing-by-mouth status and the increased risk of bleeding.

3. The answer is 3.
Postoperatively, extending the client's chin while placing him on his side and supporting the back with a pillow is the correct intervention until the client regains consciousness. The jaw thrust maneuver is appropriate for a client with respiratory obstruction. During the immediate postopertive period, turning the client every 10 minutes is inappropriate. Postoperative clients are rarely, if ever, placed in the prone position.

4. The answer is 2.
When evaluating a client's urinary elimination status, assessing intake and output is key. The nurse should note the time and amount of the last voiding and amount of urine present in the indwelling urinary catheter if one has been inserted. Keeping the side rails up at all times maintains the client's safety. Monitoring the client's vital signs aids in early detection of changes indicating possible complications such as hemorrhage. Inspecting the surgical wound is important to prevent infection. None of these interventions addresses the client's urinary status.

5. The answer is 4.
The client is exhibiting fear and anxiety. The nurse's best response in this situation is to

stand by her side and quietly ask her to describe what she is feeling. Doing so focuses on her feelings. Using therapeutic communication allows the client to express fear or grief. Squeezing the client's hand and telling her that there is nothing to be afraid of is nontherapeutic and belittles her fear or emotion. Checking the client's name band and asking the anesthesiologist to give her a sedative also is nontherapeutic, because the nurse is avoiding her expression. Letting the client cry and telling others to leave her alone is nontherapeutic because these actions may heighten her anxiety and fear.

6. The answer is **1.**
Cosmetic surgeries, by definition, are most often optional; they are done totally at the client's discretion. Elective surgery refers to procedures that are scheduled at the client's convenience (e.g., cyst removal, repair of scars or simple hernia, vaginal repair). Required surgery is warranted for conditions necessitating intervention within a few weeks (e.g., cataract surgery, thyroid disorders). Urgent or imperative surgery is indicated for a problem requiring intervention within 24 to 48 hours (e.g., some cancers, acute gallbladder infection, appendicitis, kidney stones).

7. The answer is **1.**
For informed consent to be valid, the client must be a mentally competent adult or an emancipated minor. If these requirements cannot be met, a responsible relative or guardian should sign for the client. Teaching the client would be inappropriate until the legality of the client's situation was assessed. If confusion makes the client unteachable, the nurse also should report this information. Inserting a bladder catheter is usually done after the client is anesthetized to minimize pain. It is not a priority at this time. Administering preoperative medication should not be done until the client's legal status is clear and legally valid informed consent is obtained.

8. The answer is **1.**

Typically, in the PACU, vital signs are monitored every 5 minutes x 3 and then every 15 minutes. The PACU nurse can take the vital signs more often if necessary, but not at any less frequent intervals.

9. The answer is **2.**
The main rationale for wearing specific operating-room attire and covering the hair and shoes is to protect the client from infection by eliminating outside environmental hazards, such as dust and pollutants. A "totally" sterile environment is impossible to achieve. Nonstatic clothes no longer are required, because nonexplosive gases are used in the operating room. The client, not the staff, is being protected here.

10. The answer is **4.**
Increased temperature may indicate a systemic infection and should be reported to the health care provider. An odor may indicate a wound infection and should be reported. A normal postoperative wound should be dry and intact. Typically, a postoperative wound is cleaned with soap and water daily. The client should not wait until the follow-up visit in 2 weeks to clean the wound.

11. The answer is **1.**
Applying sequential compression devices helps to promote venous blood return to the heart, thereby decreasing the risk of DVT. The client should be encouraged to perform passive and active range-of-motion exercises to prevent venous stasis. Low-dose heparin may be ordered subcutaneously. However, I.V. heparin therapy is not routinely ordered unless DVT is diagnosed. Administration of whole blood has no effect on minimizing the risk of DVT.

12. The answer is **4.**
At this time, the client is showing early signs of hypovolemia and early shock, necessitating increased fluid. The nurse should alert the surgeon about these findings and request an order to increase the I.V. fluid rate. If symp-

toms become more severe, the surgeon has already been alerted. Continuing to monitor the client is appropriate only after the surgeon has been notified and the I.V. fluid rate has been increased. This client is experiencing a complication of surgery and needs intervention. Increasing the oxygen flow rate and placing the client in Trendelenburg's position could be appropriate later. However, these responses are not critical at this early time.

13. The answer is **3**.

Seven points of a possible 10 constitutes the minimum score required for discharge from the PACU. Any score below 7 indicates that the client is not considered stable for discharge. A score of 10 points is not necessary for discharge.

14. The answer is **2**.

Immediate nursing intervention could help prevent serious complications from atelectasis and pneumonia resulting from poor respiratory hygiene and immobility. The nurse should therefore encourage the client to turn, cough, and deep-breathe. The nurse increases the client's fluid intake to help thin secre-

tions. Obtaining ABG readings may be needed later but not at this time. ABGs also require a physician's order. The client and the head of the bed should be elevated to maximize lung volume and ease the work of breathing.

15. The answer is **1**.

When a client experiences a wound dehiscence, the wound is covered with saline dressings to protect the protruding abdominal contents, and the surgeon is notified immediately because surgery is necessary to repair the wound. Leaving the client alone, completing a head-to-toe assessment, and instituting drainage precautions are inappropriate actions. The client needs immediate intervention.

16. The answer is **10**.

According to the postanesthesia care unit—modified Aldrete score, the client is functioning at the optimal level and should receive a score of 10. The client must have a score of at least 7 to be discharged from the postanesthesia care unit.

COMPREHENSIVE TEST: QUESTIONS

1. A client arrives at the clinic for a routine physical examination. During the examination, the nurse performs an otoscopic examination. Which finding would the nurse expect as normal?
   1. Pale optic disk
   2. Pearly gray typmanic membrane
   3. Positive red reflex
   4. Tactile fremitus

2. When assessing a client's role and relationship patterns, which question would be *most* appropriate to ask?
   1. "What are your ideas about health?"
   2. "Do you have any problems with mobility?"
   3. "How would you describe your family's health?"
   4. "How would you describe your strengths and weaknesses?"

3. An elderly client has pale, cool feet and diminished pedal pulses bilaterally, absence of hair tufts on toes, and a circumscribed 3 cm ulceration on the plantar surface of the first metatarsal joint. Which pathological change would the nurse suspect as the *most* likely source of the client's problem?
   1. Obstructed lymphatic flow
   2. Deep vein thrombosis (DVT)
   3. Normal age-related changes
   4. Insufficient arterial circulation

4. An adult client has the following laboratory results: White blood cells (WBCs), 6,300/mm^3; platelets, 250,000/mm^3; serum sodium, 140 mEq/L; and serum potassium, 6 mEq/L. Which condition is present?
   1. Leukocytosis
   2. Thrombocytopenia
   3. Hyperkalemia
   4. Hypernatremia

5. Which best describes the rationale for edema of inflamed tissue with cellular injury?
   1. Transient vasodilation followed by vasoconstriction
   2. White blood cell (WBC) migration away from the injured site
   3. Increased vascular permeability with leakage of plasma fluids
   4. Irritation of nerve endings by fibrinogen

6. While receiving radiation therapy for the treatment of breast cancer, a client complains of dysphagia and skin texture changes at the radiation site. Which instruction would be *most* appropriate to suggest to minimize the risk of complications and promote healing?
   1. "Wash the radiation site vigorously with soap and water to remove dead cells."
   2. "Follow a high-protein, high-calorie diet to optimize tissue repair."
   3. "Apply cool compresses to the radiation site to reduce swelling."
   4. "Drink warm fluids throughout the day to relieve discomfort in swallowing."

7. The nurse is aware that which finding represents hyperplasia?
   1. An enlarged heart muscle on X-ray
   2. Loss of cellular substances resulting in cell shrinkage
   3. Changes in epithelial cells from habitual smoking
   4. Increased breast size during pregnancy

8. A client, admitted with complaints of fatigue and muscle weakness and taking furosemide 20 mg daily for treatment of essential hypertension, has a serum potassium level of 2.8 mEq/L. The health

care provider orders potassium chloride (KCl) 20 mEq to be added to 100 ml of dextrose 5% in water and infused I.V. over 2 hours. Which intervention should the nurse implement?

1. Teaching the client about foods high in potassium and signs and symptoms of hypokalemia
2. Calling the health care provider to clarify the order because KCl should be infused at a rate of 10 mEq/L every 4 hours
3. Observing the electrocardiogram (ECG) for characteristic waveform changes, especially peaked, narrow T waves
4. Double-checking the laboratory results because low potassium levels are common with hemolyzed specimens

9. The client is receiving heparin 25 ml/hr. The heparin bag has 20,000 units/500 ml. How many units of heparin per hour is the client receiving?

_____

10. A client complaining of lethargy and confusion during the last few days also reports a loss of appetite with nausea and vomiting over the last 2 weeks. The electrocardiogram (ECG) reveals a shortened QT interval. Which electrolyte imbalance would the nurse suspect?

1. Hypernatremia
2. Hypermagnesemia
3. Hypercalcemia
4. Hyperkalemia

11. After eating fish the previous night, a client reports severe diarrhea with passage of 15 explosive diarrheal stools in the past 10 hours. Which of the followng laboratory results would the nurse expect to find?

1. Decreased blood urea nitrogen (BUN)
2. Increased hematocrit
3. Decreased urine specific gravity
4. Elevated serum calcium levels

12. A client in acute respiratory distress who is belligerent and confused has the following arterial blood gas (ABG) results: pH, 7.55; partial pressure of arterial oxygen (Pao_2), 68 mm Hg; partial pressure of carbon dioxide (Pco_2), 38 mm Hg; and bicarbonate (Hco_3-), 29 mEq/L. Which statement would *best* explain the reason for the client's behavior?

1. The client is frightened by his breathing difficulty.
2. Metabolic alkalosis is present and causing the changes in mental status.
3. This behavior is typical for any client experiencing an acute respiratory crisis.
4. The behavior is a result of the client's respiratory acidosis.

13. A client with hypermagnesemia and a history of hiatal hernia with severe heartburn admits to taking antacids several times a day. Which nursing intervention would be *most* appropriate for this client?

1. Encouraging frequent ambulation to minimize magnesium loss from the bone
2. Instructing about the role of antacids in increasing serum magnesium levels
3. Assessing the sleep pattern for disturbances related to neuromuscular irritability
4. Monitoring for signs and symptoms of fluid volume excess from magnesium retention.

14. The nurse is aware that which nerve fiber would be responsible for transmission of sharp, piercing pain immediately after a finger is cut?

1. Type C
2. Type A-gamma
3. Type A-alpha
4. Type A-delta

15. The nurse is preparing to administer 2 ounces of an antacid. How many milliliters will the nurse prepare to administer to the client?

16. A client receiving warfarin sodium, an anticoagulant, has a prothrombin time (PT) of 22 and partial thromboplastin time of 39. The control values are PT, 12.9, and PTT, 37. The International Normalized Ratio (INR) is 2.8. Which nursing intervention would be *most* appropriate?
1. Holding the medication and assessing for bleeding
2. Administering the medication as ordered
3. Preparing to administer protamine sulfate
4. Notifying the health care provider immediately

17. A client who is very stoic refuses analgesics even when experiencing severe pain. Which nursing intervention would be *most* appropriate?
1. Staying with the client and holding his hand for as long as he needs support
2. Using patient-controlled analgesia (PCA) or transcutaneous electrical stimulation (TENS)
3. Administering the analgesic crushed in food without letting the client know it is in there
4. Waiting to provide pain relief measures until the client specifically requests relief

18. For a client with a history of angina, which intervention should the nurse teach the client to do *first* if he develops chest pain at home?
1. Taking sublingual nitroglycerin (NTG) and lying down
2. Performing mild breathing and range-of-motion exercises
3. Taking an extra-long-acting nitrate tablet immediately
4. Sitting down and relaxing using guided imagery or distraction

19. During the initial interview of a client with a history of moderate to severe emphysema who is now in acute respiratory distress, he reports that he continues to smoke regularly, mows the lawn weekly, and refuses to use oxygen in front of his friends. Which nursing diagnosis would the nurse use to address these behaviors?
1. Anticipatory grieving
2. Disturbed body image
3. Ineffective coping
4. Impaired social interaction

20. The nurse is aware that to maintain acid-base balance in the body, the lungs play a primary role in controlling which components?
1. Arterial oxygen and blood urea
2. Arterial oxygen and cholesterol
3. Arterial carbon dioxide and serum albumin
4. Arterial carbon dioxide and pH

21. When planning the care of a client with a pneumothorax, which finding would the nurse expect to assess in the lung on the affected side?
1. Expanded due to the intake of atmospheric air
2. Collapsed due to disturbed negative pressure in the pleural space
3. Expanded due to altered lung pressures
4. Collapsed due to disturbed positive pressures

22. Following a mitral valve replacement 2 days ago, a client's electrocardiogram reveals premature ventricular contractions (PVCs). Which complication would the nurse assess for in the client?
1. Significant increase in cardiac workload
2. Ventricular tachycardia or ventricular fibrillation
3. Development of a myocardial infarction (MI)
4. A decrease in heart rate and blood pressure

23. The nurse finds a female client who is scheduled for coronary artery bypass grafting in the morning sitting in her room and crying. The client states, "I won't be able to work and do all the things that I usually do for a while after surgery. My poor husband. I'll be such a burden to him." Which nursing diagnosis would be most appropriate for this client?
1. Impaired verbal communication
2. Compromised family coping
3. Deficient knowledge
4. Ineffective role performance

24. For the client with intermittent claudication resulting from chronic arterial occlusive disease, which outcome should be addressed when planning nursing interventions?
1. Improving venous return from the involved extremity
2. Decreasing the need for opioid analgesics
3. Preventing edema in the extremities
4. Increasing circulation to the extremities

25. When assessing an elderly client, the nurse notes an edematous left leg that is warm to touch with palpable pedal pulses and an open, wet superficial ulcer with an irregular border above the medial malleolus surrounded by thick, coarse, brown pigmented skin. Based on these findings, which pathological change would the nurse suspect as the possible cause of the ulcer?
1. Prolonged pressure
2. Venous stasis
3. Arterial occlusion
4. Lymphedema

26. Which instruction is *most* important to provide when discharging a client from the emergency department following a penetrating foot injury?
1. "Call the health care provider at the first signs of any red streaks appearing on the foot or leg."
2. "Refrain from crossing the legs at the knee or the ankle."
3. "Avoid smoking until the entire wound is no longer open to the air."
4. "Watch for signs and symptoms of anaphylaxis from the tetanus toxoid."

27. On the first postoperative day following an above-the-knee amputation, the client exhibits hypotension, tachycardia, and tachypnea along with a 2.8″ (7 cm) area of red drainage on the distal portion of the bulky stump dressing. Which interpretation *best* explains the basis for these findings?
1. Normal response to recovery from general anesthesia
2. Early response to pain indicating a need for analgesia
3. Initial response to bleeding at the stump necessitating frequent assessment
4. Early respiratory complications requiring vigorous deep breathing exercises

28. The nurse is calculating intake and output for a client with a three way bladder irrigation for a transurethral resection of the prostate. The client has received 1,000 ml I.V., two 100 ml I.V. piggyback, and is allowed nothing by mouth at this time. The total bladder irrigation instilled is 2,000 ml and the client's output is 3,100 ml. What is the client's intake and urinary output in milliliters for this shift?

_____

29. The nurse questions a client just beginning treatment with antihypertensive agents for essential hypertension about his usual stressors and coping mechanisms. Which scientific rationale best describes the reason for this line of questioning?
1. The major cause of essential hypertension is exposure to stress.
2. Measures to reduce stress are part of any treatment regimen for hypertension.

3. Descriptions of personal stress levels will help the client relax.
4. Stress must be reduced before any teaching and learning can occur.

30. Which instruction about antacid therapy should be included in the discharge teaching plan for a client with a healing peptic ulcer?
1. "Continue the antacids as ordered, even if you feel better."
2. "Take the antacids with your other medications."
3. "Avoid magnesium antacids if a heart problem develops."
4. "Take your antacids with your meals."

31. Following a client's acute episode of ulcerative colitis, the nurse would evaluate large bowel intestinal function by assessing which data?
1. Pain relief after eating
2. Evidence of adequate nutrient absorption
3. Passage of soft, formed stool
4. Absence of belching and acid reflux

32. Which complication should the nurse be alert for in a client diagnosed with ulcerative colitis?
1. Portal hypertension
2. Ascites
3. Vomiting
4. Anorexia

33. The nurse is aware that which factor is the most common precipitating factor associated with the development of diabetic ketoacidosis (DKA)?
1. Overeating
2. Infection
3. Missed insulin dose
4. Psychological stress

34. Which instruction should be included in the teaching plan for a client with diabetes and an open foot ulcer?
1. "Clean the foot with soap and water and watch for signs of infection."

2. "Soak the foot daily in hot water and apply a compression bandage."
3. "Clean the foot with soap and water and apply iodine to the ulcer."
4. "Elevate the foot and apply heat to the area."

35. The nurse is preparing to administer meperidine 12.5 mg and promethazine 25 mg to a client complaining of pain. The medication comes in meperidine 25 mg/1 ml and promethazine 50 mg/1 ml. How many milliliters of medication will the nurse administer to the client?

36. Following a thyroidectomy, the client experiences hemorrhage. The nurse would prepare for which emergency intervention?
1. I.V. administration of calcium
2. Insertion of an oral airway
3. Creation of a tracheostomy
4. I.V. administration of thyroid hormone

37. Which clinical manifestation should the nurse expect in a client diagnosed with primary open-angle glaucoma?
1. Gradual loss of peripheral vision
2. Cloudy-appearing lens
3. Lack of eye pain or redness
4. Complaints of floating spots

38. When preparing a teaching plan for a client with impotence, the nurse should address which scientific rationale when identifying nursing interventions?
1. The incidence of impotence decreases with age.
2. Impotence typically begins suddenly.
3. The cause of impotence may be organic or psychogenic.
4. Dietary factors play a major role in impotence.

39. The nurse is aware that hemorrhage is a major complication following a prostatectomy because of which condition?
1. Pressure on the incision
2. Deep vein thrombosis (DVT)

3. Urinary tract obstruction
4. Infection

40. When discussing testicular self-examination, which instruction should the nurse include in the client teaching?
1. "Tenderness is an early sign of testicular cancer."
2. "The testes should feel smooth and oval shaped."
3. "Masses are difficult to feel with this examination."
4. "A firm, pea-sized lump may be normal."

41. Which statement best explains the scientific rationale for performing urinary catheterization on a client following an abdominal hysterectomy if she is unable to void within 8 hours?
1. Temporary atony may result from surgical manipulation in the area.
2. The bladder is removed along with the uterus.
3. Infection from surgery interferes with the client's ability to void.
4. Surgically induced menopause impairs the client's urinary function.

42. When discussing allergic contact dermatitis, the nurse should address which topic when teaching the client?
1. That the reaction to the allergen occurs immediately upon exposure
2. That chemical irritants are the primary offenders
3. That the rash is typically localized to one area
4. That the intensity of the reaction varies with the allergen

43. When planning the care of a client with rheumatoid arthritis (RA) who is worried about her condition deteriorating and an increasing inability to care for family members, which intervention should the nurse implement *first*?
1. Teaching the client about the disease and how it progresses

2. Making referrals for assistance with home activities
3. Providing emotional support for the client and her family
4. Assessing the client's physical, emotional, and environmental needs

44. Which intervention would be *most* appropriate when caring for a client experiencing an acute exacerbation of asthma who is dyspneic and irritable?
1. Elevating the head of the bed to ease breathing
2. Having the client breathe into a paper bag
3. Withholding fluids to prevent aspiration
4. Administering an antitussive agent

45. According to the American Burn Association (ABA), which burn injury is the appropriate classification for a second-degree burn in an adult involving more than 25% of the total body surface area (TBSA)?
1. Minor
2. Moderate uncomplicated
3. Major
4. Full-thickness

46. Which intervention must be implemented *first* during the initial assessment of a client with a major burn injury?
1. Eliminating the source of the burn
2. Ensuring a patent airway
3. Inserting a nasogastric tube
4. Treating for burn shock

47. Using the Parkland formula, how much fluid replacement would the nurse administer over 24 hours for a client weighing 70 kg with burns totaling 50% of the total body surface area (TBSA)?
1. 1,400 ml
2. 3,500 ml
3. 7,000 ml
4. 14,000 ml

48. The client is 8 hours postinserstion of a left lower anterior chest tube. When assessing the client, the nurse notes that there is no flucutation in the water-seal chamber. Which interventions should the nurse implement? (Select all that apply.)
1. Stripping the chest tube distal to proximal insertion site
2. Assessing the client's respiratory status
3. Notifying the health care provider that the lungs have re-expanded
4. Determining if the tubing is kinked or has dependent loops
5. Increasing the wall suction
6. Instructing the client to turn, cough, and deep-breathe

49. The nurse would suspect which signs and symptoms in a client diagnosed with myasthenia gravis?
1. Nuchal rigidity and positive Kernig's sign
2. Fatigue and difficulty in coordination
3. Muscular rigidity and resting tremor
4. Extreme muscular weakness after activity and ptosis

50. Which teaching should be included initially in the care plan for a client who develops constipation following a craniotomy?
1. The need for a sodium-restricted diet
2. The need for daily enemas
3. The need for a high-fiber diet
4. The need for stimulant laxatives

51. When ambulating a client following surgical removal of a protruded intervertebral lumbar disk, the nurse should implement which intervention?
1. Maintaining proper body alignment
2. Administering analgesia after walking
3. Providing a cane for support
4. Immobilizing the head and neck

52. Which nursing intervention should be included in the care plan for a client who sustained a moderate concussion and demonstrates a Glasgow Coma Scale grade of 7?
1. Administering prescribed osmotic diuretics
2. Maintaining the client in a supine position
3. Instituting a program of stimulation
4. Minimizing client movement in bed

53. When assessing a client with a spinal cord injury, the nurse notes loss of motor control and sensation below waist level and loss of bowel and bladder control. Which spinal cord level should the nurse expect the injury to be below?
1. C4
2. C8
3. T12
4. S1

54. For the client receiving miotic agents for the treatment of glaucoma, about which visual alteration should the nurse warn the client?
1. Impaired near vision
2. Photophobia
3. Impaired night vision
4. Diplopia

55. Which assessment finding would alert the nurse to the possibility of hemorrhage following intraocular surgery?
1. Elevated temperature
2. Diplopia
3. Visual floaters
4. Eye pain

56. A client using an over-the-counter nasal decongestant spray reports unrelieved and worsening nasal congestion. Which teaching should the nurse discuss with the client?
1. Switching to a stronger dosage of the medication
2. Discontinuing the medication for a few weeks
3. Using the spray more frequently

4. Combining the spray with an oral decongestant

57. Which nursing diagnosis is the priority for the client with a perforated eardrum?
1. Deficient knowledge related to general ear care and hearing protection
2. Disturbed sensory/auditory perception related to hearing loss
3. Risk for infection related to perforation
4. Acute pain related to vertigo and vomiting

58. Which intervention would be *most* important prior to discharging a client who underwent a total laryngectomy?
1. Making a referral to a support group
2. Providing medical identification explaining resuscitation needs
3. Instructing about measures for constipation
4. Teaching about precautions for showering and shampooing

59. Which assessment data should alert the nurse to the possibility of a fat embolism in a client with multiple fractures?
1. Hematuria
2. Mental status changes
3. Sudden fever
4. Fracture site discoloration

60. When preparing a client for magnetic resonance imaging (MRI), which intervention should the nurse implement?
1. Administering the prescribed preoperative medication
2. Scrubbing the injection site for 15 minutes using aseptic technique
3. Having the client remove any jewelry and asking about metal implants
4. Assessing for allergies to shellfish and iodine-containing substances

61. After the application of a long-arm cast, a client complains of deep, throbbing pain that is out of proportion to the injury. His capillary refill is diminished and his nailbeds are cyanotic. Which intervention should the nurse implement?
1. Notifying the health care provider immediately and preparing to bivalve the cast
2. Cutting a window in the cast over the elbow area and checking for infection
3. Elevating the casted arm, applying ice, and monitoring hourly for changes
4. Administering the prescribed analgesic and notifying the health care provider

62. Which nursing diagnosis would be the *highest* priority in the immediate postoperative period for a client with a below-the-knee-amputation?
1. Disturbed body image related to loss of a body part
2. Risk for infection related to disrupted skin integrity
3. Chronic pain related to phantom limb sensation
4. Ineffective tissue perfusion related to hemorrhage

63. The nurse would determine that the client is accepting the loss of an amputated limb when he exhibits which behavior?
1. Looking at, touching, and caring for the residual limb
2. Inviting friends and family members to visit
3. Inquiring about methods to alleviate pain
4. Expressing desire to go home and resume work

64. Which best describes the pathophysiology associated with portal hypertension?
1. Obstructed blood flow through the liver
2. Ascitic fluid movement back to the venous system
3. Rupture of esophageal varices
4. Obstructed bile flow through the common bile duct

65. A client is 4 hours postoperative abdomino-peritoneal resection with sigmoid colostomy. He is complaining of rectal pain that ranks 8 on a scale of 1 (no pain) to 10 (worst pain). Which interventions should the nurse implement? (Select all that apply.)

1. Assessing the abdominal incision
2. Medicating the client as ordered
3. Notifying the health care provider that the stoma is pink
4. Assessing the client's blood pressure and pulse
5. Assisting the client with distraction to help the pain
6. Encouraging the client to sit on the side of the bed

66. Which explanation *best* describes why the nursing diagnoses of disturbed body image and situational low self-esteem would apply to a client with ascites?

1. A grossly distended abdomen may make the client feel obese.
2. Yellow-tinged skin may make the client feel self-conscious.
3. Fecal incontinence may cause embarrassment.
4. Muscle wasting may cause weakness and mobility problems.

67. After obtaining 3 L of fluid from a client via paracentesis, the nurse would be alert for which complication?

1. Respiratory distress
2. Encephalopathy
3. Bleeding from the site
4. Vascular collapse

68. Which outcome statement *best* indicates the effectiveness of treatment to reduce the aggravating factors for cholelithiasis?

1. The client maintains intake and output within normal parameters.
2. The client reports no pain following ingestion of a low-fat meal.
3. The client demonstrates serum albumin levels within the acceptable range.

4. The client exhibits improvement on ultrasonagraphy.

69. Which statement best explains the rationale for administering meperidine rather than morphine for pain relief to a client with acute pancreatitis?

1. "Meperidine provides more prolonged analgesia than morphine."
2. "Morphine causes spasms of Oddi's sphincter; meperidine doesn't."
3. "Meperidine is less addicting than morphine."
4. "Morphine may cause liver dysfunction; meperidine doesn't."

70. Which instruction is crucial to include in the teaching plan of a client who is scheduled to receive peritoneal dialysis at home to prevent complications?

1. "Consume a high-sodium meal after the procedure."
2. "Increase the dextrose in the dialysis solution each day."
3. "Use strict aseptic technique throughout the procedure."
4. "Add heparin to the dialysis solution every other day."

71. After hemodialysis, the nurse would assess the client for bleeding because of which rationale?

1. Excessive amounts of urea in the blood
2. Heparin administration during dialysis
3. Increased platelet activity during dialysis
4. Increased hematocrit secondary to fluid removal

72. Which dietary recommendation would be appropriate for the care plan of a client with chronic renal failure?

1. Increased protein intake
2. Decreased potassium intake
3. Increased phosphorus intake
4. Decreased caloric intake

73. Which nursing diagnosis would be *most* appropriate for a client with chronic renal failure whose spouse, upon reporting that the client has been confused, irritable, and paranoid, states that she has been thinking about a divorce?
1. Noncompliance related to missed visits for follow-up
2. Situational low self-esteem related to loss of kidney function
3. Anxiety related to dialysis procedure
4. Interrupted family processes related to effects of the disease

74. An obese client is diagnosed with gastroesophageal reflux disease (GERD). Which topics should the nurse include in her discharge teaching? (Select all that apply.)
1. The importance of elevating the foot of the bed
2. The importance of lying down for two hours after eating
3. The need to follow a low-fiber, bland diet
4. The importance of avoiding food or drink 2 hours before bedtime
5. The importance of taking prescribed medications, which may include antacids and proton-pump inhibitors
6. The importance of losing weight

75. When preparing to administer a platelet transfusion, which factor should be considered when developing the care plan?
1. Platelets should be infused over 3 to 4 hours.
2. Active bleeding is the sole indication for transfusion.
3. Fever may affect the incremental count after transfusion.
4. Hemoglobinuria and hives indicate an allergic reaction.

76. Following induction chemotherapy 10 days ago, a client complains of fatigue and general malaise. His temperature is 101.4° F (38.6° C) and his white blood cell (WBC) count reveals the following: neutrophils, 300/mm³; hemoglobin, 10.5 g/dl; hematocrit, 31.5%; and a platelet count of 35,000 μl. Which intervention should the nurse implement *first*?
1. Calling the health care provider to report the findings
2. Administering acetaminophen to reduce the fever
3. Continuing monitoring every 4 hours for changes
4. Moving the client to a semi-private room

77. Which scientic rationale should be considered when planning the care of a young adult client with a hemoglobin of 6 g/dl and hematocrit of 25.3% who complains of feeling increasingly run-down and tired over the past several weeks?
1. The client will be very symptomatic because of the low hemoglobin.
2. Hematocrit, rather than hemoglobin level, is the best indicator of anemia.
3. Pallor should be assessed on the palms of the hands.
4. Rapid transfusion of packed red blood cells (RBCs) is necessary.

78. A client is diagnosed with peripheral arterial occlusive disease. Which instructions should the nurse include in her discharge teaching? (Select all that apply.)
1. "Perform scrupulous foot care daily."
2. "Apply a heating pad to both legs daily."
3. "Keep your feet elevated above heart level as much as possible."
4. "Stop activity when intermittant claudication occurs."
5. "Avoid nicotine and caffiene."
6. "Wear knee-high stockings."

79. Which statement would indicate that the client needs additional teaching about preventing a sickle cell crisis?
1. "I'll use my relaxation techniques if I feel stressed."
2. "I won't drink any alcohol."
3. "I'll make sure to rest frequently."
4. "I'll exercise strenuously every day."

80. Which nursing intervention would be the *most* effective in protecting the client with a decreased white blood cell (WBC) count from nosocomial infection?
1. Monitoring closely for signs of infection
2. Placing the client in isolation
3. Performing meticulous handwashing
4. Restricting the client's visitors

81. The nurse is aware that which of the following terms correctly denotes the type of hearing loss that results from a large amount of dry, hard wax in the ear canal?
1. Conductive
2. Perceptive
3. Sensorineural
4. Impacted

82. Which assessment data would alert the nurse to institute safety precautions for an elderly client diagnosed with heart failure and mild depression who is ambulatory?
1. Use of cathartics
2. Chronic depression
3. Excessive diuresis
4. Slowed ambulation

83. Which statement indicates that an elderly client with a stroke and right lower extremity paralysis understands the measures necessary to prevent pressure ulcers?
1. "I'll shift my weight while sitting in the wheelchair and examine my right foot every day."
2. "I'll spend the day in a reclining chair and apply lotion to my right leg every 4 hours."
3. "I'll wear my support stockings daily, and my daughter will give me a good back rub every night."
4. "I'll sit on an rubber inflatable ring in my wheelchair and wear comfortable, non-skid shoes on my feet."

84. Which outcome would be *most* appropriate for a terminally ill elderly female client with cachexia and limited mobility?
1. The client will verbalize that she is free from pain.
2. The client will demonstrate an ability to eat independently.
3. The client will remain free from skin breakdown.
4. The client will exhibit acceptance of the diagnosis.

85. When administering small doses of opioids to a client with a major burn, the nurse would select which route of administration?
1. I.V.
2. I.M.
3. Subcutaneous
4. Oral

86. The nurse instructs a client admitted to the emergency department following an automobile accident in which he sustained an abdominal injury to lie down on a stretcher. Which is the scientific rationale for the nurse's instructions?
1. To decrease abdominal pain and distention
2. To decrease risk of intra-abdominal clot dislodgment
3. To facilitate peristaltic activity of the intestines
4. To decrease risk of peritoneal infection

87. Following a bee sting, a client who develops shortness of breath and hives on his face and neck receives an epinephrine injection. Which assessment data would indicate that the epinephrine was effective?
1. Easier breathing
2. Reduced pain at the sting site
3. Drowsiness
4. Increased itching

88. Which intervention should the nurse implement *first* when beginning preoperative teaching?

1. Assessing the client's knowledge base related to the surgical procedure
2. Using a standardized preoperative teaching plan for consistency
3. Describing the possible risks of the surgical procedure
4. Having the client read the printed instructional booklet

89. Which topic would be most important to include in the postoperative teaching for the client scheduled for a vaginal hysterectomy?
1. Pelvic muscle strengthening exercises
2. Lower-extremity exercises and deep breathing
3. Availability of support persons
4. Use of a bedpan and call light

90. On the first day following a partial thyroidectomy, a client develops hypotension, tachycardia, tachypnea, swelling around the dressing, and whispered speech. Which complication should the nurse suspect?
1. Pulmonary embolism
2. Internal bleeding
3. Septic shock
4. Electrolyte imbalance

91. Following a cholecystectomy 2 days ago, a client complains of upper abdominal pain and bloating after eating solid food. Vital signs are stable but bowel sounds are hypoactive and abdominal distention is evident. Which intervention should the nurse implement *first?*
1. Application of a hyperthermia pad
2. Administration of an antiemetic
3. Insertion of a rectal tube
4. Administration of an opioid analgesic

92. Which assessment data would the nurse expect to see in a client with acute respiratory distress syndrome (ARDS)?
1. Deficient ventilation and perfusion lung scans
2. Increased anterior-posterior chest diameter

3. Bilateral pulmonary infiltrates on chest X-ray
4. Positive sputum culture

93. Five hours after a chest tube is inserted for a hemothorax, the nurse would expect which finding in the water seal chamber of the drainage device?
1. Vigorous bubbling
2. Level fluctuating with breathing
3. Bloody drainage
4. Absence of water movement

94. The nurse is caring for a client on the telemetry unit when the client goes into ventricular fibrillation. Which interventions should the nurse implement? (Select all that apply.)
1. Performing synchronized cardioversion at 50 joules
2. Assessing airway, breathing, and cardiovascular status
3. Calling a code and starting cardiopulmonary resuscitation
4. Defibrillating the client at 200 joules
5. Preparing to insert a cardiac pacemaker
6. Administering the antidysrhythmic medication, adenosine, via I.V. push

95. Which assessment findings would further support the diagnosis of a myocardial infarction (MI) in a client complaining of chest pain?
1. Jugular vein distention (JVD) and hepatomegaly
2. Fever and petechiae over the chest area
3. Nausea, vomiting, and cool, clammy skin
4. Pericardial friction rub and absent apical impulse

96. Which intervention is appropriate when administering digoxin to a client with heart failure?
1. Holding the drug if the radial pulse is below 60 beats per minute
2. Not administering the drug if the

digoxin level is 1.4 ng/ml
3. Administering the drug if the client's apical pulse is 84 beats per minute
4. Giving the drug if the client's potassium level is 3 mEq/L

97. Which statement indicates that the client with a permanent pacemaker understands the instructions about pacemaker failure?
1. "If I should feel lightheaded, I should stop what I'm doing and take a nitroglycerin tablet."
2. "I should check my incision and call the doctor if it looks red or swollen or becomes tender."
3. "I should take my pulse daily, and it should be irregular after my 2-mile walk."
4. "I'll call my doctor if I have any episodes of dizziness, weakness, or irregular pulse."

98. Which assessment data would the nurse expect to assess in a client with cholelithiasis?
1. Cramping pain in the right upper quadrant after a high-fat meal
2. Abdominal tenderness with back pain and hepatomegaly
3. Right lower quadrant pain at McBurney's point
4. Acute epigastric pain following a spicy meal

99. Which indication is the rationale for administering an antacid to a client with peptic ulcer disease?
1. To decrease hydrochloric acid production
2. To neutralize stomach acidity
3. To coat the gastric mucosa
4. To increase pepsin production

100. For the client experiencing excessive diarrhea secondary to ulcerative colitis, which signs and symptoms would warrant immediate nursing intervention?
1. Moist mucous membranes and a serum sodium level of 137 mEq/L
2. Intake equaling output for 8 hours and a serum calcium level of 9 mg/dl
3. Negative Trousseau's sign and a serum magnesium level of 2.0 mEq/L
4. Tented skin turgor and a serum potassium level of 3.1 mEq/L

101. Which discharge instruction should be included in the teaching plan for the client with a hiatal hernia?
1. "Consume a low-fiber diet."
2. "Recline after eating."
3. "Avoid bending at the waist."
4. "Eat three large meals every day."

102. Which would be an appropriate outcome for the client diagnosed with a sexually transmitted disease (STD)?
1. The client exhibits increased lymphadenopathy.
2. The client reports a decrease in sexual activity.
3. The client states pain and discharge have decreased.
4. The client states his partner needs no treatment.

103. A client with Crohn's disease is prescribed prednisone. Which statement by the client indicates that the nurse's teaching has been successful?
1. "I should take this medication after each loose bowel movement."
2. "I should stop the medication if I develop moon face."
3. "I will gradually reduce the dosage as ordered."
4. "I will need to stay on the medication for the rest of my life."

104. Which statement would be the nurse's best response to a family member asking questions about a client's transient ischemic attack (TIA)?
1. "I think you should ask the health care provider. Would you like me to call him for you?"
2. "The blood supply to the brain has de-

creased, causing permanent brain damage."

3. "It is a temporary interruption in the blood flow to the brain."

4. "TIA means a transient ischemic attack."

105. Which clinical findings would the nurse expect to assess in a client with a serum potassium level of 3.1 mEq/L?

1. Anorexia, fatigue, and muscle cramping

2. Tetany, positive Chvostek's sign, and seizures

3. Hot flushed skin, diaphoresis, and hypotension

4. Headache, drowsiness, and tachypnea

106. Which signs and symptoms would the nurse expect to find in a client with acute appendicitis?

1. Anorexia and dull left lower quadrant pain

2. Abdominal distention and diarrhea

3. Steatorrhea and weight loss

4. Pain at McBurney's point and mild fever

107. Which question would be *most* important to ask of a family member who had just witnessed a client's seizure?

1. "Why didn't you call for help sooner?"

2. "How do you feel after seeing this seizure?"

3. "Can you tell me how long the seizure lasted?"

4. "Did you say something to upset the client?"

108. A client diagnosed with chronic obstructive pulmonary disease is receiving prednisone, a glucocorticoid. Which instructions should the nurse include in her discharge teaching? (Select all that apply.)

1. "Discontinue the medication if weight gain, moon face, or buffalo hump occur."

2. "The medication must be tapered off prior to discontinuing it."

3. "Inject the medication into the abdominal wall subcutaneously daily."

4. "Take the medication on an empty stomach."

5. "Wear a medic-alert braclet while on this medication."

6. "The medication may mask infection."

109. Which statement by the client indicates a successful teaching plan about femoral cardiac catheterization?

1. "I will be asleep during the procedure so I won't feel anything."

2. "After the procedure, I will be able to walk to the bathroom with help."

3. "When the doctor injects the dye, I may feel hot and flushed."

4. "I will have to keep my arm perfectly still after the test."

110. Which term correctly describes the type of stool passed with a sigmoid colostomy?

1. Liquid

2. Semisoft

3. Formed

4. Pastelike

COMPREHENSIVE TEST: ANSWERS

1. The answer is **2.**
An otoscopic examination uses an otoscope to inspect the external canal and middle ear, specifically the tympanic membrane and its landmarks. Normally, the tympanic membrane appears pearly gray and intact. A pale optic disk is an abnormal finding during an ophthalmoscopic examination of the eyes. A positive red reflex is a normal finding with an ophthalmoscopic examination, not an otoscopic examination. Tactile fremitus is an abnormal finding when the chest is palpated.

2. The answer is **4.**
Asking about strengths and weaknesses assesses self-concept, one of the factors associated with role and relationship patterns. The client's ideas about health refer to the client's health beliefs, one aspect associated with health promotion and protection patterns. Asking about mobility and the family's health are aspects associated with health and illness patterns.

3. The answer is **4.**
The manifestations listed are indicative of insufficient arterial circulation. Other signs include delayed capillary refill in the toes; thin, shiny, dry scaling skin of the lower extremities; and toughened nails. Obstructed lymphatic flow would result in lymphedema evidenced by nonpitting edema, a dull heavy sensation, marked limb enlargement, and roughened skin without ulcerations. DVT would be manifested as edema (usually unilateral), pain in the calf muscle on foot dorsiflexion, calf or thigh tenderness and, possibly, a low-grade fever. Normal age-related changes would include thickening of the nails, dry wrinkled skin, possibly diminished extremity pulses, and sparse graying hair, but no ulcerations.

4. The answer is **3.**
The client's serum potassium level is elevated above the normal range of 3.5 to 5.5 mEq/L, indicating hyperkalemia. The client's WBC count is within the normal range, not increased as it would be in leukocytosis. The client's platelet level also is within the normal range, not decreased as it would be in thrombocytopenia, and his serum sodium level is normal, not increased as it would be with hypernatremia.

5. The answer is **3.**
Edema of inflamed tissue with cellular injury results from increased vascular permeability and leakage of plasma fluids. With cellular injury, transient vasoconstriction occurs first, followed by vasodilation resulting in an increase in vascular permeability. WBCs migrate to the site of the injury, not away from it. The release of chemical mediators, such as histamine, irritate nerve endings, causing pain, not swelling.

6. The answer is **2.**
A high-protein, high-calorie diet provides additional nutrients to promote tissue repair and healing. Vigorous washing with soap and water could easily damage the friable skin at the radiation site. The area should be washed with water only, and patted dry. Applying cool compresses to the radiation site causes vasoconstriction, thus impairing healing. Drinking warm fluids most likely would increase rather than decrease the discomfort in swallowing.

7. The answer is **4.**
Hyperplasia involves an increase in the number of cells in an organ or tissue, often related to hormonal influences. An example of hyperplasia is the increase in breast size that occurs during pregnancy. An enlarged heart indicates hypertrophy, an increase in cell size resulting in an increase

in organ size, such as from an increase in functional demand. Cell shrinkage indicates atrophy, often the result of inadequate nutrition or a decrease in workload. Epithelial cell changes secondary to smoking are an example of metaplasia resulting from a reversible change in one adult cell type, such as epithelial cells and replacement by another cell type.

8. The answer is **1**.

Furosemide is a loop diuretic that commonly causes potassium depletion. Thus, the client needs instructions about foods high in potassium to minimize the risk for hypokalemia. Additionally, the client needs instructions about the signs and symptoms of hypokalemia so that if any occur, the client can notify the health care provider to institute prompt treatment and prevent dangerously low serum potassium levels. When KCl is administered I.V., the rate of infusion should be 10 mEq per hour, not every 4 hours. The ECG should be monitored, but because the client has hypokalemia, flattened T waves, ST segment depression, and prominent U waves would be seen. Peaked, narrow T waves are associated with hyperkalemia. Also, hyperkalemia, not hypokalemia, results from hemolysis.

9. The answer is **1,000**.

To determine how many units of heparin per hour the client is receiving, the nurse must solve the equation: 20,000 units/500 ml = x units/25 ml/hr. Cross multiplication gives 500 ml (x units) = 50,000 units/ml/hour. Then, to solve for x, divide 50,000 units/ml/hour by 500 ml.

10. The answer is **3**.

The client's complaints and history, along with the ECG changes, strongly suggest hypercalcemia. The client's complaints of lethargy may indicate hypernatremia. However, more commonly, the client would complain of thirst and present with dry skin and mucous membranes. Plus, hyper-

natremia does not cause ECG changes. The client's complaints of lethargy and confusion may indicate hypermagnesemia. However, a shortened QT interval is characteristic for hypercalcemia. Nausea is associated with hyperkalemia, but the client most likely would also be experiencing some muscle weakness and paresthesias. Additionally, the ECG would reveal tall, narrow, peaked T waves along with a shortened QT interval if his serum potassium level was between 5.5 and 7.8 mEq/L.

11. The answer is **2**.

Because the client is experiencing severe diarrhea, he is losing large amounts of water along with some electrolytes. Therefore, he would be most likely to develop a fluid volume deficit. Most likely, the nurse would see an increased hematocrit because the red blood cells are contained within a relatively smaller plasma fluid volume. Also, the BUN and urine specific gravity would be increased, not decreased. Serum calcium levels reveal nothing about the client's fluid status. Elevated serum calcium levels are associated with excessive calcium intake, prolonged immobilization, renal failure, thiazide diuretic therapy, and hyperparathyroidism.

12. The answer is **2**.

Based on the ABG results, the client is experiencing metabolic alkalosis because the pH and HCO_3- levels are elevated. Metabolic alkalosis also results in mental status changes, such as belligerence and confusion. Also, the client is hypoxic, as evidenced by the low Pao_2, further contributing to the client's mental status changes. Although clients with acute respiratory distress may be anxious and frightened, more information would be needed to determine if this was the cause of the client's behavior. Also, behavioral changes are not typical findings expected in response to a respiratory crisis. Making such an assumption could lead the nurse to ignore the underlying physiologic cause. If the client was experiencing respiratory acidosis, the pH would be below 7.35 and the Pco_2 would be elevated above 45 mm Hg.

13. The answer is **2.**
Because many antacids contain magnesium, frequent or indiscriminate use of antacids may lead to high magnesium levels in the body. Therefore, the client needs instructions about the use of antacids and their role in contributing to hypermagnesemia. Encouraging frequent ambulation would aid in minimizing the loss of calcium, not magnesium, from the bone. Assessing for sleep pattern disturbances associated with neuromuscular irritability would be appropriate for the client with hypomagnesemia. Monitoring for manifestations of fluid volume excess would be appropriate if the client were retaining sodium.

14. The answer is **4.**
Type A-delta fibers transmit pain faster than type C fibers. Transmission over type A-delta fibers results in sharp, piercing pain. Type C fibers are responsible for the transmission of aching and burning pain. Type A-alpha, beta, and gamma fibers transmit touch, pressure, heat, cold, and movement impulses.

15. The answer is **60.**
One ounce is equal to 30 ml. Therefore, the nurse will prepare to administer 60 ml to the client.

16. The answer is **2.**
When a client is receiving warfarin, the PT value should be 1.5 to 2 times the control value. The INR should be between 2 to 3. The client's INR value is therapeutic, so the medication should be administered as ordered. There is no need to hold the medication or notify the health care provider. AquaMEPHYTON (Vitamin K) is the antidote for warfarin overdose. Protamine sulfate is the antidote for heparin.

17. The answer is **1.**
Staying with the client and holding hands offers support and empathy and conveys a sense of acceptance to the client. Additionally, these measures are noninvasive, commonly accepted by most clients, and may help to decrease stress and anxiety associated with the pain experience. PCA is an invasive treatment and requires the client's cooperation for effectiveness. Although TENS is a noninvasive, non-pharmacologic technique, the patient may refuse this as well. Administering the analgesic without the client's knowledge violates the client's rights. Waiting to provide pain relief measures until requested by the client ignores the client's needs.

18. The answer is **1.**
Immediate action is necessary, so the client should take a sublingual NTG tablet (a fast-acting nitrate that improves circulation) and lie down as soon as the angina begins. Lying down and resting decrease myocardial oxygen demand. Together, these actions help decrease the pain of angina. Exercise increases myocardial oxygen demand and exacerbates angina. Long-acting nitrates do not provide the immediate relief needed in this situation. Although sitting down and relaxing may decrease the myocardial oxygen demand, they have no effect on improving coronary circulation.

19. The answer is **3.**
The client is reporting behaviors that are detrimental to his condition in an attempt to consciously or unconsciously refuse to admit or accept responsibility for his illness. Usually, this is a sign of ineffective coping. Grieving over the loss of his health, as opposed to anticipatory grieving, is very likely a part of this client's emotional response. However, it would not lead to these behaviors. No evidence is presented in the scenario to support problems with body image or social interaction.

20. The answer is **4**.

The lungs work to maintain acid-base balance by controlling carbon dioxide (CO_2) and carbonic acid (H_2CO_3) excretion. CO_2 combines with water to form H_2CO_3, which in turn dissociates to form bicarbonate and hydrogen ions. This reaction determines the pH of arterial blood and the acid-base balance of the body. CO_2 is blown off or conserved to compensate for changes in the acid–base balance. Although the lungs do control oxygen (O_2) intake and gas exchange, O_2 is not a primary mechanism or regulator for acid-base balance. Cholesterol is not involved with acid-base balance, and the lungs have no control over cholesterol. The kidneys regulate urea and albumin.

21. The answer is **2**.

Pneumothorax refers to a collapsed lung that occurs when the pleura is incised or penetrated, allowing atmospheric air to rush into the pleural space. Normally, the pressure within the pleural space is negative to permit the lungs to expand. When atmospheric air enters, this negative pressure is disturbed, causing the lung to collapse on the affected side. The lung will not expand.

22. The answer is **2**.

In a client with a cardiac history, evidence of PVCs — indicative of increased automaticity of the ventricular muscle — could lead to possible lethal arrhythmias, such as ventricular tachycardia or ventricular fibrillation. PVCs are not associated with a significant increase in cardiac workload, MI, or a decrease in heart rate and blood pressure.

23. The answer is **4**.

The client is verbalizing her concerns about her role and her increased dependence on her husband after the surgery. Therefore, ineffective role performance is the most appropriate nursing diagnosis. No evidence is presented in the scenario to lead the

nurse to believe that there is impaired verbal communication or compromised family coping. More information would be needed to arrive at these nursing diagnoses. The client's statements about activity limitations imply that she has some knowledge about the postoperative course. Further investigation is needed to determine if she needs additional teaching.

24. The answer is **4**.

In chronic arterial occlusive disease, pain results from tissue ischemia. Interventions are planned to increase circulation to the extremities, thereby reducing the ischemia. Arterial, not venous, circulation is involved with chronic occlusive arterial disease. Improving venous return or preventing edema would have no effect on the ischemic pain. Although nonopioid pain relief is preferred because of the chronic nature of the disease, the pain associated with chronic arterial occlusive disease may be severe and require opioid analgesics, often in combination with other measures.

25. The answer is **2**.

The ulcer described is characteristic of a venous stasis ulcer. Venous stasis ulcers commonly occur around the ankles, especially the medial malleolus, are accompanied by edema and stasis dermatitis (the thick, coarse, brown pigmented skin), and have irregular, uneven borders. Ulcers from prolonged pressure vary in size and depth, ranging from an area of redness (stage I) to full thickness skin loss and major tissue destruction (stage IV). The presence of palpable pulses and a warm extremity indicate arterial circulation is intact. Therefore, arterial occlusion would not be the cause of the ulcer. Typically, arterial ulcers are found on the toe, heel, or over bony prominences with cool or cold skin and possibly gangrene surrounding the ulcer. Lymphedema results from obstructed lymphatic flow evidenced by nonpitting edema and roughened skin without ulceration or cellulitis.

26. The answer is **1**.
The appearance of red streaks indicates lymphadenitis and evidence of a spreading infection. The client should call the health care provider because further treatment is necessary. Not crossing the legs will aid in venous return, but foot edema is not as serious a threat to health as a spreading infection. Avoiding smoking is always an important health consideration. However, its effects are not as immediate as those of the spreading infection. Signs and symptoms of anaphylactic shock would most likely occur immediately after the administration of tetanus toxoid while the client is still in the health care facility.

27. The answer is **3**.
Blood pressure, pulse, and respiratory rate changes along with evidence of blood on the dressing are indicative of bleeding at the residual limb, one of the most common postamputation complications. Recovery from anesthesia usually is accompanied by a return to baseline vital signs, which are not known in this case. Although pain can alter a client's vital signs, no other indications of pain are presented in the scenario. Plus, the red area on the dressing is unrelated to pain. Early respiratory complications following surgery, such as atelectasis, are often accompanied by other findings such as an elevated temperature.

28. The answer is **intake, 1,200; output, 1,100.**
To determine the client's intake, the nurse must add the two I.V. piggyback administrations (200 ml total) with the I.V. administration (1,000 ml) to reach a sum of 1,200 ml. To obtain the client's urinary output, the nurse must subtract the bladder irrigation (2,000 ml) from the total output (3,100 ml) to reach a sum of 1,100 ml.

29. The answer is **2**.
The treatment of hypertension involves many aspects, one of which is stress reduction. Stress is considered one of the risk factors for the development of essential hypertension. Questioning the client about his usual stressors and coping mechanism aids in developing a client-specific teaching plan. The cause of essential hypertension is unknown. Having the client describe personal stress levels may or may not aid in relaxation. However, information about the client's stressors is important to help plan appropriate teaching strategies. Also, each client responds differently to stress, which may or may not interfere with learning. For this client, teaching must focus on helping him understand the problem and treatment alternatives to promote his active involvement in the therapeutic regimen.

30. The answer is **1**.
Antacids act to decrease the acidity and should be continued even if the client's symptoms subside or he feels better. Antacids should be taken 1 hour before or 2 hours after meals to be most effective. Because antacids alter the acid content of the stomach, they should not be taken with other medications because they can interfere with the absorption of the other medications. The sodium, not the magnesium, content of the antacid is of concern for the client with a cardiac problem.

31. The answer is **3**.
The large intestine functions primarily to absorb water from the intestinal contents and to eliminate the wastes as stool. Proper large intestinal function would be indicated by the passage of soft, formed stool. Pain relief after eating is suggestive of a duodenal ulcer. Evidence of adequate nutrient absorption would indicate proper small intestine function. Belching and acid reflux are associated with hiatal hernia.

32. The answer is **4.**

Anorexia and weight loss are common complications of ulcerative colitis. Portal hypertension and ascites will be seen with liver disorders. Vomiting is not a usual complication of ulcerative colitis.

33. The answer is **2.**

Infection is a physical stressor that causes an increase in the secretion of stress hormones, insulin resistance, and increased need for insulin. It is the most frequent cause of DKA. Overeating, a missed insulin dose, and psychological stress may contribute to hyperglycemia, but not DKA.

34. The answer is **1.**

The client who has diabetes and an open foot ulcer needs to clean the foot daily with soap and water, pat it dry, and monitor the ulcer for signs and symptoms of infection. The client with diabetes has an increased risk of infection resulting from the inability of the granulocytes to respond to infection. The existence of an open ulcer further contributes to this risk. Because of macroangiopathy and neuropathy, the client with diabetes is at risk for injury from impaired circulation and sensation. Thus, any extremes of temperature, including soaks in hot water or applications of heat, should be avoided to prevent possible burns. A compression bandage would further compromise circulation and interfere with frequent ulcer assessment. Iodine is potentially damaging to the tissues and also should be avoided.

35. The answer is **1.**

The nurse will administer 0.5 ml of meperidine (12.5 mg is half 25 mg) and 0.5 ml of promethazine (25 mg is half of 50 mg). Therefore, the total amount of medication is 1 ml.

36. The answer is **3.**

Following a thyroidectomy, postoperative hemorrhage may cause compression of the trachea, necessitating an emergency tracheostomy to maintain airway patency. Calcium and thyroid hormone may be administered postoperatively, but these agents are unrelated to the hemorrhage. Insertion of an oral airway would be ineffective in maintaining airway patency because the compression from the hemorrhage is below the airway insertion site.

37. The answer is **1.**

With primary open-angle glaucoma, the client generally has no early symptoms. As the disease progresses, the client experiences blurred vision, diminished accommodation, gradual loss of peripheral vision (tunnel vision), mild eye aching, and halos around lights as intraocular pressure increases. A cloudy lens and lack of eye pain or redness are commonly associated with cataracts. Floating spots suggest retinal detachment.

38. The answer is **3.**

Impotence, the inability to achieve or maintain an erection, is the result of numerous organic and psychogenic causes. The pathologic processes are diverse, but commonly involve decreased blood flow to the penis, altered nerve conduction, or decreased hormonal secretion. The incidence of impotence increases with age. Impotence may be partial or full, intermittent or constant, transient, selective for partners, and of sudden or gradual onset. Although dietary factors may conceivably play a role in a physiologic disease leading to impotence, they are not a primary or major consideration.

39. The answer is **3.**

The prostatic bed is a highly vascular area. Following surgery, clots form that may obstruct urinary drainage, leading to urinary retention and increased pressure on this highly vascular area, subsequently causing hemorrhage. Pressure on the incision typically results in pain, not hemorrhage. DVT and infection are not usually associated with hemorrhage.

40. The answer is **2.**

When performing a testicular self-examination, the testes should feel smooth and oval shaped without any masses. Tenderness or pain on palpation is not commonly associated with testicular cancer. In fact, testicular cancer is more commonly associated with a painless enlargement of the scrotum. Generally, testicular masses are easy to detect. A palpable, firm testicular mass may suggest testicular cancer.

41. The answer is **1.**

With a hysterectomy, the area around the bladder typically undergoes surgical manipulation. This causes edema and nerve trauma, possibly leading to temporary atony. Therefore, if the client is unable to void within 8 hours, urinary catheterization is performed to prevent urinary retention. The bladder is not removed along with the uterus in this procedure. Infection is a possibility following surgery but it is not a reason for catheterization. Rather, urinary catheterization may increase the client's risk for infection. Surgically induced menopause occurs with a hysterectomy only if the client's ovaries also were removed. However, this does not impair a client's urinary function.

42. The answer is **4.**

With allergic contact dermatitis, the allergen determines the intensity and range of the allergic reaction. The reaction involves a delayed hypersensitivity requiring a latent period ranging from several days to years. Many substances can produce allergic contact dermatitis, including exposure to poison ivy, topical medications, cosmetics, soaps, and industrial chemicals. The extent of the rash depends on the allergen and exposure; it may be localized or generalized.

43. The answer is **4.**

Although all the options are plausible for the client with RA, the first step is to assess the client's needs. Then, appropriate and necessary interventions can be planned to meet these needs. Without a thorough assessment of the client's needs, the other interventions, such as teaching, referrals, and emotional support, will be ineffective.

44. The answer is **1.**

For the client experiencing an acute exacerbation of asthma who is dyspneic and irritable, the nurse should elevate the head of the bed to ease the work of breathing and allow for maximum lung expansion. Typically, respiratory acidosis is present in clients with acute asthma. Breathing into a paper bag is inappropriate because doing so would increase the client's carbon dioxide level, which is already elevated because of the bronchoconstriction and air-trapping. Fluids are encouraged rather than withheld to liquefy secretions. An expectorant, not an antitussive agent, would be used to aid in moving the secretions.

45. The answer is **3.**

According to the ABA, major burn injuries are defined as those involving second-degree burns covering more than 25% of the TBSA in adults or 20% of the TBSA in children, or those involving third-degree burns of 10% or more of the TBSA in any client. Minor burn injuries involve second-degree burns covering less than 15% of the TBSA in adults or less than 10% of the TBSA in children. Moderate uncomplicated burn injuries are defined as second-degree burns over 15% to 25% of the TBSA in adults or 10% to 20% of the TBSA in children, or third-degree burns of more than 10% of TBSA without involvement of special care areas. Full-thickness burn injuries involve the epidermis, dermis, and underlying subcutaneous tissue.

46. The answer is **1.**

Before any other action can be taken, the source of the burn injury must be eliminated. The airway patency is ensured, any associated injuries are assessed and treated, and then burn shock is treated. Once these actions are instituted, other measures may follow, such as inserting an I.V. line, nasogastric tube, and urinary catheter and caring for the wounds.

47. The answer is **4.**
To calculate fluid replacement using the Parkland formula, the nurse would multiply 4 ml of lactated Ringer's solution by the percentage of TBSA by the client's body weight in kilograms. This would give the total fluid requirement for 24 hours postburn. In this scenario, the calculation would be: $4 \times 50 \times 70$, which equals 14,000 ml in the first 24 hours. One-half of this total, or 7,000 ml, would be given in the first 8 hours postburn; one-fourth of the total, or 3,500 ml, would be given in the second 8 hours; and the last one-fourth, 3,500 ml, in the third 8 hours. 1,400 ml would be an insufficient amount for fluid replacement.

48. The answers are **2, 4, 6.**
At 8 hours postinsertion, the chest tube must be occluded. Therefore, the nurse should assess the client's respiratory status to make sure that he is breathing, determine if the chest tube is kinked or has dependent loops, and have the client turn, cough, and deep-breathe to expel possible any clots in the tubing. The nurse should milk (not strip) the tubing; stripping the tubing may cause lung wall damage. Increasing wall suction will not unclog the chest tube. Usually, at 8 hours postinsertion, the lungs have not re-expanded, so no health care provider notification is necessary.

49. The answer is **4.**
Myasthenia gravis, a disorder affecting the neuromuscular transmission of the voluntary muscles of the body, results in extreme muscular weakness after activity and ptosis, along with diplopia and dysphonia. Fatigue and difficulty in coordination would be indicative of multiple sclerosis. Nuchal rigidity and positive Kernig's sign would be indicative of meningitis. Muscular rigidity

and resting tremor would be indicative of Parkinson's disease.

50. The answer is **3.**
Because of the client's craniotomy, straining on defecation should be avoided to prevent increasing intracranial pressure. Therefore, ensuring an adequate intake of fluids and high-fiber foods is the initial step in preventing or easing constipation. Additionally, a stool softener may be ordered to prevent straining. If these measures are ineffective, then enemas and mild laxatives may be used. However, enemas typically would not be given daily. Sodium restriction would not impact the client's bowel function.

51. The answer is **1.**
Following surgical removal of a protruded intervertebral lumbar disk, the nurse should maintain the client in proper body alignment while he is in bed and also while he is ambulating. Additionally, the client should wear well-fitting, skid-free shoes and loose objects should be removed from the client's path. If the client is experiencing pain, analgesics should be administered 15 to 30 minutes prior to ambulating to ensure effectiveness of the analgesic and to prevent pain while ambulating. A cane would only be needed if the client has another mobility problem or has footdrop. Immobilizing the head and neck is done for spinal cord injuries.

52. The answer is **1.**
The client with a Glasgow Coma Scale of 7 has suffered a severe head injury. To help maintain cerebral perfusion and prevent increased intracranial pressure, osmotic diuretics are given to decrease cerebral edema, noxious stimuli are reduced or eliminated, and the head of the bed is elevated to 30 degrees. Because of the severity of the client's condition, the client needs to be turned on a regular schedule while in bed to maintain skin integrity.

53. The answer is **3.**

With a spinal cord injury below the level of T12, the client would exhibit loss of motor control and of sensation below the waist and loss of bowel and bladder control. With an injury below C4, the client would exhibit loss of motor and sensory function from the neck down, including independent respiratory function and bowel and bladder control. Injury below the level of C8 would be evidenced as loss of motor control and sensation to parts of the arms and hands and loss of bowel and bladder control. With injury to S1, there would be loss of motor control and sensation in parts of the thighs and legs.

54. The answer is **3.**

Miotics are used to treat glaucoma because these agents lower intraocular pressure by constricting the pupil and promoting the outflow of aqueous humor. Pupil constriction results in impaired night vision. Mydriatics may impair near vision or cause photophobia (increased sensitivity to light) because of pupil dilation. Diplopia or double vision should not occur with eye medications.

55. The answer is **4.**

Following intraocular surgery, complaints of eye pain are indicative of increased intraocular pressure secondary to hemorrhage. Temperature elevations may occur as a manifestation of an inflammatory response. Diplopia is common following cataract surgery when one eye has a lens and the other doesn't. Visual floaters are symptoms of retinal detachment.

56. The answer is **2.**

Prolonged use (3 to 5 days) of nasal decongestant sprays can lead to rebound congestion, relieved by discontinuing the spray for 2 to 3 weeks. Continuing the medication alone or in combination with an oral decongestant or increasing the dosage or frequency would only worsen this phenomenon.

57. The answer is **3.**

The eardrum acts as a protective membrane, separating the external canal from the middle ear. When perforated, this protection is lost and the client is at increased risk for suppurative otitis media. With perforation, the client may or may not experience hearing loss or pain. General ear care and hearing-protection measures are usual health promotion areas and are not specific to a perforated eardrum.

58. The answer is **4.**

After a total laryngectomy, the client has a permanent tracheostomy. Thus, the client needs teaching about how to protect the opening from water and particulate matter during such activities as showering and washing the hair. Although referral to a support group is important and helpful, it is not essential that it be completed prior to discharge. Although the client should carry medical identification for special needs and should receive an explanation regarding the loss of strength with Valsalva's maneuver, these interventions are not as essential as those for self-care safety in activities of daily living.

59. The answer is **2.**

Mental status changes, such as confusion, irritability, restlessness, disorientation, stupor, and coma, are indicative of hypoxemia and are often the first sign of systemic fat embolism. The symptoms may begin subtly, with rapid onset of respiratory, cardiovascular, and other systemic symptoms depending on the location of the fat embolus. Hematuria, fever, and discoloration of the fracture site are not associated with fat embolism. Bruising and ecchymosis may be present at the fracture sites secondary to the injury.

60. The answer is **3.**

A client undergoing MRI is exposed to an extremely strong magnetic field. Therefore, it is imperative to have the client remove all jewelry and to check about the status of any electrical, magnetic, or mechanical implants, such as staples, clips, pins, or pacemakers. MRI is not invasive; therefore, preoperative medication is not required. However, this does not imply that teaching is not necessary. The test also does not involve any injections, so scrubbing is inappropriate. The test does not involve a contrast medium, so an allergy history is not necessary. However, it is always good practice to check about a client's allergies.

61. The answer is **1.**
The client's complaints of pain out of proportion to the injury along with the decreased capillary refill and cyanotic nailbeds suggest compartment syndrome, a condition caused by either a decrease in the compartment size or an increase in the compartment contents. In such a case, the nurse should notify the health care provider immediately and prepare for releasing the compression by bivalving the cast, cutting dressings, or performing a fasciotomy. Cutting a window and checking for infection, elevating the casted arm, or administering an analgesic would be inappropriate measures at this time because the client needs immediate pressure relief inside the cast.

62. The answer is **4.**
In the immediate postoperative period for the client with an amputation, the risk of hemorrhage from a loosened ligature is the most threatening complication. With hemorrhage, ineffective tissue perfusion occurs. Disturbed body image, risk for infection, and chronic pain are all possible nursing diagnoses, applicable during the postoperative period. However, none are of as high a priority as ineffective tissue perfusion.

63. The answer is **1.**
Following a limb amputation, a client typically experiences disturbed body image and must learn to accept the loss and a new image. The nurse must work closely with the client, build a trusting relationship, and

encourage the client to look at, feel, and care for the residual limb. Once the client has accomplished these tasks, he is on the way to accepting the loss and beginning to build a new self-image. Inviting family and friends to visit, asking about pain-relief methods, and expressing a desire to go home and resume work could apply to the client. However, they are not specific to the nursing diagnosis of disturbed body image and acceptance of the loss of a body part.

64. The answer is **1.**
Portal hypertension refers to the elevated pressure in the portal vein associated with resistance to blood flow through the porta hepatis. Cirrhosis or mechanical obstruction leads to obstruction of the portal venous flow through the liver. Ascites and esophageal varices result from portal hypertension. Obstructed bile flow would lead to jaundice.

65. The answers are **2, 4.**
The nurse should rule out surgical complications, such as hemorrhage, by assessing the client's blood pressure and pulse. The nurse also should medicate the client immediately because the client is only 4 hours postoperative. The client will not have an abdominal incision with this surgery (rectal dressing). The nurse would be concerned if the stoma was purple, not pink. The client needs medication, not distraction, at 4 hours postoperative. Sitting on the side of the bed will not help the client's pain.

66. The answer is **1.**
Clients commonly associate a distended abdomen with obesity. With ascites, the abdomen is distended, possibly grossly distended. Ascites does not cause jaundice although the two often occur together. Ascites is not typically associated with fecal incontinence or muscle wasting.

67. The answer is **4.**
The removal of large amounts of fluid, such

as 2 to 3 L, via paracentesis may lead to acute fluid shifting and hypotension, subsequently leading to vascular collapse. Respiratory distress is uncommon following this procedure. Paracentesis removes fluid but does not alter the ammonia levels or protein status; therefore, encephalopathy is not a complication. Bleeding from the site may occur, but this is the result of needle puncture, regardless of the amount of fluid removed.

68. The answer is **2.**
For the client with cholelithiasis, ingestion of a high-fat meal commonly results in pain. Therefore, a low-fat diet may be prescribed in an attempt to control or decrease the episodes of pain. If this treatment is effective, typically the client will report that pain is absent after ingestion of such a meal. Maintaining intake and output within normal parameters is appropriate for any client and provides no evidence for evaluating the factors associated with cholelithiasis. Serum alkaline phosphatase levels, not albumin levels, would be evaluated for the client with cholelithiasis. Plus, this outcome does not focus on the aggravating factors. Improvement on ultrasonography is appropriate for the client with cholelithiasis; however, this outcome does not address the effectiveness of treatment to reduce aggravating factors.

69. The answer is **2.**
Morphine, unlike meperidine, causes spasms of Oddi's sphincter, which may aggravate pancreatitis and increase pain. Meperidine's duration of action is slightly less than that of morphine. Both drugs have approximately the same potential for addiction. Morphine is not associated with liver dysfunction.

70. The answer is **3.**
Because insertion of the peritoneal dialysis catheter provides an opening for organisms to enter the body, the client is at risk for infection and peritonitis. Therefore, it is crucial that the client receive instructions in the use of strict aseptic technique throughout the procedure. Sodium intake is not related to dialysis. However, in most cases, a special diet will be ordered for the client because of his underlying renal problems. Typically, the dialysis solutions are premixed and the amount of dextrose in the solution is related to the fluid removal. Heparin also may be added to the solutions to help prevent fibrin clots. However, the drug plays no role in preventing infection.

71. The answer is **2.**
During hemodialysis, heparin is added to dialyzer blood to prevent clotting in the dialyzer. As a result, the client's blood becomes anticoagulated, increasing the risk for bleeding. Following hemodialysis, urea levels are typically decreased. Platelet activity is not affected by hemodialysis. Although hematocrit may be increased following hemodialysis, this would not contribute to bleeding.

72. The answer is **2.**
For the client with renal failure, typical dietary recommendations would include: decreased protein intake, decreased sodium and potassium intake, and high-calorie foods of simple sugars and carbohydrates. The majority of clients experience hyperphosphatemia, requiring the use of phosphate-binding agents, so increased phosphorus in the diet would be avoided.

73. The answer is **4.**
The spouse in this situation is verbalizing problems directly associated with the effects of the client's chronic renal failure that are affecting the marital relationship and causing a disruption. Therefore, interrupted family processes is the most appropriate nursing diagnosis. Although noncompliance, situational low self-esteem, and anxiety are possible nursing diagnoses for the client with renal failure, no evidence is

presented in the scenario to support any of these.

74. The answers are **4, 5, 6.**

GERD is excessive reflux of hydrochloric acid in the esophagus. The nurse should instruct the patient to sit up after all meals for at least 2 hours. The nurse also should impart to the client the importance of abstaining from food and drink 2 hours before bedtime, taking prescribed medications, and losing weight, if appropriate. The head of the bed (not the foot of the bed) should be elevated, and the nurse should encourage a low-fat, high-fiber diet. A bland diet will not help GERD.

75. The answer is **3.**

Fever, infection, alloimmunization from previous transfusions, bleeding, autoimmune destruction, and hypertension may result in poor incremental increases in the count following a platelet transfusion. Platelets should be infused as rapidly as tolerated, usually 4 units every 30 to 60 minutes. Platelets may be used in selected instances to prevent bleeding. Hemoglobinuria is a manifestation of a hemolytic transfusion reaction, whereas hives, generalized pruritus, wheezing, and anaphylaxis (rare) indicate an allergic reaction.

76. The answer is **1.**

The client's blood count reveals a severely depressed WBC count with neutrophils less than $500/mm^3$, indicating neutropenia. Fever and infection in a client with neutropenia can be rapidly fatal if broad-spectrum antibiotic therapy is not instituted immediately. Thus, the health care provider needs to be called immediately so that appropriate treatment can be started. Once the health care provider has been notified, acetaminophen may be given and the nurse should monitor the client frequently, but more often than every 4 hours. Additionally, the client should be moved to a private room (the location should allow for fre-

quent monitoring) and placed on reverse isolation.

77. The answer is **3.**

Color changes associated with anemia are best assessed where capillary beds are superficial and pigmentation is abnormal. These areas include the nailbeds, hard palate, lips, palms of the hands, soles of the feet, and conjunctivae. A client may exhibit few symptoms if the onset of anemia was gradual and adequate cardiopulmonary compensation has occurred. Because hematocrit may be affected by the client's hydration status (plasma volume) and red blood cell size, it is not the best indicator of anemia. Too rapid an infusion of packed RBCs in a client exhibiting few symptoms and, subsequently, compensation for the anemia may result in circulatory overload.

78. The answers are **1, 4, 5.**

The client with peripheral arterial occlusive disease has decreased arterial blood to the lower extremities, which results in leg pain (intermittent claudication). Therefore, when pain occurs, the client should stop all activity. The client also should perform scrupulous foot care daily and abstain from nicotine and caffeine, which cause vasoconstriction, further decreasing blood to the lower extremities. Never apply heat to the area, it can lead to paresthesia and tissue damage. Feet should be kept in a dependent position to increase peripheral blood flow. Wearing knee-high stockings can cause constriction, further impeding arterial blood flow.

79. The answer is **4.**

Strenuous physical activity, including strenuous exercise, is contraindicated for a client with sickle cell anemia because the physiologic stress that it creates can precipitate a crisis. Relaxation techniques are helpful in controlling emotional stress, which may precipitate a crisis. Alcohol consumption and fatigue also are contributing factors to a sickle cell crisis. Therefore, frequent rest periods and avoiding alcohol are helpful in preventing a crisis.

80. The answer is **3.**
The most important and effective measure to prevent nosocomial infections, especially in a client with a decreased WBC count, is to perform meticulous hand-washing before, during, and after caring for him. Observing for signs of infection also is important, but prevention is the priority. Isolating the client may be used in some institutions if the client's WBC count (neutrophils) drops below a specified level. Family members who are ill should be restricted from visiting the client. However, other family members who are in good health may visit the client as long as they, too, perform proper handwashing.

81. The answer is **1.**
A large amount of dry, hard wax in the ear canal refers to impacted cerumen, the leading cause of conductive hearing loss. With this type of hearing loss, sound is unable to be transmitted through the canal to the tympanic membrane. Sensorineural or perceptive hearing loss involves the middle or inner ear. Impacted is not a type of hearing loss.

82. The answer is **3.**
The client with heart failure typically receives diuretic therapy leading to diuresis and volume depletion. As a result, the client may experience orthostatic hypotension, becoming dizzy and lightheaded when arising. This places the client at risk for falling. Cathartics may cause problems with elimination, but unless they were overused or abused (leading to electrolyte imbalances), they would not increase the client's risk of falling. Depression and slowed ambulation are not typically associated with an increased risk of falling and the need for safety precautions.

83. The answer is **1.**
Regular position changes and weight shifts can help prevent pressure ulcer formation. The skin of the affected extremity should be inspected daily because altered sensation may leave the client unaware that an injury has occurred. Applying lotion to the skin prevents dryness. However, if applied too frequently, it may exacerbate skin breakdown. The use of support stockings aids in venous return and a back rub is comforting. However, neither helps to prevent pressure ulcers. Sitting on an inflatable ring can impair tissue perfusion. The rubber also can impair moisture evaporation from the skin, predisposing the client to skin breakdown.

84. The answer is **3.**
A terminally ill elderly client with cachexia is nutritionally depleted and at very high risk for skin breakdown. In addition, the client has limited mobility, further contributing to her risk for skin breakdown. Therefore, remaining free from skin breakdown would be the most appropriate outcome. Freedom from pain may be an appropriate outcome for a terminally ill client, but more information would be needed to determine if this is appropriate. The most important aspect about the client's ability to eat is not her independence in doing so. Rather, the focus is on ensuring an adequate intake. Acceptance of the diagnosis may or may not be appropriate because some clients with cancer never completely accept what is happening to them.

85. The answer is **1.**
A client with a major burn is in shock and often in severe pain. Therefore, the route providing the quickest onset of action — the I.V. route — should be used. As a result of shock, the client's peripheral circulation is poor, thus contraindicating use of the I.M. and subcutaneous routes. Clients with major burns also commonly develop paralytic ileus and, as such, receive nothing by mouth.

86. The answer is **2**.

For the client who has sustained an abdominal injury, the primary rationale for having him lie down is to minimize activity, thereby preventing intra-abdominal clots from dislodging, which could resulting in hemorrhage. Lying down also may help to decrease pain (although not the primary reason for lying down), but it has no effect on distention. Lying down and, subsequently, bedrest and immobility would decrease peristaltic activity. Bedrest has no effect on whether or not the client develops a peritoneal infection.

87. The answer is **1**.

The client is exhibiting an allergic reaction to the bee sting. Epinephrine acts as a bronchodilator to ease the client's breathing. It has no effect on pain and will not cause drowsiness or increase itching.

88. The answer is **1**.

Before beginning any teaching program, the nurse must first assess the client's knowledge base. Doing so allows the nurse to identify the client's teaching needs, avoid repetition of areas the client is already familiar with, and identify and correct any misconceptions or misinformation that the client might have. Once this is completed, the nurse may use a standardized teaching plan that has been adapted to the client's specific needs. Explaining the possible risks of surgery is the responsibility of the health care provider. Written instructional information may be used to supplement the teaching plan. However, it does not take the place of teaching.

89. The answer is **2**.

Use of the lithotomy position for a vaginal hysterectomy predisposes the client to deep vein thrombosis (DVT). Additionally, atelectasis from surgery also may occur. Thus, the client needs instructions on lower-extremity exercises to minimize the risk of DVT. She also needs instruction on deep-breathing exercises to prevent atelectasis.

Pelvic muscle strengthening exercises are inappropriate unless the client has difficulty with controlling urination; the health care provider would order these exercises. Availability of support persons, although important, is less of a priority when compared with the client's risk for complications from the surgery. Use of the bedpan and call light should be part of the client's orientation to the hospital room.

90. The answer is **2**.

The client is exhibiting signs and symptoms of hypovolemic shock along with edema at the surgical site. These would suggest internal bleeding. Pulmonary embolism typically is evidenced by chest pain and hemoptysis. In septic shock, the client's skin would be warm and flushed or cool and clammy, and his temperature would be elevated. Since only a partial thyroidectomy was performed, electrolyte imbalance is unlikely because not all of the parathyroid glands were disrupted.

91. The answer is **3**.

The signs and symptoms exhibited by the client suggest abdominal flatus, a common event with eating solid foods at this point in the client's recovery. The client should be encouraged to ambulate to aid in moving and expelling the gas. Additionally, a rectal tube may be used to aid in expulsion. A hyperthermia pad will have no effect on the passage of flatus. An antiemetic is not indicated because the client is not experiencing nausea or vomiting. An opioid analgesic would slow peristalsis, leading to an increase in gas accumulation and abdominal distention.

92. The answer is **3**.

ARDS is a clinical syndrome characterized by pulmonary edema and a progressive decrease in arterial oxygen content. It is always secondary to another illness or injury. Typically, the chest X-ray shows bilateral pulmonary infiltrates. Deficient ventilation and perfusion lung scans are seen with pulmonary embolism. Increased anterior-posterior chest diameter occurs with emphysema. A positive sputum culture indicates an infection.

93. The answer is **2.**
Five hours after insertion, water level fluctuation should occur with inspiration and expiration. This typically continues until the lung is fully inflated. If vigorous bubbling occurs, the nurse should suspect an air leak. Bloody drainage should appear in the drainage chamber, not the water seal chamber. If the water level doesn't fluctuate, the nurse should assess the chest tube for kinks or clots.

94. The answers are **2, 3, 4.**
Ventricular fibrillation is a life-threatening dysrhythmia. The nurse should call a code; assess the client's airway, breathing, and cardiovascular status; and defibrillate him up to three times starting at 200 joules. Synchronized cardioversion would be indicated for ventricular tachycardia. A cardiac pacemaker is for sinus bradycardia or asystole. Adenosine is for supraventricular tachycardia.

95. The answer is **3.**
Common clinical manifestations of an MI include radiating chest pain; diaphoresis; cool, pale skin; nausea and vomiting; dyspnea with or without crackles; syncope; and restlessness. JVD and hepatomegaly are signs of heart failure. Fever and chest area petechiae indicate endocarditis. Pericardial friction rub and absent apical impulse suggest pericarditis.

96. The answer is **3.**
Digoxin should be administered if the client's apical, not radial, pulse rate is above 60 and below 100 beats per minute. If the client's apical pulse is outside this range, then the drug is withheld and the health care provider is notified. A digoxin level of 1.4 ng/ml is within the normal range of 0.5 to 2 ng/ml. Hypokalemia, evidenced by a serum potassium level below 3.5 mEq/L, would increase the client's risk for digoxin toxicity, so the drug should not be given until the potassium level is back within normal range.

97. The answer is **4.**
If pacemaker failure occurs, the client will exhibit signs and symptoms of heart failure, such as dizziness, weakness, or an irregular pulse. If the client experiences lightheadedness, he should notify the health care provider immediately. Checking the incision for signs and symptoms of infection is appropriate, but an incisional infection would not lead to pacemaker failure. Any irregular pulse should be brought to the health care provider's attention immediately.

98. The answer is **1.**
With cholelithiasis, the client typically experiences episodic cramping pain in the right upper quadrant after a high-fat meal with the pain radiating to the right shoulder. Additional manifestations include nausea and vomiting, fat intolerance, fever, and leukocytosis. Abdominal tenderness with back pain and hepatomegaly suggest liver failure. Right lower quadrant pain at McBurney's point is typical of appendicitis. Acute epigastric pain following a spicy meal is associated with peptic ulcer disease.

99. The answer is **2.**
Antacids are given for acute epigastric pain secondary to peptic ulcer disease. The antacid neutralizes the acid in the stomach, decreasing the pH to prevent erosion of the mucosal lining. Histamine receptor antagonists decrease the stimulus for hydrochloric acid production. Mucosal protectant agents produce an ulcer-adherent complex that hastens healing by coating the mucosal lining. Pepsin is an enzyme and is not affected by the action of antacids.

100. The answer is **4**.

The client is losing large amounts of fluid and electrolytes through his stool. Tented skin turgor and hypokalemia (serum potassium level below 3.5 mEq/L) indicate a fluid volume deficit secondary to diarrhea requiring intervention. Moist mucous membranes, a serum sodium level of 137 mEq/L, equal intake and output, a serum calcium level of 9 mg/dl, negative Trousseau's sign, and a serum magnesium level of 2.0 mEq/L are within normal parameters.

101. The answer is **3**.

For the client with a hiatal hernia, teaching focuses on measures to decrease activities that increase intra-abdominal pressure, such as bending at the waist, lifting heavy objects, and straining to defecate. Additionally, the client should eat a high-fiber diet to avoid constipation and straining. The client should be encouraged to sit up after eating to prevent acid reflux. Small, frequent, bland meals are recommended.

102. The answer is **3**.

For the client with an STD, appropriate outcomes would focus on a decrease in the signs and symptoms of the disease, such as a decrease in pain and discharge. Lymphadenopathy should decrease. The client should abstain from sexual activity until there is evidence of disease cure or control. In addition, the client's partners should receive treatment.

103. The answer is **3**.

Prednisone, a corticosteroid, must be taken directly as ordered and should be discontinued gradually with dosage tapering, not stopped abruptly, to prevent adrenal crisis. After prolonged therapy, adrenal insufficiency may develop if the medication is stopped abruptly. Prednisone is typically taken daily, not after each loose bowel movement. Moon face is an adverse effect of the drug, but it is not a reason for discontinuing the medication. Prednisone is ordered for acute exacerbations of Crohn's disease and is not indicated as lifelong therapy because the drug will suppress adrenal gland function.

104. The answer is **3**.

With a TIA, there is a temporary interruption in the blood flow to the brain, typically lasting from seconds to hours. This interruption causes transient neurologic deficits that clear completely within 12 to 24 hours. This response is easiest for a layperson to understand. Telling the family member to ask the health care provider is inappropriate. The nurse is capable and able to explain what a TIA is. Saying that the blood supply to the brain has decreased, causing permanent brain damage, is inaccurate. Stating that TIA means a transient ischemic attack provides the family member with no information.

105. The answer is **1**.

The client's serum potassium level is decreased, indicating hypokalemia. Common clinical manifestations of hypokalemia include anorexia, fatigue, muscle cramping, paresthesia, and electrocardiogram changes. Tetany, positive Chvostek's sign, and seizures are associated with hypocalcemia. Hot flushed skin, diaphoresis, and hypotension are indicative of hypermagnesemia. Headache, drowsiness, and tachypnea may be seen with metabolic acidosis.

106. The answer is **4**.

The manifestations of acute appendicitis include acute abdominal pain, usually in the right lower quadrant (McBurney's point); rebound tenderness; nausea and vomiting; and a low-grade fever. Anorexia, dull left lower quadrant pain, distention, diarrhea, steatorrhea, and weight loss are not associated with acute appendicitis.

107. The answer is **3**.

The most important question is to ask the family member to provide details about the seizure, such as how long it lasted, which body parts were affected, or whether the client noticed an aura. This information provides valuable clues for understanding the seizure activity and planning care. Asking why he did not call for help sooner or whether he said something to upset the client is condescending and attempts to assign blame for the seizure. Asking him how he feels after seeing the seizure may be important at a later time once information about the seizure has been obtained.

108. The answers are **2, 5, 6.**

Prednisone is an oral medication that may cause a decrease in adrenal gland production. Therefore, the medication must be tapered off. Prednisone also may mask infection, and the client should wear a medic-alert bracelet to alert all health care providers that he is taking the medication. Adverse effects of prednisone include weight gain and moon face, but the client should continue taking the medication even if these effects develop. The client should take the medication orally, not by subcutaneous injection. The client should take the medication with food to decrease gastric upset.

109. The answer is **3.**

During a cardiac catheterization using the femoral artery, the client may experience a hot, flushed feeling and some chest discomfort when the dye is injected. The client will be awake during the procedure and will be maintained on strict bed rest for 8 to 12 hours following the procedure to prevent arterial bleeding. Because the femoral artery is being used, the client will be required to keep the leg, not the arm, perfectly straight after the test.

110. The answer is **3.**

With creation of a sigmoid colostomy, the rectum and part of the descending colon are removed. However, enough of the colon remains so that the stool passed is formed, the same consistency as that eliminated through the rectum prior to the surgery. Liquid stool is characteristic of an ileostomy. Semisoft and pastelike stool would be characteristic of ostomies created higher than the descending colon.

BIBLIOGRAPHY

American Association of Critical Care Nurses. *Core Curriculum for Critical Care Nurses,* 5th ed. Philadelphia: W.B. Saunders Co., 1998.

Ackley, B.J., and Ladwig, G.B., eds. *Nursing Diagnosis Handbook: A Guide to Planning Care,* 6th ed. St. Louis: Mosby-Year Book, Inc., 2004.

American Cancer Society. *Cancer Facts and Figures 2004.* Atlanta: American Cancer Society, 2004.

Barkauskas, V.H., et al., eds. *Health and Physical Assessment,* 3rd ed. St. Louis: Mosby-Year Book, Inc., 2001.

Bickley, L.S., and Szilagyi, P.G. *Bates' Guide to Physical Examination and History Taking,* 8th ed. Philadelphia: Lippincott Williams & Wilkins, 2003.

Bullock, B.L., and Henze, R.L. *Focus on Pathophysiology.* Philadelphia: Lippincott Williams & Wilkins, 2000.

Carpenito-Moyet, L.J. *Nursing Diagnosis: Application to Clinical Practice,* 10th ed. Philadelphia: Lippincott Williams & Wilkins, 2003.

Cohen, B.J., and Wood, D.L. *Memmler's Structure and Function of the Human Body,* 7th ed. Philadelphia: Lippincott Williams & Wilkins, 2000.

Dambro, M.R. *Griffith's 5-Minute Clinical Consult, 2004.* Philadelphia: Lippincott Williams & Wilkins, 2004.

Devita, V.T., Jr., et al., eds. *Cancer: Principles and Practice of Oncology,* 6th ed. Philadelphia: Lippincott Williams & Wilkins, 2001.

Doenges, M.E., et al. *Nursing Care Plans: Guidelines for Individualizing Patient Care,* 5th ed. Philadelphia: F.A. Davis Co., 2002.

Fischbach, F.T. *A Manual of Laboratory and Diagnostic Tests,* 7th ed. Philadelphia: Lippincott Williams & Wilkins, 2004.

Freeman, J.B., et al. *Pharmacologic Basis of Nursing Practice,* 6th ed. St. Louis: Mosby-Year Book, Inc., 2000.

Harkness, G.A. *Medical-Surgical Nursing Total Patient Care,* 10th ed. St. Louis: Mosby-Year Book, Inc., 2001.

Karch, A. *2004 Lippincott's Nursing Drug Guide.* Philadelphia: Lippincott Williams & Wilkins, 2004.

Kumar, V, et al. *Robbins Basic Pathology,* 7th ed. Philadelphia: W.B. Saunders Co., 2003.

Lehne, R.A. *Comprehensive Cardiac Care,* 8th ed. Philadelphia: W.B. Saunders, Co., 2001.

Lewis, S.M., et al, eds. *Medical-Surgical Nursing: Assessment and Management of Clinical Problems,* 6th ed. St. Louis: Mosby-Year Book, Inc., 2004.

Miller, C.A. *Nursing for Wellness in Older Adults: Theory and Practice,* 4th ed. Philadelphia: Lippincott Williams & Wilkins, 2004.

Morton, P.G., et al., eds. *Critical Care Nursing: A Holistic Approach,* 8th ed. Philadelphia: Lippincott Williams & Wilkins, 2005.

North American Nursing Diagnosis Association. *Nursing Diagnoses: Definitions and Classifications 2003-2004.* Philadelphia: North American Nursing Diagnosis Association, 2003.

Nursing2005 Drug Handbook, 25th ed. Philadelphia: Lippincott Williams & Wilkins, 2005

Pagana, K.D., and Pagana, T.J. *Diagnostic Testing and Nursing Implications: A Case Study Approach,* 6th ed. St. Louis: Mosby-Year Book, Inc., 2003.

Porth, C.M., and Kunert, M.P. *Pathophysiology: Concepts of Altered Health States,* 6th ed. Philadelphia: Lippincott Williams & Wilkins, 2002.

Rankin, S.H., and Stallings, K.D. *Patient Education: Principles and Practice,* 4th ed. Philadelphia: Lippincott Williams & Wilkins, 2001.

Rosdahl, C.B., and Kowalski, M., eds. *Textbook of Basic Nursing,* 8th ed. Philadelphia: Lippincott Williams & Wilkins, 2002.

Sahrmann, S. *Diagnosis and Treatment of Movement Impairment Syndromes.* St. Louis: Mosby-Year Book, Inc., 2002.

Schiff, E.R., et al., eds. *Schiff's Diseases of the Liver,* 9th ed. Philadelphia: Lippincott Williams & Wilkins, 2003.

Smeltzer, S.C., et al., eds. *Brunner and Suddarth's Textbook of Medical-Surgical Nursing,* 10th ed. Philadelphia: Lippincott Williams & Wilkins, 2003.

Society of Gastroenterology Nurses and Associates. *Gastroenterology Nursing: A Core Curriculum,* 3rd ed. Chicago: Society of Gastroenterology Nurses and Associates, 2003.

Timby, B.K., and Smith, N.E. *Introductory Medical-Surgical Nursing,* 8th ed. Philadelphia: Lippincott Williams & Wilkins, 2003.

U.S. Department of Health and Human Services. *The Seventh Report of the Joint National Committee on Detection, Evaluation, and Treatment of High Blood Pressure.* Washington, D.C.: U.S. Department of Health and Human Services, 2003. Available at: *www.nhlbi.nih.gov/guidelines/hypertension/jncintro.htm.* Last accessed July 16, 2004.

Weber, J., and Kelley, J. *Health Assessment in Nursing,* 2nd ed. Philadelphia: Lippincott Williams & Wilkins, 2003.

Woods, S.L., et al., eds. *Cardiac Nursing,* 5th ed. Philadelphia: Lippincott Williams & Wilkins, 2005.

APPENDIX A:
REFERRAL ORGANIZATIONS

Alcoholics Anonymous
Phone: 212-870-3400
Web site: *www.alcoholics-anonymous.org*

Alzheimer's Association
Phone: 1-800-272-3900
Web site: *www.alz.org*

Alzheimer's Disease Education and Referral Center
Phone: 1-800-438-4380
Web site: *www.alzheimers.org*

American Association of Diabetes Educators
Phone: 1-800-338-3633
Web site: *www.aadenet.org*

American Association of Kidney Patients
Phone: 1-800-749-2257
Web site: *www.aakp.org*

American Cancer Society
Phone: 1-800-ACS-2345
Web site: *www.cancer.org*

American Diabetes Association
Phone: 1-800-342-2383
Web site: *www.diabetes.org*

American Foundation for the Blind
Phone: 1-800-232-5463
Web site: *www.afb.org*

American Heart Association
Phone: 1-800-242-8721
Web site: *www.americanheart.org*

American Liver Foundation
Phone: 1-800-465-4837
Web site: *www.liverfoundation.org*

American Lung Association
Phone: 212-315-8700
Web site: *www.lungusa.org*

American Parkinson Disease Association
Phone: 1-800-223-4399
Web site: *www.apdaparkinson.org*

American Social Health Association
Phone: 919-361-8400
Web site: *www.ashastd.org*

American Society for Reproductive Medicine
Phone: 205-978-5000
Web site: *www.usrm.org*

American Thyroid Foundation
Phone: 703-998-8890
Web site: *www.thyroid.org*

Amputee Coalition of America
Phone: 1-888-267-5669
Web site: *www.amputee-coalition.org*

ALS (Amyotrophic Lateral Sclerosis) Association
Phone: 818-880-9007
Web site: *www.alsa.org*

Arthritis Foundation
Phone: 1-800-283-7800
Web site: *www.arthritis.org*

Asthma and Allergy Foundation of American
Phone: 1-800-727-8462
Web site: *www.aafa.org*

Centers for Disease Control and Prevention (CDC)
Phone: 1-404-639-3534
Web site: *www.cdc.gov*

CDC National Prevention Information Network
Phone: 1-800-458-5231
Web site: *www.cdcnpin.org*

Crohn's and Colitis Foundation of America
Phone: 1-800-932-2423
Web site: *www.ccfa.org*

Endometriosis Association
Phone: 414-355-2200
Web site: *www.endometriosisassn.org*

Epilepsy Foundation
Phone: 1-800-332-1000
Web site: *www.epilepsyfoundation.org*

Glaucoma Foundation
Phone: 212-285-0080
Web site: *www.glaucomafoundation.org*

Glaucoma Research Foundation
Phone: 1-800-826-6693
Web site: *www.glaucoma.org*

Guillain-Barré Syndrome Foundation International
Phone: 610-667-0131
Web site: *www.gbsfi.com*

International Foundation for Functional Gastrointestinal Disorders
Phone: 1-888-964-2001
Web site: *www.iffgd.org*

Intestinal Disease Foundation
Phone: 1-877-587-9606
Web site: *www.intestinalfoundation.org*

Les Turner Amyotrophic Lateral Sclerosis Foundation
Phone: 1-888-257-1107
Web site: *www.lesturnerals.org*

Lighthouse International
Phone: 1-800-829-0500
Web site: *www.lighthouse.org*

Lupus Foundation of America
Phone: 202-349-1155
Web site: *www.lupus.org*

MedicAlert
Phone: 1-888-633-4298
Web site: *www.medicalert.org*

Mended Hearts
Phone: 1-888- 432-7899
Web site: *www.mendedhearts.org*

Multiple Sclerosis Association of America
Phone: 1-800-532-7667
Web site: *www.msaa.com*

Multiple Sclerosis Foundation
Phone: 1-800-225-6495
Web site: *www.msfacts.org*

Myasthenia Gravis Foundation of America
Phone: 1-800-541-5454
Web site: *www.myasthenia.org*

National Association of People with AIDS
Phone: 202-898-0414
Web site: *www.napwa.org*

National Cancer Institute
Phone: 1-800-422-6237
Web site: *www.cancer.gov*

National Eye Institute
Phone: 1-301-496-5248
Web site: *www.nei.nih.gov*

National Foundation for Infectious Diseases
Phone: 301-656-0003
Web site: *www.nfid.org*

National Graves' Disease Foundation
Phone: 828-877-5251
Web site: *www.ngdf.org*

National Hemophilia Foundation
Phone: 1-800-424-2634
Web site: *www.hemophilia.org*

National Hypertension Association
Phone: 212-889-3557
Web site: *www.nathypertension.org*

National Injury Prevention Foundation: ThinkFirst
Phone: 1-800-844-6556
Web site: *www.thinkfirst.org*

National Institute on Deafness and Other Communication Disorders
Phone: 1-800-241-1044
Web page: *www.nidcd.nih.gov*

National Institute of Diabetes & Digestive & Kidney Diseases
Phone: 1-800-860-8747 (diabetes); 1-800-891-5389 (digestive); 1-800-891-5390 (kidney)
Web site: *www.niddk.nih.gov*

National Institute of Neurological Disorders and Stroke
Phone: 1-800-352-9424
Web page: *www.ninds.nih.gov*

National Kidney Foundation
Phone: 1-800-622-9010
Web site: *www.kidney.org*

National Multiple Sclerosis Society
Phone: 1-800-344-4867
Web site: *www.nmss.org*

National Osteoporosis Foundation
Phone: 202-223-2226
Web site: *www.nof.org*

National Parkinson Foundation
Phone: 1-800-327-4545
Web site: *www.parkinson.org*

National Rehabilitation Information Center for Independence
Phone: 1-800-346-2742
Web site: *www.naric.com*

National Spinal Cord Injury Association
Phone: 1-800-962-9629
Web site: *www.spinalcord.org*

National Stroke Association
Phone: 1-800-787-6537
Web site: *www.stroke.org*

Prevent Blindness America
Phone: 1-800-331-2020
Web site: *www.preventblindness.org*

Project Inform
Phone: 415-558-8669
Web site: *www.projinf.org*

Self Help for Hard of Hearing People
Phone: 301-657-2248
Web site: *www.hearingloss.org*

Sickle Cell Disease Association of America
Phone: 1-800-421-8453
Web site: *www.sicklecelldisease.org*

Smokenders
Phone: 1-800-828-4357
Web site: *www.smokenders.com*

United Ostomy Association
Phone: 1-800-826-0826
Web site: *www.uoa.org*

Wound, Ostomy, and Continence Nurses Society
Phone: 1-888-224-9626
Web site: *www.wocn.org*

ADDITIONAL ORGANIZATIONS

Healthfinder (provides information about prevention of many disease processes)
Web page: *www.healthfinder.gov*

MedWebPlus (an Internet-based health science index)
Web page: *www.medwebplus.com*

National Institutes of Health
Phone: 301-496-4000
Web page: *www.nih.gov*

Occupational Health Research (provides information systems, training, and technical support nationwide for hospitals and clinics)
Phone: 1-800-444-8432
Web page: *www.employeehealth.com*

United States National Library of Medicine
Phone: 1-888-346-3656
Web page: *www.nlm.nih.gov*

APPENDIX B: GLOSSARY OF TERMS

Abduction Movement of a limb away from the body.

Adduction Movement of a limb toward the axis of the body.

Akinesia An abnormal state of motor and psychic hypoactivity or muscular paralysis.

Albuminuria Suffix meaning a "(specified) condition characterized by excess serum proteins in the urine."

Allen's test A test for the patency of the radial artery after insertion of an indwelling monitoring catheter. The client's hand is formed into a fist while the nurse compresses the ulnar artery. Compression continues while the fist is opened. If blood perfusion through the radial artery is adequate, the hand should flush and resume normal pinkish coloration.

Angioedema An acute, painless dermal, subcutaneous, or submucosal swelling of short duration. It involves the face, neck, lips, larynx, hands, feet, genitalia, or viscera. It may result from food or drug allergy, infection, or emotional stress, or it may be hereditary. Treatment depends on the cause. For severe forms, subcutaneous injections of epinephrine, intubation, or tracheotomy may be necessary to prevent respiratory obstruction. Prevention depends on the identification and avoidance of causative factors.

Anuria The cessation of urine production or a urinary output of less than 100 ml per day. Anuria may be caused by kidney failure or dysfunction, a decline in blood pressure below that required to maintain filtration pressure in the kidney, or an obstruction in the urinary passages. A rapid decline in urinary output, leading ultimately to anuria and uremia, occurs in acute renal failure.

Arteriosclerosis A common arterial disorder characterized by thickening, loss of elasticity, and calcification of arterial walls. It results in a decreased blood supply, especially to the cerebrum, heart, and lower extremities.

Arthralgia Joint pain.

Ataxia An abnormal condition characterized by an impaired ability to coordinate movement. A staggering gait and postural imbalance are caused by a lesion in the spinal cord or cerebellum that may be the sequela of birth trauma, congenital disorder, infection, degenerative disorder, neoplasm, toxic substance, or head injury.

Aura A sensation, such as light or warmth, that may precede an attack of migraine or an epileptic seizure.

Azotemia Retention of excessive amounts of nitrogenous compounds in the blood. This toxic condition is caused by failure of the kidneys to remove urea from the blood and is characteristic of uremia.

Bradykinesia An abnormal condition characterized by slowness of all voluntary movement and speech, such as caused by parkinsonism, other extrapyramidal disorders, and certain tranquilizers.

Brudzinski's sign An involuntary flexion of the arm, hip, and knee when the neck is passively flexed. It occurs in clients with meningitis.

Bruit An abnormal blowing or swishing sound or murmur heard while auscultating a carotid artery, organ, or gland, such as the liver or thyroid. The specific character of the bruit, its location, and the time of its occurrence in a cycle of other sounds are all of diagnostic importance.

Bulla A thin-walled blister of the skin or mucous membranes greater than 1 cm in diameter, containing clear, serous fluid.

Bursitis An inflammation of the bursa, the connective tissue structure surrounding a joint. Bursitis may be precipitated by arthritis, infection, injury, or excessive or traumatic exercise or effort. The chief symptom is severe pain of the affected joint, particularly on movement.

Cachexia General ill-health and malnutrition, marked by weakness and emaciation, usually associated with severe disease, such as tuberculosis or cancer.

Cardiomyopathy Any disease that affects the structure and function of the heart.

Carotenemia The presence of high levels of carotene in the blood, which results in an abnormal yellow appearance of the plasma and skin. The conjunctivae are not discolored.

Carpal tunnel syndrome A common painful disorder of the wrist and hand, induced by compression on the median nerve between the inelastic carpal ligament and other structures within the carpal tunnel. It is often seen in cumulative trauma to the wrist. The median nerve innervates the palm and the radial side of the hand; compression of the nerve causes weakness, pain with opposition of the thumb, and burning, tingling, or aching, sometimes radiating to the forearm and shoulder joint. Pain may be intermittent or constant and is often most intense at night.

Conjunctivitis Inflammation of the conjunctiva, caused by bacterial or viral infection, allergy, or environmental factors. Red eyes, thick discharge, sticky eyelids in the morning, and inflammation without pain are characteristic results of the most common cause, bacteria. This cause may be found by microscopic examination or bacteriologic culture of the discharge.

Cor pulmonale Enlargement of the heart's right ventricle caused by primary lung disease. It eventually results in right ventricular hypertrophy and then right ventricular failure. Pulmonary hypertension associated with this condition is caused by some disorder of the pulmonary parenchyma or of the pulmonary vascular system between the origin of the left pulmonary artery and the entry of the pulmonary veins into the left atrium. Chronic cor pulmonale commonly increases the size of the right ventricle, which cannot accommodate an increase in pressure as easily as the left ventricle. In some clients, however, the disease also increases the size of the left ventricle.

Decerebrate posture The position of a client who is comatose in which the arms are extended and internally rotated and the legs are extended with the feet in forced plantar flexion. This position indicates a problem between the cerebrum and lower portions of the central nervous system.

Decorticate posture The position of a client who is comatose in which the upper extremities are rigidly flexed at the elbows and at the wrists. The legs also may be flexed. This position indicates a lesion in a mesencephalic region of the brain. In some instances, the posture may be produced by applying a painful stimulus to a comatose client.

Diplopia Double vision caused by defective function of the extraocular muscles or a disorder of the nerves that innervate the muscles.

Dyscrasia Pertaining to an abnormal condition of the blood or bone marrow, such as leukemia, aplastic anemia, or prenatal Rh incompatibility.

Dyskinesia An impairment of the ability to execute voluntary movements. Tardive dyskinesia is caused by an adverse effect of prolonged use of phenothiazine medications in elderly clients or those with brain injuries.

Dyspareunia An abnormal pain during sexual intercourse. It may result from abnormal conditions of the genitalia, dysfunctional psychophysiologic reaction to sexual union, forcible coition, or incomplete sexual arousal. Dyspareunia is also associated with hormonal changes of menopause and lactation, which result in drying of the vaginal tissues, as well as with endometriosis. Painful adhesions around the vagina and ligaments may result, decreasing their flexibility during intercourse.

Dysphagia Difficulty in swallowing, commonly associated with obstructive or motor disorders of the esophagus. Clients with obstructive disorders, such as esophageal tumor or lower esophageal ring, are unable to swallow solids but can tolerate liquids. Persons with motor disorders, such as achalasia, are unable to swallow solids or liquids. Diagnosis of the underlying condition is made through barium studies, the observed clinical signs, and evaluation of the client's symptoms.

Dysuria Painful urination, usually caused by a bacterial infection or obstructive condition in the urinary tract. The client complains of a burning sensation when passing urine, and laboratory examination may reveal the presence of blood, bacteria, or white blood cells. Dysuria is a symptom of such conditions as cystitis, urethritis, prostatitis, urinary tract tumors, some gynecologic disorders, and use of certain medications such as opiates.

Ecchymosis Bluish discoloration of an area of skin or mucous membrane caused by the extravasations of blood into the subcutaneous tissues as a result of trauma to the underlying blood vessels or fragility of the vessel walls.

Ectropion Eversion, most commonly of the eyelid, exposing the conjunctival membrane lining of the eyelid and part of the eyeball.

Entropion Turning inward or turning toward, usually a condition in which the eyelid turns inward toward the eye.

Epispadias A congenital defect in which the urethra opens on the dorsum of the penis at some point proximal to the glans. Urinary incontinence occurs because the urinary sphincters are defective, restricting healthy sexual function. The corresponding defect in women, in which the urethra opens by the separation of the labia minora and a fissure of the clitoris, is rare.

Erythema Redness or inflammation of the skin or mucous membranes that is the result of dilation and congestion of superficial capillaries. Examples of erythema are nervous blushes and mild sunburn.

Erythropoiesis The process of erythrocyte production involving the maturation of a nucleated precursor into a hemoglobin-filled, nucleus-free erythrocyte that is regulated by erythropoietin, a hormone produced by the kidney.

Eversion A turning outward or inside-out, such as a turning of the foot outward at the ankle.

Exophthalmos An abnormal condition characterized by a marked protrusion of the eyeballs, usually resulting from the increased volume of the orbital contents caused by a tumor; swelling associated with cerebral, intraocular, or intraorbital edema or hemorrhage; paralysis of or trauma to the extraocular muscles; or cavernous sinus thrombosis. It may also be caused by an endocrine disorder, such as hyperthyroidism or Graves' disease; varicose veins within the orbit; or injury to orbital bones.

Extension A "straightening" movement allowed by certain joints of the skeleton that increases the angle between two adjoining bones, such as extension of the leg, which increases the posterior angle between the femur and the tibia.

Flaccid Weak, soft, and flabby; lacking normal muscle tone, such as flaccid muscles associated with peripheral neuritis, poliomyelitis, and early stroke.

Flatulence The presence of an excessive amount of air or gas in the stomach and intestinal tract, causing distention of the organs and in some cases mild to moderate pain.

Flexion A movement allowed by certain joints of the skeleton that decreases the angle between two adjoining bones, such as bending the elbow, which decreases the angle between the humerus and the ulna.

Fremitus A tremulous vibration of the chest wall that is primarily palpated during physical examination.

Goiter An enlarged thyroid gland, usually evident as a pronounced swelling in the neck. The enlargement may be associated with hyperthyroidism, hypothyroidism, or normal levels of thyroid function. It may be cystic or fibrous, containing nodules or an increased number of follicles. The goiter may surround a large blood vessel, or a part of the enlarged gland may be situated beneath the sternum or in the thoracic cavity.

Heberden's nodes An abnormal cartilaginous or bony enlargement of a distal interphalangeal joint of a finger, usually occurring in degenerative diseases of the joints.

Hematopoiesis The normal formation and development of blood cells in the bone marrow. In severe anemia and other hematologic disorders, cells may be produced in organs outside the marrow (extramedullary hematopoiesis).

Hematuria Abnormal presence of blood in the urine. It is symptomatic of many renal diseases and disorders of the genitourinary system.

Hemoptysis Coughing up of blood from the respiratory tract. Blood-streaked sputum often is present in minor upper respiratory infections or bronchitis. More profuse bleeding may indicate *Aspergillus* infection, lung abscess, tuberculosis, or bronchogenic carcinoma, in which exsanguination (blood loss) is caused by erosion of the pulmonary vessels by the tumor.

Hemorrhoid A varicosity in the lower rectum or anus caused by congestion in the veins of the hemorrhoidal plexus.

Hernia Protrusion of an organ through an abnormal opening in the muscle wall of the cavity that surrounds it. A hernia may be congenital, may result from the failure of certain structures to close after birth, or may be acquired later in life as a result of obesity, muscular weakness, surgery, or illness.

Hiatal hernia Protrusion of a portion of the stomach upward through the diaphragm. The major difficulty in symptomatic clients is gastroesophageal reflux, the backflow of the acid contents of the stomach into the esophagus.

Hirsutism Excessive body hair in a masculine distribution pattern as a result of heredity, hormonal dysfunction, porphyria, or medication. Treatment of the specific cause usually stops growth of more hair.

Homonymous hemianopia Blindness or defective vision in the right or left halves of the visual fields.

Hydrocele An accumulation of fluid in any saclike cavity or duct, specifically in the tunica vaginalis testis or along the spermatic cord. The condition is caused by inflammation of the epididymis or testis or by lymphatic or venous obstruction in the cord.

Hyperkinesis A syndrome affecting children, adolescents, and adults characterized by short attention span, hyperactivity, and poor concentration. The symptoms may be mild or severe and are associated with functional deviations of the central nervous system without signs of major neurologic or psychiatric disturbance. The people affected are usually of normal or above average intelligence. Other symptoms include impairment in perception, conceptualization, language, memory, and motor skills; decreased attention span; increased impulsivity; and emotional lability. Also known as *attention deficit disorder.*

Hyperreflexia Increased reflex reactions (to bend back).

Hypospadias A congenital defect in which the urinary meatus is on the underside of the penis. Incontinence does not occur because the sphincters are not defective. The opening may be off-center or anywhere along the underside of the penis or on the perineum. A corresponding defect in women is rare but recognized by the location of the urinary meatus in the vagina.

Inflammation The protective response of body tissue to irritation or injury. Inflammation may be acute or chronic; its cardinal signs are redness, heat, swelling, and pain, often accompanied by loss of function. The process begins with a transitory vasoconstriction, then is followed by a brief increase in vascular permeability. The second stage is prolonged and consists of sustained increase in vascular permeability, exudation of fluids from the vessels, clustering of leukocytes along the vessel walls, phagocytosis of microorganisms, deposition of fibrin in the vessel, disposal of the accumulated debris by macrophages and, finally, migration of fibroblasts to the area and development of new, normal cells. The severity, timing, and local character of any particular inflammatory response depend on the cause, the area affected, and the condition of the host. Histamine, kinins, and various other substances mediate the inflammatory process.

Inversion An abnormal condition in which an organ is turned inside out, such as a uterine inversion.

Ischemia A decreased supply of oxygenated blood to a body organ or part. The condition is often marked by pain and organ dysfunction, as in ischemic heart disease. Some causes of ischemia are arterial embolism, atherosclerosis, thrombosis, and vasoconstriction.

Kernig's sign A diagnostic sign for meningitis marked by a loss of the ability of a supine client to completely straighten the leg when it is fully flexed at the knee and hip. Pain in the lower back and resistance to straightening the leg constitute a positive Kernig's sign. Usually the client can extend the leg completely when the thigh is not flexed on the abdomen.

Kussmaul's breathing Abnormally deep, very rapid sighing respirations that are characteristic of diabetic ketoacidosis.

Laryngitis Inflammation of the mucous membrane lining the larynx, accompanied by edema of the vocal cords with hoarseness or loss of voice, occurring as an acute disorder caused by a cold, irritating fumes, sudden temperature changes, or as a chronic condition resulting from excessive use of the voice, heavy smoking, or exposure to irritating fumes. In acute laryngitis, there may be a cough, and the throat usually feels scratchy and painful.

Leukorrhea A white discharge from the vagina. Normally, vaginal discharge occurs in regular variations of amount and consistency during the course of the menstrual cycle. A greater-than-usual amount is normal in pregnancy, and a decrease is to be expected after delivery, during lactation, and after menopause. Leukorrhea is the most common reason women seek gynecologic care.

Lyme disease An acute, recurrent inflammatory infection transmitted by a tickborne spirochete, *Borrelia burgdorferi*. The disease is spread by two species of deer ticks, *Ixodes dammini* and *I. pacificus*. An early sign of an infection is the appearance of a red macule at the site of the bite, although the erythema migrans feature may not be observed until 3 days to 1 month later, when many clients do not recall receiving a tick bite. The bite site may expand to form concentric circles in a "bull's eye" pattern. About half of untreated Lyme disease clients develop multiple skin lesions due to movement of the spirochetes through the circulatory system. Knees, other large joints, and temporomandibular joints are most commonly involved, with local inflammation and swelling. Chills, fever, headache, malaise, and erythema chronicum migrans (an expanding annular, erythematous skin eruption) often precede the joint manifestations. Occasionally, cardiac conduction abnormalities, aseptic meningitis, and Bell's palsy are associated conditions. Symptoms appear in recurrent episodes, lasting usually about 1 week, at intervals of 1 to several weeks, declining in severity over a 2- or 3-year period.

Malaise A vague, uneasy feeling of body weakness, distress, or discomfort, often marking the onset of and persisting throughout a disease.

Mastitis An inflammatory condition of the breast, usually caused by streptococcal or staphylococcal infection.

Myalgia Diffuse muscle pain, usually accompanied by malaise. Also called *myoneuralgia*.

Nuchal rigidity A resistance to flexion of the neck, a condition seen in clients with meningitis.

Nystagmus Involuntary, rhythmic movements of the eyes; the oscillations may be horizontal, vertical, rotary, or mixed.

Oliguria A diminished capacity to form and pass urine, less than 500 ml in every 24 hours, so that the end products of metabolism cannot be excreted efficiently. It is usually caused by imbalances in body fluids and electrolytes, renal lesions, or urinary tract obstruction.

Opisthotonus A prolonged, severe spasm of the muscles causing the back to arch acutely, the head to bend back on the neck, the heels to bend back on the legs, and the arms and hands to flex rigidly at the joints.

Orthopnea An abnormal condition in which a person must sit or stand to breathe deeply or comfortably. It occurs in many disorders of the cardiac and respiratory system, such as asthma, pulmonary edema, emphysema, pneumonia, and angina pectoris.

Osseous Bony; consisting of or resembling bone.

Pallor An unnatural paleness or absence of color in the skin.

Papilledema Edema of the optic disk, visible on ophthalmoscopic examination of the fundus of the eye, caused by an increase in intracranial pressure. The meningeal sheaths that surround the optic nerves from the optic disk are continuous with the meninges of the brain; therefore increased intracranial pressure is transmitted forward from the brain to the optic disc in the eye to cause edema.

Paralytic ileus A decrease in or absence of intestinal peristalsis. It may occur after abdominal surgery or peritoneal injury or may be associated with severe pyelonephritis, ureteral stone, fractured ribs, myocardial infarction, extensive intestinal ulceration, heavy-metal poisoning, porphyria, retroperitoneal hematomas — especially those associated with fractured vertebrae, or any severe metabolic disease. The most common overall cause of intestinal obstruction, paralytic ileus is mediated by a hormonal component of the sympathoadrenal system.

Paresthesia Any subjective sensation, experienced as numbness, tingling, or a "pins and needles" feeling. Paresthesias often fluctuate according to such influences as posture, activity, rest, edema, congestion, or underlying disease. When experienced in the extremities, it is sometimes identified as acroparesthesia.

Petechiae Tiny purple or red spots appearing on the skin as a result of tiny hemorrhages within the dermal or submucosal layers. Petechiae range from pinpoint to pinhead size and are flush with the surface.

Photophobia Abnormal sensitivity to light, especially by the eyes. The condition is prevalent in albinism and various diseases of the conjunctiva and cornea and may be a symptom of such disorders as measles, psittacosis, encephalitis, Rocky Mountain spotted fever, and Reiter's syndrome.

Polycythemia An increase in the number of erythrocytes in the blood that may be primary or secondary to pulmonary disease, heart disease, or prolonged exposure to high altitudes, or may be idiopathic.

Polyp A small tumorlike growth that projects from a mucous membrane surface.

Pronation 1. Assumption of a prone position, in which the ventral surface of the body faces downward. 2. (of the arm) The rotation of the forearm so that the palm of the hand faces downward and backward. 3. (of the foot) The lowering of the medial edge of the foot by turning it outward and through abduction movements in the tarsal and metatarsal joints.

Pruritus The symptom of itching, an uncomfortable sensation leading to the urge to scratch. Scratching may result in secondary infection. Some causes of pruritus are allergy, infection, jaundice, chronic renal disease, lymphoma, and skin irritation.

Ptosis An abnormal condition of one or both upper eyelids in which the eyelid droops because of congenital or acquired weakness of the levator muscle or paralysis of the third cranial nerve. Partial ptosis and a small pupil may be caused by an unusual hematologic disorder of the sympathetic part of the autonomic nervous system.

Pulsus paradoxus An abnormal decrease in systolic pressure and pulse wave amplitude during inspiration. The normal fall in pressure is less than 10 mm Hg, and an excessive decline may be a sign of tamponade, adhesive pericarditis, severe lung disease, advanced heart failure, and other conditions.

Pyuria The presence of white blood cells in the urine, usually a sign of an infection in the urinary tract.

Rhabdomyolysis A paroxysmal, potentially fatal disease of skeletal muscle characterized by myoglobulinuria. It is also associated with acute renal failure in heatstroke.

Rinne test A method of distinguishing conductive from sensorineural hearing loss. The test may be performed with tuning forks of 256, 512, and 1024 cycles. The base of the vibrating fork is placed against the client's mastoid bone. While one ear is tested, the other is masked. When the client no longer hears the sound, the time in seconds is noted, and the fork is positioned about a $1/2''$ (1.3 cm) from the ipsilateral external auditory meatus. The time that sound is heard is noted. Air-conducted sound should be heard twice as long as bone-conducted sound after bone conduction stops. In sensorineural loss, the sound is heard relatively longer by air conduction; in conductive hearing loss, the sound is heard longer by bone conduction.

Scalene muscles One of a group of four muscles arising from the cervical vertebrae with insertions on the first or second rib.

Seborrheic keratosis Any skin lesion in which there is overgrowth and thickening of the corni-fied epithelium.

Shingles An acute infection caused by reactivation of the latent varicella zoster virus, which main-ly affects adults. It is characterized by the development of painful vesicular skin eruptions that follow the underlying route of cranial or spinal nerves inflamed by the virus.

Sjögren's syndrome An immunologic disorder characterized by deficient moisture production of the lacrimal, salivary, and other glands, resulting in abnormal dryness of the mouth, eyes, and other mucous membranes. Atrophy of the salivary glands results in dental disorders and loss of taste and odor sensations. When the lungs are affected, the dryness increases susceptibility to pneumonia and other respiratory infections.

Steatorrhea Greater-than-normal amounts of fat in the feces, characterized by frothy, foul-smelling fecal matter that floats (as in celiac disease), some malabsorption syndromes, and any condition in which fats are poorly absorbed by the small intestine.

Supination 1. One of the kinds of rotation allowed by certain skeletal joints, such as the elbow and the wrist joints, which allow the palm of the hand to turn up. 2. The position of lying on the back, face up.

Telangiectasis Permanent dilation of groups of superficial capillaries and venules. Common caus-es are actinic damage, atrophy-producing dermatoses, rosacea, elevated estrogen levels, and collagen vascular diseases.

Tenosynovitis Inflammation of a tendon sheath caused by calcium deposits, repeated strain or trauma, high levels of blood cholesterol, rheumatoid arthritis, gout, or gonorrhea. In some instances, movement yields crackling noise over the tendon.

Tinnitus A subjective noise sensation, often described as ringing, heard in one or both ears. It may be a sign of acoustic trauma.

Varicocele A dilation of the pampiniform venous complex of the spermatic cord. The varicocele forms a soft, elastic swelling that can cause pain. It is most common in men ages 15 to 25 and affects the left spermatic cord more often than the right. It is usually more pronounced and painful in the standing position.

Vertigo A sensation of instability, giddiness, loss of equilibrium, or rotation, caused by a distur-bance in the semicircular canal of the inner ear or the vestibular nuclei of the brainstem. The sensation that one's body is rotating in space is called *subjective vertigo*, whereas the sensation that objects are spinning around the body is called *objective vertigo*.

Vitiligo A benign acquired skin disease of unknown cause, consisting of irregular patches of vari-ous sizes, totally lacking in pigment, and often having hyperpigmented borders. Exposed areas of skin are most often affected.

Weber's test A method of screening auditory acuity. It is especially useful in determining whether defective hearing in an ear is a conductive loss caused by a middle-ear problem or a sen-sorineural loss resulting from a disorder in the inner ear or auditory nerve system. The test is performed by placing the stem of a vibrating 256-Hz tuning fork in the center of the person's forehead, or the midline vertex. The loudness of the sound is equal in both ears if hearing is nor-mal. If the person has a sensorineural loss in one ear, the unaffected ear perceives the sound as louder. When conductive hearing loss is present, the sound is louder in the affected ear because it does not hear ordinary background noise conducted through the air and receives only vibra-tions by bone conduction.

INDEX

i refers to an illustration; t refers to a table.

i refers to an illustration; t refers to a table.

i refers to an illustration; t refers to a table.

i refers to an illustration; t refers to a table.

i refers to an illustration; t refers to a table.

i refers to an illustration; t refers to a table.

i refers to an illustration; t refers to a table.

i refers to an illustration; t refers to a table.

i refers to an illustration; t refers to a table.

Perioperative nursing *(continued)*
  in intraoperative period, 581-583
  in preoperative period, 577-581
Perioperative period
  assessment during, 577-578
  client goals for, 578-579
  health care team in, 575-576
  medications for, 585t
  nursing diagnoses for, 578
  outcome evaluation of, 580-581
  phases of, 575
Peripheral circulation
  assessment of, 20-21, 157-158
  in elderly client, 21
  functions of, 156-157
  signs and symptoms of altered function of,
    157
  structures of, 154-156, 154i, 155i
Peripheral nervous system
  pain impulses and, 71-72, 71i
  structure and function of, 335-336, 336t
Peripheral vascular disorders, 160-179. *See also*
    specific disorder.
  goals for management of, 158
  implementing interventions for, 158-159
  medications for, 162-164t
  nursing diagnoses for, 158
  outcome evaluation of, 159-160
  risk factors for, 157
Peripheral vascular system, review of, for health
    history, 6
Peritoneojugular shunting, 443
Peritoneum, 187
Peritonitis, 201-203, 202i
Permanent pacemakers, 144-146
Perthes' test, 169
Petit mal seizures, 349-350
pH, 50
Phantom pain, 74, 174. *See also* Pain.
Pharyngitis, 395-396
Pharynx, 88i, 391, 392, 392i
Phimosis, 266-267
Phlebography, 158
Phosphate-binding agents, 469t

Phosphorus
  deficiency of, 61
  excess of, 61-62
Physical examination, 8-28. *See also specific*
    body part or system.
  assessment techniques for, 9
  general appearance in, 10
  general principles of, 8-9
  height and weight in, 10
  vital signs in, 9-10, 10t
Pituitary gland, 217, 218i, 219i
  dysfunction of, 222-223, 226-227
Plasma
  composition of, 489
  function of, 491-492
Plasma proteins, 489, 491-492
Plasminogen, 492
Platelet aggregation, 494
Platelets. *See also* Thrombocytes.
  aggregates of, in lungs as transfusion compli-
    cation, 520
  normal values for, 29t
  transfusion of, 518-519t
Plethymography, 158
Pleura, 89
Pleural effusion, 104
Pleural rub, 19t
Pleur-Evac system, 105, 106i
Pneumococcal vaccination, 281
Pneumonia, 94-95
Poisoning with ingested agents, 209-210
Pons, 333, 333i
Portal hypertension, 440, 442i, 443, 443i
Position sense, 384
Postanesthesia care unit chart, 584i
Posterior pituitary dysfunction, 223, 226-227
Postoperative period
  immediate
    assessment in, 583
    client goals for, 583
    implementing interventions for, 583, 584i,
      585-586
    nursing diagnoses for, 583
    outcome evaluation of, 586

i refers to an illustration; t refers to a table.

i refers to an illustration; t refers to a table.

i refers to an illustration; t refers to a table.

i refers to an illustration; t refers to a table.

NOTES

NOTES

About the CD-ROM

Lippincott's Review Series CD-ROMs provide a convenient way to assess readiness for academic tests and licensure exams. More than 200 carefully selected, multiple choice and alternate-format questions are provided for study and simulated testing.

Minimum system requirements

- Windows 98
- Pentium 166
- 128 MB RAM
- 8 MB of free hard-disk space
- SVGA monitor with High Color (16-bit)
- CD-ROM drive
- Mouse

Installation

Place the CD in your CD-ROM drive. After a few moments, the installation process will automatically begin. If the installation process doesn't automatically begin, click on the Start button and select Run. At the command line, type D:\setup.exe. (*Note:* The letter D represents the CD-ROM drive. If your drive is designated by a different letter, use your drive letter instead.) Click OK. Follow the installation instructions.

Technical support

For technical support, call toll-free 1-800-638-3030, Monday through Friday, 8:30 a.m. to 5 p.m. Eastern Time. You may also write to Lippincott Williams & Wilkins Technical Support, 351 W. Camden Street, Baltimore, MD 21201-2436, or e-mail us at techsupp@lww.com.